A TEXTBOOK OF
DENTAL BIOCHEMISTRY

A TEXTBOOK OF
DENTAL BIOCHEMISTRY
THIRD EDITION

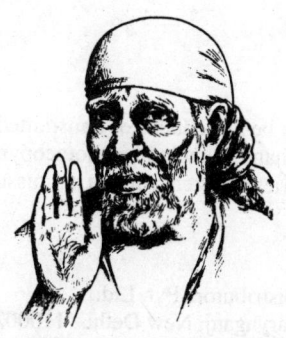

S.P. Singh

Ph.D, FACBI, Former WHO Fellow-
Texas A & M University, Texas, U.S.A.
Nominated by Government of India for Commonwealth Medical Fellowship- 1983
Professor and Head, Department of Biochemistry,
MLB Medical College, Jhansi- 284128, U.P.
and
Chief Consultant in Biochemistry,
MLB Medical College Associated Hospital, Jhansi

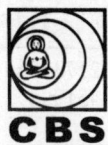

CBS

CBS Publishers & Distributors Pvt. Ltd.

New Delhi • Bengaluru • Chennai • Kochi • Kolkata • Mumbai
Hyderabad • Nagpur • Patna • Pune • Vijayawada

ISBN: 978-81-239-1719-1

First Edition: 2000
Reprint: 2002, 2003, 2004
Second Edition: 2004
Reprint: 2005, 2006
Third Edition: 2009
Reprint: 2011, 2016

Published by:
Satish Kumar Jain for CBS Publishers & Distributors Pvt. Ltd.,
4819/XI Prahlad Street, 24 Ansari Road, Daryaganj, New Delhi - 110002
delhi@cbspd.com, cbspubs@airtelmail.in • www.cbspd.com
Ph.: 23289259, 23266861, 23266867 • Fax: 011-23243014

Corporate Office: 204 FIE, Industrial Area, Patparganj, Delhi - 110 092
Ph: 49344934 • Fax: 011-49344935
E-mail: publishing@cbspd.com • publicity@cbspd.com

Branches:
• *Bengaluru:* 2975, 17th Cross, K.R. Road, Bansankari 2nd Stage,
  Bengaluru - 70 • Ph: +91-80-26771678/79 • Fax: +91-80-26771680
  E-mail: cbsbng@gmail.com, bangalore@cbspd.com
• *Chennai:* No. 7, Subbaraya Street, Shenoy Nagar, Chennai - 600030
  Ph: +91-44-26681266, 26680620 • Fax: +91-44-42032115
  E-mail: chennai@cbspd.com
• *Kochi:* Ashana House, 39/1904, A.M. Thomas Road, Valanjambalam,
  Ernakulum, Kochi • Ph: +91-484-4059061-65
  Fax: +91-484-4059065 • E-mail: cochin@cbspd.com
• *Kolkata:* 6-B, Ground Floor, Rameshwar Shaw Road, Kolkata - 700014
  Ph: +91-33-22891126/7/8 • E-mail: kolkata@cbspd.com
• *Mumbai:* 83-C, Dr. E. Moses Road, Worli, Mumbai - 400018
  Ph: +91-9833017933, 022-24902340/41 • E-mail: mumbai@cbspd.com

Representatives:

• Hyderabad: 0-9885175004   • Nagpur: 0-9021734563
• Patna: 0-9334159340   • Pune: 0-9623451994
• Vijayawada: 0-9000660880

Printed at:
J.S. Offset Printers, Delhi

By
the grace and kind blessings
of
Peetambara Peeth, Datia (M.P.)
&
Lord Shri Shirdi Sai Baba
{ Kopargaon - Manmad (Maharashtra) }

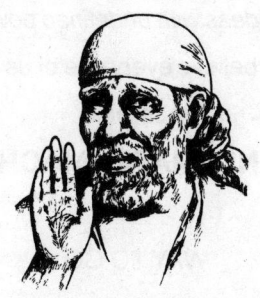

&
Lord Satya Sri Sai Baba
(Puttaparti-Bangalore)

Dedicated

to

Chandi Mata - Machail

J & K State

Goddess with undefined power

I believe every one of us

must visit

CHANDI MATA - MACHAIL

WAY TO GO

Jammu

↓

210 Km (One day journey by bus)

Bhadarwah
(Village : CHANOTE)

↓

90 Kms (One day journey by bus)

Kishtwar

↓

65 Kms (One day journey by bus)

Gulab-Garh (District-Padar)

↓

(on foot) 30 kms

Machail

Note - Best time to visit from July- Sept

{ YATRA starts on every 18th of August and returns

on 28th of August (11 days programme)}

In 2007 nearly 80,000 people participated in the yatra

PREFACE AND ACKNOWLEDGEMENTS TO THE THIRD EDITION

It gives me great pleasure in bringing out **third edition** of this book, credit goes to the students/ readers who are liking this book because of simple english, salient features in the boxes, etc.

To write a book is not an easy task which even becomes an uphill task to write a text book while sitting at Jhansi where power (electricity) cut ranges from 6-12 hours a day for the last five years or so. This scenario is not changing. Under these abnormal conditions, to accomplish such a work where deep concentration is wanted and required is not at all easy.

Anyway, I am doing this work for the students' cause and am sharing in this book my views of teaching and research experience of more than 34 years.

In this edition, besides the addition of some new chapters, new material has been added in almost every chapter so as to enhance and update the knowledge of the students. At the end of this book, new tables have been given with sound interpretations. Even though, more suggestions from the students and the readers shall be most welcomed as before as knowledge is not a domain of any individual one. **A man is a real man who shares his views and dissipates his/her knowledge.**

While completing this book, the encouragement rendered to me by my wife Dr. (Smt.) Manju Singh, Reader in History, Bundelkhand Postgraduate College, Jhansi, Sons- Er. Vikrant Singh (Tata Motors Limited, Area Manager, Ukraine) and Er. Vijyant Singh, M.Tech (U.K.), daughter-in-laws Charu Singh and Radha Singh; pets Pasha & Jini cannot be forgotten and underestimated at any cost.

In the last, I am really indebted to Sri Satish Kumar Jain, Sri Vinod Kumar Jain, Sri Sonu Jain- all proprietors respectively of firm M/s CBS Publishers and Distributors, New Delhi and other officers/workers who all pushed me like anything of the same firm.

While writing book, different kinds of ideas come, some of them stay, whereas the rest go away. When I had finished my almost full work of composing, idea came to my mind to write a new separate chapter on **Biochemistry - the Yoga and the Health;** therefore, I did the same in the larger interest of the students and the readers.

Lastly, I am heartily highly obliged to **Mr. Prakash Sahu,** Compositor of the firm **'Akancha Computers', 390, Sadar Bazar, Jhansi** for beautiful computer work.

On the eve of Birth Anniversary i.e.   **- S.P. Singh**
6th February of my wife Dr. (Smt.) Manju Singh,
Reader in History, Bundelkhand Post Graduate
College, Jhansi., U.P.

PREFACE TO THE SECOND EDITION

Thanks a lot to the students and teachers who are seeing something in the **'Manual of Practical Biochemistry'** which has compelled me to bring out 5th edition of the same.

I would further highly appreciate new ideas/suggestions of the students/teachers from my inner corner of heart. One brain is insufficient in front of so many brains **and no one is complete in knowledge and ideas.**

I am ever indebted to my wife Dr. (Smt.) Manju Singh, Reader in History, Bundelkhand Post Graduate College, Jhansi; Sons Er. Vikrant and Er. Vijyant and daughter-in-law Smt. Charu Singh who all stood by me in difficult hours in this gigantic work.

I shall further fail in my duties if I do not express my feelings to my real well wishers i.e. Mr. K.V. Srivastava, Mr. S.S. Shukla, Mr. Khalak Singh, Mr. Chinta Mani - all of the Department of Biochemistry and Mr. Vishan Lal (Librarian), Er. S.S. Chaturvedi (Civil Engineer), and Er. V.N. Pathak (Electrical Engineer) all of this college - I can not forget the new ideas of Dr. Ajai Bhargava, Reader and Head, Biochemistry Department, Dental College, Gwalior (M.P.), Dr. Anurag Srivastava, Demonstrator in Biochemistry (a thorough gentelman) and Shri Sudhir Arora, M/s English Book Depot, Sadar Bazar, Jhansi.

I believe the revised **second edition** shall fulfill the syllabi of B.D.S. course of various Indian Universities and those of neighbouring countries like Nepal, Bangladesh, Pakistan, Afganistan, Burma, Bhutan and Gulf, Countries.

I am also ever grateful to the blessings of **Lord Shri Shirdi Sai Baba (Kopar Gaon, Maharashtra) & Shri Satya Sai Baba (Puttaparti, Andhra Pradesh)** without whose blessings and inspiration, **such works to complete is altogether impossible and just like dreams.**

I am also grateful to Shri Prakash Sahu **"Akancha Computer" Sadar Bazar, Jhansi** for beautiful computer work, Shri Satish Kumar Jain, Shri Vinod Kumar Jain, Shri B.M. Singh, Shri B.M. Sharma (Senior Marketing Executive), Shri Nayar and Shri Dharam Veer - all of the firm M/S C.B.S. Publishers & Distributors, 11, Darya Ganj, New Delhi for helping and encouraging me to bring out this new edition at an early date.

Knowledge is for spread, therefore, we must contribute it liberally and open heartedly.

- S.P. Singh

PREFACE TO THE FIRST EDITION

It is assumed that first edition of **'A Text Book of Dental Biochemistry'** will prove to be invaluable one to the students of B.D.S., and M.D.S. because several new topics have been included in it keepint in mind the need of the day. In this way, students shall get majority of topics of allied branches at one place.

There is still scope of addition of new topics in this book for which ideas from the students and the teachers are always most welcome. Students and the learned teachers may always act as a honourable **'judge'** for this pious work and they are the **'keys'** for opening the locks of the doors of the 'Educations' which in fact has got no boundary.

I feel highly indebted heartily to Prof. P.L. Shukla, former, Principal & Dean, B.R.D. Medical College, Gorakhpur (U.P.) who employed me as a teacher in medical faculty at the stinct of his childhood friend Late Dr. S.N. Singh, the then Professor and Head, Department of Geology, Lucknow University, Lucknow and rather also encouraged me whole heartedly for this pious profession of a 'teacher'. In this way, perhaps, I have completed my duty by writing 7 books for students' fraternity besides teaching them.

5th september 1999
(The Teachers' Day)

- S.P. Singh

CONTENTS

CONTENTS

BIOCHEMICAL ABBREVIATIONS

Ac	: Acetate		1,25 DHCC	: 1,25 dihydroxy cholecalciferol
Ac CoA	: Acyl coenzyme A		DMD	: Duchenne muscular dystrophy
A	: Adenine		DNP	: 2, 4 - dinitrophenol
ACD bottle	: Acid citrate dextrose bottle		DPN^+	: Diphosphopyridine nucleotide, oxidized
ALD	: Aldolase			
AIDS	: Acquired immune deficiency syndrome		$DPNH_2$	: Diphosphopyridine nucleotide, reduced
AMP	: Adenosine monophosphate (adenylic acid)		DNA	: Deoxyribonucleic acid
			DOC	: Deoxycorticosterone
ADP	: Adenosine diphosphate		DOPA	: Dioxyphenylalanine or Dihydroxyphenylalanine
ACE	: Angiotensin converting enzyme			
ACP	: Acid phosphatase		EDTA	: Ethylene diamine tetra acetic acid
ALT	: Alanine transaminase (previously GPT)		EAA	: Essential amino acids
			EFA	: Essential fatty acids
AST	: Aspartate transaminase (previously GOT)		FA	: Folic Acid
			FAD	: Flavin adenine dinucleotide
ATP	: Adenosine triphosphate		FDP	: Fructose 1, 6-diphosphate
ADPR	: Adenosine diphosphate ribose		FH_2	: Dihydro folic acid
ATPase	: Adenosine triphosphatase		FH_4	: Tetrahydro folic acid
AT-10	: Dehydrotachysterol (antitetany compound- 10)		FMN	: Flavin mono nucleotide
			FAO	: Food and Agriculture Organization
AZT	: Azidothymidine the only drug effective against AIDs, this is going to be marketed in India by 'Cipla' under the name of 'Zidovir'		GC-MS	: Gas Chromatograph-Mass spectrometer
			GA	: Glyceraldehyde
			GPx	: Glutathione peroxidase
BCG	: Bacillus Calmette and Guerin		GSH	: Glutathione (reduced form)
BMR	: Basal metabolic rate		GSSG	: Glutathione (oxidized form)
CF	: Citrovorum factor (folinic acid)		γ-GT	: γ- glutamyl transferase
CoA	: Coenzyme A		G	: Guanine
CoA SH	: Coenzyme A reduced		GMP	: Guanosine monophosphate (guanylic acid)
C	: Cytosine			
CMP	: Cytosine monophosphate (cytidylic acid)		GDP	: Guanosine diphosphate
			GTP	: Guanosine triphosphate
CDP	: Cytosine diphosphate		GDH	: Glucose dehydrogenase
cDNA	: Complementary DNA		GLDH	: Glutamate dehydrogenase
CT	: Computed tomography		GnRH	: Gonadotropin- releasing hormone
CTP	: Cytosine triphosphate		HbCO	: Carboxy(Carbon monoxy) hemoglobin
cTnT	: Cardiac troponin T			
Cal	: Calorie, large (kilocalorie)		HBsAG	: Hepatitis B surface antigen i.e., Australia antigen
ChE	: Choline esterase			
CPK	: Creatine phosphokinase		HBV	: Hepatitis B virus
DAP	: Dihydroxyacetone phosphate		HPLC	: High performance liquid
DFP	: Diisopropyl fluorophosphate			

	chromatography
HIV	: Human immuno-deficiency virus
IAA	: Iodoacetate
I	: Inosine
ICD	: Isocitrate dehydrogenase
IMP	: Inosine monophosphate (Inosinic Acid)
IDP	: Inosine diphosphate
ITP	: Inosine triphosphate
KG	: α- Ketoglutarate
LTs	: Leukotrienes
Mb	: Myoglobin
MB	: Methylene blue
MRI	: Magnetic resonance imaging
NMN	: Nicotinamide mononucleotide
NAD^+	: Nicotinamide adenine dinucleotide (older name is DPN^+, also known as Co I)
$NADP^+$	: Nicotinamide adenine dinucleotide phosphate (older name is TPN^+, also known as Co II)
NPN	: Non protein nitrogen
OAA	: Oxaloacetate
OD	: Optical density
PABA	: Para amino benzoic acid
PBI	: Protein bound iodine
PEP	: Phosphoenolpyruvate
3-PGA	: 3- Phosphoglyceric acid
PGE_2	: Prostaglandin E_2
Pi	: Inorganic phosphate
PP	: Pyrophosphate
PKU	: Phenylketonuria
POMC	: Pro-opio melanocortin
PSA	: Prostate specific antigen (semenogelase)
RNA	: Ribonucleic acid
RNAse	: Ribonuclease
R-5-P	: Ribose-5-Phosphate
R.Q.	: Respiratory Quotient
SOD	: Superoxide dismutase
SRP	: Signal recognition particle
STH	: Somatotropic hormone
TCA	: Trichloroacetic acid
THAM	: Tris (hydroxymethyl) aminoethane
TPP	: Thiamine pyrophosphate

TPN^+	: Triphosphopyridine nucleotide (oxidized form)
$TPNH_2$	: Triphosphopyridine nucleotide (reduced form)
U	: Uracil residue
UMP	: Uridine monophosphate (uridylic acid)
UDP	: Uridine diphosphate
UTP	: Uridine triphosphate
UDPG	: Uridine diphosphoglucose
UDPGal	: Uridine diphosphogalactose
USP	: United States Pharmacopoeia
WHO	: World Health Organization
XMP	: Xanthosine monophosphate
Xyl	: Xylose
Xul	: Xylulose

AMINO ACIDS

Ala	: Alanine
Arg	: Arginine
Val	: Valine
His	: Histidine
Leu	: Leucine
Ile	: Isoleucine
Met	: Methionine
Pro	: Proline
Phe	: Phenylalanine
Trp	: Tryptophan
Asp	: Aspartic acid
Asn	: Asparagine
Gln	: Glutamine
Glu	: Glutamic acid
Gly	: Glycine
Ser	: Serine
Thr	: Threonine
Thx	: Thyroxine
Tyr	: Tyrosine
Cys-SH	: Cysteine
Cys-S-	: 1/2 Cystine
Lys	: Lysine

HORMONES

ACTH	: Adrenocorticotrophic hormone
FSH	: Follicle stimulating hormone
GH	: Growth hormone
HCG	: Human chorionic gonadotropin

ICSH	: Interistitial cell stimulating hormone	UV	: Ultraviolet
LH	: Luteinizing hormone	VDM	: Vasodepressor material
LTH	: Leuteotrophic hormone	HRP	: Horseradish peroxidase
MSH	: Melanocyte stimulating hormone	TMB	: Tetra methyl benzidine
PTH	: Parathyroid hormone	Eukaryotes	: Mammalian cells
TSH	: Thyroid stimulating hormone	Prokaryotes	: Bacteria
T_3	: Triiodothyronine	NEPH	: Nephelometry
T_4	: Tetraiodothyronine (thyroxine)	REP	: Radio electrophoresis
		RU	: Radio uptake
		CC	: Column Chromatography
		RIA	: Radio-immunoassay

MISCELLANEOUS

AHG	: Antihemophilic globulin	CLIA	: Chemiluminescence immunoassay
BAL	: British anti- lewisite	ELISA	: Enzyme linked Immunosorbent assay
IR	: Infrared		
PRPP	: Phosphoribosyl pyrophosphate	HAA	: Haem agglutination assay

BIOCHEMISTRY - THE 'YOGA' AND THE HEALTH

Do some 'Yoga' daily atleast half an hour and advise others also for the same after the age of 20 years atleast as the body's biochemistry starts deteriorating very gradually. Increase its time after the age of 40 years to atleast one hour. It will keep the body's biochemistry fit and in order and will keep you away from a doctor.

'Yoga' is a complete science of Ancient Indian system of Medicine which is more than 5,000 years old whereas the present more prevalent system of allopathic medicine is nearly 200 years old only.

Plus points of allopathic system of Medicine are that it is of great value in completely curing diseases caused due to bacteria/microorganisms; in surgical/accidental (traumatic)/emergency cases, whereas the 'yoga' system of medicine has got the capability to cure incurable diseases permanently. If 'yoga' and ancient system of medicine i.e., Ayurvedic are used simultaneously for curing a disease then the results are quicker but it's not always advisable to take Ayurvedic pills. 'Yoga' alone is a very good system of medicine which to a greater extent can cure innumerable diseases/ disorders of human beings permanently whereas there is no such permanent cure of such diseases in allopathic system. To name such incurable diseases, following are the few examples:

1. Blood pressure (Hypertension)
2. Hypercholesterolaemia/hypertri-glyceridaemia
3. Obesity (reduction in weight)
4. Parkinson's disease
5. Polio
6. Alzheimer's disease
7. Heart- aliments
8. Psoriasis
9. Asthma
10. Hyperacidity
11. Piles
12. Joint problems like ankylosis, prolapse disc, lumbago (pain in the lumbar region), cervical and lumbar spondylosis, osteo- arthritis, rheumatoid arthritis, gout, arthralgia (pain in joints), frozen shoulders, sprains, etc.
13. Bronchitis
14. Atherosclerosis
15. SLE (partially)
16. Tumours
17. Cancers (to some extent, Ist stage only)
18. Anaemia
19. Mysthenia gravis
20. Diabetes mellitus

21. Hyperthyroidism
22. Baldness
23. Greyish of hairs
24. Varicose veins
25. Fibroids in the uterus
26. Deafness
27. Muscular dystrophy
28. For gain in body weight
29. Neurological disorders
30. Depression
31. Epilepsy
32. Scleroderma
33. Leucoderma
34. Eye sight
35. Glaucoma
36. Osteoporosis
37. Constipation
38. Ulcers in the gastrointestinal tract
39. Spinal problems
40. Renal problems
41. Psychic problems
42. Sharpness of the wisdom
43. Paralysis
44. Insomnia
45. Vitality
46. Respiratory problems, etc.

■ **The science of 'Yoga' demands regularity, sincerity, dedication and time.**

■ Duration of time in performing 'Yoga' has got more meaning.

■ By the application of 'Yoga', one can lead a long smooth life, may be hundred years or more as there are examples of Indian Rishis and Munis having longevity as much as 150 years or so. What 'Yoga' does to the biochemistry of human beings?

■ It brings out proper synchronisation and balance of various hormones **(endocrine system)** and enzymes of our system which play innumerable vital role in thousands of biochemical reactions of our body.

■ It reactivates and re-energises cells of our system.

■ It regenerates cells.

■ It checks degeneration process which is mainly associated with the advancing age.

■ It reactivates various organs like pancreas, lungs, etc.

■ It brings out inhalation of proper quantity of oxygen.

■ It keeps the biochemistry of the body fit and in order which one can realise and come across the consequences in one's own life.

Credit for revolution in 'Yoga' in the present era goes to the untiring efforts of **Param Pujya yogi swami Ram Dev Ji Maharaj of Haridwar of Uttranchal state whose dream is first to see every Indian healthy and then the human race round the globe.**

Although, this science of 'Yoga' is not the new one but 'Yogi ji' is solely responsible for bringing awareness in the masses.

He deserves 'Bharat Ratna' while alive. Govt. of India must confer upon him this prestigious award. He has awaken all of us. We were really sleeping for more than fifty years like 'Kumkhkaran' (brother of Rawan) of 'Ramayana Age'. **He emphasizes mainly on three 'yogic exercises', namely :**

(i) **Anulom - Vilom,**

(ii) **Kapalbhati, and**

(iii) **Bhastrika**

BIOCHEMISTRY TODAY

Biochemistry, these days is treated to be the most important subject of life-sciences whether medical sciences or plant-sciences. Nearly 70 years ago, this subject was in infancy but now it is deep rooted and possesses an unique position because it is said to be the foundation of the modern medicine on which it is erected.

> **The word 'Biochemistry' is very broad in its meaning which may be defined as the study of different chemical processes going on in the body at molecular level, no matter it's a plant or animal body.**
>
> Besides, it also deals with the nature of the chemical constituents of the living organisms; the functions and transformations of such chemical entities in the biological systems and also with the chemical and energetic changes associated with such transformations during the course of activity.
>
> Day by day, its applicability in the field of life sciences is going on increasing and it is being utilized for the benefit of mankind and plant kingdom as well.

The history of biochemistry as it is in the present form is not very old. Most of the work in the field of biochemistry has been carried out in the last half-century. In this period of development, it is being increasingly recognized as an essential discipline among the life- sciences. In some of the advanced Western countries, there are full fledged independent institutes of biochemistry but unfortunately there is even not a single separate full fledged independent institute of biochemistry in India because of the want of which our country is lagging behind as far as *biochemical sciences* are concerned. Unfortunately our country has neither got a separate *'Institute of Biochemistry'* nor *'Biochemical Engineering';* whereas now the time is fully mature to establish such an independent institute in India so that we could keep pace with the Western world. Although, we have some good institutes of Science and Technology like **Central Drug Research Institute at Lucknow; Industrial Toxicology Research Centre at Lucknow; National Institute of Immunology at New Delhi; National Institute of Nutrition at Hyderabad; Centre for Food & Technological Research Institute at Mysore; Indian Institute of Science at Bangalore; Centre for Biochemical Technology at New Delhi; National Chemical Laboratory at Pune; Indian Institute of Chemical Technology at Hyderabad; Bhabha Atomic Research Centre at Trombay (Mumbai); Tata Institute of Fundamental Research at Mumbai; All India Institute of Medical Sciences at New Delhi; Centre for Cellular and Molecular Biology at Hyderabad, Centre for DNA Finger**

Printing & Diagnostics at Hyderabad; National Brain Research Centre at Manesar (Haryana); Institute of Genomics & Integrative Biology at New Delhi; International Centre for Genetic Engineering & Biotechnology at New Delhi etc, which have got very good well equipped biochemistry sections. Scientists and doctors are working whole heartedly round the clock at these centres to make 'science' more approachable and meaningful to the mankind. We have some eminent biochemists in India like *Prof G.P. Talwar, Padam Shree (Ex-Professor & HOD, Department of Biochemistry, AIIMS, New Delhi & ex-*Director, National Institute of Immunology, New Delhi), and at present Director, Talwar Research Foundation, New Delhi, whose team has so far been able to publish wonderful research papers in the field of 'Immunology' in world class journals and still working on several projects like "developing peptide based vaccine for **Plasmodium vivax malaria**" etc; Dr Lalji Singh, Director, Centre for Cellular and Molecular Biology, Hydera-bad; whose team is working on several projects related to **DNA finger printing** technology, uses of various biochemical techniques/ applications in forensic sciences, etc., for e.g., in establishing parentage problems/issues, etc. *Professor D. P. Burma,*Ex-Prof. and H.O.D.of Biochemistry, Institute of Medical Sciences, B.H.U.,

CBT	: New Delhi
CDRI	: Lucknow
CFTRI	: Mysore
CCMB	: Hyderabad
ITRC	: Lucknow
ICGEB	: New Delhi
IGIB	: New Delhi
IISc	: Bangalore
IICT	: Hyderabad
NCL	: Pune
NII	: New Delhi
NIN	: Hyderabad
TIFR	: Mumbai
CDFD	: Hyderabad
NBRC	: Manesar (Haryana)

Varanasi, now a days settled at Calcutta is a worker on *Nucleic Acids (Ribosomologist); Prof P.P. Singh,* Ex-Head of the Department of Biochemistry, R.N.T. Medical College, Udaipur is a worker on **Urolithiasis**; *Prof T.N. Pattabiraman,* Ex-Head of the Department of Biochemistry, Kasturba Medical College, Manipal, is an *Enzymologist; Prof. B.C. Harinath, Ex-*Head of the Department of Biochemistry, Mahatma Gandhi Institute of Medical Sciences, Sevagram (Wardha, Maharashtra), is an *Immunologist* of repute and high profile. Dr P.M. Bhargava, Ex- Director, CCMB, Hyderabad is a Biochemist of repute who is working with his team on several projects of National interest.; Dr G.K. Khullar, Professor & Head, Biochemistry Department, P.G.I., Chandigarh is a Biochemist of repute working on **'designing polymer based novel drug carriers for Experimental Tuberculosis;** Professor Balaram, Chairman, Division of Biological Sciences, Indian Institute of Science, Bangalore is a Biochemist of repute working on several projects of human interest; Dr. K. Taranath Shetty, Professor and Head Department of Biochemistry, NIMHANS, Bangalore, is a Biochemist of repute working on several projects related to **neurobiochemistry;** Dr V. S. Chauhan, Director, International Centre for Genetic Engineering & Biotechnology, New Delhi whose team is working on hereditary and allied disorders; Dr Samir Brahmachari, Director, Institute of Genomics & Integrative Biology, New Delhi whose team is working on **'Genome Project'** and allied topics; Dr Sandeep Basu, Director, National Institute of Immunology, New Delhi whose team is working in developing vaccines for various disorders; Dr P. N. Tandon, Director, National Brain Research Centre whose team is working on several projects of brain chemistry and **Dr Seyed E Hasnain,** Director, Centre for DNA Finger Printing & Diagnostics, Hyderabad whose team is working on several topics of human interest.

We are having **National Institute of Nutrition at Hyderabad,** an institute of its type in whole of Asia which is dedicated towards the inventions of cheaper sources of proteins, vitamins, etc. and also trying to evolve cheaper vegetable/plant substitutes of animal proteins for the vegetarians as in our country quite a sizable population is vegetarian and in the Western world too quite a good number of people conscious to health and obesity are now a days turning to vegetarianism. This institute also attracts young doctors having aptitude for research in medicine; institute is also dedicated in quality research work in bringing out solution of the diseases being caused due to the deficiency of vitamins and hormones, also involved in the search of good cheaper easily available sources of calories so that the poorer around the world may be benefited. Besides, **institute is also doing work as to how sufferers of certain diseases like diabetes mellitus, kwashiorkor, marasmus, protein energy malnutrition (PEM),etc. may get rid of such fierceful diseases / states.** Institute is also looking after various interests of pregnant and lactating women with special reference to poverty.

CFTRI (Mysore), is also looking after the interest of the good health of the people of the globe with special reference to pure drinking water, beverages, adulterations (trend of adulteration is on increase day by day in some countries like India where the punishment for the adulterators, if at all existing is either of mild nature or nil) etc. Adulteration in edibles/ beverages like sweets, oils, spices, condiments, milk, medicines, flour, and a number of variety of preparations which are used in daily routine by the human beings and the animals has become a common thing now-a-days. **Adulteration is the mother of so many diseases and a perfect sound 'Nation' can not be footed so long the adulterators are alive.** Therefore, the Governments should be very strict in dealing with such adulterators.

C.D.R.I. (Lucknow) is also dedicated towards the search of newer, safer, potent drugs having no or lesser toxicity.

I.T.R.C. (Lucknow) is likewise dedicated in studying various aspects of toxicity to mankind with special reference to pollutants, gases, adulteration of toxic substances like lead, cadmium, cobalt etc. i.e., non-permitted (banned) colours etc, to the edibles. They are also working to see the effect of poisonous gases/materials etc. on the health of factory/industry workers.

NII (New Delhi) is dedicated towards the synthesis of newer vaccines of certain diseases. They are also doing work towards the synthesis of *'birth control vaccine';* it shall be the most revolutionary day in the history of science. It shall be a laurel not only to the Indian Scientists but to the entire scientific community of the world. *Prof. G.P. Talwar,* Ex-Head of the Department of Biochemistry, All India Institute of Medical Sciences, New Delhi and at present Director, Talwar Research Foundation, New Delhi is engaged for more than last two decades towards the synthesis of birth control vaccine. One such group from Mumbai, besides some groups from the Western world are also engaged for the same cause. These days, control of the explosion of the population is the ever biggest challenge before the entire scientific community of the world.

A lot of work is being done both on basic and applied fields of biochemistry in order to make it more useful and viable for the benefit of mankind and understanding the secrets of life. The discipline has so far established an unique position in the field of medicine because of the fact that it is forming a **major tool in explaining the development of disorders and diseases in the body;** that is why, one finds sophisticated latest update biochemical instruments like **PCR, gas liquid chromatography, atomic absorption spectrophotometer, autoanalysers, radioisotope laboratory, tissue culture laboratory, etc.** in the well established good departments/sections/units of biochemistry. The knowledge of biochemistry has been able to pinpoint the exact site of the disorder and to give a clue towards the line of treatment in most of the diseases. **The new offshoot of biochemistry i.e. genetic engineering is flourishing like anything in the Western advanced countries like U.S.A., U.K., Germany, France, Japan, etc. which may bring solution of several disorders like those of hereditary disorders and other incurable diseases, the treatment of which is not possible at the moment. Scientists and doctors are working day and night in these countries to synthesize genes responsible for various genetic defects but unfortunately in our own country, this science is still lagging behind. It is a cause of serious concern to the Government of India.**

Hereditary diseases, which are considered to be incurable at present might be easily controlled or treated satisfactorily in the near future by simply changing the nature of the particular gene(s) responsible for the causation of such disease(s). **Attempts are being made to synthesize genes biochemically. Success in this field is bound to bring revolutionary, miraculous changes in the world of life-sciences.** Genes are the carriers of hereditary characters. After the synthesis of newer genes, it might be quite possible to produce off-springs of ones own choice. Suppose, then, if someone wishes a wrestler, or an athlete or a gymnast or a tall fellow, or a very intellectual one, it would be quite possible to have it. This also means that the usage of genes for the betterment of mankind may also be misused by someone; hence, care must be taken for its 'use' and not 'misuse'; therefore the Governments must enact some law(s) in future for the use of **'genes'** and the power of its usage should never be vested in a single hand (single doctor), rather in a board comprising of atleast 5-7 highly qualified specialists of that field.

Dr Har Gobind Khorana, India born Chemist, turned into a Biochemist, nowadays settled in U.S.A. (a permanent citizen of U.S.A at present) is working for more than a quarter century on DNA and the synthesis of genes for which he was awarded the most prestigious award i.e. *"Nobel Prize"* in the year 1968.

The knowledge of biochemistry is also being extensively used in the field of diagnosis of diseases. Estimations of the levels of biogenic compounds and enzymes in the circulating blood/CSF/urine have been proved to be of valuable guidance to the Physicians/Surgeons in making the diagnosis of diseases, for instance, blood sugar level gets elevated in diabetes mellitus, blood urea and creatinine levels get raised in nephritis, serum calcium level gets elevated in hyperthyroidism and gets decreased in infantile tetany, serum inorganic phosphorus gets decreased in rickets, serum cholesterol level gets elevated in nephrosis, diabetes mellitus, obstructive jaundice, myxoedema and xanthomatosis and may be decreased in *hyperthyroidism*, level of enzyme acid phosphatase gets increased in the carcinoma of prostate glands, serum glutamic oxaloacetic transaminase (GOT) and creatine phosphokinase (CPK or CK) levels get elevated in myocardial infarction, and so on.

Certain qualitative tests in urine, e.g. for the detection of sugar, protein, bile pigments, bile salts, blood, chyle, etc. are of great importance to the Physicians/ Surgeons in making proper diagnosis. Besides qualitative tests, certain quantitative tests in urine like that of the estimation of total proteins in a 24 hrs urine sample is of diagnostic value in cases of nephrotic syndrome.

Estimations of hormones in serum are of equally great diagnostic value, e.g. the estimations of T_3 and T_4 are most reliable means of confirming the diagnosis of hyperthyroidism or hypothyroidism. Highly specific and sensitive radioimmunoassays are used to measure serum T_3 and T_4 concentrations. In thyrotoxic states, serum TSH concentration is almost always low or undetectable.

NORMAL RANGE
T_4 : 4 -12 µg/dl
T_3 : 80-100 ng/dl
TSH: Less than 5 µU/ml

This is of little diagnostic value, since most assays can not distinguish between normal and subnormal values. Measurement of serum TSH is the best means of distinguishing between untreated hypothyroidism of thyroid origin, in which the values are invariably increased, and pituitary or hypothalamic hypothyroidism, in which the values are usually undetectable or within the normal range.

Certain diseases are merely controlled by using specific enzyme inhibitors or activators. Recent studies have proved that the medicines mostly act by influencing certain enzyme or enzyme systems. The same also holds true for hormones. Structure activity relationships have been established in most of the cases. Such studies are covered in the field of *biochemical pharmacology*. After ascertaining the site of action and the structure responsible for a particular activity, it has now become possible to synthesize newer medicines having lesser toxicity and greater beneficial effects.

Radioisotopes are of great use in certain types of diseases like malignancies (cancers) of different origin of various organs/tissues. Isotopes of cobalt, iodine, etc. are used satisfactorily with very good results in different types of early diagnosed cancers by the radiophysicists under the guidance/ consultation of Physicians/Surgeons treating such patients. In our country, establishment of radioisotope laboratory requires clearance by the *Bhabha Atomic Research Centre (BARC), Trombay* as one must take all kinds of precautions in the handling of radioisotopes. All staff members connected with such a laboratory must be well versed with the *"Radiation Hazards"*, which are otherwise very fatal and injurious to the humans, many times more fatal than the X-Rays.

Disposal of the used radioactive material is also a cause of great concern. This material must be disposed as per the guidelines and instructions laid down by BARC, Trombay. All kinds of wares i.e: plasticwares/glasswares etc. being used for the estimation purposes or therapy purposes or otherwise should not be used for routine work, hitherto must be disposed safely. **Radioactive material, if handled casually, may otherwise kill the normal healthy cells, may also cause *'mutation'* which may even persist in the off-springs (1-2-3 generations).**

CHAPTER 1

CARBOHYDRATES

> We are very important for the human beings as we are the driving force (petrol) for them. We are polyhydroxy aldehydes or ketones or their derivatives. To achieve us is very easy and we are inexpensive but teeth should take care of us, especially the infants and the children. When you eat us like other things and do not brush, we get accumulated in the interspaces of teeth, thus invite bacteria to grow which results in caries, a fierceful disease. We have storehouses in the body like liver, muscles, etc.

Introduction

The class of substances known as carbohydrates is comprised of a large number of relatively heterogenous compounds. They are especially prominent constituents of plants, but also do occur and serve important functions in animals.

Carbohydrates

‖

carbon + hydrogen + oxygen

or

carbon + hydrogen + oxygen + nitrogen + sulphur

They are found in abundance in plant kingdom in the form of cellulose and starch; besides are also found in abundance in animal kingdom as well in the form of glucose or glycogen or chondroitin sulphates, etc.

Carbohydrates serve as the chief source of energy in the food of humans and many other animals. As is evident from the name itself, these are generally the compounds of carbon, hydrogen and oxygen but the higher carbohydrates have also been found to possess nitrogen and sulphur in their structures.

Carbohydrates may be defined as polyhydroxy-aldehydes or polyhydroxy-ketones or derivatives of them. Their molecular weight ranges from less than 100 to well over 1 million and in general are, white solids, sparingly soluble in organic solvents but soluble in water except for some high molecular weight carbohydrates.

Classification

For convenience, carbohydrates may be classified into three major groups (Table 1.1) namely :

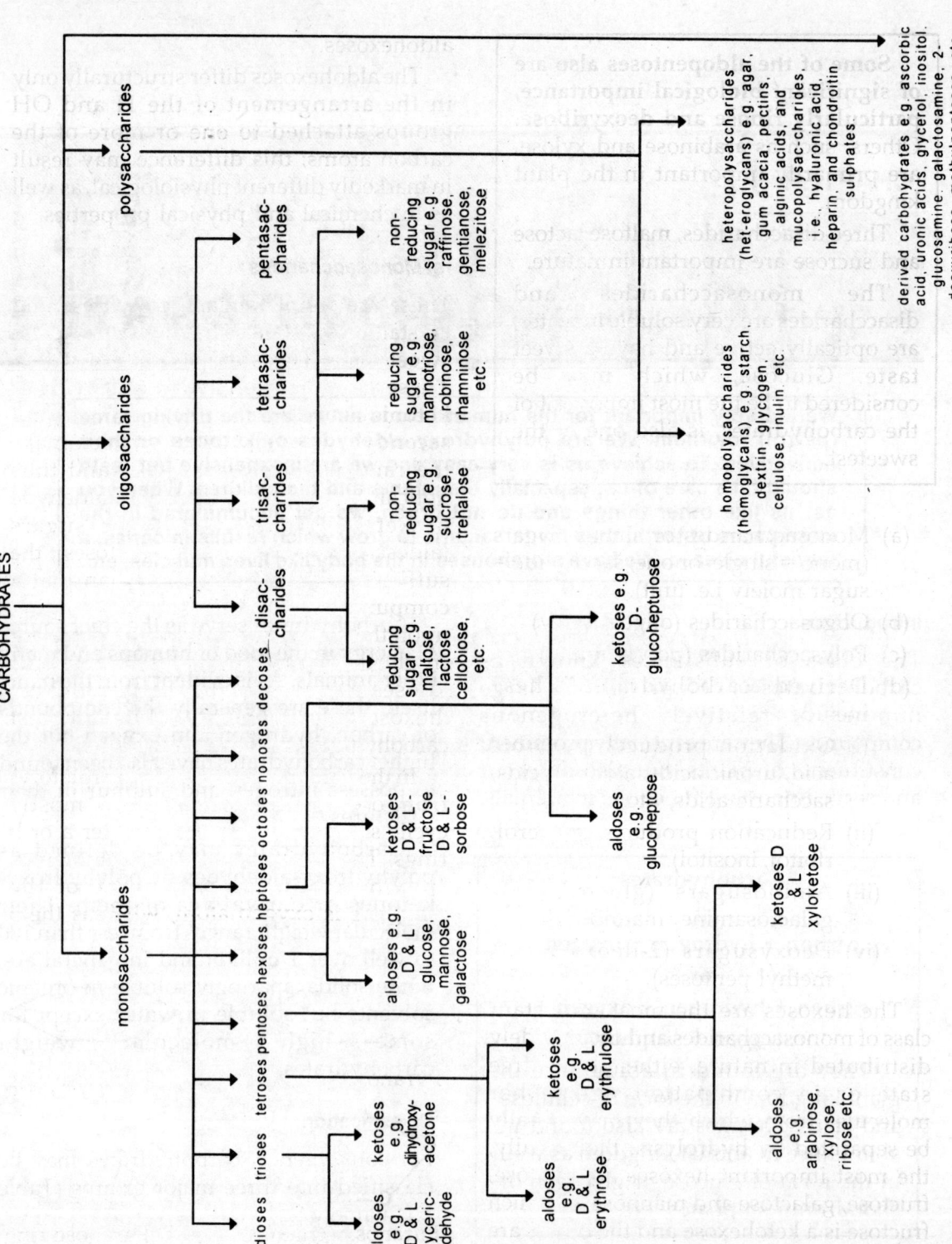

Table 1.1 : Classification of Carbohydrates

Some of the aldopentoses also are of significant biological importance, particularly ribose and deoxyribose. Others, such as arabinose and xylose, are primarily important in the plant kingdom.

Three disaccharides, maltose lactose and sucrose are important in nature.

The monosaccharides and disaccharides are very soluble in water, are optically active and have a sweet taste. Glucose, which may be considered to be the most important of the carbohydrates, is also one of the sweetest.

(a) Monosaccharides or simple sugars (mono = single or one; saccharide = sugar moiety i.e. unit).

(b) Oligosaccharides (oligo= a few)

(c) Polysaccharides (poly = many)

(d) Derived carbohydrates; these include :

  (i) Oxidation products (ascorbic acid, uronic acids, aldonic acids, saccharic acids, etc.)

  (ii) Reducation products (glycerol, ribitol, inositol).

  (iii) Aminosugars (glucosamine, galactosamine, mannosamine).

  (iv) Deoxysugars (2-deoxyribose, methyl pentoses).

The hexoses are the most important class of monosaccharides and occur widely distributed in nature, either in the free state or in combination with other molecules from which they may usually be separated by hydrolysis. Biologically, the most important hexoses are glucose, fructose, galactose and mannose, of which fructose is a ketohexose and the others are aldohexoses.

The aldohexoses differ structurally only in the arrangement of the H and OH groups attached to one or more of the carbon atoms; this difference may result in markedly different physiological, as well as in chemical and physical properties.

(a) Monosaccharides

These are simple sugars, colourless and crystalline substances having more or less sweet taste. Thess are soluble in water. **These are either polyhydric aldehydic or ketonic alcohols having both primary and secondary alcoholic groups** which make the carbon atoms asymmetric and thus optically active. The presence of aldehyde or ketone groups i.e. aldose sugars (aldoses) and ketone sugars (ketoses); the suffix- ose can be taken to mean that a compund is a carbohydrate. Depending upon the number of carbon atoms present in the molecule, these are named as 'dioses', 'trioses', 'tetroses', 'pentoses', 'hexoses' etc. (Table 1.2). The simplest carbohydrate is glycolaldehyde.

In the nature mostly 'D' (dextrorotatory) from occurs. Sugars may show mostly cyclic structures. They form either a or b rings. The 6 membered ring is known as "pyranose" ring in which one of the members is oxygen atom, whereas the 5

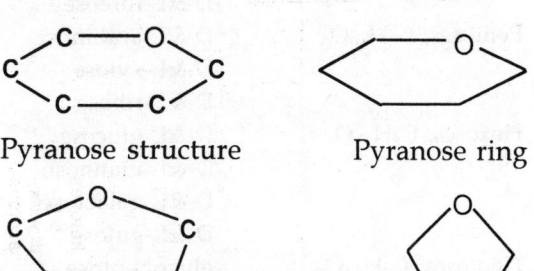

Pyranose structure   Pyranose ring

Furanose structure   Furanose ring

membered ring is known as "furanose" ring. Again one member of the furanose ring is oxygen atom. The sugars, by virtue of their alcoholic group can form esters with acids, all the free hydroxy group being replaceable. In the biological systems, the alcoholic groups at position "6" or "1" are found to be most reactive.

Being aldehydes or ketones, they can readily reduce copper, bismuth or silver solutions. They can condense with hydroxylamine or phenylhydrazine forming oximes and osazones.

The important sugars belonging to monosaccharides are **glucose (dextrose), fructose (levulose),** mannose, galactose, ribose, ribulose, xylose, xylulose, erythrose, sedoheptulose, glyceraldehyde, dihydroxyacetone etc.

If the primary alcoholic group of the monosaccharides is oxidized to -COOH; the acid formed is known as " uronic acid" such as glucose forms glucuronic acid, galactose forms galacturonic acid etc. Such uronic acids are found in mucoproteins.

$$
\begin{array}{cccc}
H - C = O & & H - C = O \\
| & & | \\
H - C - OH & & HO - C - H \\
| & & | \\
CH_2OH & & CH_2OH
\end{array}
$$

D-glyceric aldehyde   L-glyceric aldehyde

All the D-aldose sugars may be considered as the derivatives of D-glyceric aldehyde and all the L-aldose sugars as the derivatives of L-glyceric aldehyde.

$$
\begin{array}{cccc}
H - C = O & & H - C = O \\
| & & | \\
H - C - OH & & HO - C - H \\
| & & | \\
H - C - OH & & H - C - OH \\
| & & | \\
CH_2OH & & CH_2OH
\end{array}
$$

D- erythrose   D-threose

Table 1.2 : Classification of monosaccharides

General formula $C_2 (H_2O)_2$	Aldoses	Ketoses
Dioses, $C_2H_4O_2$	Glycolaldehyde	
Trioses, $C_3H_6O_3$	D-&L*-glycerose or glyceric aldehyde	dihydroxyacetone
Tetroses, $C_4H_8O_4$	D-&L-erythrose	erythrulose
	D-&L-threose	
Pentoses, $C_5H_{10}O_5$	D-&L-arabinose	D-&L-xyloketose
	D-&L-xylose	
	D-&L-ribose	
Hexoses, $C_6H_{12}O_6$	D-&L-glucose	D-&L-fructose
	D-&L-mannose	D-&L-sorbose
	D-&L-galactose	
	D-&L-gulose	
Heptoses, $C_7H_{14}O_7$	glucoheptose	D-glucoheptulose
	mannoheptose	L-glucoheptulose

Levorotatory

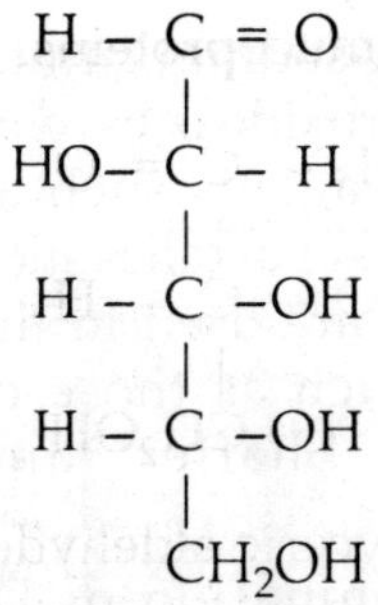

```
  H – C = O              H – C = O              H₂– C = O
      |                      |                      |
 HO– C – H              H – C –OH                  C = O
      |                      |                      |
  H – C –OH              H – C –OH             HO– C – H
      |                      |                      |
  H – C –OH              H – C –OH              H – C –OH
      |                      |                      |
    CH₂OH                  CH₂OH                 H – C –OH
 D-arabinose             D-ribose                  |
                                               H₂– C –OH
                                                D-fructose
```

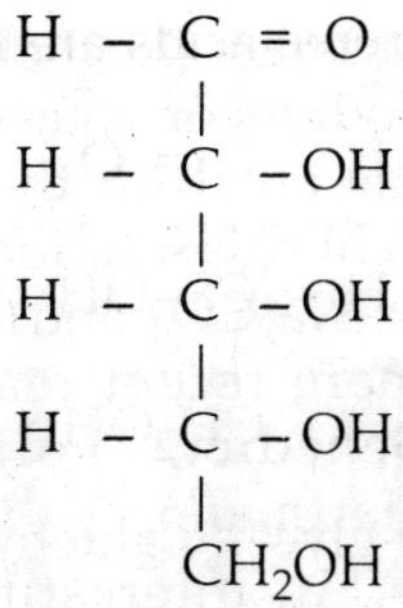

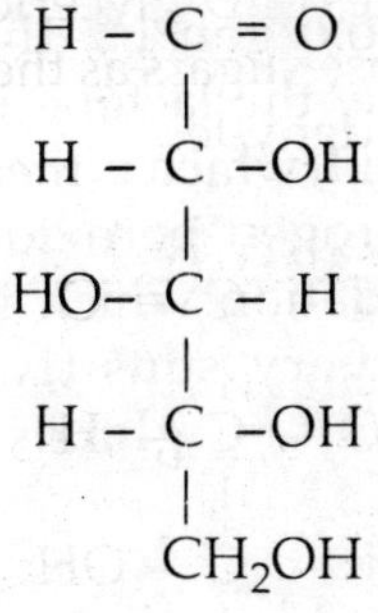

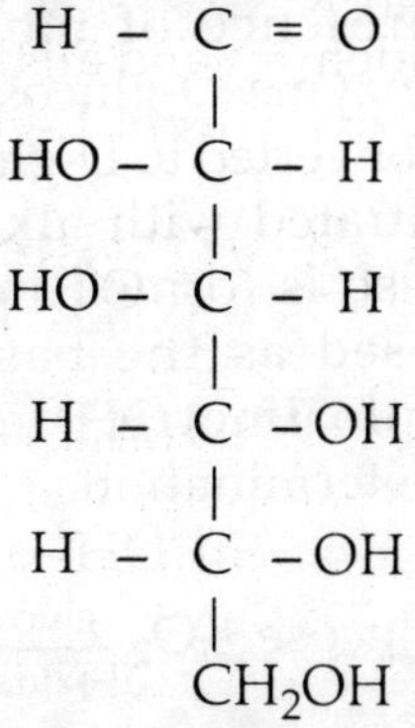

```
  H – C = O              H – C = O
      |                      |
  H – C –OH             HO – C – H
      |                      |
 HO– C – H             HO – C – H
      |                      |
  H – C –OH              H – C –OH
      |                      |
    CH₂OH               H – C –OH
  D-xylose                  |
                          CH₂OH
                        D-glucose
```

osazones:

Phenylhydrazine and substituted hydrazones react with the monosaccharides and other carbohydrates containing a free sugar group to form hydrazones and osazones. With few exceptions, the hydrazones are soluble and difficult to isolate. On the other hand, osazones of different sugars are relatively insoluble and crystallize in beautiful and characteristic forms.

```
  H – C = O              H – C = O
      |                      |
  H – C –OH             HO – C – H
      |                      |
 HO– C – H             HO – C – H
      |                      |
 HO– C – H              H – C –OH
      |                      |
  H – C –OH              H – C –OH
      |                      |
    CH₂OH                  CH₂OH
 D-galactose            D-mannose
```

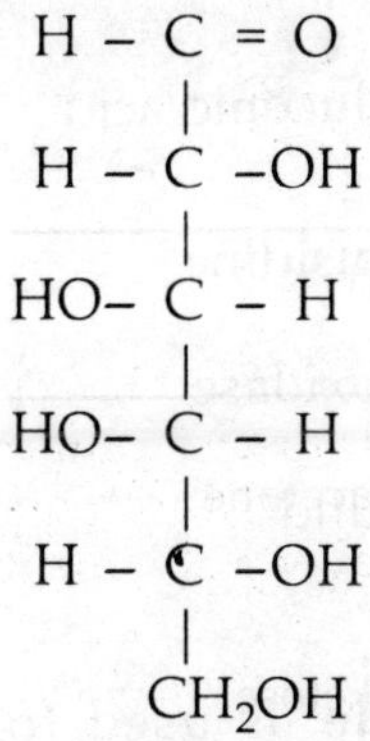

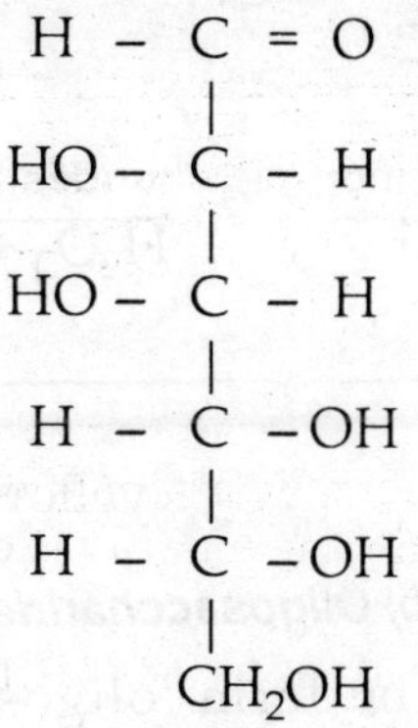

Some important reactions of monosaccharides are as mentioned below:

1. Reactions of monosaccharides characteristic of the aldehyde and ketone group. Reaction with hydrazines to form hydrazones and

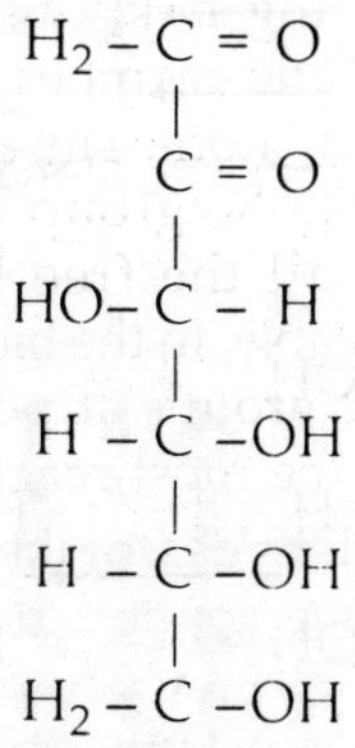

2. Monosaccharides react with hydrogen cyanide to form cyanhydrins.

3. Monosaccharides react with hydroxylamine to form oximes.

4. Reduction to form sugar alcohols: Both aldoses and ketoses may be reduced to the corresponding polyhydroxy alcohols. This may be accomplished with sodium amalgam, or better, electrolytically or by hydrogen under high pressure in the presence of a catalyst. Thus, the alcohols formed from glucose, mannose and fructose are as follows:

D- glucose $\longrightarrow$ D - sorbitol

D-mannose $\longrightarrow$ D - mannitol

D-fructose $\longrightarrow$ D-mannitol, D-sorbitol

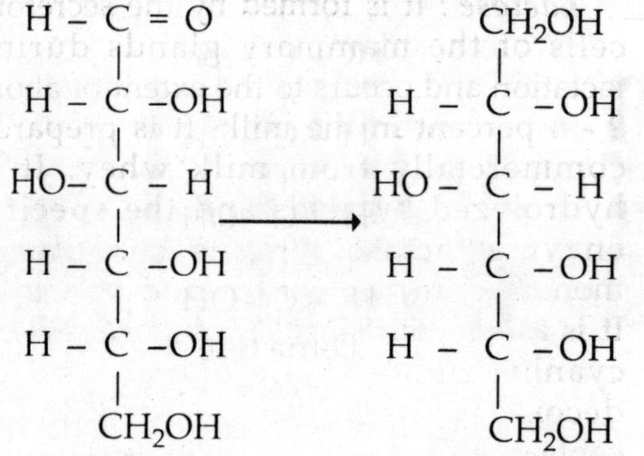

$$
\begin{array}{ccc}
H - C = O & & CH_2OH \\
| & & | \\
H - C -OH & & H - C -OH \\
| & & | \\
HO - C - H & \longrightarrow & HO - C - H \\
| & & | \\
H - C -OH & & H - C -OH \\
| & & | \\
H - C -OH & & H - C -OH \\
| & & | \\
CH_2OH & & CH_2OH \\
\text{D-glucose} & & \text{D-sorbitol}
\end{array}
$$

5. Monosaccharides get oxidized to form sugar acids, for example:

$$\text{D-glucose} \xrightarrow{\text{bromine water}} \text{D-gluconic acid}$$

6. Reducing action of sugars in alkaline solution:

Determination of sugars

All the sugars that contain free sugar group undergo enolization and various other changes when placed under alkaline solution. The enediol forms of the sugars are highly reactive and are easily oxidized by oxygen and other oxidizing agents. This means that these sugars in alkaline solution are very powerful reducing agents. They readily reduce oxidising ions such as Ag^+, Hg^{++}, Bi^{+++}, Cu^{++} and $Fe(CN)_6^{---}$ and the sugars are odixized to complex mixture of acids. This reducing action of sugars in alkaline solution is utilized for both the qualitative and quantitative determination of sugars. Reagents containing Cu^{++} ions are most commonly used. These are generally alkaline solutions of cupric sulphate containing sodium potassium tartarate (Rochelle salt) or sodium citrate. Sodium or potassium hydroxide is used as the alkali in the older reagents such as Fehling's solution; but weaker alkalies such as Na_2CO_3 and $NaHCO_3$ are used in the more recent reagents, such as those of Benedict, Folin and Shaffer and Hartmann.

An interesting determination of D-glucose is based upon its quantitative oxidation to D-gluconolactone in the presence of molecular oxygen by the enzyme D-glucose oxidase. the lactone is converted to D-gluconic acid, which is then titrated with alkali. Hydrogen peroxide also is formed in the oxidation which is used as the basis of a very sensitive colorimetric method for glucose determination.

$$\text{glucose} + O_2 \xrightarrow[\text{oxidase}]{\text{glucose}} \text{gluconolactone} + H_2O_2$$

$$\downarrow + H_2O$$

$$\text{D- gluconic acid}$$

$$H_2O_2 + o - \text{dianisidine}$$

$$\downarrow \text{peroxidase}$$

$$\text{yellow compound}$$

(b) Oligosaccharides

The term 'oligosaccharide' is used for compounds made up by the condensation of 2-10 molecules of simple sugars. The important carbohydrates of this group are sucrose, maltose, lactose and raffinose. These are distinguished from each other by nomenclature such as disaccharides, tri, tetra and pentasaccharides. On hydrolysis such saccharides give simple sugars. These may be regarded as the products of condensation of two or more sugars with the elimination of water. These have a general formula $C_n(H_2O)_{n-1}$. In general the reducing disaccharides are less potent as reducing agents than monosaccharides.

Disaccharides: The following tabulation gives the better known disaccharides with their component monosaccharides. Those possessing a free sugar group, are reducing sugars and give reactions characteristic of monosaccharides.

Disaccharides $C_{12}H_{22}O_{11}$	Constituent Monosaccharides
I **Reducing sugars**	
(a) Maltose	glucose+glucose
(b) Lactose	glucose+galactose
(c) Cellobiose	glucose+glucose
II **Non-reducing sugars**	
(a) Sucrose	glucose+fructose
(b) Trehalose	glucose+glucose

Of the above, maltose, lactose and sucrose are the most important examples of disaccharides.

Maltose: It is composed of two glucose units (Fig. 1.1) and is formed when the enzyme amylase or diastase hydrolyzes starch. It is a product of the action of salivary amylase (ptyalin) and pancreatic amylase (amylopsin) upon starch during the process of digestion. It is also formed as an intermediate product in the acid hydrolysis of starch and is an important constituent of corn syrups, which are

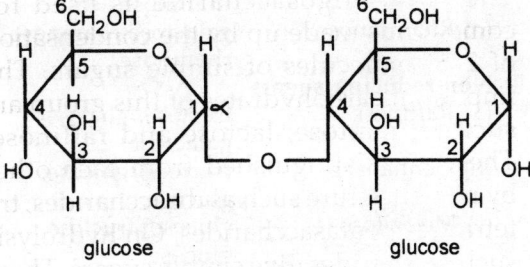

Fig 1.1 : Maltose

prepared by partial hydrolysis of starch with dilute acids. Enzyme maltase hydrolyzes it to glucose.

Lactose : It is formed by the secretory cells of the mammary glands during lactation and occurs to the extent of about 2 - 6 percent in the milk. It is prepared commercially from milk whey. It is hydrolyzed by acids and the **specific enzyme lactase** into its constituent monosaccharides, glucose and galactose. It is a reducing sugar, forms osazones, a cyanhydrin, and an oxime, and is decomposed by alkali. It accordingly contains a free sugar group in its structure (Fig 1.2).

It is of interest to know that the human milk differs from cow's milk in containing, in addition to regular lactose, **other oligosaccharides, such as L-fucosyl lactose.**

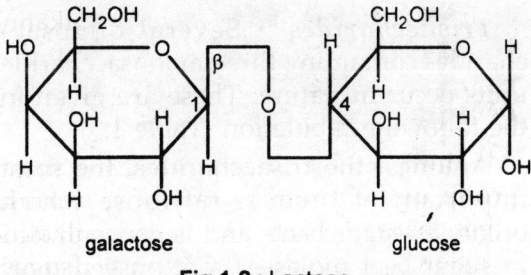

Fig 1.2 : Lactose

Sucrose: It occurs especially in the juices of plants such as sugar beets, sugar cane, sorghum, sugar maple and pineapple and in smaller quantities in the juices of many other plants. Ripe fruits are rich in sucrose. It is by far the most abundantly distributed of the sugars.

Hydrolysis of sucrose (Fig. 1.3) by dilute acids or enzyme invertase or sucrase produces one molecule each of glucose and fructose.

Sucrose is not a reducing sugar, is relatively stable towards the action of alkali, and in general does not give the reactions characteristic of the sugar group. When surcose in heated to about 200°C, it loses water and forms a brown amorphous mass called "Caramel". Surcose is readily fermented by yeast. It is first split into glucose and fructose by invertase, and the monosaccharides are then fermented by the zymase system of enzymes.

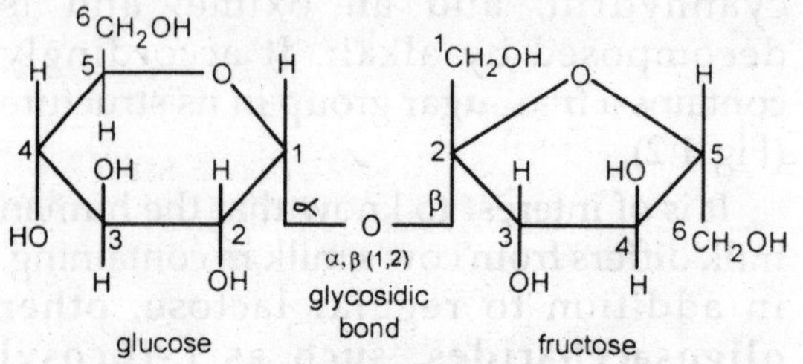

Fig. 1.3 : Surcose

Trisaccharides : Several oligosaccharides containing three monosaccharide units occur in nature. These are given in the following tabulation (Table 1.3) :

Amongst the trisaccharides, the most important of them is raffinose which occurs in sugar beets and is concentrated in sugar beet molasses. Cottonseed meal contains about 7 percent of raffinose. It is also frequently found in higher plants and fungi. It is hydrolyzed by enzymes of the gastrointestinal bacteria of herbivorous animals and serves as food for these animals whereas it is not well utilized as food by the human beings. Raffinose is fermented by yeast.

(c) Polysaccharides

Carbohydrates composed of ten or more monosaccharide units are generally classified in the category of "polysaccharides". Their molecules are colloidal in size. They may be considered as condensation polymers in which the monosaccharides (or their derivatives such as the amino sugars and uronic acids) are joined together by glycosidic linkages. Another term for the polysaccharides is the "glycans". The plysaccharides such as starches, glycogen and cellulose, which are made up of a single kind of monosaccharide, are called "homoglycans" i.e. homopolysaccharides and the polysaccharides composed of two or more kinds of monosaccharides (or their derivatives) , such as the **mucopolysaccharides**, are called as **"heteroglycans"** i.e. heteropolysaccharides made up of mannose and xylose are called as **"mannans"** and **"xylans"** respectively etc.

Some polysaccharides contain units that are derivatives of the monosaccharides, for example, chitin is made up of the amino sugar glucosamine and hyaluronic acid is composed of glucuronic acid and glucosamine.

Table 1.3 : Classification of trisaccharides

Trisaccharides	Constituent monosaccharides with order of linkage
I Reducing sugars	
(a) Mannotriose	galactose, galactose, glucose
(b) Robinose	galactose, rhamnose, rhamnose
(c) Rhamninose	galactose, rhamnose, rhamnose
II Non-reducing sugars	
(a) Raffinose	fructose, glucose, galactose
(b) Gentianose	fructose, glucose, glucose
(c) Melezitose	glucose, fructose, glucose

Polysaccharides

```
                Polysaccharides
        ┌───────────────┴───────────────┐
        ▼                               ▼
Homopolysaccharides
Heteropolysaccharides
(Starch, glycogen,          Agar, pectins, alginic
cellulose, etc.)                    acids, etc.)
```

Since the monosaccharide units of polysaccharides are joind together by glycosidic linkage, the polysaccharides are readily hydrolyzed by mineral acids but are resistant to alkaline hydrolysis.

The polysaccharides are hydrolyzed by the group or enzymes called "polysaccharidases". Important examples of polysaccharides include starch, glycogen, cellulose, dextrins, inulin etc. their molecules are so large that they can't be obtained in the form of true solution. **They give colloidal solutions except cellulose, which is insoluble.** Determination of their molecular weight reveals that a particular type of compound may have different molecular weights and shapes. Polysaccharides such as cellulose, starch, glycogen and dextrins are made up of many D-glucose units They can be readily hydrolyzed to glucose by boiling with dilute acids except cellulose which is hydrolyzed by strong acids only. The polysaccharide **inulin is a compound made up of fructose units exclusively.**

Homopolysaccharides

Starches

These occur widespread as reserve carbohydrate in tubers such as potatoes, in grains and seeds, in many fruits and in the rhizomes and pith of plants. Native starches are a mixture of two types of compounds that are separable from each other and are named as amylose and amylopectin.

The enzymes which hydrolyze starch are known as the **'amylases'.** The animal amylases are represented by **ptyalin of saliva and amylopsin of pancreatic juice.**

Starches generally contain 80-90% amylopectin and the remaining i.e. 10-20% amylose. Both the amylose and amylopectin are hydrolyzed by acid to D-glucose. Partial acid hydrolysis gives complex mixtures of dextrins, maltose and glucose.

Amylose

Molecule of amylose consists of many glucose units joined together through a-

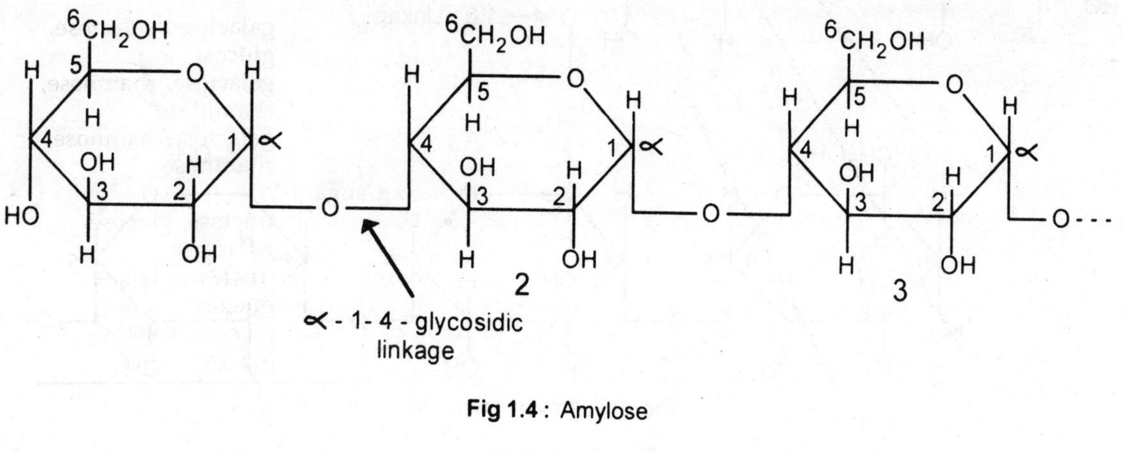

α - 1- 4 - glycosidic linkage

Fig 1.4 : Amylose

glycosidic linkage, chiefly as found in maltose. The glucose units of amylose are linked in the unbranched chain. The amylose structure (Fig. 1.4) may be considered as an expanded maltose structure with a free sugar group on one end.

Amylose may be easily hydrolyzed by acids to D-glucose. Partial acid hydrolysis gives complex mixtures of dextrins, maltose and glucose. Starches generally contain 10-20 percent amylose, though in a few instances the amylose content is higher. The amylose extracted from starch grains is a mixture of molecules of different sizes. Amylose fractions with molecular weights from 4,000 to 4,00,000 have been obtained. It gives a characteristic colour reaction with iodine. **It produces a blueblack colour with iodine solution.** The color disappears upon heating the solution and reappears upon cooling.

Amylopectin

Like that of amylose molecule, it too consists of many glucose units joined together through α-glycosidic linkage, chiefly as found in maltose. Its molecule also contains chains of glucose units like that of amylose and also has branches of these glucose chains linked through the 6-OH of glucose in the following manner:(Fig. 1.5).

Amylopectin is also easily hydrolyzed by acids to D-glucose units. Partial acid hydrolysis yields complex mixtures of dextrins, maltose and glucose. Starches generally contain 80-90 percent amylopectin. Its molecules differ from amylose molecules not only in possessing many branched chains, but also in being larger. The molecular weight of amylopectins apparently vary from 50,000 to about 1000,000. **It gives a characteristic violet to red-violet colour with iodine solution. As with amylose, the colour disappears upon heating the solution and reappears upon cooling.**

Glycogen

It is the carbohydrate reserve of animals.

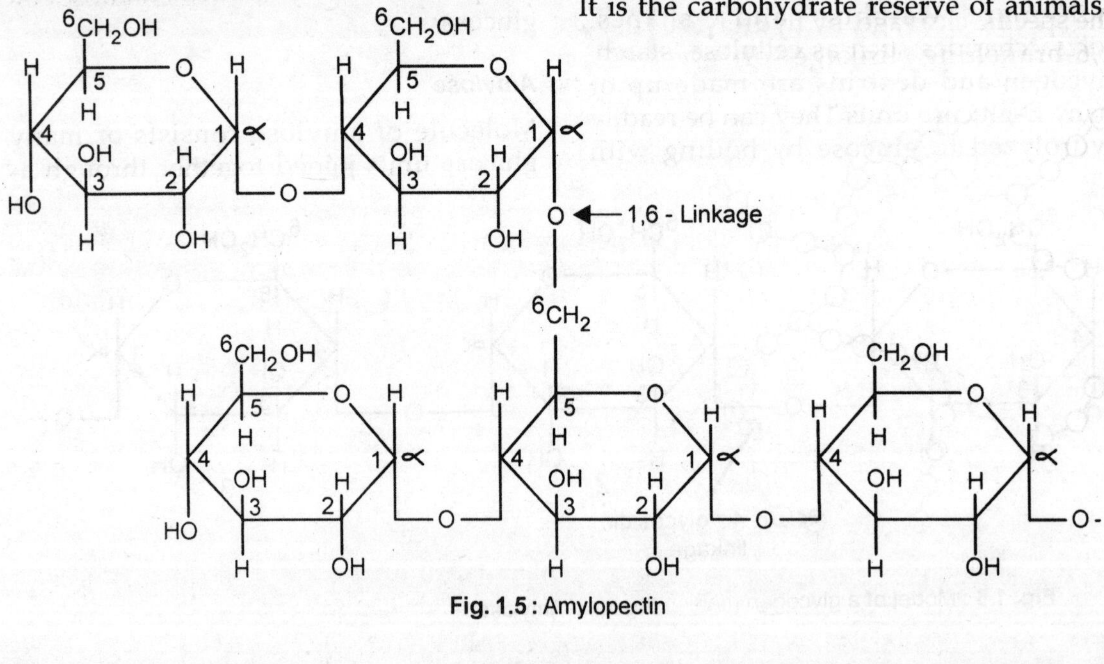

Fig. 1.5 : Amylopectin

It is stroed chiefly in the liver and muscles. It is also found in the plants which have no chlorophyll content such as fungi and yeast. Its structure is similar to that of amylopectin in that it is a branched molecule. It has been found to have 7 to 12 glucose residues per non- reducing end group and hence it is even more highly branched. Molecular weights ranging from 270,000 to 100 millions have been reported. It is readily soluble, **its solution is opalescent and gives a red-brown or red colour with iodine solution.** It yields D-glucose upon complete hydrolysis. Its structure may be represented as shown in (Fig. 1.6) Where each bead of chain represents a glucose molecule.

Biochemically, glycogen is one of the most important substances in the body. Liver glycogen is broken down to glucose and passed into the blood stream for use by the tissues. **Muscle glycogen is a source of energy for muscle contraction. Mollusks such as oysters and clams are usually rich in glycogen.**

Amylo- 1-6-glucosidase is involved in the specific cleavage, by hydrolysis, of the 1,6-branching linkage of glycogen,

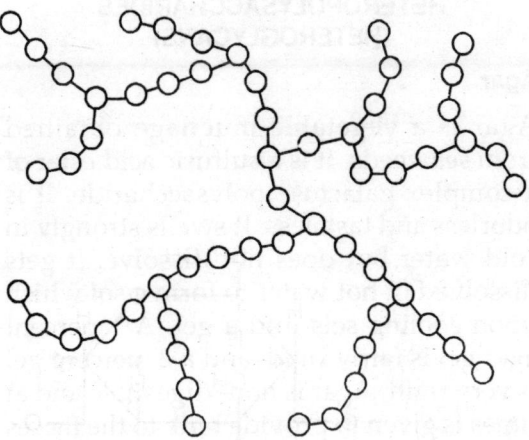

Fig. 1.6 : Model of a glycogen molecule

releasing free glucose. The combined action of the phosphorylase and the amylo 1,6-glucosidase results in the liberation of glucose- 1-phosphate and glucose. Indeed, the ratio of these two defines the extent of branching in a glycogen (or amylopectin) molecule.

Cellulose

Cellulose is the chief constituent of the fibrous parts of the plants and consequently is the most abundant organic material in nature. The cellulose content of flax, ramie and cotton amounts from 97 to 99 percent, while the content in wood varies from 41 to 53 percent. cereal straws contain from 30 to 43 percent cellulose. Thus, it is the most abundant **structural polysaccharide of plant kingdom. It does not occur in animal body.**

Although usually considered to be only a plant product, **cellulose (tunicin) is also found in certain marine animals.**

Cellulose yields D-glucose as the final product of hydrolysis. It is resistant to hydrolysis and requires the action of strong acids. Various bacteria and other lower froms possess enzymes called **cellulases,** capable of hydrolyzing cellulose. The snail produces a cellulase that completely hydrolyzes cellulose to glucose. **Since cellulase remains absent in the animal digestive juices, hence cellulose is not utilized in the human alimentary canal. However, the intake and consumption of cellulose via diet is not harmful hitherto very useful because it provides roughage to the faecal matter and may prevent one from being the victim of colon cancer etc.**

Contrarily, herbivorous animals utilize cellulose as food by virtue of the action of gastrointestinal bacteria and fungi which split it into glucose and other utilizable products.

Partial hydrolysis of cellulose by acids yields a mixture of cellodextrins, various oligosaccharides, cellobiose and glucose.

Studies seem to indicate that cellulose is a linear polysaccharide consisting of β-1,4 linked glucose units. The M.W. of cellulose samples varies from 200,000 to 2,000,000. It is insoluble in water. It does not give characteristic colour with iodine solution.

Cellulose may be nitrated to form nitrocellulose which is of much importance in the manufacture of explosive celluoid and other substance. Cellulose acetates are used in making photographic films, rayon and various plastic materials.

Dextrins

Partial hydrolysis of starch by acids, or α- and β- amylase, produces substances known as "dextrins", These substances consist of a very complex mixture of molecules of different sizes and structures and are known as amylodextrins, erythrodextrins and achrodextrins. **Amylodextrin** gives **blue colour** with iodine, **erythrodextrin** gives **reddish-brown colour** whereas **achrodextrin does not give any colour**. Their reducing property is feeble and they have got faint

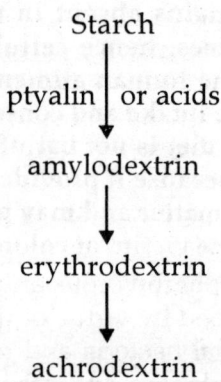

Starch

ptyalin | or acids

amylodextrin

erythrodextrin

achrodextrin

sweet taste. They are generally soluble in water and produce sticky solutions and hence are used as adhesives and binders. All dextrins have free sugar groups and accordingly reduce alkaline copper solotions and give other sugar reactions.

Dextrins occur in the leaves of all starch producing plants, and in honey etc. They are important constituents of various food products such as corn syrups.

Inulin

It is a polysaccharide which exclusively contains **D-fructose units.** It occurs as the reserve carbohydrate in the tubers of chicory, Jerusalem artichoke, dahlia and in the bulbs of onion and garlic. It is a white, more or less crystalline powder. It is very easily hydrolyzed by acids. It is not hydrolyzed by amylase **but is split by inulinase.**

Inulin is used as a source of commercial fructose. It is also administered to animals in the studies of glomerular membrane filtration rates. It is not hydrolyzed by any of the enzymes of the gastrointestinal tract and is not utilized as food.

HETEROPOLYSACCHARIDES (HETEROGLYCANS)

Agar

Agar is a vegetable mucilage obtained from seaweeds. It is a sulfuric acid ester of a complex galactose polysaccharide. It is odorless and tasteless. It swells strongly in cold water but does not dissolve. It gets dissolved in hot water to form a sol which upon cooling sets into a gel. A 1 percent agar gel is fairly rigid, and a 2 percent gel is very rigid. Agar is non- digestible and at times is given to provide bulk to the faeces in the treatment of constipation.

Gum Acacia or Gum Arabic

The vegetable gums are carbohydrate materials containing hexoses or pentoses or both in glycosidic union and a carbohydrate acid group. It is one of the most important and best- known gum. Gum arabic appears to be the salt of a high polymer of arabic acid which upon complete hydrolysis yields galactose, arabinose, rhamnose and glucuronic acid.

Gum arabic is used in the preparation of pharmaceuticals, in confections, and as an adhesive.

Pectins

"Pectin" is the term used to represent the substance or substances which in the presence of sugar and the proper acid concentration causes the formation of jellies. It occurs in abundance in nature and is found especially in the pulp of citrus fruits; apples, carrots, beets, etc. Commercial pectin is generally prepared from lemons or apples. When soluble, pectin is boiled with dilute acid, it is slowly hydrolyzed to pectic acid and methyl alcohol.

Large amounts of pectin are used in the fruit conserving industry and for other purposes.

"Pectin" is a group term and a number of different pectins are known today, some of which are insoluble and useless for gelation.

Alginic Acids

Alginic acids consist chiefly of linear polymers of D-mannuronic acid units. Its molecular weights range from 50,000 to 1,85,000. These are found in many marine algae and in giant kelp, which is a commercial source. Large amounts are used as emulsifier and smoothing agents in food industries.

Mucopolysaccharides (Glycosaminoglycans)

These are referred to as the substances which are composed of amino sugar and uronic acid units as the principal components, through some are chiefly made up of amino sugar and monosaccharide unit without the presence of uronic acid. The hexosamine present is generally acetylated.

Mucopolysaccharides are essential components of tissues. They may be combined with proteins as mucoproteins or mucoids. Important examples of mucopolysaccharides include hyaluronic acid, heparin and the chondroitin sulphates.

Hyaluronic acid

It is found in vitreous humour, synovial fluid, skin, umbilical cord and other sources. It appears to serve as an integral part of the gel- like ground substance of connective and other tissues and as lubricant and shock absorbent in joints. It acts as an intercellular cement. It is a viscous, high molecular weight (several million) polysaccharide consisting of chains of N-acetylglucosamine and glucuronic acid residues. **Hyaluronidase** is a the enzyme which hydrolyzes it into its constituents, This enzyme is widely distributled in microorganisms and mammalian tissues (Fig 1.7).

Heparin

It is a blood anticoagulant which is found in liver, lung, thymus, spleen and blood. It is a polymer of D-glucosamine and D-glucuronic acid. The amino groups and some of the hydroxyl groups remain combined with sulphuric acid. The

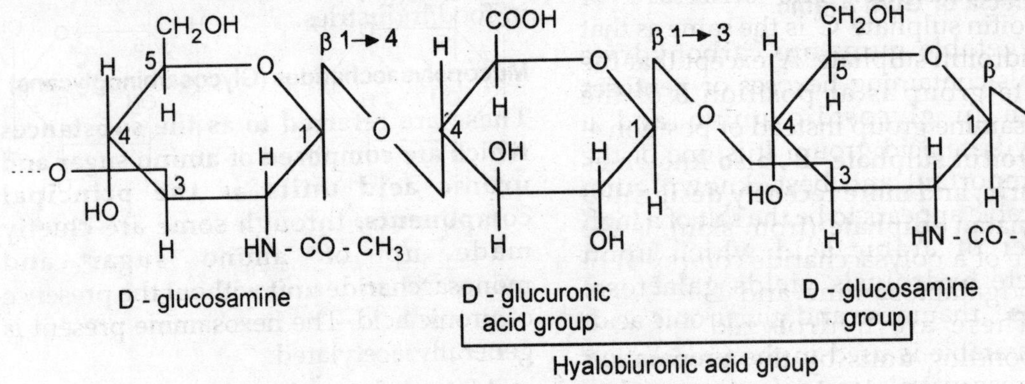

Fig. 1.7 : Repeating units in hyaluronic acid structure

molecular weight of heparin appears to be in the range of 17,000 to 20,000. **It is strongly acidic due to the presence of sulphuric acid group and readily forms salts. It inhibits the transformation of prothrombin to thrombin, preventing the conversion of fibrinogen to fibrin, which is catalyzed by thrombin. The probable repeating units are as follows (Fig.1.8):**

Chondroitin sulphates

These are among the principal mucopolysaccharides (**proteoglycans**) in the ground substance of mammalian tissues and cartilage, and occur combined with proteins. Three kinds of chondroitin sulphate have been isolated so far and named as A, B and C. Out of them, **chondroitin sulphate 'A' remains chiefly**

present in the following:

(a) Cartilage,

(b) Adult bone,

(c) Cornea, etc.

Chondroitin sulphate 'B' remains chiefly present in:

(a) Skin

(b) Heart valves

(c) Tendons, etc.

Chondroitin sulphate 'C' remains chiefly present in:

(a) Cartilage

(b) Tendons, etc.

The basic structure of chondroitin sulphate 'A' consists of repeating unit of N-acetyl galactosamine and glucuronic acid with esterified sulphate at position 4

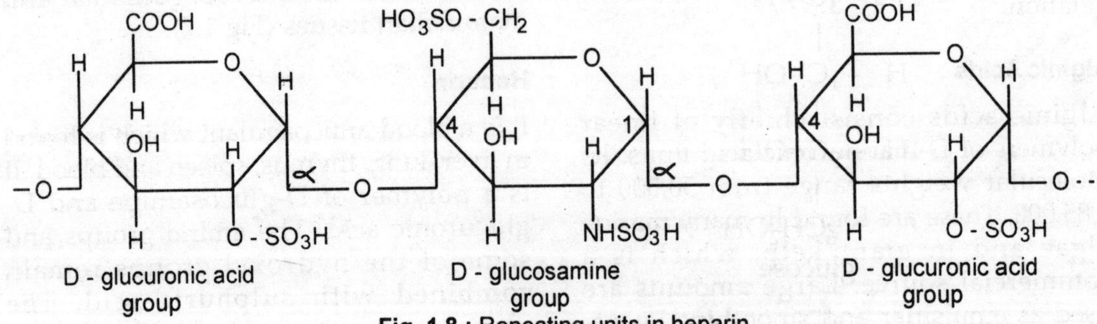

Fig. 1.8 : Repeating units in heparin

of galactosamine. The structure of chondroitin sulphate 'C' is the same as that of chondroitin sulphate 'A' except that the sulphate group is at position 6 of the galactosamine group instead of position 4. **Chondroitin sulphate `B', also known as β- heparin, and more recently designated as dermatan sulphate** (from skin), is the sulphate of a polysaccharide composed of N-acetylgalactosamine and L-iduronic acid. These are hydrolyzed to their corresponding units by the mammalian enzyme named as hyaluronidase.

MUTAROTATION, ANOMERS, EPIMERS

The α-and β-forms of glucose spontaneously undergo interconversion (mutarotation) in water (Fig. 1.9). α-D-glucose and β- D- glucose differ only in the conformation of the hydroxyl group on carbon atom number 1. **These and other pairs of sugar molecules that differ only in this respect are termed as anomers.**

Such isomers which differ only in the configuration of a single carbon atom are termed as "epimers". Examples of epimeric pairs include those of glucose-mannose and glucose-galactose. Glucose and

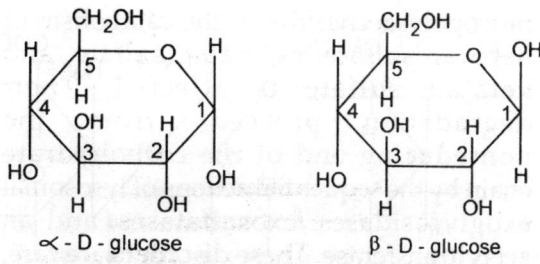

Fig. 1.9 : Two conformations of D-glucose

mannose are epimers with respect to carbon atom 2; whereas glucose and galactose are epimers with respect to carbon atom 4.

MUCOPOLYSACCHARIDOSES

Mucopolysaccharidosis (MPS) encompasses disorders in which undegraded or partly degraded glycosaminoglycans accumulate in the lysosomes of many tissues owing to a deficiency of specific lysosomal enzymes. **These disorders, with the exception of Hunter's syndrome, which is an X-linked trait, are inherited in the autosomal recessive manner. All of the deficient enzymes are acid hydrolases except the acetyltransferase in Sanfilippo's syndrome type C.** In

$$
\begin{array}{ccc}
_1CHO & _1CHO & _1CHO \\
| & | & | \\
H -_2C{-}OH & H0 -_2C{-} H & H -_2C{-}OH \\
| & | & | \\
HO -_3C{-} H & HO -_3C{-} H & HO-_3C{-} H \\
| & | & | \\
H -_4C{-}OH & H -_4C{-}OH & HO-_4C{-} H \\
| & | & | \\
H -_5C{-}OH & H -_5C{-}OH & H -_5C{-}OH \\
| & | & | \\
_6CH_2OH & _6CH_2OH & _6CH_2OH \\
glucose & mannose & galactose
\end{array}
$$

mucopolysaccharidoses, the catabolism of heparan sulfate, dermatan sulfate, and keratan sulfate is affected. Their degradation proceeds from the nonreducing end of the carbohydrate chain by the sequential actions of lysosomal exoglycosidases, exosulfatases, and an acetyltransferase. These disorders are rare; collectively, they may occur 1 in 20,000 live births. Since proteoglycans are widely distributed in human tissues, the syndromes can affect a wide variety of tissues; thus, the clinical features vary considerably. All types are characterised by reduced life expectancy except a few.

These (Table 2.4) are the hereditary disorders caused due to the absence/deficiency of certain enzymes of the metabolism of mucopolysa-ccharides leading to the accumulation of certain mucopolysaccharide(s) in one or the other tissue(s) of the body; there are atleast seven types of such disorders out of which two are of paramount importance, **namely Hurler's syndrome and Hunter's syndrome.**

Table 2.4 : Different types of Mucopolysaccharidoses

Sl. No.	Name of disorder	Affected compound (s)	Enzyme defect	Clinical manifestations	Age of onset
1.	Hurler's syndrome (Mucopolysaccha-ridose -I)	Dermatan sulphate (DS) and Heparan sulphate(HS)	α-L-Iduronidase	Corneal opacity, deafness, claw hands, stubby fingers, hepatomegaly, spleenomegaly, severe mental retardation. Urine contains DS & HS	1 year
2.	Hunter's syndrome (MPS-II)	Dermatan sulphate & Heparan sulphate	L-Iduronate sulphatase	Same as in (1); usually no corneal opacity. Urine contains DS & HS	1 year
3.	MPS-III A Sanfilippo A syndrome	Heparan sulphate	Sulphamidase	Coarse facies, hypertrichosis, HS in urine, mild hepatomegaly, progressive spastic quadriparesis, severe mental retardation	2 - 3 years
4.	MPS-III B Sanfilippo B syndrome	Heparan sulphate	α- N - Acetyl glucosaminidase	HS excreted in urine. Rest same as in (3)	2 - 3 years

CHAPTER 2

LIPIDS

We do not have affinity with water but have with organic solvents. We make the food palatable and delicious. We are somewhat costly. We are found in many food oils/ seeds/ pulses and other innumerable eatables. In excess, we make you run to the doctor, hence use us with full precautions. We have store houses in the body like subcutaneous tissue, omentum, adipose tissue, etc. We can disfigure your body if consumed in excess.

Lipids are the organic compounds that are poorly soluble in water but quite soluble in organic solvents such as the structural components of cell membranes, as storage forms of energy, as metabolic fuel and as emulsifying agents. Surprisingly, four of the vitamins (A, D, E and K) are lipids. In addition, the prostaglandins, substances that stimulate smooth muscle contractions and function in intracellular regulatory processes, are lipid derivatives. The transport of lipids through the blood plasma is an extremely important subject from the standpoint of health, because the abnormalities in these processes are thought to be a major factor in the development of coronary artery diseases which are on the increase throughout the globe. **Obesity results from the storage of execssive amounts of lipids in the** body. Such common diseases like diabetes mellitus, obstructive jaundice, pancreatitis, and hypothyroidism have associated plasma lipid transport abnormalities. In addition, there are a number of rare inherited diseases, known as the lipid storage diseases or lipidoses. For instance Tay-Sach's disease, Niemann-Pick disease, Gaucher's disease, Fabry's disease, Farber's disease, etc.

To summarize, lipid is a term used to describe a group of fats and fatlike substances that constitute a major portion of tissue components and a major foodstuff.

Properties of Lipids

Lipids have the following important properties:

(A) Hydrolysis

Triglycerides can be hydrolyzed by acids, alkalies or enzymes for e.q. lipase which act on triglycerides and give a mixture of glycerol and free fatty acids as shown below:

$$\begin{array}{l}
CH_2OCOC_{15}H_{31} \\
| \\
CHOCOC_{15}H_{31} \xrightarrow{\text{lipase}} \\
| \\
CH_2OCOC_{15}H_{31} \\
\text{tripalmitin}
\end{array} \quad \begin{array}{l}
CH_2OH \\
| \\
CHOH + 3\, C_{15}H_{31}\,COOH \\
| \qquad\qquad \text{palmitic acid} \\
CH_2OH \\
\text{glycerol}
\end{array}$$

(B) Saponification

Hydrolysis of triglycerides by alkali forms soap as shown below; this phenomenon is termed as saponification. Sodium and potassium soaps are soluble in water and are used as emulsifying agents. Calcium, magnesium and barium soaps are insoluble.

$$\begin{array}{l}
CH_2OCOR_1 \\
| \\
CHOCOR_2 \xrightarrow{\text{3NaOH}} \\
| \\
CH_2OCOR_3 \\
\text{triacylglycerol}
\end{array} \quad \begin{array}{l}
CH_2OH \\
| \\
CHOH + 3\,RCOO.Na \\
| \qquad\qquad \text{soap} \\
CH_2OH \\
\text{glycerol}
\end{array}$$

The number of mg of KOH required to completely saponify 1g of the oil or fat is termed as saponification number.

(C) Halogenation

Unsaturated fatty acids present in triglycerides accept halogens such as iodine (I_2) at the double bond., This process is known as halogenation. Iodine number is a measure of the degree of unsaturation of a fat which is defined as the number of gram of iodine that combines with 100 g of fat. **Higher the iodine number- higher the degree of unsaturation of fatty acids present in the fat.**

(D) Rancidity

Naturally occurring fats particularly from animal sources, on storage in the presence of moist air give unpleasant smell and develop a characteristic taste and odour which is due to the partial hydrolysis of fats which are further oxidised into aldehydes and ketones. This process is termed as rancidity. **Certain antioxidants such as vitamin C, E can prevent oxidation of fats and therefore the development of rancidity.**

Functions of lipids

There are numerous functions of lipids in the animal body. They play vital functions in the body which may be remembered as given in Table 2.1.

Table 2.1 : Functions of lipids

Sl. No.	Lipid	Function(s)
1.	Fatty acids	Metabolic fuel, building blocks for other lipids
2.	Prostaglandins	Intracellular modulators
3.	Glyceryl esters	
	(a) Acylglycerols	Fatty acid storage, metabolic intermediates
	(b) Phospho-glycerides	Membrane structure
4.	Sphingolipids	
	(a) Sphingomyelin	Membrane structure
	(b) Glycosphingo-lipids	Membranes, surface antigens
5.	Sterol derivatives	
	(a) Cholesterol	Membrane and lipoprotein structure

Sl. No.	Lipid	Function(s)
(b)	Cholesterol esters	Storage and transport
(c)	Bile acids	Lipid digestion and absorption
(d)	Steroid hormones	Metabolic regulation
(e)	Vitamin D	Calcium and Phosphorus metabolism
6.	Terpenes	
(a)	Vitamin A	Vision, epithelial integrity
(b)	Vitamin E	Lipid antioxidant
(c)	Vitamin K	Blood coagulation

LIPOTROPIC FACTORS

These are the substances which facilitate mobilisation of fats from the liver. These include choline, betaine, methionine and inositol. These are required for the conversion of triglycerides to phospholipids and thus help in normal transport and utilisation of lipids, especially in liver.

The deficiency of lipotropic factors results in increased fat content of liver called fatty liver.

Biological significance/ functions of lipids

There are numerous very important vital function of lipids in the animal body:

1) Lipids play an important role in the diet by helping in the absorption of fat soluble vitamins, i.e. A, D, E, and K.
2) Lipids are the principal energy yielding substances as they have high calorific value.
3) They are found in nervous tissue.
4) Lipids stored in the adipose tissue and else where are a direct and potential source of energy.
5) Lipids present in subcutaneous tissue and around certain organs act as insulating material.
6) Lipids in the form of **lipoproteins.,** are the important cellular constituents and occur in cell membrane, mitochondria and cytoplasm. Lipoproteins also help in the transportation of lipids in blood.
7) Prostaglandins which have numerous functions in the body, are the derivatives of fatty acid.

Isolation of Lipids from Tissue

The chloroform- methanol (2:1) solvent introduced by Folch for lipid extraction has largely replaced the older well-known ethanol- ether (3:1) solvent introduced by Bloor.

Classification of Lipids

There is no single internationally accepted system of classification for the lipids. However, generally accepted classification is given in Table 2.2.

Simple Lipids

These are the esters of fatty acids with certain alcohols. They are usually further classified according to the nature of the alcohols, as follows:

Fats and Oils

These are the esters of fatty acids and glycerol. If they are solid at room temperature, then they are known as fats and if liquid at room temperature, then they are termed as oils.

Fatty acids. Fatty acids found in fats and other lipids are of various types. Some of them, like palmitic acid ($CH_3(CH_2)_{14}.COOH$) and stearic acid ($CH_3(CH_2)_{16}.COOH$) are straightchain

Table 2.2 : Classification of Lipids

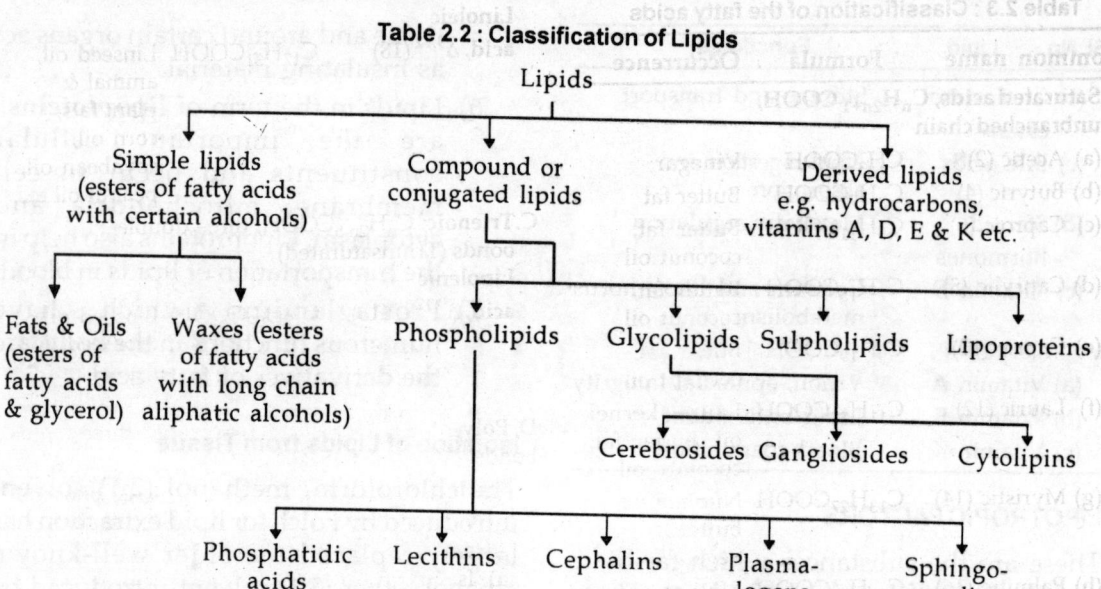

saturated acids belonging to the acetic acid series, and have the general formula $C_nH_{2n}O_2$. Others are unsaturated and have one more double bonds in their molecules. Thus, oleic acid ($C_{18}H_{34}O_2$) has one double bond in its molecule, linoleic acid ($C_{18}H_{32}O_2$) has two double bonds, and linolenic acid ($C_{18}H_{30}O_2$) has three. In addition to the above types of acids, some lipids contain hydroxy acids, both saturated and unsaturated and dicarboxylic acids. Thus, castor oil contains an unsaturated hydroxy acid, ricinoleic acid ($C_{18}H_{32}O_3$). Certain cyclic saturated and unsaturated fatty acids are likewise also found in nature (Table 2.3).

Saturated fatty acids

They are generally represented by the general formula $C_nH_{2n}O_2$ or $C_nH_{2n+1}COOH$. Physical properties of the saturated fatty acids depend upon their molecular weights. Whereas those fatty acids that contain ten carbon atoms or fewer in their molecules are liquids at room

temperature, the remainder are solids whose melting points rise which increasing molecular weight. The liquid acids are also known as **volatile fatty acids,** since they may be distilled with steam, whereas the others, the **nonvolatile acids,** are carried over by steam distillation only in traces or not at all. Fatty, acids with four carbon atoms or fewer are miscible with water in all proportions. As the length of the carbon chain increases beyond this. The solubility rapidly decreases to zero. The important examples of straight chain **saturated fatty acids** found in nature as constituents of lipid molecules include **butyric, caproic, caprylic, capric, lauric, myristic, palmitic, stearic etc.** (Table 2.3).

Unsaturated fatty acids

These are characterized by the presence of one or more double bonds in the molecle. They have been classified in accordance with the number of double bonds and named by reference to the parent hydrocarbon, the position of the

Table 2.3 : Classification of the fatty acids

Common name	Formula	Occurrence
1. Saturated acids, $C_nH_{2n+1}COOH$, unbranched chain		
(a) Acetic (2)*	CH_3COOH	Vinegar
(b) Butyric (4)	C_3H_7COOH	Butter fat
(c) Caproic (6)	$C_5H_{11}COOH$	Butter fat, coconut oil
(d) Caprylic (8)	$C_7H_{15}COOH$	Butter fat, coconut oil
(e) Capric (10)	$C_9H_{19}COOH$	Butter fat, coconut oil
(f) Lauric (12)	$C_{11}H_{23}COOH$	Laurel kernel oil, butter fat, coconut oil
(g) Myristic (14)	$C_{13}H_{27}COOH$	Nutmeg fat, butter, vegetable fats
(h) Palmitic (16)	$C_{15}H_{31}COOH$	Most vegetable & animal fats
(i) Stearic (18)	$C_{17}H_{35}COOH$	Most vegetable & animal fats
(j) Arachidic acid (20)	$C_{19}H_{39}COOH$	Peanut oil
(k) Behenic acid (22)	$C_{21}H_{43}COOH$	Rapeseed oil, peanut oil
(l) Lignoceric acid (24)	$C_{23}H_{47}COOH$	Cerebrosides, sphingomyelin, peanut oil.

II, Unsaturated fatty acids

A. **Monoethenic, $C_nH_{2n-1}COOH$, one double bond (Monounsaturated)**

(a) **Paimitoleic,** Δ^9 (16)	$C_{15}H_{29}COOH$	⎫
(b) **Oleic acid,** Δ^9 (18)	$C_{17}H_{33}COOH$	⎬ Animal and vegetable fats
(c) **Erucic acid** Δ^{13}(22)	$C_{21}H_{41}COOH$	
(d) **Nervonic acid** Δ^{15} (24)	$C_{23}H_{45}COOH$	⎭

B. **Dienoic, $C_nH_{2n-3}COOH$, two double bonds (Diunsaturated)**

*number of carbon atoms in the fatty acid molecule

Linoleic acid, $\Delta^{9,12}$ (18) $\quad C_{17}H_{31}COOH \quad$ Linseed oil, animal & plant fats, corn oil, soyabean oil, peanut oil etc.

C. **Trienoic, $C_nH_{2n-5}COOH$, three double bonds (Triunsaturated)**

Linolenic acid, $\Delta^{9,12,15}$ (18) $\quad C_{17}H_{29}COOH \quad$ Linseed oil, rapeseed oil, soyabean oil, liver oil etc.

D. **Polyenoic, $C_nH_{2n-7}COOH$, more than three double bonds. (Many unsaturations)**

Arachidonic acid, $\Delta^{5,8,11,14}$ (20) $\quad C_{19}H_{31}COOH \quad$ Fats, phospholipids etc.

III. Branched-chain acids

(a) Isobutyric acid (4)	C_3H_7COOH	Waxes
(b) Tuberculostearic acid (19)	$C_{18}H_{37}COOH$	Wax of tubercle bacillus

IV. Hydroxy acids

(a) Cerebronic acid (24)	$C_{23}H_{46}(OH)COOH$	⎫
(b) Ricinoleic acid (18)	$C_{17}H_{32}(OH)COOH$	⎬ Animal and vegetable fats
(c) Hydroxy-nervonic Acids (24)	$C_{23}H_{44}(OH)COOH$	⎭

V. Cyclic acids

(a) Chaulmoogric acid	*R-$(CH_2)_{12}$-COOH	seed oils
(b) Hydnocarpic acid	*R-$(CH_2)_{10}$-COOH	seed oils

* Where R is

$$CH = CH \diagdown$$
$$| \qquad\qquad >C - $$
$$CH_2 - CH_2 \diagup H$$

double bond or bonds in the chain being indicated by a number referred to the carboxyl carbon atom as number one.

Nomenclature of fatty acids

Carbon atoms are numbered from the carboxyl carbon (carbon No. 1). The carbon atom adjacent to the carboxyl carbon (No.2) is also known as α- carbon. Carbon atom No.3 is the β-carbon, and the end methyl carbon is known as a ω-carbon or **n-carbon**. Various conventions are in use for indicating the number and position of the double bonds; for e.g., Δ^9 indicates a double bond between carbon atoms 9 and 10 of the fatty acid. The ω- 9 indicates a double bond on the 9th carbon counting from the ω-carbon atom. Widely used conventions to indicate the number of carbon atoms, the number of the double bonds, and the positions of the double bonds are prevalent. To cite an example, see the structure of oleic acid.

Oleic (C_{18}) $C_{18}H_{34}O_2$

$$18 : 1; 9 \text{ or } \Delta^9 \, 18 : 1$$

$$\overset{18}{C}H_3-\overset{17}{C}H_2-\overset{16}{C}H_2-\overset{15}{C}H_2-\overset{14}{C}H_2-\overset{13}{C}H_2-\overset{12}{C}H_2-\overset{11}{C}H_2-\overset{10}{C}H$$

$$= \overset{9}{C}H(CH_2)_7 \overset{1}{C}OOH$$

OR

$$\overset{\omega(n)\,2}{C}H_3-\overset{3}{C}H_2-\overset{4}{C}H_2-\overset{5}{C}H_2-\overset{6}{C}H_2-\overset{7}{C}H_2-\overset{8}{C}H_2-\overset{9}{C}H_2-CH_2$$

$$\overset{10}{=} CH(CH_2)_7 \overset{18}{C}OOH$$

In animals, additional double bonds are introduced only between the existing double bond e.g., ω9, ω6, or ω3 and the carboxyl carbon, leading to three series of fatty acids known as the ω9, ω6 and ω3 families, respectively.

Some unsaturated fatty acids of physiologic and nutritional importance are as given below:

Number of carbon atoms and position of double bonds	Series	Common name
Monoenoic acids (one double bond)		
16 : 1; 9	ω 7	Palmitoleic
18 : 1; 9	ω 9	Oleic
22 : 1; 13	ω 9	Erucic
Dienoic acids (2 double bonds)		
18 : 2 ; 9, 12	ω 6	Linoleic
Trienoic acids (3 double bonds)		
18 : 3; 6, 9, 12	ω 6	γ - Linolenic
18 : 3; 9, 12, 15	ω 3	α - Linolenic

[Other nutritionally important ω-3 (omega-3) fatty acids include Eicosapentaenoic acid and Docosahexaenoic acid which are obtained from fish oils]

Tetraenoic acids (4 double bonds)		
20 : 4; 5, 8, 11, 14	ω 6	Arachidonic

Triglycerides (Neutral fats)

The neutral fats (triglycerides) are

$$
\begin{array}{ccccc}
CH_2OH & & HO.OC.C_3H_7 & & CH_2.O.CO.C_3H_7 \\
| & & | & & | \\
CHOH & + & HO.OC.C_3H_7 & \longrightarrow & CH.O.CO.C_3H_7 \quad + \; 3H_2O \\
| & & | & & | \\
CH_2OH & & HO.OC.C_3H_7 & & CH_2.O.CO.C_3H_7 \\
\text{glycerol} & & \text{butyric acid} & & \text{tributyrin} \\
& & \text{(3 moles)} & & \text{(a triglyceride)}
\end{array}
$$

General formula for a fat is

$$
\begin{array}{c}
CH_2.O.CO.R_1 \\
| \\
CH.O.CO.R_2 \\
| \\
CH_2.O.CO.R_3
\end{array}
$$

where R_1, R_2 and R_3 may be derived from the same or different fatty acids.

important because the bulk (as much as 90 per cent) of the lipid material stored in the adipose tissue of the body is **neutral fat** and represents a concentrated form of energy stored until required for metabolic purposes.

Glycerol reacts with one molecule of fatty acid to form a **monoglyceride**, with two molecules to form a **diglyceride** and with three to form a **triglyceride** as shown on page 22.

Compound or Conjugated Lipids

These are the esters of fatty acids which, upon hydrolysis, yield other substances in addition to the fatty acids and an alcohol. Some important members of this group are:

1. Phospholipids (Phosphatides)

Lipids which upon hydrolysis, yield fatty acids, phosphoric acid, sometimes, but not always, glycerol and a nitrogenous base. These are subdivided into the following groups:

(A) Phosphatidic acids: Lipids which when hydrolyzed yield one molecule each of glycerol and phosphoric acid and two molecules of fatty acids of which one is probably saturated and the other unsaturated.

(B) Lecithins: These are the lipids containing fatty acids, phosphoric acid, glycerol, and the nitrogenous base choline.

The saturated fatty acids present in lecithin molecules include palmitic and stearic acids while the unsaturated fatty acids present include oleic, linoleic, linolenic and arachidonic acids. Lecithins are widely distributed in animal tissues for instance brain, liver, blood, cardiac

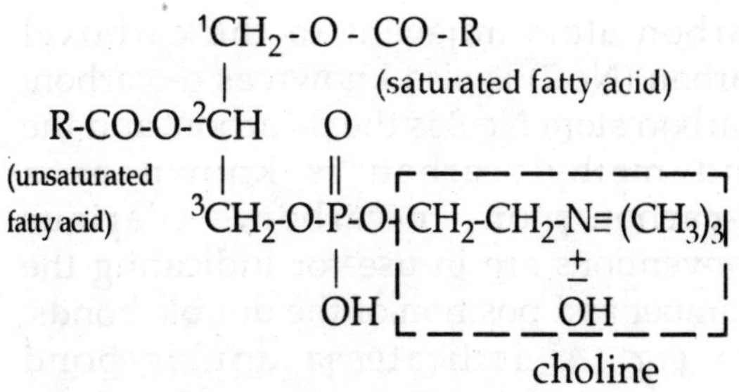

$$^1CH_2\text{-}O\text{-}CO\text{-}R \quad \text{(saturated fatty acid)}$$

$$R\text{-}CO\text{-}O\text{-}^2CH$$

(unsaturated fatty acid) $^3CH_2\text{-}O\text{-}P\text{-}O\text{-}[CH_2\text{-}CH_2\text{-}N\equiv(CH_3)_3]$

$$OH \qquad OH$$

choline

α - Lecithin

muscles etc., they are also found in vegetable sources e.g. plant seeds etc.

Lecithins when purified are waxy white substances but soon become brownish when exposed to air and light, owing to autoxidation and decomposition. They are soluble in ordinary fat solvents like ethanol, ether etc. but not in acetone. **Large quantities of soyabean lecithins are used these days as emulsifying and smoothing agents in the food industry.**

Lecithins are hydrolyzed by boiling with alkalies and dilute mineral acids and also by the corresponding enzymes i.e. **lecithinases (phospholipases).** The nature of hydrolysis depends upon the kind of phospholipase acting. Scientist **'Hanahan' has shown that lecithinase A (phospholipase A) found in certain snake venoms (cobra, cotton mouth moccasin, vipers), poisons of scorpions and bees,and various mammalian tissues, specifically hydrolyzes off the fatty acid to form lysolecithins. The lysolecithins so formed are very powerful hemolytic agents which rapidly hemolyze blood erythrocytes, and are considered to be responsible for harmful physiological effects of venoms containing phospholipase A.**

$$
\begin{array}{c}
\quad\quad\quad O \\
\quad\quad\quad \| \\
H_2C - O - C - R \\
| \\
HO - C - H \\
| \quad\quad\quad O \\
| \quad\quad\quad \| \\
H_2C - O - P - O - CH_2.\ CH_2.\ \overset{+}{N}\ (CH_3)_3 \\
| \\
O
\end{array}
$$

L-α-Lysolecithin

Four kinds of lecithinases i.e. A, B, C and D are known today which are very specific in nature. These are found in different vegetables, mammalian tissues and microorganisms.

(C) Cephalins. Lipids which upon hydrolysis yield fatty acids, glycerol, phosphoric acid, and either the nitrogenous base ethanolamine

$$
\begin{array}{c}
CH_2 - O - CO - R \\
| \\
R-CO-O-CH \\
| \quad\quad\quad O \\
| \quad\quad\quad \| \\
{}^{3}CH_2 - O - P - O\ \overline{\underline{[CH_2.CH_2.NH_2]}} \\
| \quad\quad\quad\quad\quad\quad \text{ethanolamine} \\
OH
\end{array}
$$

α-Cephalin

(L-α-Phosphatidyl ethanolamine)

(colamine) or the amino acid serine. Lipids of uncertain structures which contain inositol, fatty acids, phosphoric acid, ethanolamine, and possibly galactose and tartaric acid have also been included in this class.

Cephalins contain the saturated fatty acid called stearic acid and the unsaturated fatty acids, oleic, linoleic and arachidonic acids. They are found in various animal tissues e.g. brain, liver, egg yolk, erythrocytes and cardiac muscles and are also found to be present in various plant sources i.e. plant seeds etc. Cephalins, like lecithins, are hygroscopic solids and are decomposed on exposure to air. These are insoluble in alcohol and acetone, but soluble in ether.

The cephalins are hydrolyzed by boiling with alkalies and dilute mineral acids. Lecithinase A from snake venom hydrolyzes cephalins to form Iysocephalins which are similar to the lysolecithins formed from lecithins.

(D) Plasmalogens. These on hydrolysis yield one molecule each of aliphatic aldehyde, fatty acid, glycerol, phosphoric acid, and a nitrogen containing base (ethanolamine or choline). These contribute to an appreciable proportion (about 10 percent) of the phospholipids of muscles and brain. Cardiac muscles and erythrocytes also contain plasmalogens.

(E) Sphingomyelins. These on hydrolysis yield a nitrogenous base sphingosine, a single fatty acid molecule, phosphoric acid, and choline, but *no glycerol*. These are soluble in hot ethanol, but not in ether, acetone or cold ethanol. They are found in brain, liver, blood, cardiac muscles etc.

2. Glycolipids

As the name indicates, these are the complex lipids containing carbohydrate in combination with long chain aliphatic acids or alcohols.

(A) Cerebrosides. Lipids which contain carbohydrate (galactose or glucose), one fatty acid, and sphingosine, but no phosphoric acid or glycerol. The fatty acids of the cerebrosides chiefly are lignoceric, behenic, and palmitic acids.

CH$_3$(CH$_2$)$_{12}$ – CH = CH – CH – CH – CH$_2$ – O – C
sphingosine group

fatty acid residue ⟶ R

H-C-OH

HO-C-H

HO-C-H

H-C

CH$_2$OH

D-galactosyl group

Cerebroside

Various cerebrosides have been obtained from brain and nerves which are differentiated from each other by the presence of other fatty acids they possess. Such fatty acids are cerebronic acid, lignocerie acid, nervonic acid, and oxynervonic acid.

These are found in large amounts in the white matter of brain and in the myelin sheaths of nerves. In smaller quantities, they appear to be very widely distributed in animal tissues. **Large amounts of the cerebrosides accumulate in the liver and spleen in Gaucher's disease- a rare hereditary disease of lipid metabolism. This disease was for the first time noticed by the scientist Gaucher in a patient in whom the splenic pulp was replaced entirely by large pale cells, which now are known after his name as "Gaucher Cells". These cells are found particularly in spleen, brain, and bone marrow.**

(B) Gangliosides. These arc related to the cercbrosides and contain sphingosine, long-chain fatty acids, hexoses (usually galactose or glucose) and neuraminic acid (sialic acid). These are rich in carbohydrates. Brain gangliosides are known to be complex one.

Gangliosides have been isolated from nerve cells, spleen and red blood cell stroma. **Large amounts of it are found in the brain in cases of Tay-Sachs disease and Niemann-Pick disease (diseases of lipid metabolism).**

(C) Cytolipins. These lipids contain fatty acids, sphingosine, glucose and galactose.

3. Sulpholipids

Lipid material containing sulphur has long been known to be present in the tissues, examples being liver, kidney, brain, salivary glands, testicles, tumors etc. It's most abundantly found to be present in the white matter of the brain. In composition, these are similar to the cerebrosides except for the fact that sulphuric acid is present as cerebronic acid ester.

4. Lipoproteins

They are the complex compounds made up of two moieties i.e., lipids and proteins, hence the name given to them as lipoproteins. Since lipids are insoluble in water, they can not be transported as such in plasma, therefore, they form complex with proteins to form lipoproteins. The protein moiety of lipoproteins is called **apolipoprotein** or **apoprotein**. The important sites for their synthesis are liver and intestine repectively.

5. Apolipoproteins

The apolipoproteins associated with lipoprotein particles serve as structural components of the lipoproteins, provide recognition sites for cell surface receptors and serve as activation for the enzymes involved in lipoproteins metabolism. **Various apolipoproteins are divided into different classes from A to H. Most of the classes have subclasses like apo A-I, apo**

AII, apo B-100, apo B-48, apo C-I, apo C-II, apo C-III, apo D, apo E, apo Lp (a), apo J, etc.

Depending upon the density [by ultracentrifugation (Table 2.3) or electrophoresis technique(Fig 2.1)], the lipoproteins in plasma have been classified into five major types which are important physiologically and are useful in the clinical diagnosis. These are as follows:

1. **Chylomicrons.**
2. Very low density lipoproteins **(VLDL)** or pre- beta lipoproteins.
3. Intermediate density lipoproteins **(IDL)** or broad- beta lipoproteins.
4. Low density lipoproteins **(LDL)** or beta- lipoproteins; and
5. High density lipoproteins **(HDL)** or alpha lipoproteins.

The lipoproteins are generally abbreviated as Lp.

Besides, the free fatty acids **(FFA)** or nonesterified fatty acids **(NEFA)** remain bound to albumin which although not lipoproteins are important lipid fractions in serum.

Chemical composition and density or various lipoproteins are given in Table 2.4.

Table2.4 : Density and composition of lipoproteins

Lipoproteins (Lp) (%)	Density (g/L)	Proteins (%)	Total lipids
Chlomicrons	< 0.96	1 - 2	98-99
VLDL	0.96-1.006	7 - 10	90-93
IDL	1.006-1.019	11	89
LDL	1.019-1.063	21	79
HDL	1.063 - 1.21	40	60

Derived Lipids

Derived lipids are substances formed during the hydrolysis of simple or compound lipids which still retain the properties of this class of compound.

1. Fatty Acids: Saturated and unsaturated acids.

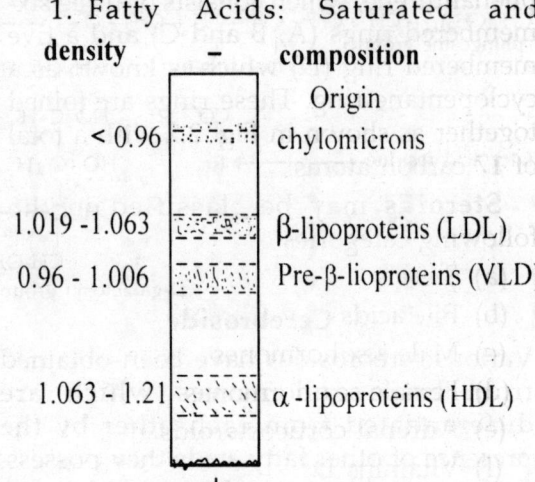

Fig. 2.1 : Separation of plama lipoproteins by electrophoresis

Hyperlipidemia currently is receiving considerable attention of the scientists because **it has been positively correlated with atherosclerotic cardiovascular disease,** which has a high mortality and morbidity rate.

2. Alcohols: Compounds of high molecular weight but not glycerol. These may be classified as follows:
   (A) Aliphatic alcohols such as cetyl, stearyl and myricyl alcohols.
   (B) Sterols which contain the phenanthrene nucleus (cholesterol, ergosterol, sitosterol and stigmasterol).

Steroids

A large number of compounds found in nature belong to the. class of compounds known as steroids. These have the parent nucleus named as perhydrocyclopentano-phenanthrene, which consists of three six-membered rings (A, B and C) and a five membered ring (D) which is known as a cyclopentane ring. These rings are joined together as shown in Fig. 2.2 with a total of 17 carbon atoms.

Steroids may be classified in the following categories:

(a) Sterols
(b) Bile acids
(c) Male sex hormones
(d) Female sex hormones
(e) Adrenal corticosteroids
(f) Vitamins D
(g) Saponins
(h) Cardiac glycosides

Sterols

The best known of the sterols is cholesterol, In the animal kingdom, the most abundant steroid is the sterol called as cholesterol. It remains present in all animal cells and is particularly abundant in nervous tissue. It is not found in vegetables and plant tissues. Because of its abundance, its historical

interest and its clinical importance to man, it will be considered in some detail over here.

As early as 1815, **Chevreul** gave the name cholesterine to a white waxy material that could be isolated **from gallstones.** It was later identified as an alcohol stable to boiling with strong alkali. Fatty acid esters of the alcohol were also isolated from certain tissues.

Cholesterol, literally means bile solid-alcohol; derives its name from the fact that it was first isolated from human gallstones, of which it is generally the chief component. The amount of cholesterol in animal tissues varies widely. It is particularly abundant in brain, nerve tissue, adrenal glands and egg yolk. Dry white matter of brain contains about 14 per cent of cholesterol, and spinal cord 10-15 per cent. Scientist Bloor, an authority on lipids gives the percentage values (Table 2.5) for the average cholesterol content of dry tissues.

Cholesterol is usually accompanied by dihydrocholesterol and 7-dehydrocholesterol. It has the structure as shown in Fig. 2.3.

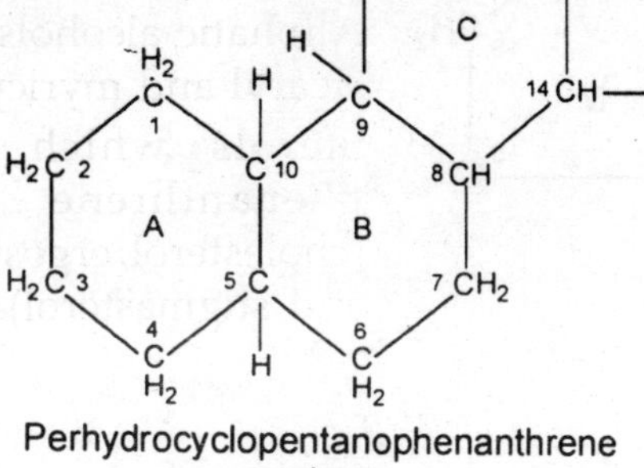

Perhydrocyclopentanophenanthrene
nucleus

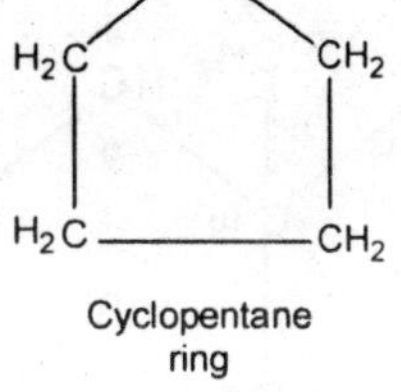

Cyclopentane
ring

Fig. 2.2 : Structures of perhydrocyclopentanophenanthrene and cyclopentane rings

Table 2.5 : Percentage of cholesterol in dry tissues

Sl.No.	Tissue	%
1.	White matter of brain	14.00
2.	Gray matter of brain	6.00
3.	Kidney	1.60
4.	Spleen	1.50
5.	Skin	1.30
6.	Liver	0.93
7.	Mammary glands	0.70
8.	Whole blood	0.65
9.	Smooth muscle.	0.55
10.	Diaphragm	0.35
11.	Skeletal muscle	0.25

Cholesterol generally crystallizes as white, shining rhombic plates. It melts at $149°$-$150°C$. It is tasteless and odourless. It is insoluble in water, acids and alkalies, somewhat soluble in soap solutions and much more soluble in the solution of bile salts. It is readily soluble in ether, benzene, chloroform, petroleum ether, carbon bisulfide and acetone. It is also readily soluble in hot alcohol, but only slightly soluble in cold alcohol. It dissolves readily in oleic acid and liquid fats. It is commercially produced from the spinal cords of the cattle. It may be readily prepared in the laboratory by extraction from gallstones or brain tissue with the help of organic solvents.

Since cholesterol is a poor conductor of electricity and has a high dielectric value, it's a good insulator against electric discharge. Possibly, as an abundant constituent of brain, nerves and spinal cord, it functions as an insulating covering of impulse generating and transmitting structures. It is well established that brain and nerve impulses are electrial in character.

On account of the presence of a double bond, cholesterol gives the addition reactions characteristic of unsaturated compounds. The addition of hydrogen produces dihydrocholesterol. This substance occurs along with cholesterol in animal tissues. Cholesterol takes up halogens at the double bond to form cholesterol dihalides.

Upon oxidation, it gives various ketones, hydroxy compounds and acids, the products depending upon the oxidizing agents and conditions used.

Cholesterol is the best known and most

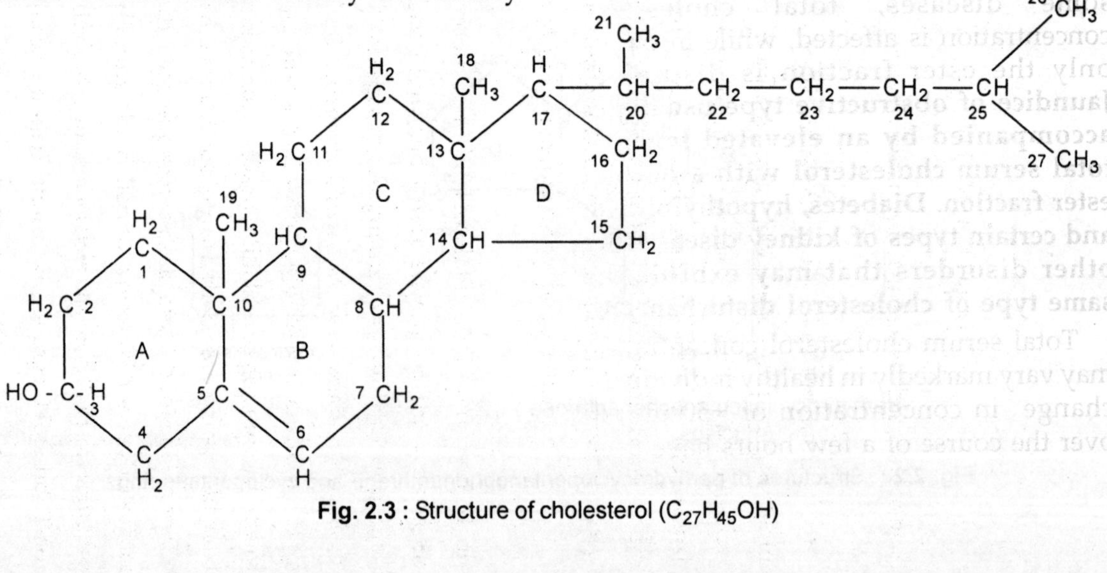

Fig. 2.3 : Structure of cholesterol ($C_{27}H_{45}OH$)

widely determined lipid and is an important intermediate in the synthesis of steroid hormones. In the blood it occurs both in the free and esterified forms. The latter form is a mixture of many cholesterol esters, each of which has a different fatty acid bound in ester linkage to cholesterol at the OH group. Usually, only the *total* cholesterol concentration is of clinical interest but occasionally separate estimation of the free and esterified forms is of value to the clinicians. The normal range of cholesterol esters is between 70 and 75% of the total with free cholesterol making up the remaining 25 to 30%. **The normal range of the concentration of cholesterol in the serum is from 150 to 200 mg/dl. In normal infants and children lower values of cholesterol are found in the serum whereas higher values are found in normal older persons. The concentration of total cholesterol gets elevated in several diseases like nephrosis, diabetes mellitus, and hypothyroidism. Low values may be found in hyperthyroidism, malnutrition, Gaucher's disease and acute hepatitis.** However, the increase usually is not clinically diagnostic of these diseases. In some diseases, total cholesterol concentration is affected, while in others only the ester fraction is disturbed. **Jaundice of obstructive type usually is accompanied by an elevated level of total serum cholesterol with a normal ester fraction. Diabetes, hypothyroidism and certain types of kidney diseases are other disorders that may exhibit the same type of cholesterol disturbance.**

Total serum cholesterol concentration may vary markedly in healthy individuals; change in concentration of ±50 mg/dl over the course of a few hours have been noted.

Since, the liver cells esterify cholesterol, infectious hepatitis cirrhosis and most types of liver damage are accompanied by a decreased percentage of cholesterol esters. Only the ester percentage is significant, not the absolute ester concentration.

In the recent years interest in lipid metabolism has increased tremendously, primarily as a result of possible relationship between lipid metabolism and atherosclerosis.

Other Animal Sterols: A number of sterols closely related to cholesterol are found in various tissues. 7-dehydrocholesterol is a precursor of vitamin D_3. Skin is a good source of both Δ^7- cholesterol (lathosterol) and 7 - dehydrocholesterol. Desmosterol (24-dehydrocholesterol) and several methlyderivatives such as lanosterol and agnosterol have been isolated from skin lipids and are recognised as intermediates in cholesterol biosynthesis. Lanosterol and agnosterol are also present in wool lipids.

7 - Dehydrocholesterol

Δ^7 - Cholesterol, lathosterol

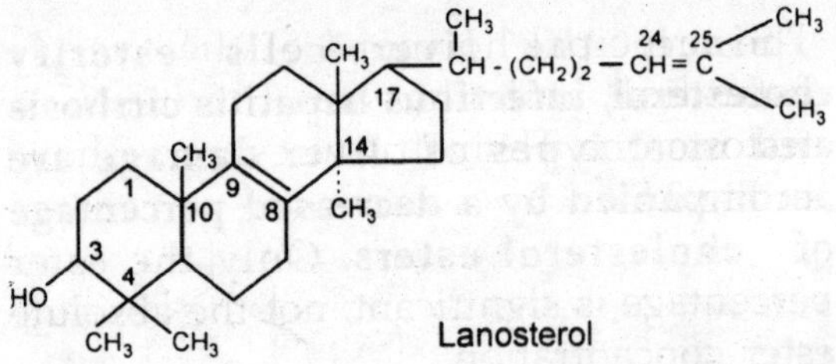

Lanosterol

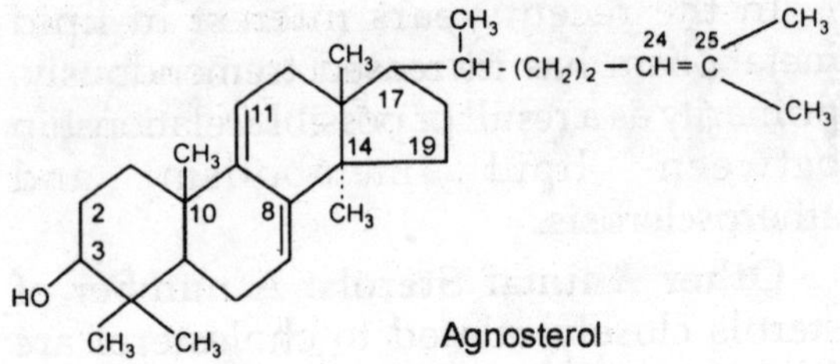

Agnosterol

Sterols of Yeast and Fungi: Mycosterols

Important examples of this category are two:

(a) Ergosterol

(b) Zymosterol

Ergosterol. This sterol is the principal sterol of fungi and yeast and is classed as a mycosterol. **Its name derives from the fact that it was first discovered in ergot bodies which are formed on rye and other cereal plants diseased with ergot fungi. It is produced commercially in large quantities from certain strains of yeast.**

It is an important substance because when irradiated with ultraviolet light, a series of substances is formed which even includes calciferol (vitamin D_2) and tachysterol, from which another member of the vitamin D group, dihydrotachysterol is derived.

Sterols of Higher Plants: Phytosterols

Imortant examples of this category are the following (Table 2.6):

Table 2.6 : Sterols and their occurrence

Sl.No.	Sterol	Formula	Occurrence
1.	Cholesterol	$C_{27}H_{45}OH$	All animal cells
2.	Dihydro-cholesterol	$C_{27}H_{47}OH$	Accompanies cholesterol
3.	7 -Dehydro-cholesterol	$C_{27}H_{43}OH$	Skin, brain, other tissues
4.	Coprostanol	$C_{27}H_{47}OH$	Feces
5	β-Equistanol	$C_{30}H_{53}OH$	Urine of pregnnancy
6.	Sitosterols	$C_{29}H_{49}OH$	Lipids of higher plants
7.	Stigmasterol	$C_{29}H_{47}OH$	Soya & calabar beans
8.	Brassicasterol	$C_{29}H_{47}OH$	Rapeseed oil
9.	Spinasterol	$C_{27}H_{45}OH$	Spinach, alfalfa
10.	Ergosterol	$C_{28}H_{43}OH$	Ergot, yeast
11.	Zymosterol	$C_{27}H_{43}OH$	Yeast
12.	Fucosterol	$C_{29}H_{47}OH$	Algae

(a) Stigmasterol. **This sterol occurs especially in calabar and soybean oils. It is of interest hccause it can be convelted in the laboratory into the hormone of the corpus luteum progesterone.**

(b) Sitosterols. These are generally found in the oils of higher plants, being especially abundant in wheat germ oil. Seven sterols of this group have been reported.

Sterols and their Occurrence

Table 2.5 indicates certain important sterols with their occurrence:

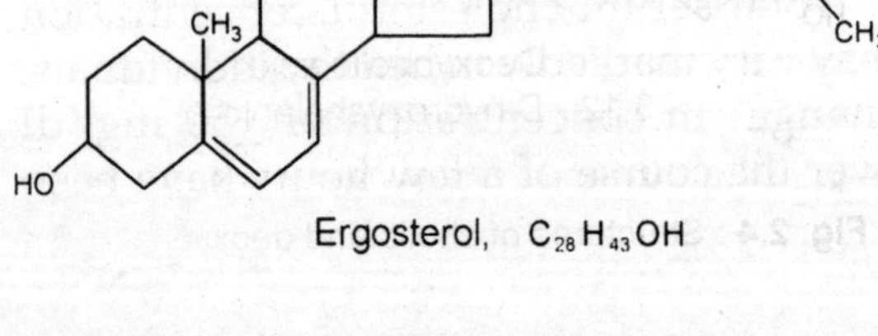

Ergosterol, $C_{28}H_{43}OH$

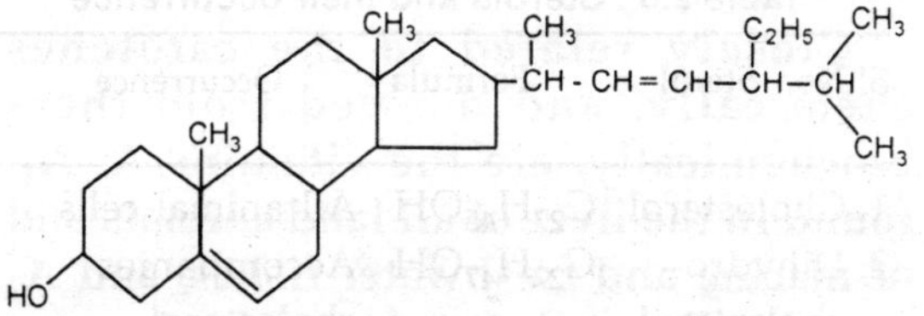

Stigmasterol, $C_{29}H_{47}OH$

Bile Acids

Human bile contains three different bile acids cholic, deoxycholic, and chenodeoxycholic acids.

Deoxycholic acid is microbial in origin and is absorbed from intestinal contents. The bile acids are present largely as derivatives of glycine and taurine. The bile acids differ from the sterols because of the *trans* relationship of its OH group at the 3- carbon to the angular CH_3 group. Structures of some of the bile acids are as given in Fig. 2.4.

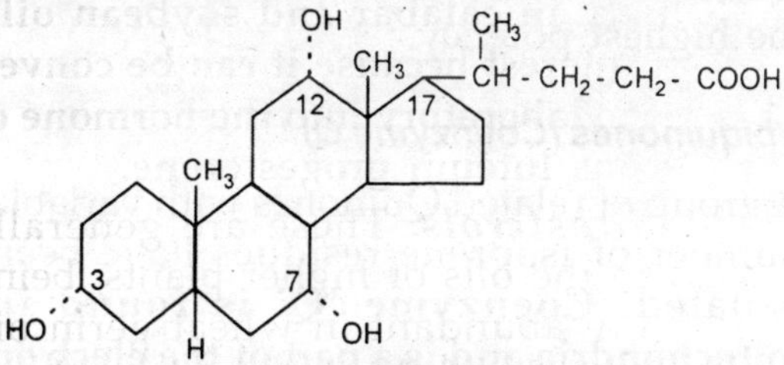

Cholic acid
3,7,12 - Trihydroxycholanic acid

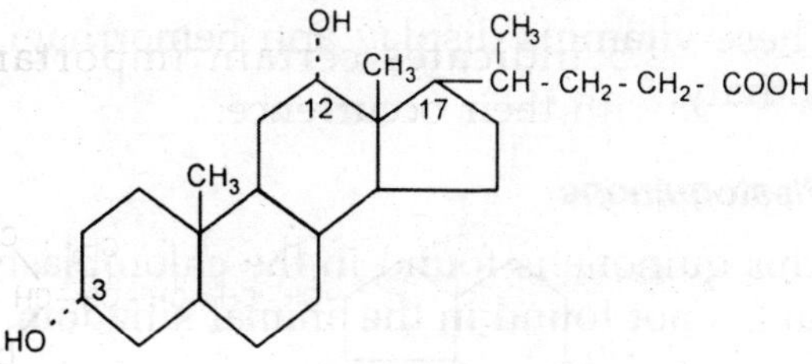

Deoxycholic acid
3,12 - Dihydroxycholanic acid

Fig. 2.4 : Structures of cholic and deoxycholic acids

Sex hormones

The principal hormone of the ovary is estradiol and that of the testis is testosterone. Their structures are as shown in Fig 2.5.

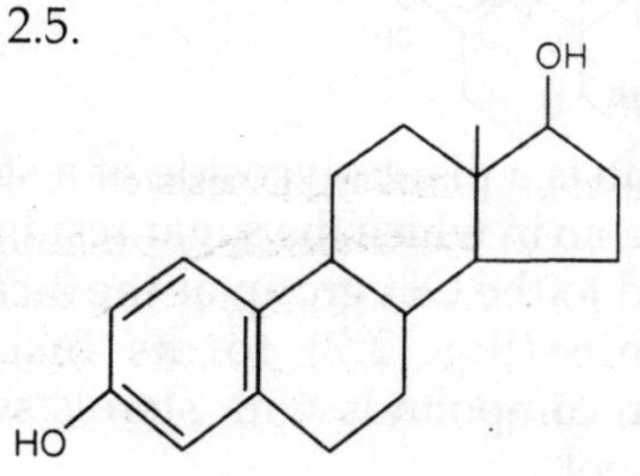

Estradiol

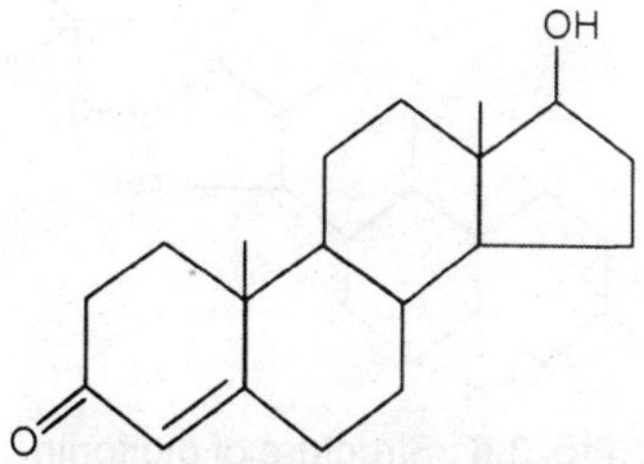

Testosterone

Fig. 2.5 : Estradiol and testosterone

Adrenal Corticosteroids

The adrenal cortex synthesizes a number of steroids of metabolic importance. One of the very important of these is corticosterone (Fig 2.6).

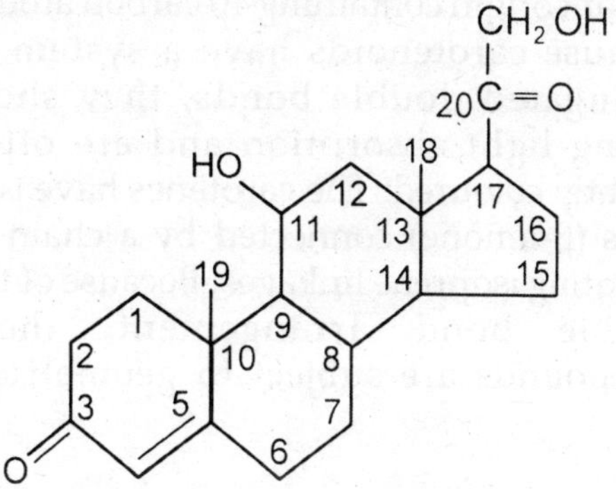

Fig. 3.5 : Structure of corticosterone

Vitamin D

Irradiation with ultraviolet light converts a number of sterols to compounds with vitamin D activity.

Saponins

Digitonin is a plant glycoside of a steroid-digitogenin in which the sugar residues are attached to the OH group at the 3-carbon. Digitonin (Fig. 2.7) forms insoluble addition compounds with sterols such as cholesterol.

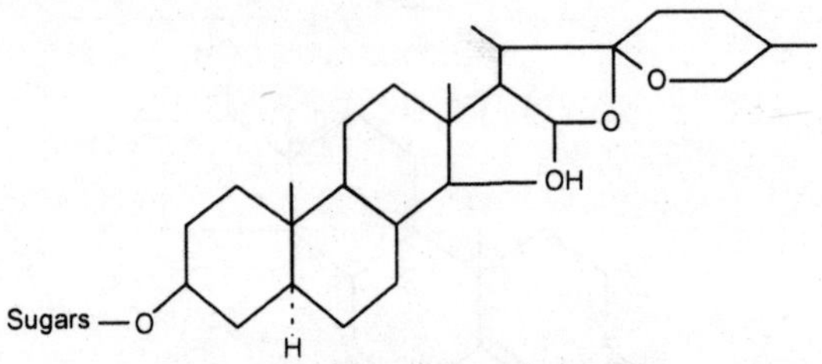

Fig. 3.6 : Structure of digitonin

Cardiac glycosides

These compounds have therapeutic applications. Strophanthin is a glycoside of the steroid strophanthidin.

Carotenoids and Vitamin A

Carotenoids are isoprenoid hydrocarbons of plant origin containing 40 carbon atoms. Because carotenoids have a system of conjugated double bonds, they show strong light absorption and are often brightly coloured. The carotenes have two rings (β-ionone) connected by a chain of repeating isoprene linkages. Because of the double bond arrangement, these compounds are subject to geometrical isomerism.

Closely related to the carotenes chemically, and derived from them biochemically, are the vitamins A, A_1, found in the liver of all land animals and of marine and freshwater fishes; and A_2 found in liver oils from some fresh water fishes. Metabolic intermediates of vitamin A occur in the form of aldehydes - the retinines. (For details, consult chapter on vitamins).

Vitamin E and the Quinones

These compounds bear close similarities in their structures, and it has been suggested that their biological functions (in cellular oxidation) may also be related.

Tocopherols (Vitamin E)

Several forms of this compound are known to possess biological activity as an antisterility factor in rats. The α-variety has the highest potency.

Ubiquinones (Coenzyme Q)

A group of related Quinones with variable number of isoprene residues have been isolated. **Coenzyme 'Q' is found in mitochondria and is a part of the electron transport mechanism.**

Phylloquinones (Vitamin K)

These vitamins display anti hemorrhagic activity.

Plastoquinone

This quinone is found in the chloroplasts and is not found in the animal kingdom.

Vitamin D

Irradiation with ultraviolet light converts
a number of sterols to compounds with

CHAPTER 3

CHEMISTRY OF AMINO ACIDS, PROTEINS AND IMMUNOGLOBULINS

> We are very complex substances having large molecular weights and are
> expensive of all the foodstuffs and found in innumerable eatables. We have
> the wonderful unimaginable properties like involvement in (i) blood clotting
> (ii) hereditary transmission (iii) transport of O_2 and CO_2 (iv) defence
> (antibodies) (v) enzymes (vi) cementing substances (vii) buffers and many
> more.
>
> There will come no end in ours inventions and our contribution in various
> physiological/ biochemical/ metabolic processes will remain everlasting.

Chemistry of Amino acids

Normally occurring amino acids are those
amino acids which contain (i) amino
group and (ii) carboxyl group in the carbon
atom and are represented by the following
general formula:

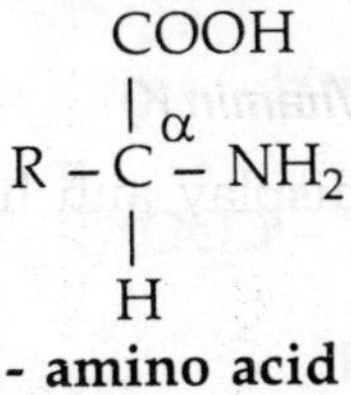

$$\begin{array}{c} COOH \\ | \\ R - \overset{\alpha}{C} - NH_2 \\ | \\ H \end{array}$$

α - amino acid

*All amino acids (structures as given ahead)
found in living systems i.e. plant and animal
proteins are L -α - amino acids (derived
from L-glyceraldehyde). In nature, glycine
is the only amino acid which is optically
inactive and cannot be resolved into D -*

or L - form because of symmetry on the α
- carbon atom. Rest amino acids are
optically active.

The configuration of L - α - amino acid
is

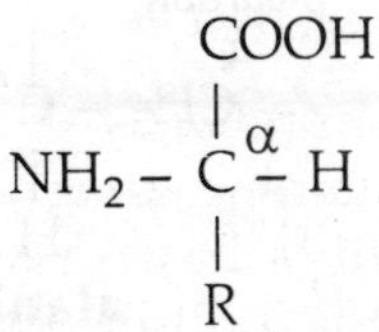

$$\begin{array}{c} COOH \\ | \\ NH_2 - \overset{\alpha}{C} - H \\ | \\ R \end{array}$$

L- amino acid

Classification of the Amino acids

Amino acids have been classified in many
ways. They can either be classified
:according to the presence of (a) acidic,
basic, or neutral groups or due to the
presence of (b) polar groups, non-polar
groups, sulphur containing groups,

aromatic groups, heterocyclic ring, branched chain, etc. in their structures.

It is as metioned in Table 3.1, i.e.,

1. Aliphatic amino acids,
2. Aromatic amino acids, and
3. Heterocyclic amino acids

Table 3.1 : Classification of Amino Acids

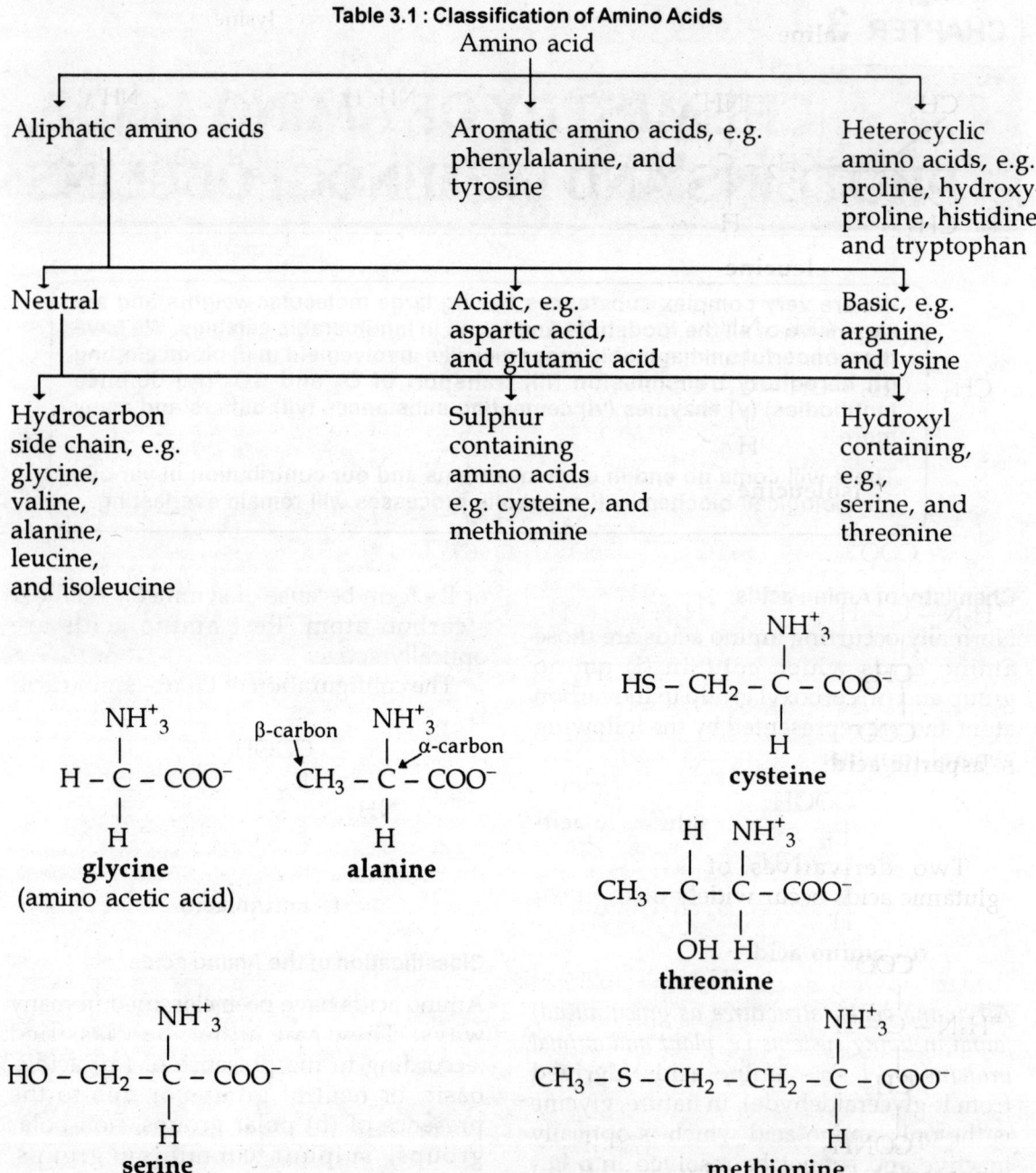

$$\begin{matrix} CH_3 & & NH^+_3 \\ & \diagdown & | \\ & CH - C - COO^- \\ & \diagup & | \\ CH_3 & & H \end{matrix}$$
valine

$$H_2N - CH_2 - CH_2 - CH_2 - CH_2 - \overset{\displaystyle NH^+_3}{\underset{\displaystyle H}{C}} - COO^-$$
lysine

$$\begin{matrix} CH_3 & & NH^+_3 \\ & \diagdown & | \\ & CH - CH_2 - C - COO^- \\ & \diagup & | \\ CH_3 & & H \end{matrix}$$
leucine

$$H_2N - \overset{\displaystyle NH}{\overset{\displaystyle ||}{C}} - \overset{\displaystyle H}{\overset{\displaystyle |}{N}} - CH_2 - CH_2 - CH_2 - \overset{\displaystyle NH^+_3}{\underset{\displaystyle H}{C}} - COO^-$$
arginine

$$CH_3 - CH_2 - \overset{\displaystyle CH_3}{\overset{\displaystyle |}{C}}H - \overset{\displaystyle NH^+_3}{\underset{\displaystyle H}{C}} - COO^-$$
isoleucine

$$\begin{matrix} & NH^+_3 \\ & | \\ CH_2 - C - COO^- \\ | & | \\ S & H \\ | \\ S & NH^+_3 \\ | & | \\ CH_2 - C - COO^- \\ & | \\ & H \end{matrix}$$
cystine

$$\langle\!\!\bigcirc\!\!\rangle - CH_2 - \overset{\displaystyle NH^+_3}{\underset{\displaystyle H}{C}} - COO^-$$
phenylalanine

$$\begin{matrix} COO^- \\ | \\ {}^+H_3N - C - H \\ | \\ CH_2 \\ | \\ COO^- \end{matrix}$$
aspartic acid

$$\begin{matrix} COO^- \\ | \\ {}^+H_3N - C - H \\ | \\ CH_2 \\ | \\ CH_2 \\ | \\ COO^- \end{matrix}$$
glutamic acid

$$HO - \langle\!\!\bigcirc\!\!\rangle - CH_2 - \overset{\displaystyle NH^+_3}{\underset{\displaystyle H}{C}} - COO^-$$
tyrosine

Two derivatives of aspartic and glutamic acids occur widely distributed:

$$\begin{matrix} COO^- \\ | \\ {}^+H_3N - C - H \\ | \\ CH_2 \\ | \\ CONH_2 \end{matrix}$$
asparagine (Asn)

$$\begin{matrix} COO^- \\ | \\ {}^+H_3N - C - H \\ | \\ CH_2 \\ | \\ CH_2 \\ | \\ CONH_2 \end{matrix}$$
glutamine (Gln)

$$\langle\!\!\bigcirc\!\!\rangle\!\!\overset{\displaystyle C - CH_2 - \overset{\displaystyle NH^+_3}{\overset{\displaystyle |}{C}} - COO^-}{\underset{\displaystyle \underset{H}{N}}{\overset{\displaystyle |}{CH}}}\quad\quad\quad\quad H$$
tryptophan

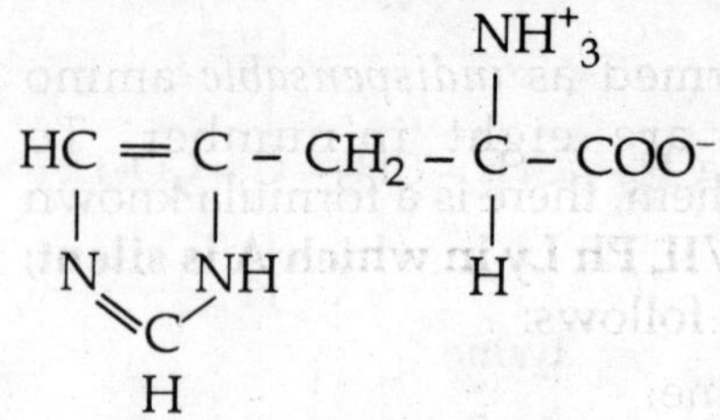

$$HC = \overset{\overset{\displaystyle NH_3^+}{|}}{C} - CH_2 - \overset{\overset{\displaystyle}{|}}{\underset{\underset{\displaystyle}{|}}{C}} - COO^-$$

histidine

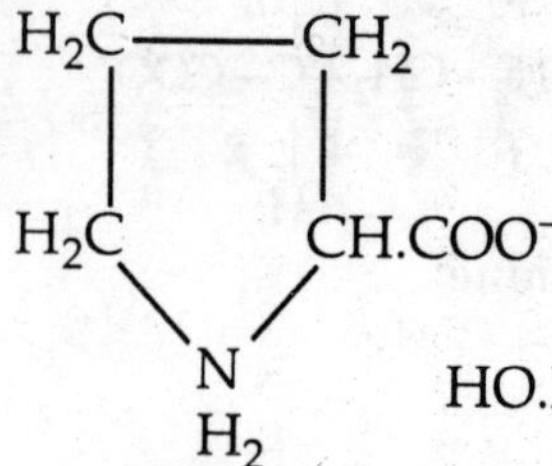

proline

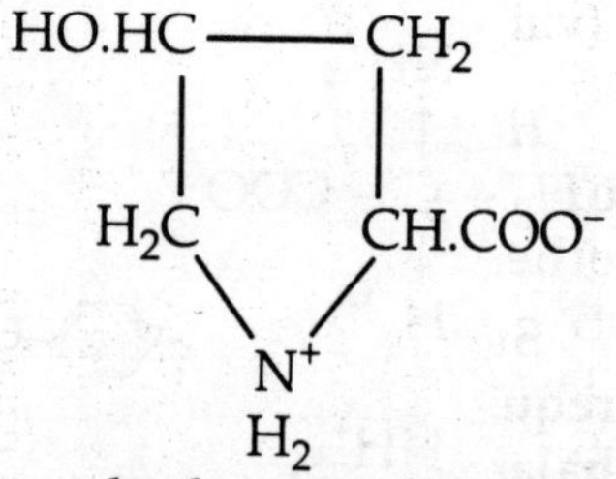

hydroxyproline

Following are some of the important amino acids which are found in special sources whose structural formulae are as given below. These amino acids so called **special amino acids** do not occur in proteins but they may play some as yet unknown part in biosynthesis.

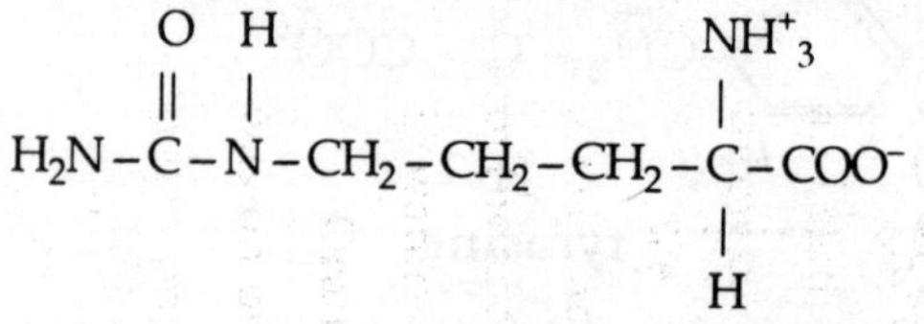

$$H_2N - \overset{\overset{\displaystyle O}{||}}{C} - \overset{\overset{\displaystyle H}{|}}{N} - CH_2 - CH_2 - CH_2 - \overset{\overset{\displaystyle NH_3^+}{|}}{\underset{\underset{\displaystyle H}{|}}{C}} - COO^-$$

citrulline
(in watermelon juice, liver)

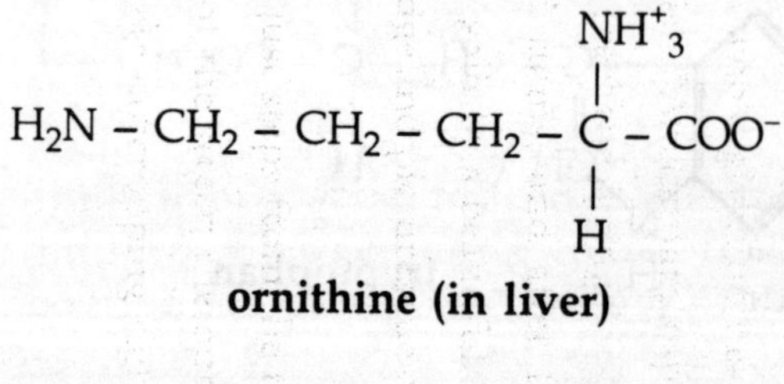

$$H_2N - CH_2 - CH_2 - CH_2 - \overset{\overset{\displaystyle NH_3^+}{|}}{\underset{\underset{\displaystyle H}{|}}{C}} - COO^-$$

ornithine (in liver)

$$H_3N^+ - CH_2 - CH_2 - COO^-$$
β - alanine
(constituent of vitamin pantothenic acid)

$$H_3N^+ - CH_2 - CH_2 - CH_2 - COO^-$$
γ - aminobutyric acid
(in plants, brain, and other animal tissues)

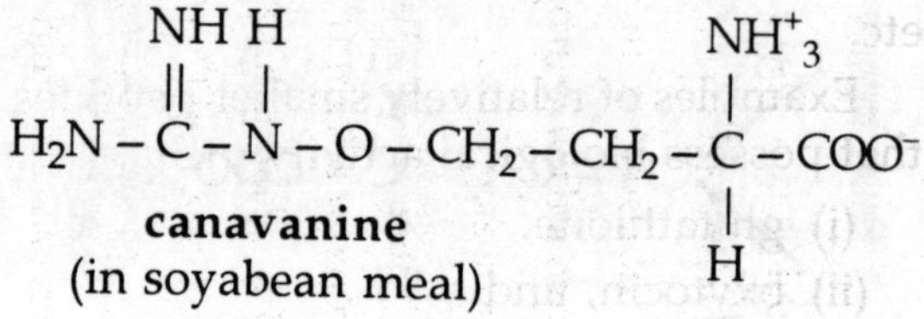

$$H_2N - \overset{\overset{\displaystyle NH}{||}}{C} - \overset{\overset{\displaystyle H}{|}}{N} - O - CH_2 - CH_2 - \overset{\overset{\displaystyle NH_3^+}{|}}{\underset{\underset{\displaystyle H}{|}}{C}} - COO^-$$
canavanine
(in soyabean meal)

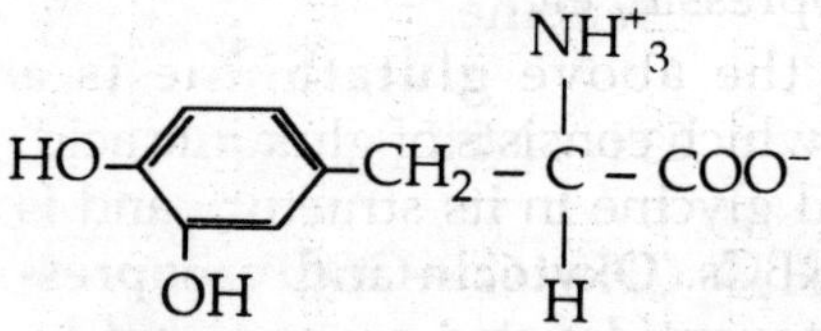

dihydroxyphenylalanine (DOPA)
(in sprouts and seedlings of velvet bean)

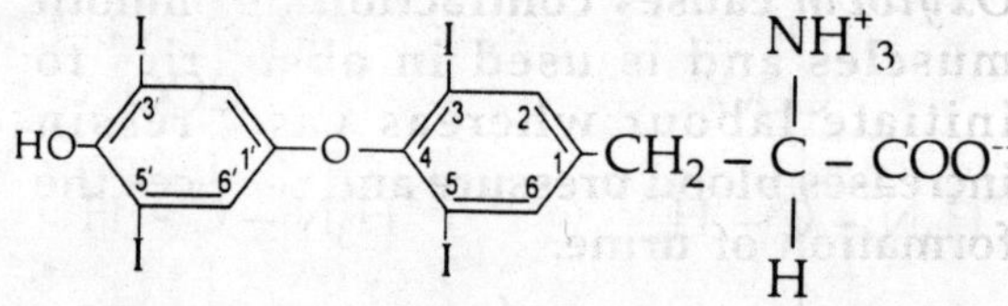

thyroxine
3, 5, 3′, 5′ - tetraiodothyronine, T_4 (in thyroid gland)

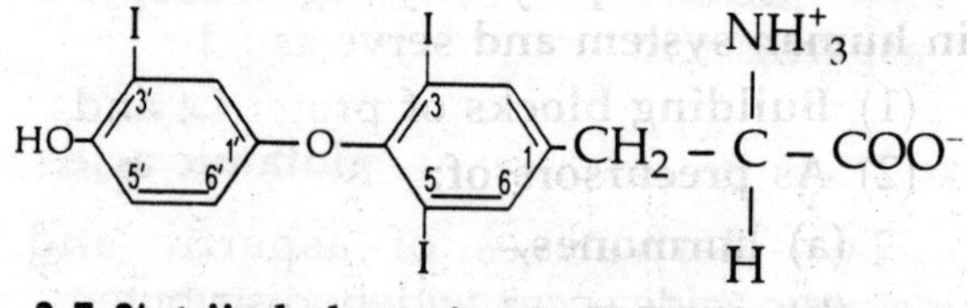

3, 5, 3′ - triiodothyronine, T_3 (in thyroid gland)

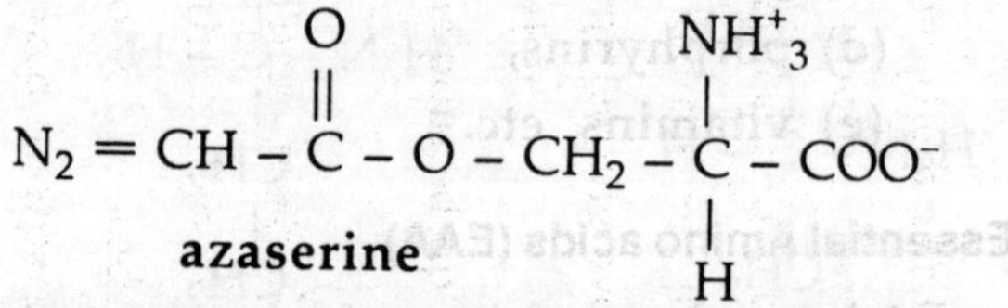

$$N_2 = CH - \overset{\overset{\displaystyle O}{||}}{C} - O - CH_2 - \overset{\overset{\displaystyle NH_3^+}{|}}{\underset{\underset{\displaystyle H}{|}}{C}} - COO^-$$
azaserine
(from a streptomyces sp.; an antibiotic and an anticancer agent; inhibitor of nucleic acids synthesis)

Besides the regular 20 amino acids, there are number of special amino acids which are found in free or combined form but do not occur in protein molecules, these include triiodothyronine (T_3), tetraiodothyronine (T_4), ornithine, citrulline, β-alanine, γ - aminobutyric acid, etc.

Examples of relatively smaller peptides that possess biological activity include:

(i) glutathione,

(ii) oxytocin, and

(iii) vasopressin, etc.

Out of the above **glutathione is a** *tripeptide* which consists of glutamic acid, cystine and glycine in its structure and is found in RBCs. **Oxytocin and vasopressin are** *octapeptides* **and are secreted by the posterior part of the pituitary gland,** each is made up of 8 amino acids. *Oxytocin* **causes contraction of smooth muscles and is used in obstetrics to initiate labour whereas vasopressin increases blood pressure and reduces the formation of urine.**

Functions of of Amino acids

Amino acids play very important role in human system and serve as :

(1) **Building blocks of proteins, and**

(2) **As precursors of:**

    (a) **hormones,**

    (b) **purines,**

    (c) **pyrimidines,**

    (d) **porphyrins,**

    (e) **vitamins, etc.**

Essential Amino acids (EAA)

EAA are those amino acids which are not synthesized in the body and hence have to be provided in the diet. They are also termed as *indispensable* amino acids and are eight in'number. To remember them, there is a formula known as **M A TTVIL Ph Ly in which A is silent;** these are as follows:

(i) Leucine,

(ii) Isoleucine,

(iii) Valine

(iv) Methionine

(v) Tryptophan

(vi) Phenylalanine

(vii) Lysine, and

(viii) Threonine

Histidine **is treated under the category of 'Essential' in case of infants, otherwise semiessential.**

Sufficient amounts of EAA are required to maintain the proper nitrogen balance. Deficiency of one or more EAA in the diet affects the synthesis of proteins resulting failure in the growth of the child, negative nitrogen balance in the adults and fall in the levels of plasma proteins and hemoglobin.

Semiessential Amino Acids: Are those amino acids which are required half-heartedly by the body for proper growth and development, these include:

(i) Arginine

(ii) Tyrosine

(iii) Cystine

(iv) Glycine

(v) Serine and

(vi) Histidine

Non-essential Amino Acids

These are not required by the body but are synthesized by the body and include aspartic acid, glutamic acid, proline, hydroxyproline, etc. These are derived from the carbon skeletons of carbohydrates and lipids metabolism or from the transformation of essential amino acids.

Nitrogen Balance

The ratio of:

$$\frac{\text{Intake of N}}{\text{Output of N}} =$$

1, i.e., nitrogen equilibrium. Normal adults are in nitrogen equilibrium.

> 1, i.e., Positive Nitrogen Balance, e.g., pregnancy, convulsions and growth.

< 1, i.e., Negative Nitrogen Balance, e.g., malnutrition and certain wasting diseases where there is tissue breakdown.

Ionic properties of Amino Acids:

The amphoteric (property of behaviour either as an acid or a base) properties of amino acids account for their separation of electrophoresis on paper at pH 6.0 (Fig. 3.1).

The amphoteric nature of α - amino acids determines that, in the absence of other acids or bases, the carboxyl and amino groups are both ionized fully to give rise to the term zwitterion

```
COO⁻           CH₃            NH₃⁺
 |              |              |
CH₂            CH.NH₃⁺        (CH₂)₄
 |              |              |
CH.NH₃⁺        COO⁻           CH.NH₃⁺
 |             Alanine         |
COO⁻                          COO⁻
Aspartic                      Lysine
acid
```

(German zwitter = hybrid or hermaphrodite). This kind of nature may

be understood as follows:

negatively charged isoionic positively charged

$$\downarrow \qquad \downarrow \qquad \downarrow$$

point of application of the mixture

Fig. 3.1 : To show pattern of electrophoresis

Separation of Amino acids by Ion-Exchange Chromatography

In addition to permitting the separation of amino acids by electrophoresis, their ionic properties also permit their separation by ion exchange chromatography. Ion exchange is performed using a resin to which positivelycharged groups (anion-exchange resin) or negatively charged groups (cation exchange resin) are covalently bound and thus immobilized.

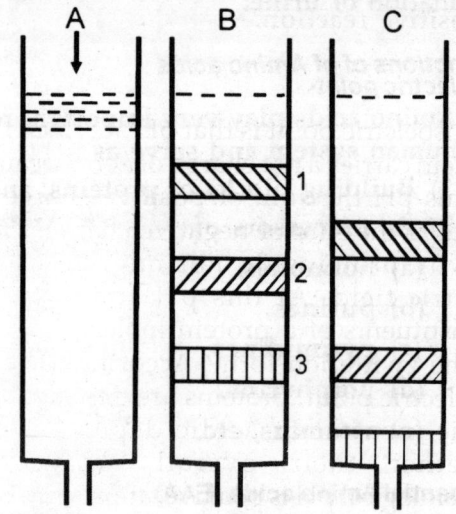

Fig. 3.2 : Principle of column chromatography. Material applied at top of column (A) gets separated into three components (B and C)

Ions passed down a column of such a resin bind competitively to the charged groups. Principle of ion-exchange chromatogrpahy has been shown as in (Fig. 3.2):

The peptide bond

This bond is formed by the interaction of two amino acids with the elimination of water between the NH_2 and COOH groups as shown below.

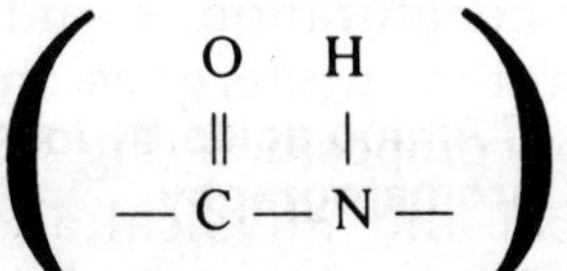

$$\left(\begin{array}{c} O \quad H \\ \parallel \quad | \\ -C-N- \end{array} \right)$$

The Biuret Reaction

Biuret has the formula $NH_2CONHCONH_2$, and is a simple substance containing a peptide bond. **When *Biuret* is treated with $CuSO_4$ in alkaline solution, a purple colour is produced. This is known as the *Biuret Reaction*. All proteins give a positive reaction.**

Isoelectric point

The isoelctric point is that pH at which the protein carries a net charge of zero because at this pH the sum of positive charge is equal to the sum of negative charge. That is why proteins do not migrate in an electric field. At this pH amino acids (constituents of a protein molecule) exist in the zwitterion form. According to the isoelectric point, proteins are described as basic, neutral or acidic depending or whether their overall charge at physiological pH is positive, approximately zero, or negative. lsoelectric points of some Common proteins are as follows:

High Performance Liquid Chromatography (HPLC)

This is the most latest kind of chromatography in which an instrument named as *Bio-Rad* protein *Chromatography system* is used. **By this technique, separation of a variety of peptides may be done, for example:**

  (i) Oxytocin
  (ii) Met-Enkephalin
  (iii) TRH
  (iv) α - Endorphin
  (v) α - MSH
  (vi) β - Endorphin
  (vii) Angiotensin II
  (viii) Substance P
  (ix) LHRH,
  (x) Neurotensin, etc.

The technique depends upon the use of microfine column matrixes to give high resolution rapidly.

α₁ Antitrypsin (AT) and its role in Emphysema

The predominant component of the α_1 - globulin band consists of a protein named as α_1-**antitrypsin (AT)**. It has been wrongly named because it is active against elastase rather than trypsin and is a member of a group of **Serine Proteinase**

Protein	Isoelectric point
Serum albumin	4.7
α_1, - Globulin	2.0
γ_2, - Globulin	5.8
Fibrinogen	5.8
Hemoglobin	7.2
Pepsin	1.0
Insulin	5.4
Cytochrome	9.8
Lysozyme	11.1

Inhibitors or, Serpins.

In normal young, the destructive power of enzyme elastase released from the neutrophils in checked by AT. **Cigarette smoking increases the number and activity of lung neutrophils and consequently the amount of enzyme elastase.** Moreover, oxidation reduces the protection afforded by a given amount of circulating AT.

α_1- antitrypsin is less active after oxidation; elastase then causes tissue breakdown and loss of elasticity ih the lungs vis-a-vis *emphysema*. **It means that smoking leads to tendency to emphysema.**

Proteins

Proteins may be defined as extremely complex nitrogen containing organic compounds which are polymers of amino acids and possess high molecular weight. Amino acids present in the protein molecules remain linked to each other with the help of a special linkage known as a peptide linkage (– CO – NH –).In addition to carbon, hydrogen and oxygen, proteins invariably contain nitrogen and generally sulphur also.

Proteins have also been found to contain phosphorus, iron, copper, iodine, manganese, zinc and other elements.

Denaturation

A protein is said to be a native protein if its amino acid composition and stereochemical structures remain unchanged from the natural state. These properties control all the functions of a protein, whether solubility in dilute salt solutions, proteolytic activity, oxygen carrying capacity, or whatever it may be. These characteristics are altered and the

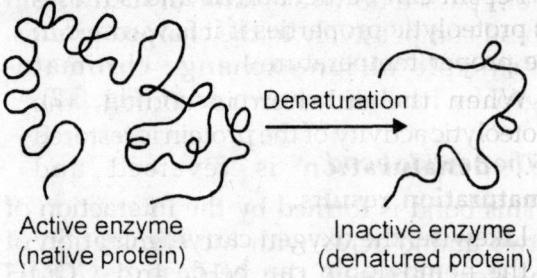

Active enzyme
(native protein)

Denaturation

Inactive enzyme
(denatured protein)

Fig. 3.3 : Representation of denaturation of a protein

process of denaturation is said to occur when a protein undergoes changes in structure or composition (Fig 3.3).

Chemical and physical agents that cause these changes are called denaturing agents. Their action involves the splitting of some or all the protein cross linkages with their possible reformation, in some cases, to cause a rearrangement of the peptide chains.

Denaturation may be caused by the following:

1. Heat
2. Mineral acids and alkalies
3. Shaking or stirring
4. Grinding
5. Ultraviolet radiations
6. Ultrasonic waves
7. Neutral Chemical agents, etc.

Renaturation

Denatured proteins may, however, under certain conditions, be restored to proteins with many of the properties of the original protein. This process is known as 'renaturation'. It appears, however, that renaturation seldom results in the complete restoration of the denatured protein to its original state.

Pepsin can be denatured and so loses its proteolytic properties if it is warmed to the proper temperature.

When the solution is cooled, the proteolytic activity of the protein is restored i.e., **denaturation** is reversed and **renaturation results.**

Likewise, the oxygen carrying capacity of the hemoglobin can be destroyed by denaturing with salicylate. On reversal, the restored hemoglobin is very similar to the original untreated hemoglobin.

Classification of Proteins

Proteins have been classified on the basis of their composition as follows:

I Simple proteins

Simple proteins are made up of amino acids only and upon hydrolysis yield a mixture of amino acids only.

Examples

(A)	**Fibrous (insoluble) proteins**	: Also called as **scleroproteins.** They impart a supporting or protective function in the animal. These are insoluble in water.
(a)	Collagens:	Principal supporting proteins of skin, tendons and bones. They possess very large amount of hydroxyproline. They are **resistant to peptic and tryptic digestion.**
(b)	Elastins	: Found in elastic tissues like tendons and arteries. **Readily digested by trypsin and pepsin.** It contains smaller amount of hydro-

xyproline.

(c)	Keratins :	Found in animal skin, nails, horns, hoofs, hair, feathers, etc. They possess high cystine content.
(B)	**Globular : (soluble) proteins**	Are soluble proteins with definite molecular weights. Each molecule contains one or more peptide chains, held in a coiled configuration by disulfide bridges and other bonds.
(a)	Albumins:	Include ovalbumin from egg white, serum albumin from blood serum, and lactalbumin from milk. They are coagulable by heat and soluble in pure water. They are precipitated from solution by **full saturation of ammonium sulphate.**
(b)	Globulins :	Include serum globulins, lactoglobulin from mlik, thyroglobulin from thyroid gland. Also found in many plant seeds, e.g. edestin from hempseed. Are soluble in dilute salt solutions and are precipitated from solution by **half saturation of ammonium sulphate.** Coagulated by heat.
(c)	Plant proteins (glutenins, prolamins)	: Cereal proteins such as glutelins of wheat, orygenin of rice and zein of maize. Soluble in very weak acids or alkalies

but insoluble in all neutral solvents.

(d) Protamines: They are simpler polypeptides. Uncoagulable by heat and possess strong basic properties. Rich in arginine. Example is **salmine from salmon sperms.**

(e) Histones : Are soluble in water but insoluble in dilute ammonia. Rich in arginine and lysine and possess strong basic properties. Example scombrone from mackerel sperms.

(C) Denatured Proteins

When proteins are subjected to certain physical and chemical agents, they get denatured. In fact, they undergo intramolecular changes which cause changes in solubility and other properties. Soluble proteins for example albumins and globulins are converted by heat, ultraviolet light, mechanical agitation or long contact with alcohol, etc. into insoluble materials known as coagulated proteins. Such coagulated proteins are denatured one.

II Conjugated Proteins

Are those proteins which consist of protein combined with some non protein substance (the prosthetic group). They are classified according to the nature of the prosthetic group, as indicated below:

III Derived Proteins

Include those substances formed from simple and conjugated proteins. It is the least well defined of the protein groups. These are subdivided into primary derived proteins and secondary derived proteins.

1. Primary derived proteins : Slight change with little or no hydrolytic cleavage of peptide bonds.

(a) Proteans : Insoluble products, example fibrin from fibrinogen

(b) Metaproteins: Generally soluble in very

Conjugated Protein = Protein part + prosthetic group

		Prosthetic group	Example
1.	Nucleoproteins	= Nucleic acid	Virus proteins
2.	Glycoproteins and Mucoproteins	= Carbohydrate or a derivative of carbohydrate	Mucin of saliva
3.	Phosphoroteins	= Phosphoric acid	Casein of milk, ovovitellin of egg yolk.
4.	Chromoproteins	= Metalloporphyrine or some similar substance which absorbs visible light.	Haemoglobin
5.	Metalloproteins	= Metals(copper, Mn, Mg, Zn, Mo etc.)	Tyrosinase, arginase,anhydrase, xanthine oxidase, etc.
6.	Lipoproteins	= Lipids (cholesterol, phospholipids triglycerides.etc.)	Serum lipoproteins, lipoproteins of egg yolk

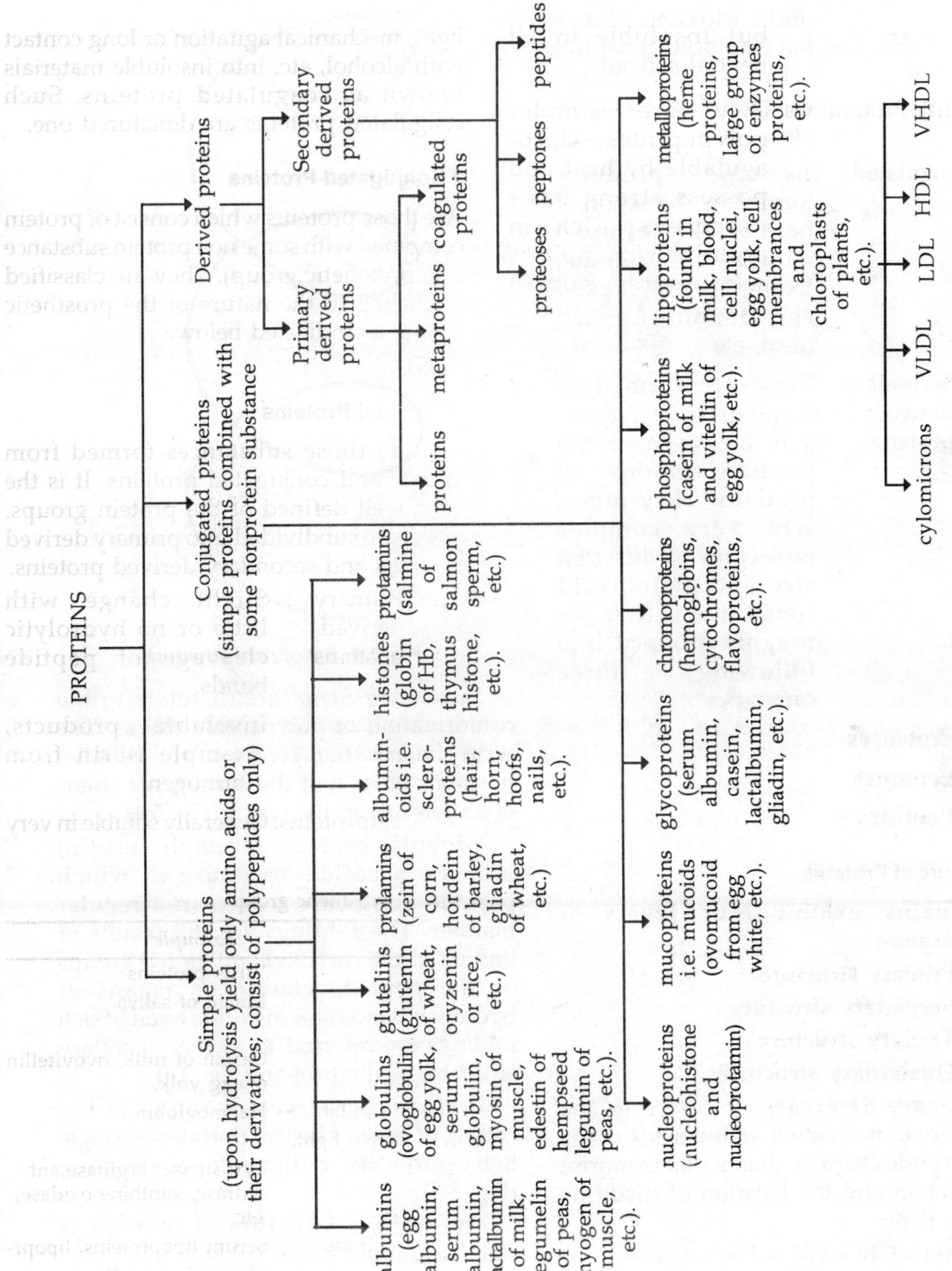

Table 3.2 : Classification of proteins

dilute acids and alkalies but insoluble in neutral solvents. Examples are acid and alkali albuminates.

(c) Coagulated : Insoluble products formed by the action of heat or alcohol upon natural proteins. Examples are cooked egg albumin, cooked meat, etc.

2. Secondary derived proteins : These are formed in the progressive hydrolytic cleavage of the peptide unions of proteins. They represent very complex molecules of different size and amino acid composition. They are roughly grouped into following three categories :

(a) **Proteoses**

(b) **Peptones**

(c) **Peptides**

Structure of Proteins

Proteins exhibit four levels of organization

1. **Primary structure**
2. **Secondary structure**
3. **Tertiary structure**
4. **Quaternary structure**

Primary Structure: It refers to the sequence of individual amino acids in the polypeptide chain or chains that comprise the protein and the location of disulfide bonds, if any.

– Ala – Gly – Gly – His – Leu –

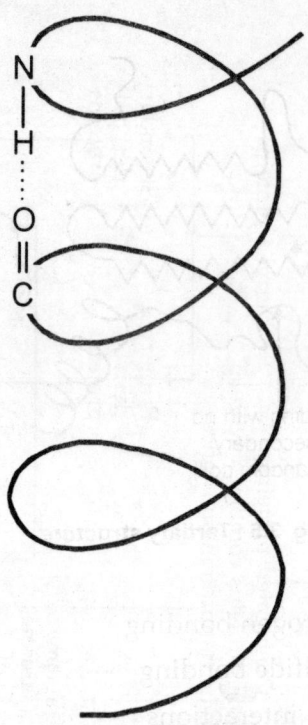

Fig. 3.4 : Secondary structure

Secondary Structure: It refers to the conformation of polypeptide chains. The term *conformation* refers to the relative positions of each of the constituent atoms of a molecule in the space (Fig. 3.4).

Globular proteins (example insulin) indicate a coiled structure in which peptide bonds are folded in a regular manner. The foldings are the results of linking of the carboxyl and amino groups of the peptide chains by means of hydrogen bonds and disulfide bonds. Such foldings are referred to as the secondary structure of the protein (Fig. 3.4).

Tertiary Structure: It refers to the coiling of several helical portions of single helix into a three dimentional structure (Fig. 3.5).

The tertiary structure of proteins is stabilised and maintained by :

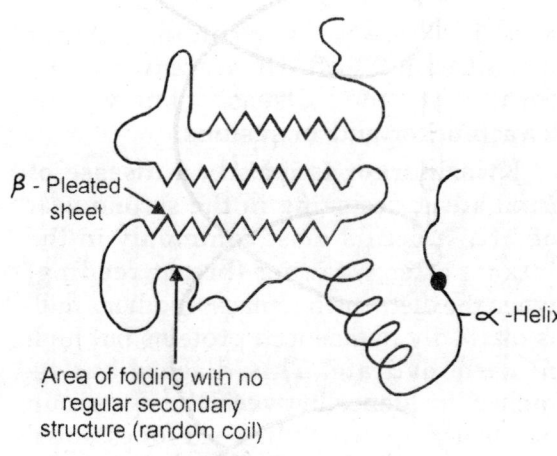

β - Pleated sheet

α -Helix

Area of folding with no regular secondary structure (random coil)

Fig 3.5 : Tertiary structure

(a) Hydrogen bonding

(b) Disulfide bonding

(c) Ionic interactions

(d) Vander Waal's forces

(e) Hydrophobic interactions

(f) Ester bonding

Example of the tertiary structure of protein is the protein of tobacco mosaic virus **(TMV)** which resembles the kernel of the corn.

Quaternary Structure

Proteins containing more than one polypeptide chain display fourth level of structural organization called **Quaternary structure**. In this type, the individual polypeptide chain is arranged in relation to each other so as to give a simple three dimensional structure on the overall protein molecule. Each polypeptide chain in such a protein is called a subunit. Depending upon the number of subunits present, such proteins are called as dimers, trimers, tetramers or polymers, etc. **Examples are haemoglobin, ferritin, etc.**

Biochemical functions/roles or biological importance of proteins

They play very important roles in the human body and are very essential substances. They play following important roles in the human body.

1. Proteins may be said as the essence of life processes.

2. All enzymes are made up of proteins.

3. Many of the hormones are proteinous in nature for example **insulin, glucagon, oxytocin, vasopressin, etc.**

4. They serve as building block units for subcellular, cellular and organic structures.

5. They act as defence against infections by way of protein antibodies.

6. They are involved in blood clotting through thrombin, fibrinogen and other protein factors.

7. Cementing substances and the reticulum which bind the cells as tissues/organs are partly made up of proteins.

8. They perform hereditary transmission by way of nucleoproteins found in the cell nucleus.

9. They act as buffers.

10. They help in the transport of oxygen and CO_2 by way of haemoglobin and certain special enzymes which are found in red blood cells.

Dietary Requirement of Proteins

Requirement of proteins of an individual depends upon the age, sex and body weight. It is as mentioned in Table 3.3

Now the chemists have reached the fact that the quantity of protein alone does not

Table 3.2 : Recommended daily dietary protein intake

Category	Description	Daily protein allowance (g)	Nature of diet
Man	Body weight 55 kg	55	
Woman	Body weight 45 kg	45	Mainly cereals and pulses NPU = 65*
Woman	2nd half of pregnancy	55	
Woman	Lactation upto 1 year	65	
Infants	0-3 months	2.3 /kg	Entirely milk NPU=75-100
Infants	3-6 months	1.8/kg	
Infants	6-9 months	1.8/kg	Milk, cereals and pulses, NPU = 65*
Infants	9-12 months	1.5/kg	
Children	1 year	17	
Children	2 years	18	
Children	3 years	20	
Children	4-6 years	22	Mostly cereals and pulses NPU = 50*
Children	7-9 years	33	
Children	10-12 years	41	
Adolescents: Boys 13-15 years		55	
Adolescents: Boys 16-18 years		60	

* The essential amino acids requirement of adults is less exacting than those of infants and children, therefore, the same dietary has a higher NPU for adults than for children.

solve the entire purpose but the **quality** of a protein has got more significance hence one must give more emphasis on the quality of a protein. **By the quality of a protein, we mean that it must comprise of essential amino acids in it.**

Deficiency Diseases

Protein deficiency is generally encountered during infancy and childhood and is known as protein- energy malnutrition **(PEM)**. There are two severe forms of the disease known as kwashiorkor and marasmus.

Kwashiorkor is mainly a disease of rural areas, occurring in the second year of life. It occurs most commonly in the infants after weaning (breast feeding) when the diet which replaces mother's milk is markedly deficient in proteins but high in carbohydrate. This disease has its highest incidence **between the age group of 1 to 4 years** when the need for essential amino acids for tissue synthesis is more.

This syndrome is characterized by growth failure, retarded development, loss of appetite, mental apathy, hypoalbuminemia leading to edema, diarrhoea, pellagrous skin lesions, low plasma amino acids, lipids, glucose and potassium levels, gastrointestinal disturbances, dermatosis, fatty liver infiltration and mental disturbances are also frequent.

Marasmus

Marasmus literally means "to waste". It results from a continued severe deficiency of both dietary proteins and the calories i.e. energy.

Marasmus is predominantly due to the **deficiency of calories**. This is usually observed in children given watery gruels (of cereals) to supplement the mother's breast milk.

It generally occurs in the children below one year of age. The symptoms include growth retardation, muscle wasting, anemia, weakness, and repeated infections. Attitude is irritable. Skin is shrunken, dry and atrophic.

A marasmic child does not show edema or decreased concentration of plasma albumin (usual level in them is 2 to 3 g/dl whereas in kwashiorkor cases it is always less than 2 g/dl) and the level of cortisol in serum gets increased in marasmic child whereas decreased in kwashiorkor ones.

Immunoglobulins

Immunoglobulins or *antibodies* are synthesized in B lymphocytes or their derivatives, plasma cells and with remarkable specificity bind to *antigenic sites* on their moelcules.

All immunoglobulins are composed of four polypeptide chains, two identical light (L) chains(MW 23,000) and 2 identical heavy (H) chains (MW 53,000-75,000) which are held together as a tetramer (L_2H_2) by disulfide bonds (Fig. 3.6). Each chain can be divided into specific regions that have structural and functional significance. The half of the *light* (L) *chain* towards the carboxyl terminus is referred to as the *constant region* (C_L), whereas the amino-terminal half is the *variable region* of the light chain (V_L). Nearly, one-quarter ofthe *heavy (H) chain* at the amino terminus is referred to as its variable region (V_H) and the remaining three quarters of the heavy chain are referred to as the constant regions (C_H1, C_H2, C_H3) of that H chain. The function of the immunoglobulin molecule that binds the specific antigen is formed by the amino-terminal portions (variable regions) of both the H and L chains i.e., the V_H and V_L regions.

As made clear in Fig. 3.6, digestion of an immunoglobulin by the enzyme papain produces 2 antigen binding fragments (Fab) and one crystallizable fragment (F_c). The area in which papain cleaves the

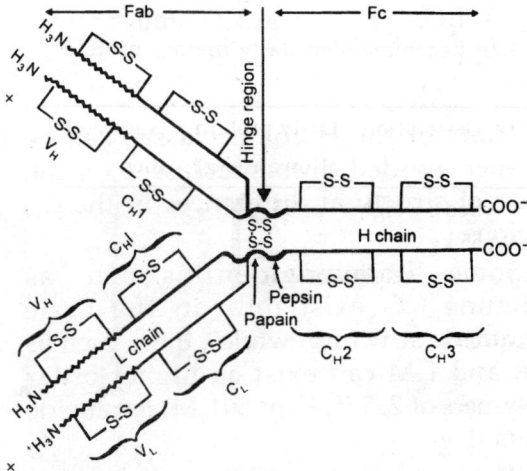

Fig 3.6 : **A simplified model for an IgG human antibody molecule showing the 4-chain basic structure and different regions. V, indicates variable region; C, the constant region, and the vertical arrow, the hinge region. Thick lines represent H and L chains; thin lines represent disulfide bonds.**

immunoglobulin molecule i.e., the region between the C_H1 and C_H2 regions is referred to as the **hinge region.**

There are two general types of light chains i.e. *kappa* (k) and *lambda* (λ). A given immunoglobulin molecule always contains two *k* or two λ light chains, never a mixture of *k* and λ. In human the *k* chains are more common than λ chains in immunoglobulin molecules.

In human, 5 classes of H chains have been found which can be easily distinguished from each other by differences in their C_H regions. The 5 classes of H chains are designated γ, α, μ, δ & ε which vary in their molecular weight ranging from 50,000 to 70,000. The μ and ε chains each have four C_H regions rather than the usual 3. The type of H chain determines the class of immunoglobulin and thus its main function. **There are five classes of immunoglobulins known so far namely:**

1. I_gG,   4. I_gD, and
2. I_gA,   5. I_gE
3. I_gM,

Many of the H chain classes can be further divided, into subclasses on the basis of structural differences in the C_H regions.

Some immunoglobulins.such as immune I_gG exist only in the basic tetrameric structure, while others such as I_gA and I_gM can exist as higher-order polymers of 2, 3 (I_gA) or 5 (I_gM) tetrameric units (Fig. 3.7).

The L and H chains are synthesized as separate molecules and are subsequently assembled within the B cell or plasma cell into mature immunoglobulin molecules,

all of which are glycoproteins in nature.

Schematic model of I_gG molecule is as shown below in Fig. 3.8.

Each immunoglobulin light chain is the product of at least 3 separate structural genes i.e., a variable region (V_L) gene, ajoining region (J) gene (bearing no relation to the J chain of I_gA or I_gM) and a constant region (C_L) gene. Each heavy chain is the porduct of at least 4 different genes i.e., a variable region (V_H) gene, a diversity region (D) gene, a joining region (J) gene and a constant region (C_H) gene. **In this way, the 'one gene, one protein' concept is no more valid.**

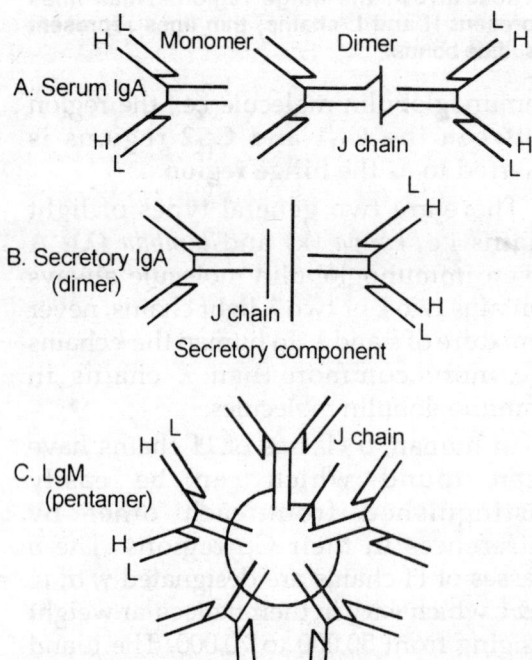

Fig. 3.7 : **Highly schematic illustration of polymeric human immunoglobulins. Polypeptide chains are represented by thick lines; disulfide bonds linking different polypeptide chains are represented by thin lines.**

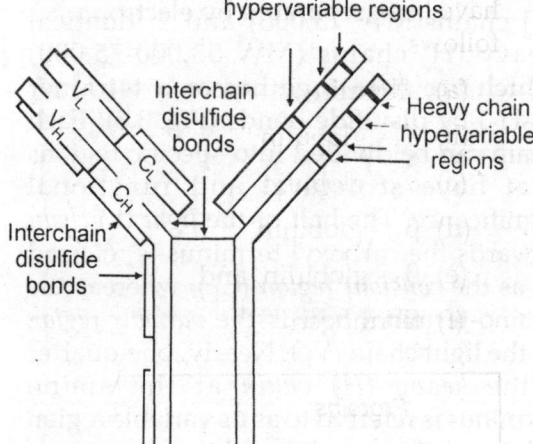

Fig. 3.8 : **Schematic model of an I_gG molecule showing approximate positions of the hypervariable regions in heavy and light chains.**

Each person is capable of generating antibodies directed against perphaps one million different antigens.

Various disorders of immunoglobulins include increased production of specific classes of immunoglobulins or even specific immunoglobulin molecules. **Hypogamma-globulinemia** may be restricted to a single class of immunoglobulin molecules (eg, I_gA or I_gG) or may involve underproduction of all classes of immunoglobulins (I_gA, I_gD, I_gE, I_gG and I_gM).

Plasma Proteins

Normal value of plasma total protein ranges from 6 to 8 gm per 100 ml of blood.

Plasma proteins include albumin, globulin and fibrinogen which can be separated from each other by:

(1) Precipitation method using varying concentrations of salts like sodium sulphate, ammonium sulphate, etc.

(2) Electrophoresis

In normal human plasma six fractions have been separated by electrophoresis as follows:

(a) albumin

(b) α_1 - globulin

(c) α_2 - globulin

(d) β_1, - globulin

(e) β_2 - globulin, and

(f) fibrinogen

Functions of Plasma Proteins

1. **Osmotic Pressure:** Plasma proteins are important in regulating water between blood and tissues, thus they help in maintaining intravascular colloid osmotic pressure.

2. *As carrier of certain metabolites:* They act as a carrier molecule for bilirubin, fatty acids, trace elements and many drugs.

3. *As buffers:* Proteins are amphoteric in nature and thus help in maintaining the pH of blood.

4. **The lipoproteins act as *carrier molecules*** for different types of lipids and lipid-soluble molecules that are not soluble in the plasma water.

5. *Some metal-binding proteins fore.g.* transferrin have the properties of globulins. and act as carriers for trace elements.

6. *As immunoglobulins:* The property of antibodies formation resides in the γ- globulin fraction of the proteins which are very important from various angles.

Proteins	Biological role
Collagen, keratins	Structural proteins
Pepsin, amylase, etc.	Enzymes
Insulin, prolactin	Hormones
Haemoglobin, ceruloplasmin	Transport proteins
Ferritin	Storage proteins
γ - globulins	Immune functions
Hormone receptors	Protein receptors

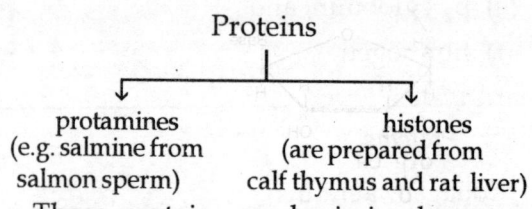

CHAPTER 4

NUCLEIC ACIDS

> We are the carriers of genetic information from one offspring to another.
> What wonderful unimaginable property? We are very complex molecules.
> Scientists are pursuing us and shall continue to pursue us till the 'universe'
> is present as we are very very complicated molecules. Many many thanks to
> the science- stalwarts like James Watson, Francis Crick, Morris Wilkins
> (forgotten man of DNA), Chargaff, etc. who dedicated their lives for us.
> 'Genome technology' is only due to us.

If any group of compounds can be said to be **'controller'** in **biochemistry, it is the nucleic acids** which are found in every living cell and these may be defined as the nitrogen containing compounds of high molecular weight, **vis-a-vis polymers of nucleotides.** These are in fact macromolecules which remain present in most of the living cells, either in the free state or combined with proteins. The nucleic acid protein complexes are known as nucleoproteins, and these can be separated into the component proteins and nucleic acids by treatment with acid or high salt concentration. For the first time, they were reported by the scientist Miescher in 1871. Proteins associated with nucleic acids fall into two major classes as mentioned below:

Proteins

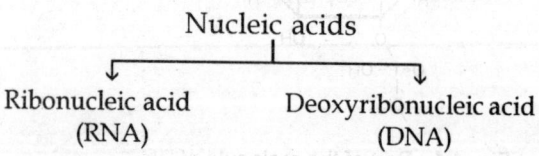

protamines (e.g. salmine from salmon sperm)

histones (are prepared from calf thymus and rat liver)

These proteins are basic in character, for example salmine which consists of 40 arginine residues out of a total of 120.

As the name suggests, nucleic acids are acidic in character at physiological pH and carry a high density of negative charge. Nucleic acids are mainly of the following two types:

Nucleic acids

Ribonucleic acid (RNA)

Deoxyribonucleic acid (DNA)

Nucleic acids may be defined as the macromolecules in which the nucleotides remain linked to each other by phosphodiester bonds between the 3' and 5' positions of the sugars.

A portion of a molecule of RNA therefore has the structure as given in Fig. 4.1 **where base can either be a purine or pyrimidine.**

Most nucleic acids are very large molecules, therefore, to show the complete formulae is rather very cumbersome. A useful form of shorthand for the structure is therefore employed which exhibits the bases present by using their first letter. The sequence of bases is extremely important so that a nucleic acid may be shown by the first letters of the bases only (Fig. 4.2).

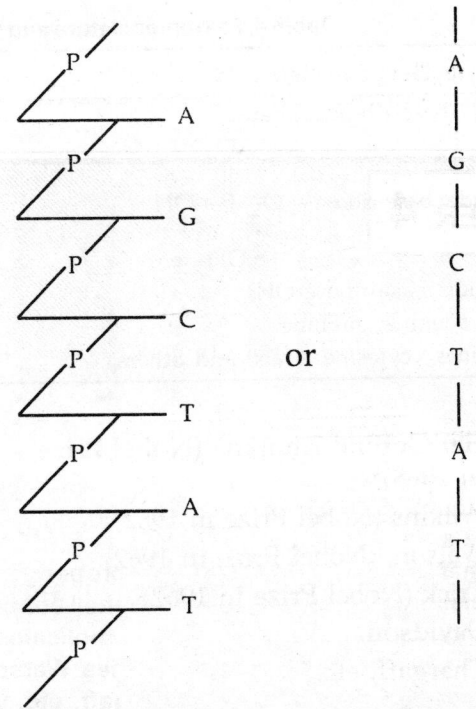

Fig. 4.2 : Shorthand notation to exhibit the base sequence of a nucleic acid

Hydrolysis of DNA and RNA under controlled conditions yields *nucleotides*, which can be regarded as the basic unit of nucleic acids just as amino acids are the basic unit of the proteins and monosaccharides of the polysaccharides. **Further hydrolysis of** *nucleotides* **yields** *nucleosides* and eventually phosphate, a sugar and number of purine and pyrimidine bases. Nomenclature and components of nucleic acids have been described in Table 4.1.

Our understanding regarding the nucleic acids has grown tremendously in the recent years. Several top scientists of the world's top laboratories are working day and night on 'nucleic acids', amongst whom good contributories are:

(i) Miescher,

(ii) A.R Todd,

O=P—OH
|
O
|
CH₂   O   Base
H   H   H   H
   O   OH
O=P—OH
|
O
|
CH₂   O   Base
H   H   H   H
   O   OH
O=P—OH
|
O
|
CH₂   O   Base
H   H   H   H
   O   OH
O=P—OH
|
O

Fig. 4.1 : Part of the molecule of RNA

Table 4.1 : Nomenclature and Components of nucleic acids

RNA (cytoplasmic nucleic acid)	DNA (nuclear nucleic acid)
Polymer: (base-rib-phosphate)$_n$	(base-deoxyrib-phosphate)$_n$
$$\text{Nucleotide : base-ribose—O—}\overset{\displaystyle O}{\overset{\displaystyle \|}{\underset{\displaystyle OH}{P}}}\text{—OH}$$	$$\text{base-deoxyrib—O—}\overset{\displaystyle O}{\overset{\displaystyle \|}{\underset{\displaystyle OH}{P}}}\text{—OH}$$
Nucleoside: base-ribose-OH	base-deoxyrib-OH
Purine : adenine, guanine	adenine, guanine
Pyrimidines : cytosine, uracil and others	cytosine, thymine

(iii) **Har Gobind Khorana (Nobel Prize in 1968)***

(iv) Wilkins (Nobel Prize in 1962)

(v) Watson, (Nobel Prize in 1962)

(vi) Crick (Nobel Prize in 1962)

(vii) Davidson,

(viii) Chargaff, etc.

Functions of the Nucleic Acids

(i) Nucleic acids are responsible for the direction of metabolism throughout the life of a cell.

(ii) They direct the synthesis of proteins.

(iii) They control the synthesis of enzymes.

(iv) They are responsible for the transfer of genetic information from one offspring to another.

(v) Nucleic acids, in fact, contribute the essential substance of the genes and the apparatus by which the genes act.

(vi) For the clinician, they are of major interest as they are undoubtedly involved in the causation of cancers **(malignancies).**

He succeeded in synthesizing the first wholly artificial gene, which contained in it 77 nucleotides. He was of Indian origin, later settled in U.S.

Chemical Composition

Nucleic acids fall into two principal classes according to the nature of the sugar they contain:

(i) the deoxyribonucleic acid, i.e., DNA which contains the sugar known as deoxyribose sugar, and

(ii) the ribonucleic acids i.e., RNAs which contain the sugar known as ribose.

RNA and DNA are polymers of nitrogenous bases, sugars, and phosphoric acid; thus

$$(\text{base-sugar-phosphate})_n$$
nucleic acid

where n is a large number.

The link between the polymer units is the phosphate diester bond as shown below:

$$- \text{sugar} - O - \overset{\displaystyle O}{\overset{\displaystyle \|}{\underset{\displaystyle \underset{OH}{|}}{P}}} - O - \text{sugar} -$$

phosphate diester bond

Nucleotides

When the phosphate diester bond gets hydrolyzed, the monomeric units of nucleic acids are separated which consist of a nitrogenous base, a sugar and a phosphate; such a unit is called as a nucleotide as shown below:

$$base - sugar - O - \overset{\overset{\textstyle O}{\|}}{\underset{\underset{\textstyle OH}{|}}{P}} - OH$$

nucleotide

Nucleotides and nucleosides are named after the bases contained in their structure, as below:

Base	Nucleoside	Nucleotide
Adenine	Adenosine	Adenylic acid
Guanine	Guanosine	Guanylic acid
Uracil	Uridine	Uridylic acid
Cystosine	Cytidine	Cytidylic acid
Thymine	Thymidine	Thymidylic acid

If the base is linked to deoxyribose, then the names are modified so that a nucleoside consisting of adenine and deoxyribose would be called deoxyadenosine. As well as the nucleotides indicated, a number of biologically important nucleotides such as adenosine di- and triphosphate (ADP and ATP), guanosine di- and triphosphate (GDP and GTP) and nicotinamide adenine

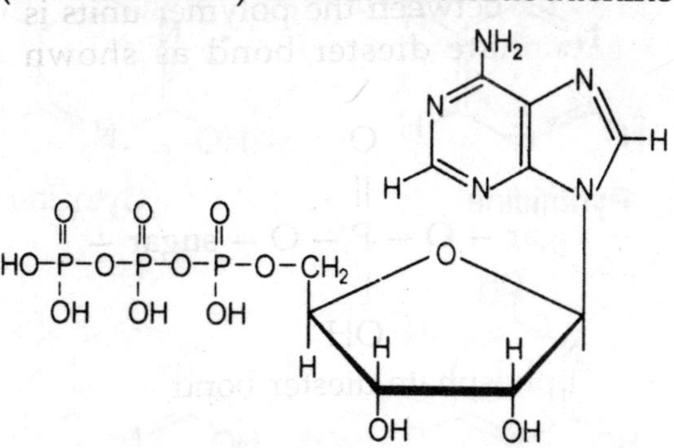

Adenosine triphosphate (ATP)

dinucleotide (NAD) are known to occur in the free state.

Nucleosides

When the ester bond between the sugar and the phosphate group in a nucleotide is hydrolyzed, a fragment consisting of a nitrogenous base and a sugar moiety is obtained which is called as a *nucleoside*,

$$base - sugar - OH$$

nucleoside

The important examples of nucleosides

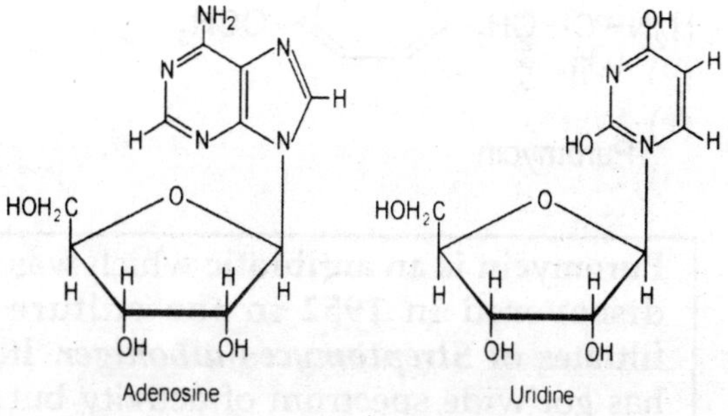

include adenosine and uridine whose structures are as given below; others are guanosine, thymidine, cytidine, etc.

Most of the bonds linking the sugar and the base are as shown above, but transfer **RNA does contain an unusual nucleotide pseudo-uridine in which ribose is linked to the uracil via the 5 position.**

Other examples of nucleosides of natural origin (not derived nom nucleic acids) include the important antibiotics like puromycin, tubercidin, nebularine, cordycepin, etc., which are derived from moulds, fungi and also from a group of compounds isolated from sponges, among which the important examples are those of spongothymidine, spongouridine, and spongosine, etc.

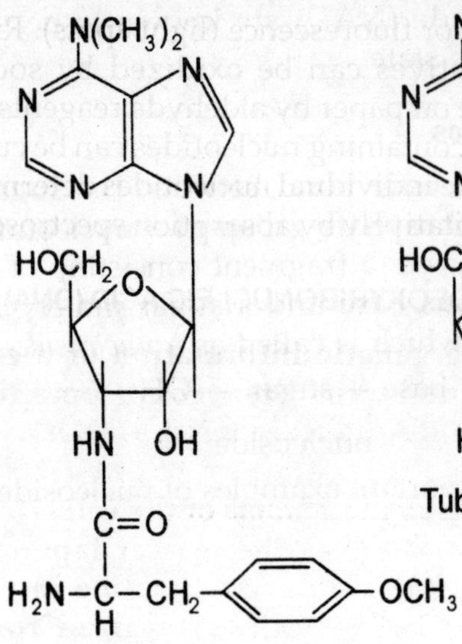

Tubercidin

Puromycin

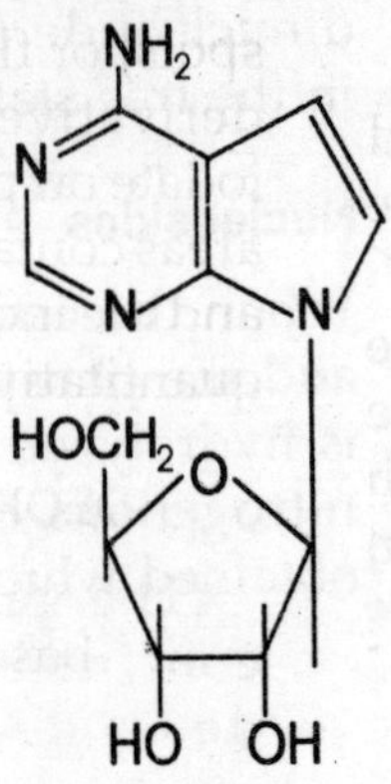

> **Puromycin is an antibiotic** which was discovered in **1952** in the culture filtrates of *Streptomyces alboniger.* It has got wide spectrum of activity but unfortunately is not being used in human beings because of its toxic nature to the mammalian cells.

Pentose Sugars

Sugars found in the nucleic acids are either D-ribose as in RNA or D-2-deoxyribose as in DNA, structure of which are as given below. The 'type' of the presence of pentose sugars in nucleic acids is the basis of its classification, **if they contain 'ribose' sugar in its structure, then they are known as ribonucleic acids and if deoxyribose then deoxyribonucleic acid.**

The structure of these sugars are as given below:

The carbon atoms on the sugars are denoted as 1', 2', etc. in order to differentiate them from the atoms of the bases.

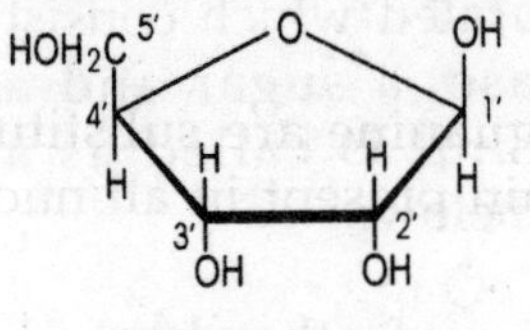

β-D-Ribofuranose 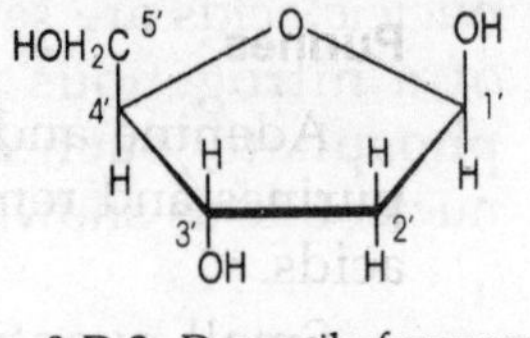   β-D-2- Deoxyribofuranose

Nitrogenous Bases

The formulae of the main nitrogenous bases found in the nucleic acids are as shown below:

Purines

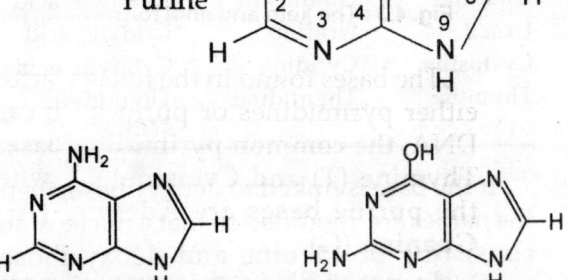

Purine

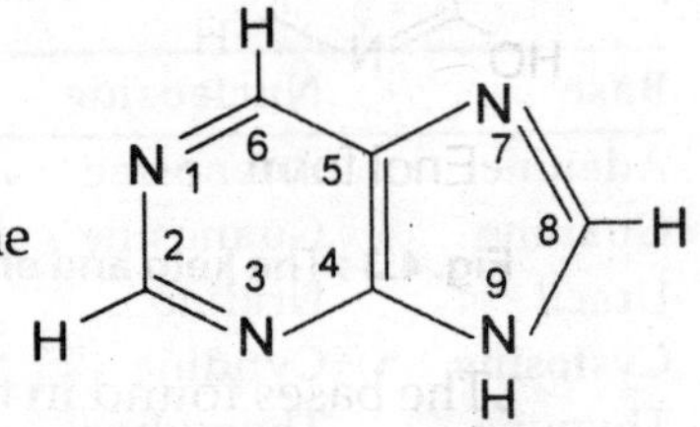

Adenine   Guanine

Pyrimidines

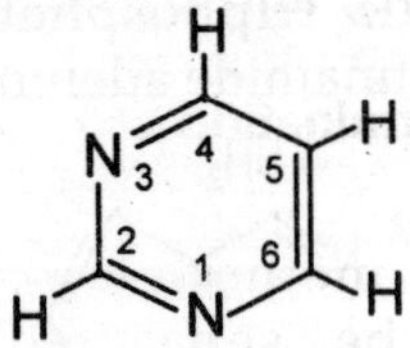

Pyrimidine 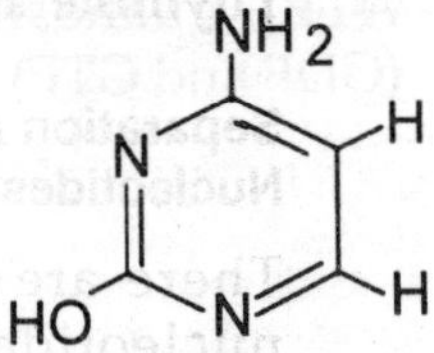   Cytosine

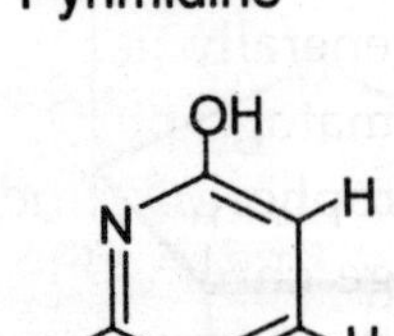

Uracil 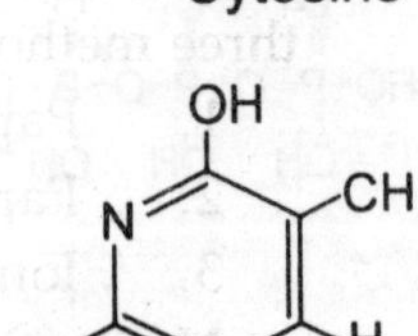   Thymine

Purines

Adenine and guanine are substituted purines and remain present in all nucleic acids.

Small quantities of other bases have been detected in nucleic acids from some sources. It should be noted that both purine and pyrimidine bases can exist in the keto or enol form (Fig. 4.3).

Enol form   **Keto form**

Fig. 4.3 : The keto and enol forms of thymine

The bases found in the nucleic acids are either pyrimidines or purines. In case of DNA, **the common pyrimidine bases are Thymine (T) and Cytosine (C); whereas the purine bases are Adenine (A) and Guanine (G).**

In case of RNAs, they generally contain only four bases namely, **the purine bases are Adenine and Guanine and the pyrimidine bases are Uracil (not Thymine as in DNA), and Cytosine.**

Separation and Determination of Nucleotides

There are various methods by which nucleotides can be separated and determined, out of which the following three methods are generally used:

1. Paper chromatography,
2. Paper electrophoresis, and
3. Ion-exchange chromatography.

Nucleotides can be identified on the developed chromatogram either by ultraviolet (UV) light absorption (dark spots) or fluorescence (light spots). Ribose derivatives can be oxidized by sodium iodate on paper by aldehyde reagents. The areas containing nucleotides can be cut out and the individual nucleotides determined quantitatively by absorption spectroscopy.

DEOXYRIBONUCLEIC ACID (DNA)

The genetic information of a cell is confined in its complement of deoxyribonucleic acid (DNA). This genetic information scientifically is known as the *genome* of the celL We may regard DNA as the master tape of the cell, the computer programme in which all the information required for the operation of the cell and its reproduction is contained. It has been studied that an *E. coli* cell is about 1 μm long; its DNA is 1 mm long. **This DNA encodes for atleast 4,000 proteins and contains many regions that regulate the expression of these proteins.**

DNA is intimately associated with the genetic material of the cell. In some microorganisms, a single strand of DNA seems to be the store for the genetic information but, in higher organisms, the DNA is present as nucleoprotein in the chromosomes. The amount of DNA in the cell of a particular species is constant, whereas the germ cells with half the number of chromosomes contain half the DNA present in other cells. **The DNA occurs almost exclusively in the nucleus and in minute quantity in the mitochondria.** It plays following *biological roles:*

Biological Roles of DNA

(i) The function of DNA is to act as a *store house of genetic information and to control the synthesis of proteins in the cell.*

(ii) *Cell replication:* Hereditary characteristics are passed on to daughter cells through replication of DNA; during cell division, the two strands of DNA get separated and free nucleotides are attached to each strand according to the *'base pairing'* rule. The nucleotides are then probably 'zipped' together by the action of a DNA polymerase to give two identical molecules of the original DNA (Fig. 4.4).

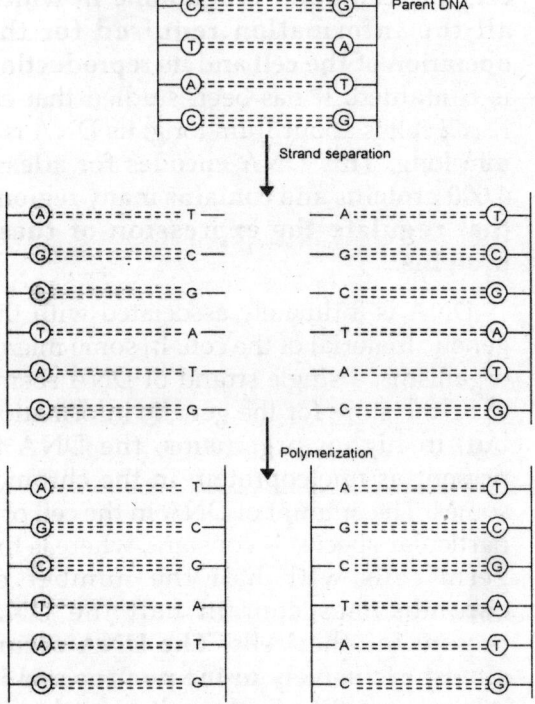

Fig. 4.4 : The replication of DNA (A, G, T and C represent the nucleotides on the newly synthesized strand of DNA)

(iii) *Control of protein synthesis:* It is now clear from a number of experiments that the sequence of bases in the nuclear DNA determines the proteins synthesized in the cytoplasm of the cell. The *'genetic code'* is such that 3 non-overlapping bases known as a *'codon "* code for each amino acid. The code is 'degenerate' in that more than one triplet may code for a particular amino acid. The DNA therefore acts in the first instance as a *'template'* on which the messenger RNA (m-RNA) gets synthesized. The m-RNA, with a complementary base sequence to the nuclear DNA, then carries the genetic message from the nucleus to the *protein synthesizing system on the ribosomes.*

Structure of DNA

For convenience, we may study the structure of DNA into three stages namely:

(a) Primary structure,

(b) Secondary structure, and

(c) Tertiary structure

(a) Primary Structure

DNA is a linear polymer (double stranded in its native state) of 21-deoxynucleotide residues which remain linked to each other by phosphodiester bonds between 3' and 5' positions of the 2'-deoxyribosyl moieties (Fig. 4.5).

The most common bases in DNA are:

(a) Adenine

(b) Thymine

(c) Guanine, and

(d) Cytosine

The *primary structure* of DNA is referred to as the linear sequence of nuleotide residues comprising the polydeoxyribonucleotide chain.

The primary structure of DNA molecules from various sources range from a few thousand residues in some viruses

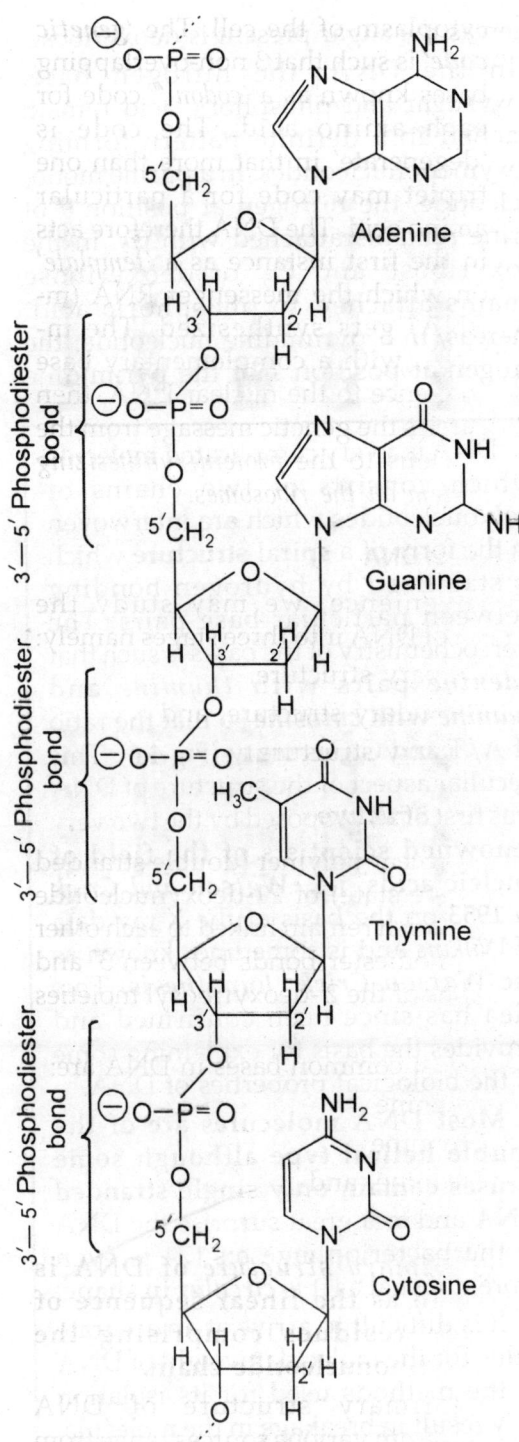

Fig. 4.5 : Covalent backbone of DNA

to 10^6 residues in bacteria to 10^9 residues in a human chromosomal DNA. A single molecule of bacterial DNA is nearly 1 mm long; whereas the length of a DNA molecule of a human chromosome is estimated to be 8.2 cm. **Molecular weights and lengths of DNA from various sources vary widely.**

Base Composition of DNA

Base composition of DNA remained unidentified after its discovery for nearly a century because of the difficulty of separating the products of DNA hydrolysis from one another. Invention of paper chromatography provided a mean to overcome this difficulty and E. Chargaff was the first scientist to determine the base composition of many species in 1950. The base composition differs widely from one species to another. Each species has a characteristic base composition but every organ of higher organisms has the same base composition. Strikingly, for every organism the ratio of pyrimidines to purines, $(A + G)/(C + T)$, is nearly unity as shown in Table 4.2.

Table 4.2: Base composition of DNA (mol %) and ratios of various components

Source	A	G	C	T	$\frac{A+T}{G+C}$	A/T	G/C	$\frac{A+G}{C+T}$
Man	30.4	19.9	19.9	30.1	1.52	1.009	1.000	1.006
Ox	29.0	21.2	21.2	28.7	1.36	1.010	1.000	1.006

The mole percent ratio of guanine to cytosine (G/C) and adenine to thymine (A/T) are also nearly unity in each case as shown above. The $(A + T)/(G + C)$ ratios, however vary widely.

(b) Secondary structure

Scientists **Watson and Crick** were responsible for deducing the structure of DNA in 1953; they were awarded Nobel

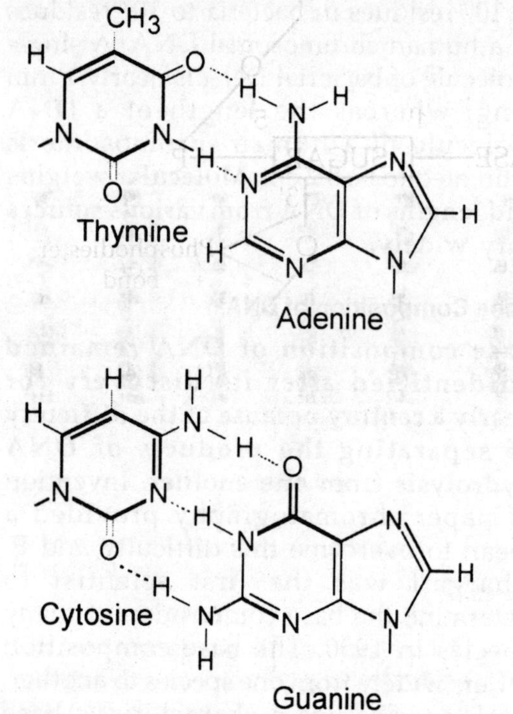

Fig. 4.6 : The pairing of bases by hydrogen bonding (-.-----) as in DNA

prize in 1962 for this brilliant discovery. One key to the structure of DNA was Chargaff's observation that purines and pyrimidines are present in DNA in eqimolar quantities.

Deoxyribonucleic acids are very complex molecules which possess a molecular weight ranging from 6-100 millions. They are elongated in shape and consist mostly of two strands which remain coiled in a parallel helical manner.

Complete hydrolysis of DNA leads to the formation of the following:

(a) Various nitrogenous bases,

(b) Sugar, and

(c) Phosphoric acid

The nitrogenous bases include both purine (adenine and guanine) and pyrimidine (cytosine and thymine);

whereas the sugar present is deoxyribose.

In the DNA, the nitrogen base, deoxysugar and phosphoric acid remain attached in a definite pattern forming deoxymononucleotides. In a purine mononucleotide, the nitrogen at position 9 of purine remains attached with C_1 in the deoxyribose and $C_{5'}$ of deoxyribose remains attached to phosphoric acid. Whereas, in a pyrimidine nucleotide, the nitrogen at position 1 of the pyrimidine

DNA is a very complicated molecule which consists of two chains of polynucleotides which are interwoven in the form of a **spiral structure** which is stabilized by hydrogen bonding between particular base pairs. The stereochemistry of the bases is such that *adenine* pairs with *thymine* and *guanine* with *cytosine* so that the ratio of A/T and G/C is unity (Fig.4.6). This peculiar aspect of the structure of DNA was first of all proposed by the **two very renowned scientists of the field of nucleic acids, i.e., Watson and Crick in 1953** on the basis of the X-ray data of *Wilkins* and is sometimes known as the *Watson-Crick hypothesis*. This idea has since been confirmed and provides the basis for explaining some of the biological properties of DNA.

Most DNA molecules are of the double helical type although some viruses contain only single stranded DNA and to a great surprise the DNA in the bacteriophage φx 174 is even more unusual as it is *circular* in shape.

It is difficult to arrive at an accurate value for the molecular weight of DNA as the methods used for its isolation may result in breakage in the molecule, but it ranges in millions.

nucleus remains attached to the C_1, of deoxyribose and $C_{5'}$ of deoxyribose remains attached to the phosphoric acid.

Each strand of DNA molecule contains large number of deoxymononucleotides (d- B-S-P) which include both pyrimidine and purine bases, namely, thymidine monophosphate (T), deoxycytidine monophosphate (dC), deoxyadenosine monophosphate (dA) and deoxyguanosine monophosphate (dG). These deoxynucleotides remain firmly attached internally in each strand by means of 3', 5'-phosphodiester bonds. Such type of bonds are formed by esterification of the hydroxyl group at position 3' of deoxyribose of one deoxymononucleotide and the hydroxyl groups at position 5' of deoxyribose in the next adjacent deoxymononucleotide to a common phosphoric acid molecule which exists in the latter deoxymononucleotide. The formation *of* such bonds has been illustrated in Figure 4.7.

The phosphoric acid of the former deoxymononucleotide remains esterified with another deoxymononucleotide existing previous to it. In this manner, a polynucleotide chain gets formed by inter-linking of large number of mononucleotides by 3', 5'-phosphodiester bonds. These polynucleotides form the DNA strand.

In different DNAs, the sequence *of* deoxymononucleotides is found to vary. The specific properties exhibited by the DNA -molecules are governed by this sequence. The two strands of DNA molecule are complementary to each other. Their base sequence is interdependent which follows the base pairing rule.

In a double-helix, formed by parallel coiling of the two strands along a longitudinal axis, the placing of the bases is such" that **adenine is placed in the**

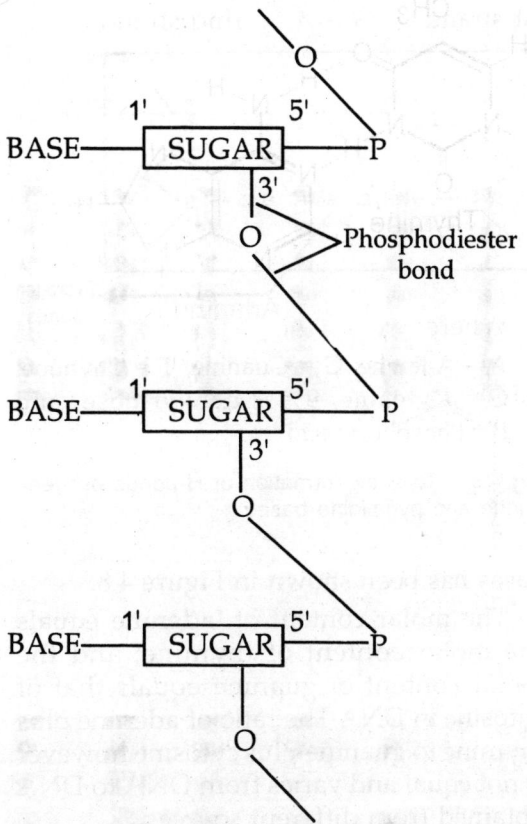

Fig. 4.7 : Formation of 3', 5'-phosphodiester linkages between mononucleotides

plane of thymine and guanine is placed in the plane of cytosine or vice versa, the so called base-pairing rule.

(c) *Tertiary structure*

The two strands are kept in position and the structure is stabilized by means *of* hydrogen bonds, each amino group being joined to a keto group, i.e., adenine to thymine, guanine to cytosine, etc. Formation of two hydrogen bonds between adenine and thymine; and three hydrogen bonds between guanine and cytosine is maximally possible. The formation of the H-bonds between such

Ist strand   IInd strand

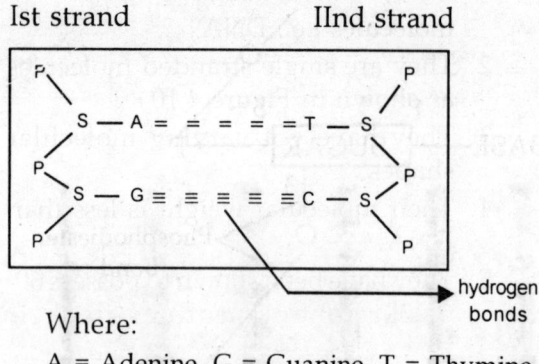

Where:

A = Adenine, G = Guanine, T = Thymine,
C = Cytosine, S = 2-deoxyribose, and
P = Phosphoric acid

Fig. 4.8 : To show formation of H-bonds between purine and pyrimidine bases

bases has been shown in Figure 4.8.

The molar content of 'adenine equals the molar content of thymine; and the molar content of guanine equals that of cytosine in DNA The ratio of adenine plus thymine to guanine plus cytosine however is not equal and varies from DNA to DNA obtained from different sources.

DNA helix consists of several million turns. The two strands of a DNA helix run parallel but in opposite directions. **The double helical structure is although quite stable but may be denatured by heat treatment or extremes of pH.** Denaturation of DNA results in uncoiling of the two strands as a result *of* which two separate chains are formed; the molecular weight also gets halved and absorbance at 260mμ (characteristic of nucleic acids) also gets increased.

DNAs are mainly present in the nucleus of the cells and are the carriers of hereditary characters. DNA can reproduce itself by the phenomenon of replication. **Genes are composed of the DNA proteins which are believed to be associated with the mechanism of**

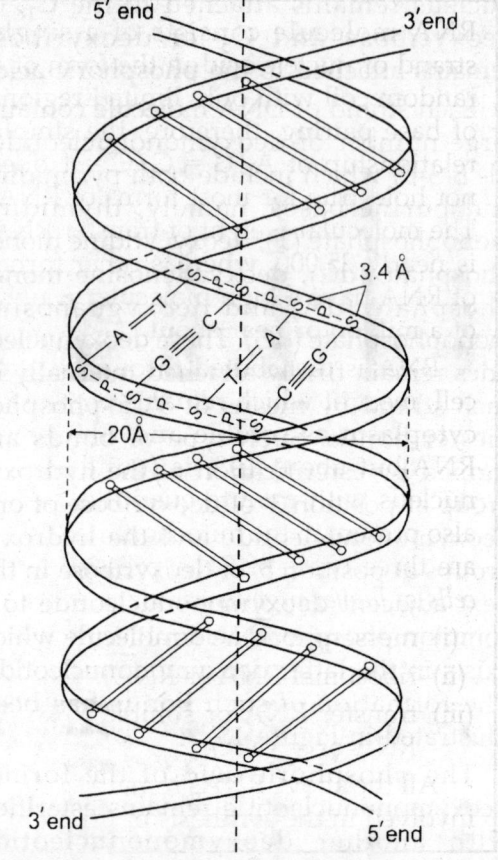

Where: (i)   P means phosphate diester
(ii) S means deoxyribose sugar
(iii) A = T is the adenine thymine pairing
(iv) G = C is the guanine cytosine pairing

Fig. 4.9 : Double helical structure of DNA

retention of memory in the brain. Viruses which infect the bacterial cells are also purely DNA-proteins. Double helical structure of DNA is as shown in Figure 4.9.

The monomeric units

When nucleic acids are subjected to complete chemical hydrolysis; they yield mixtures containing one molecule of

RNA molecule consists of a single strand of nucleic acid in the form of a random coil with only limited regions of base pairing, therefore, the simple relationship of A/U = G/C = 1 does not hold true for most forms of RNA. The molecular weight of transfer RNA is nearly 25,000, whereas other forms of RNA have a high molecular weight of a million or near about.

RNA is distributed throughout the cell, most of which remains present in cytoplasm as soluble and ribosomal RNA,but about 10% is found in the nucleus with minute quantities being also present in the mitochondria. There are three types of RNA present *in the cells of higher organisms,* viz :

(i) messenger RNA (m-RNA),

(ii) ribosomal RNA (r-RNA),

(iii) transfer RNA or soluble RNA (t-RNA or s-RNA).

All the above RNAs remain actively involved in the synthesis of protein.

phosphate, one molecule of sugar and one molecule of a mixture of heterocyclic bases. If the chemical hydrolysis is performed under milder conditions or by enzymatic means, one obtains either in equimolar mixture of Pi plus a group of nucleosides which are the N-ribo (or deoxyribo) sides of the bases, or the corresponding set of nucleotides, Which are sugar phosphate esters of the latter. Therefore, nucleotides are the true monomeric units of the nucleic acids.

RIBONUCLEIC ACIDS (RNAs)

1. The molecules of ribonucleic acids are comparatively less organized if compared to their counterpart molecules i.e., DNA.

2. They are single stranded molecules as shown in Figure 4.10

3. They have got varying molecular shapes.

4. Their molecular weight is less than DNA.

5. They have been shown to possess 60-6,000 mononucleotides in their molecules.

6. Complete hydrolysis of ribonucleic acids yields a mixture of purines, pyrimidines, sugar and phosphoric acid. The purines found in the hydrolysates are generally adenine and guanine whereas the pyrimidines are cytosine and uracil.

7. Certain purines and pyrimidines are also sometimes found in some RNAs which include:

(i) 5-methylcytosine,

(ii) 5-hydroxymethylcytosine

(iii) 1-methylguanine,

(iv) 2-methylamino-6 hydroxypurine,

(v) 6-methylaminopurine, and

(vi) 6-dimethylaminopurine.

8. *The sugar in all types of* RNAs has been identified to be a pentose sugar named as D- ribose.

9. Different mononucleotides existing ordinarily in the RNAs are:

(i) adenylic acid (A),

(ii) uridylic acid (U),

(iii) guanylic acid (G), and

(iv) cytidylic acid (C)

The sequence of these mononucleotides varies from RNA to RNA. **Different mononucleotides in a RNA strand are interlinked by the 3',5'phosphodiester bonds which are formed in a similar manner as in DNA molecules.**

Types of RNAs

At present, following four types of RNAs are known to exist:

    (a) m-RNA (messenger RNA),

    (b) t-RNA (transfer RNA) or S-RNA (soluble RNA),

    (c) r-RNA (ribosomal RNA), and

    (d) viral RNA.

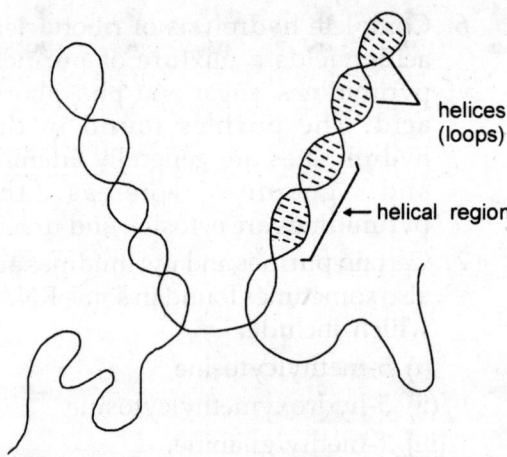

helices (loops)

← helical region

Fig 4.10 : Single stranded helical structure of a RNA molecule. The helical regions are stabilized and maintained in their shapes by A to U & G to C interactions; such interactions (bindings)are maintained by H-bonds.

(a) m-RNA

1. These nucleic acids exhibit highest molecular weight amongst all RNA.

2. Their M.W. ranges from 2-5 lacs.

3. They are highly elongated molecules.

4. They possess varying molecular shapes.

5. They are very short lived.

6. They are synthesized as a result of transcription of the DNA molecules within the nucleus and their base sequence strongly resembles to one of the corresponding DNA strand; the difference occurs only in a pyrimidine base. **In place of thymine, m-RNA contains uracil.**

7. These have been shown to contain 60-6,000 mononucleotides in their molecules.

8. **They are known as "informational molecules" which carry message from nuclear DNA to the site of protein synthesis i.e. ribosomes, informing various aminoacyl-t RNAs as to when they should add their particular amino acid residue to the growing polypeptide chain. In this way, mRNAs give signal for the synthesis of various very important substances like the enzymes, the proteins, a variety of polypeptide hormones, etc.**

9. Thus, the m-RNAs contain various

Messenger RNA

The first step in the synthesis of protein is the transfer of genetic message of the DNA to messenger RNA, the process is known as 'transcription.

The messenger RNA migrates into the cytoplasm and it is here, in association with ribosome and transfer RNA, **that the 4 letter code is converted to the 20 letter code of proteins. This stage is known as 'translation'.** Part of the DNA strand is only transcribed, so that m-RNA is smaller than the nuclear DNA. The actual molecular weight of a particular m-RNA is determined by the number of amino acid residues in the protein being synthesized, but is often of the order of a million or so. The mRNA, unlike the other forms, is metabolically unstable.

information in the form of codes which consist of nucleotide triplets (e.g., GAA, UAG, GUU, GUC, GUA, GUG etc).

(b) t- RNA or s- RNA

This is also known as soluble RNA (s-RNA); it constitutes nearly 10-20 per cent of total RNAs of the cell. Its M.W. ranges from 20,000 to 40,000 and it bears 70 to 80 mononucleotides in its molecule.

They are found in the soluble fraction of tissue homogenates after centrifugation at high speed i.e. 100,000 x g. There is evidence of the existence of atleast 21 transfer RNAs, each being specific for each naturally existing amino acid. It has been further studied that many amino-acids have more than one different t-RNA. Their main function is just to get attached with the activated amino acid and to carry it

'to the site. of protein synthesis i.e. ribosomes so that it be added to the growing polypeptide chain.

Besides the presence of regular bases i.e. adenine, guanine, uracil and cytosine, t-RNAs have been found to contain some very unusual bases like ribothymidine, dihydrouracil, inosine, dihydrouridine, pseudouridine etc., which possess an unusual linkage between the sugar ribose and the base.

The molecule of alanine-t-RNA has been fully studied which is a single stranded molecule. Its structure resembles to that of *clover-leaf* (clover is a kind of grass) and is as shown below - this has been confirmed

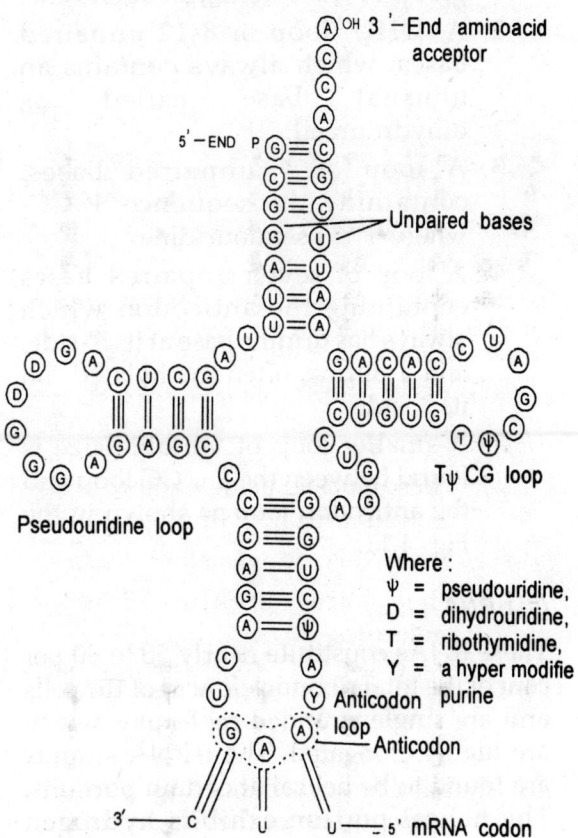

Fig. 4.11 : A possible structure of alanine-t-RNA

Transfer RNA

Each amino acid has a specific t-RNA which transfers the activated amino acid to the site of protein synthesis. Unlike the other forms of RNA, transfer ribonucleic acids have low molecular weights and are made up of relatively few nucleotides. The complete sequence of nucleotides has been determined for some t-RNA's and speculations made about the *'recognition sites'* on the molecule. There are two of these sites on each t-RNA molecule, one that identifies a particular amino acid and the other which recognizes and binds to the triplet base on the codon. This triplet of bases on the t-RNA is known as an *anti-codon*. All t-RNA's have the same terminal group of bases *CCA* and it is the adenine that reacts with the activated amino acid.

by x-ray diffraction techniques.

All transfer RNAs have been found to possess a terminal adenosine which bears a free hydroxyl group at 2' or 3' position of ribose and cytidylic acid at second and third positions (Fig. 4.11).

Studies have also revealed that t-RNA molecules have a complex structure with extensive internal base-pairing (Figure 4.11) The following points are common to all known t-RNA structures:

1. Guanosine at the 5-terminal, and the sequence of *CCA* at the 3'-terminal. The amino acid becomes attached through its carboxyl group, by an ester link to a ribose hydroxyl group of the 3'-terminal adenosine.

2. A 'DHU' loop of 8-12 unpaired bases, which always contains an unusual base called as dihydrouracil.

3. A loop of 7 unpaired bases, containing the sequence Ψ CG, where Ψ is pseudouridine.

4. A loop of seven unpaired bases containing the anticodon which always has uridine base at its 5'-side, and a purine, often methylated on its 3'-side.

5. A smaller loop of variable size is found between the T ψ CG loop and the anticodon loop as shown in the Fig. 4.11.

(c) r-RNA

These RNAs constitute nearly 50 to 60 per cent of the total ribonucleic acid of the cells and are single stranded molecules which are highly elongated. The r-RNA strands are found to be helical at certain portions. The helical portion exhibits hydrogen bonding as per base-pairing rule.

Most of the r -RNA is found to be combined with proteins in macro molecular aggregates called as ribosomes which are found in the cytoplasm and on the cytoplasmic surface of granular endoplasmic reticulum. They are also often called *cytoribosomes*. On the granular endoplasmic reticulum, 5-8 ribosomes are linked by a m-RNA strand to form a linear cluster called *polyribosome* or *polysome* (Fig. 4.12).

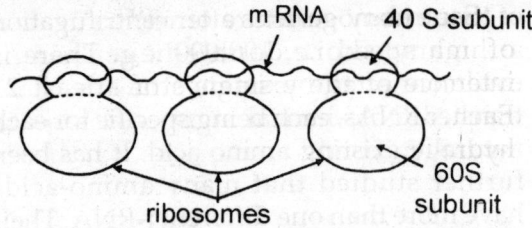

Fig. 4.12 : Polyribosome

Ribosomes may be characterized by their sedimentation constant. Ribosomes possess a sedimentation constant of 80 S and mass of 4.4×10^6 daltons. The 80 S ribosome is made up of 2 snbunits namely

---

Ribosomal RNA

Ribosomes are microscopic particles in the cell which are visible only under the electron mi croscope with a fairly uniform composition of about 60% protein and 40% RNA. These are made up of two parts which can be separated *in vitro*. In animal cells, the 80 S ribosomes consist of 60 S and 40 S sub-units of different chemical composition. Several ribosomes may be attached to a particular strand of m-RNA to form a 'polysome', rather like beads on a string.

a large subunit of 60 S and a small sub unit of 40 S.

Primary structure of r-RNA referred to the number and sequence of nucleotide (i.e., their bases). For instance, mammalian 5 S, 5.8 S, 18 S and 28 S r-RNAs consist of about 120, 160, 1900 and 4,700 bases respectively which include mainly adenine, guanine, cytosine and uracil and a few pseudouridines. Besides the major bases, some minor nitrogenous bases may also be found.

Secondary structure of r-RNA consists of many short double-helical stems interconnected by single stranded loops. Each double-helical stem is formed by hydrogen bonds.

(d) Viral-RNA

Viruses which infect the animal and plant cells are mostly ribonucleoproteins. The percentage of RNA in such viruses ranges from 1 to 44. So far, the most studied viral-RNA is that of tobacco mosaic virus (TMV). **TMV is rod like in shape,** approximately 3,000 Å in length and 170 Å in diameter.

Viral-RNAs are single stranded helical molecules which generally possess molecular weight of nearly 2.2×10^6. However, the M.W. of different types of viral-RNAs may range from 1.2×10^6 to 32×10^6. They have been found to have 6,400 mononucleotides in their molecules. Each helix has a radius of 40 Å and has

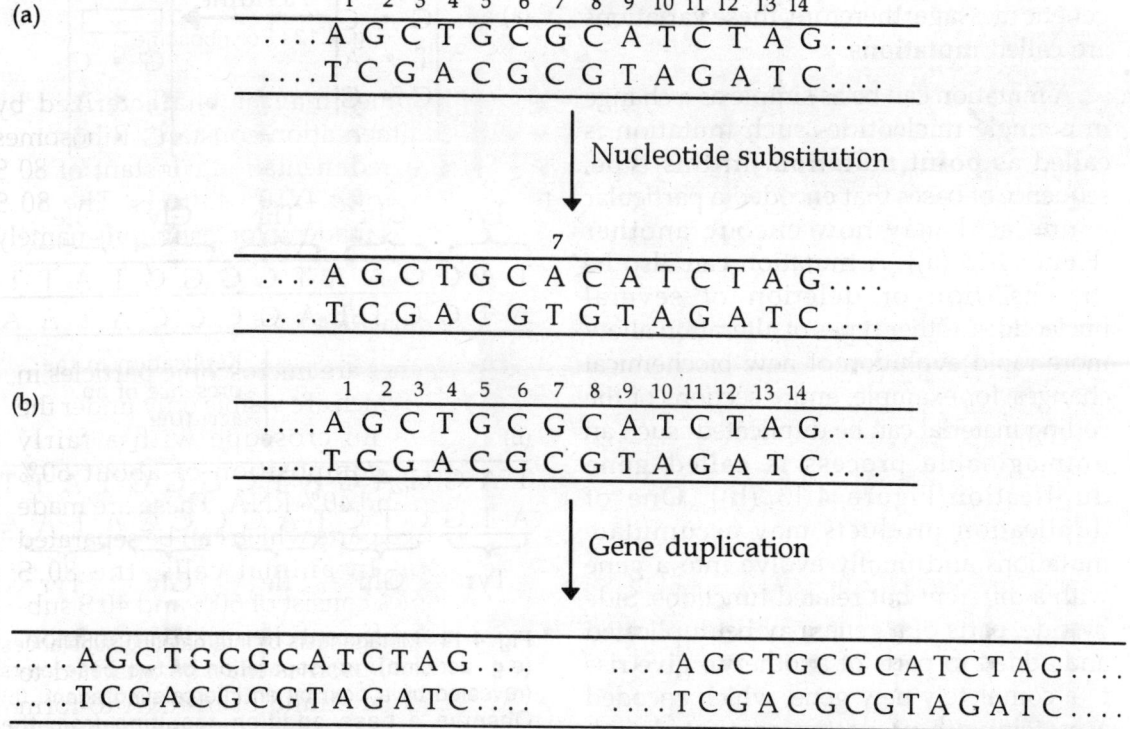

Fig 4.13 (a) & (b) : Biochemical evolution; in Figure 'a' observe a single base (nucleotide) change at position number 7 (example of a point mutation; whereas in Figure 'b' observe a clear cut duplication of a 'gene'; here two genes have evolved from one gene (example of wonderful gene evolution).

been found to contain some 49 nucleotides per turn. Adenylic acid remains present at the terminal nucleotide at each end. The fact that the RNA molecule remains covered by the protein molecule has been established. Careful separation of the protein part of viral nucleoproteins by the sophisticated latest techniques has revealed that it is the nucleic acid portion which is infective and not the protein portion.

DNA Mutation, Point Mutation, Gene Duplication

Mutation is referred to as any change in the base sequence of DNA. The most common change is a substitution, addition, rearrangement or deletion of one or more bases. Such variations in living systems are changes that alter the meaning of the genetic message; therefore, these variations are called **mutations.**

A mutation can be as simple as a change in a single nucleotide- such mutation is called as **point mutation.** In this type, sequence of bases that encoded a particular amino acid may now encode another {Figure 4.13 (a)}. A mutation can also be the insertion or deletion of several nucleotides. Other types of alteration allow more rapid evolution of new biochemical changes; for example, entire sections of the coding material can be duplicated- such an unimaginable process is called **gene duplication**{Figure 4.13 (b)}. One of duplication products may accumulate mutations and finally evolve into a gene with a different but related functions. Side by side, parts of a gene may be duplicated and added to parts of another to give rise to a completely new gene, which encoded a protein with properties associated with each parent gene. In this way gene duplication followed by specialisation has

been a complicated process in evolution which permits the generation of macromolecules having particular functions without the need to start from scratch. In this way accumulation of genes with large and complicated differences allows '**evolution**' i.e., from lower to higher organisms.

Mutagen, Mutagenesis

A **mutagen** is referred to as a physical agent or chemical reagent that causes mutations; for instance, nitrous acid reacts with some DNA bases, changing their chemistry and hydrogen bonding properties therefore, nitrous acid is called as a mutagen.

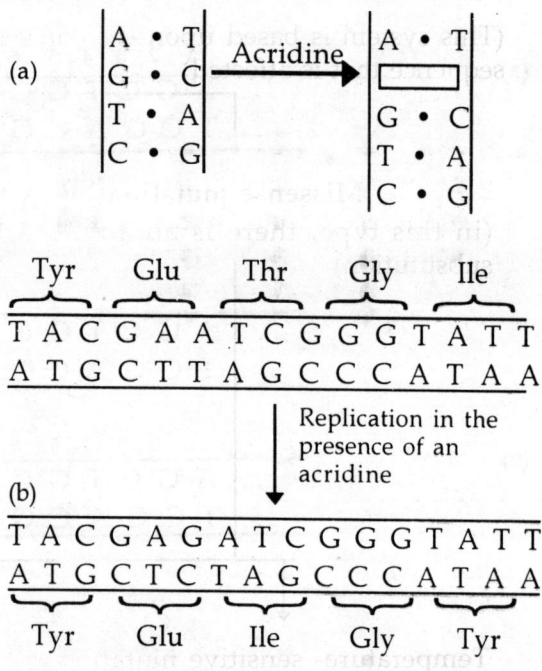

Fig. 4.14 : Mutagenesis by intercalating substances (e.g. acridine). (a) separation of two base pairs (revealed by a box) by an intercalating agent. (b) Observe a base addition resulting from the replication in the presence of an acridine. The change in the amino acid sequence read from the upper strand in groups of three bases is also shown.

Mutagenesis is referred to as the process of producing a mutation. If somehow it occurs in nature without the action of a known mutagen then it is known as **spontaneous mutagenesis** and the resulting mutations as spontaneous mutations. Contrarily, if a known mutagen is used then it is called as **induced mutagenesis.**

Types of Mutation

There are several types of mutation; for better understanding, its various types are as given in the flow diagram:

Types of mutation (Ist System)

Point mutation (in which a single base pair gets changed; it may be a base substitution, a base insertion or a base deletion, but the term most frequently used is base substitution.)

Multiple mutation {in which several (two or more) base pairs get changed}

Types of mutation (IInd System)

(This system is based upon the consequence of the change in term of the amino acid sequence that is affected)

Missense mutation

(in this type, there is an amino acid substitution)

Frame-shift mutation (this is an interesting class of mutagens which are intercalating agents, e.g., acridines. These planar molecules insert between base pairs. When replication occurs in the region of an intercalated molecule, one or both daughter strands are synthesized that either lack one or more nucleotides or have additional ones. These changes alter the reading frame of the base sequence of a gene and hence are called frame shift mutation (Figure 4.14).

Temperature- sensitive mutation i.e. Ts {in this type, the substitution produces a protein that is active at one temperature (typically 30°C) and inactive at a higher temperature (usually 40-42°C)}.

Chain termination mutation or nonsense mutation (in this type no amino acid corresponds to a new base sequence; in that case, termination of the synthesis of the protein occurs at that point. These mutations generate one of the three nonsense codons; e., UAA, UAG or UGA).

URIC ACID OF URINE, BLOOD AND TISSUES

Uric acid is the final oxidation product of the purine ring in the human beings, and is the chief nitrogenous end product in birds, lizards, snakes etc. The formula of uric acid is as follows and the type of isomerism possible is as shown below:

```
HN—CO                N=C.OH
 |   |                 |   |
OC  C—NH              C   C—NH
 |   ||    >CO ⇌ HO|| ||      >C.OH
HN—C—NH              N—C—N
Keto-form            Enol-form
```
Uric acid

Uric acid is dibasic. Monosodium and disodium salts of uric acid are known.

The quantity of urinary uric acid is related to the amount of ingested nucleoproteins and to the extent of catabolism of tissue nucleic acids and nucleotides. **Most of the uric acid (85-90%) filtered by the glomeruli is reabsorbed.**

A very important point to be remembered is that in leukemia where the destruction of leukocytes takes place rapidly, output of uric acid gets tremendously increased. This is also true in the diseases of the liver and organs rich in nucleoproteins. There is always found disturbed metabolism of uric acid in the disease 'gout', the biochemistry of which is not yet very clear. It is seen that prior to an attack of gout, the urinary output of uric acid gets somewhat decreased and after the attack, it gets increased and remains increased for several days. Uric acid forms salts with sodium, calcium, magnesium, ammonium and potassium to give corresponding urates. Uric acid

crystals may be easily distinguished in a sediment of urine sample under microscope (Figs. 4.16 and 4.17).

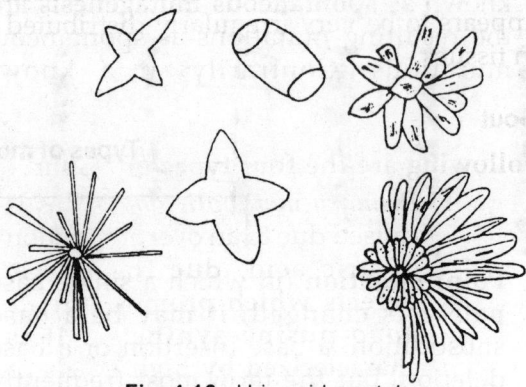

Fig. 4.16 : Uric acid crystals

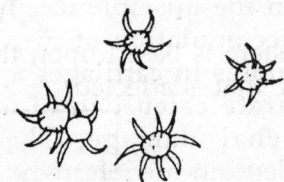

Fig. 4.17 : Ammonium urate crystals

Uric acid crystals when aggregate to form clusters, give rise to troublesome stones either in the kidneys or the bladder. The largest contribution in the formation of stones in the kidneys is that of calcium oxalate crystals; then phosphate crystals and then the least contribution is of uric acid crystals. The acid sodium urate may form clusters of needles or stellar-shaped clusters. Ammonium urate crystals are often spherical and generally covered with spikes. They are also referred to as "thorn apple" crystals (Fig. 4.14). These are usually pigmented. In addition, they may exhibit many *'bizarre'* shapes. **The range of uric acid in normal human plasma is from 2 to 6 mg per cent, averaging 4 mg%. Values for females is a little on lower**

side averaging to about 3.5 mg% than their counterparts i.e. males who have an average value of about 4.5 mg%. Red blood cells appear to contain about half as much uric acid as in plasma. Uric acid appears to be very irregularly distributed in tissues.

Gout

Following are the four types of "Gout'

1. *Primary metabolic gout:* This is caused due to an overproduction of uric acid, **due to genetic defects which promote the *de novo* purine synthesis. It is characterized by high levels of blood and urinary urates, rise in the miscible uric acid pool, accumulation of uric acid and urates in cartilages and joints, urate calculi in kidneys and renal damage.** These urate deposits are referred to as *tophi.* Such deposits in the joints provoke a painful inflammatory condition; for some reason it has been observed that the joints at the base of the big toe get especially susceptible; such a condition is known as **acute gouty arthritis.** The chronic inflammatory changes induced by the depositions of sodium urate tophi can generate **chronic gouty arthritis,** eventually resulting in the destruction of joints. The exact mechanism for the deposition of such urates is not yet clear.

2. *Secondary metabolic gout:* It **results from a secondary increase in the catabolism of purines in various states like prolonged fasting, leukaemia** and polycythaemia etc. In this type, more breakdown of tissues takes place as a result of which system gets loaded with unusually high amount of nucleotides.

3. *Primary renal gout:* **This is caused due to the failure of urate excretion by the renal tubules which is due to the genetic deficiency of the urate transport system in renal tubules.** This type of gout does not involve any over production of uric acid.

4. *Secondary renal gout:* **This results from a failure of urate elimination in the glomerular filtrate** which is due to a generalized renal failure in the kidney disorder called **glomerulonephritis.**

Effect of Diet

Excretion of uric acid continues at a rather constant rate during starvation and purine-free diet due to the so-called endogenous (tissue) purine metabolism. **The ingestion of foods high in nucleoproteins, such as glandular organs, produce a marked increase; whereas a diet of milk, eggs, and cheese (very low in purine content), causes practically no elevation in uric acid excretion.**

Treatment of Gout

The classic treatment for gout is the administration of *colchicine,* **a drug which has got the tendency to interrupt the mitosis of leucocytes** and thus prevents development of inflammation. It is believed that the inflammation is a consequence of phagocytosis of urate crystals by the leucocytes that invade the affected area.

Cancers are made up of cells that continue to divide indefinitely. Since cell division requires a net synthesis of nucleic acids, there has been considerable effect **made** to find compounds that will selectively inhibit the formation of nucleic acids and check the uncontrolled growth of cancer.

Synthetic analogs of nucleobases, nucleosides and nucleotides are widely used in medical sciences and clinical medicine. One of the most important components of the oncologist's pharmacopeia is the group of synthetic analogs of puripe and pyrimidine nucleobases and nucleosides.

The purine analog 4-hydroxypyrazolopyrimidine *(allopurinol)* is widely marketed as an inhibitor of *de novo* purine biosynthesis and of xanthine oxidase. **It is used for the treatment of hyperuricemia and gout. Nucleosides containing arabinose rather than ribose as the sugar moieties, notably cytarabine and vidarabine are used in the chemotherapy of canccr and viral infections.**

Caffeine (1,3,7 - trimethylxanthine) is found in coffee, tea and other plants; theobromine (3,7-dimethylxanthine) occurs in tea, cocoa and chocolate. Other purines are also found in plants and some of these like caffeine and theobromine have important pharmacological actions.

Nuclease may catalyze the hydrolysis specifically of DNA and RNA or they may attack both kinds of polynucleotide. These enzymes are generally of two types :

(i) *Exonucleases:* Which require a terminus at which to initiate hydrolysis, and

(ii) *Endonucleases:* Which do not require a terminus and which may attack at one or many sites within a polynucleotide.

Various compounds which promote the excretion of urate by the kidneys have been introduced as a means of controlling gout.

More recently, **a competitive inhibitor of xanthine oxidase has been developed to control gout by preventing the formation of urate** so that excess purines are excreted as hypoxanthine and xanthine; **this compound is known as** *allopurinol* and differs from hypoxanthine in the distribution of ring nitrogens. The rationale for its use is that hypoxanthine and xanthine will not precipitate in the joints. Hypoxanthine is more soluble than urate, although xanthine is not. Allopurinol also is not a completely safe drug.

Allopurinol

LESCH-NYHAN SYNDROME

Rare patients afflicted with a condition named as *Lesch-Nyhan Syndrome* may be met with once in a while; **this disease is caused by a hereditary deficiency of GMP pyrophosphorylase. This x-linked** recessive disease is peculiarly horrifying because children suffering from it mutilate (damage their own organs/body parts) themselves. Characteristically, they will bite off the tips of their own fingers or bite their lips if their hands are protected i.e. tied upon with some string/rope etc. The aggressive attacks may be of serious nature like biting of others or as age advances, may use obscene abusive language. The pathos of the affliction is accentuated by the tendency of the children to be very likeable and open, quick to laugh and capable of warm affection. The climax is that such children get sometime terrified of their own aggression; they may even scream under the cover of fear and may bite their fingers seriously. Patients suffering from this disease have a tendency to excrete large quantities of uric acid - more per unit of body mass than is seen in any other condition. Their synthesis of purines is extraordinarily rapid (of course, they also become gouty as an additional distress).

The missing enzyme i.e. GMP pyrophosphorylase is responsible for the salvage (protection from loss) of free guanine and hypoxanthine by converting them to the corresponding nucleoside monophosphates. This enzyme is found to be more active in brain, which has over 10-fold more enzyme than does the liver.

Genetic Tracing of Fatherhood

DNA finger printing technology now available in our country in various upgraded well equipped laboratories is a very good mean in establishing *paternity.*

This technology is responsible in establishing fatherhood while dealing with cases where a husband has abandoned his wife. Previously there did not exist any specific law to take action against culprits who abandoned their wives and children taking advantage of absence of any legally admissible evidence of their marriage to these women. **This technology is a 'full proof' method in establishing paternity scientifically.**

CHAPTER 5

ACIDS/BASES/BUFFERS/ HYDROGEN ION CONCENTRATION

In appearance, we appear to be small molecules and we are also not given due weightage but we are the only substances which are 'shock absorbers' that is to say we have the capability to withstand the changes in pH of body fluids. If somehow, we are incapable to withstand the changes in pH, then we create noisy scene in the body making it very uncomfortable. Therefore, our importance should never be undermined.

Protolysis of Water

Water dissociates to a small but definite extent to give H^+ and OH^- ions (dissociation or protolysis of water). The released protons (H^+) immediately join H_2O molecules to form hydronium ions (H_3O^+); even bigger ions like $H_9O_4^+$ may arise from several associated H_2O molecules. Protolysis gets increased with temperature.

pH: It is the negative logarithm of the H^+ concentration to the base 10 when the H^+ concentration is expressed in mol litre^{-1}. It is expressed as :

$$pH = -\log [H^+] = \log \frac{1}{[H^+]}$$

Thus, for pure water or neutral aqueous solution at room temperature,

$$pH = -\log [H^+] = -\log [10^{-7}] = 7$$

Sorensen's pH scale is a logarithmic scale ranging from 0 to 14 for dilute aqueous

solutions like biological fluids. pH 7 is considsered as the neutral pH. **The greater the alkalinity, the higher is the pH.** The rise or fall of pH by 1 signifies a ten fold fall or rise, respectively, in the H^+ concentration.

pH of some important biological fluids is as shown below:

Biological fluid	pH
Aqueous humour	7.3 - 7.4
Bile	6.9 - 8.6
Cerebrospinal fluid	7.3 - 7.4
Gastric juice	0.9 - 3.0
Intestinal juice	6.4 - 9.1
Intracellular fluids	6.0 - 7.1
Pancreatic juice	7.1 - 8.4
Plasma, tissue fluid	7.35 - 7.45
Saliva	5.9 - 7.2
Sweat	3.8 - 7.5
Tear	5.6 - 8.2
Urine	4.8 - 8.0

Acids, Bases and Salts

According to the proton transfer theory of Bronsted and Lowry, acids are substances which donate protons (H^+) to increase the H^+ concentration of their solutions while bases accept protons to lower the H^+ concentration.

The anion liberated by the ionization of an acid behaves as a base and is called the *conjugate base* of the acid, because it can accept a proton (H^+) by the reverse reaction to yield the original acid. In a dilute aqueous solution, an acid HA ionizes to give its conjugate base A.

$$HA + H_2O \rightleftharpoons H_3O^+ + A$$

$$\therefore Keq = \frac{[H_3O^+][A]}{[H_2O][HA]} = \frac{[H^+][A^-]}{[H_2O][HA]}$$

because H_3O^+ and H^+ have practically identical concentrations. (The bracketed terms represent molar concentrations). The mass of unaffected water is so vast so as to remain practically constant inspite of the reaction,

$$\frac{[H^+][A^-]}{[HA]} = Keq\,[H_2O] = K_a$$

Where K_a is the temperature-dependent acid dissociation constant. Its values are more conveniently expressed in terms of pK_a, called the ionization exponent of an acid.

$$pK_a = -\log K_a = \log (1/K_a)$$

The stronger the acid, the greater is its ionization and so the higher is its K_a and the lower its pK_a. A strong acid like HCl possesses a high K of the order of 10^{-3} or higher. A weak acid like carbonic acid dissociates little in solution and has a low K_a of the order of 10^{-4} or lower; at equilibrium for any weak acid HA,

$$\frac{[H^+][A^-]}{[HA]} = K_a \text{ or } [H^+] = Ka\frac{[HA]}{[A^-]}$$

$$\therefore -\log [H^+] = -\log K_a - \log \frac{[HA]}{[A]}$$

$$\text{or } pH = pK_a + \log \frac{[A^-]}{[HA]}$$

This is known as the *Henderson-Hasselbalch* equation which follows that where $[A^-] = [HA]$, pH equals pK_a

A salt ionizes in aqueous solutions so as to give an anion corresponding to the conjugate base of the parent acid and also a cation corresponding to the conjugate acid of the parent base. Aqueous solution of a salt is neutral, acidic or alkaline depending upon the acid strength of its cation and the basic strength of its anion. For instance, NH_4Cl solution is acidic because NH_4Cl ionizes into NH_4^+ (the strong conjugate acid of the weak parent base NH_3) and Cl^- (the weak conjugate base of the strong parent acid HCl); similarly other salts of strong acids and weak bases are also acidic in solution due to the same reason. Again, the aqueous solution of a salt of a weak acid and a strong alkali, e.g., Na^-propionate is alkaline in reaction because such a salt ionizes into a strong conjugate base anion (e.g. propionate ion) of the parent acid and a 'neutral' cation (e.g. Na^+). The aqueous solution of a salt of a strong acid and a strong alkali, e.g., NaCl or KCl is neutral because such a salt ionizes into a very weak conjugate base anion (e.g. Cl^-) of the strong parent acid and a 'neutral' cation (e.g. Na^+ or K^+).

Buffers

A buffer solution resists the change of pH when acids or alkalies are added to it. Generally, it contains a mixture of either a weak acid [HA] and its conjugate base (A^-) or a weak base (B) and its conjugate acid (BH^+). Because a salt (BA) ionizes to give the conjugate base (A^-) of its parent acid, the *buffer may also be constituted of a weak acid and its salt*, i.e., a mixture of HA and A^-. Besides, a mixture of two acid salts of a weak polybasic acid also serves as a buffer.

Examples of buffer solutions Include the following i.e., :

(a) Bicarbonate buffer (H_2CO_3 : $NaHCO_3$)
(b) Phosphate buffer (KH_2PO_4: Na_2HPO_4)
(c) Acetate buffer (acetic acid: Na acetate)
(d) Ammonium chloride buffer (NH_4Cl: ammonia)
(e) Glycine - HCl buffer (glycine: glycine hydrochloride)

Isoelectric pH: **It is that pH at which the protein carries a net charge of zero.** According to the isoelectric point, proteins are described as basic, neutral or acidic depending on whether their overall charge at physiological pH is positive approximately zero or negative. Isoelectric pH of some common proteins are as follows:

Proteins of blood	Isoelectric pH
γ_1 - globulin	2.0
Haptoglobin	4.1
Serum albumin	4.7
Fibrinogen	5.8

Buffers in pH regulation

Buffers have a role to minimize the pH changes in the cells and the extracellular fluids so as to maintain a constant pH in the living body.

Principal buffers of the *extracellular fluids* include the:

(i) Bicarbonate buffer,
(ii) Phosphate buffer, and
(iii) Protein buffer

and those of the *intracellular fluids* include :

(i) Phosphate buffer,
(ii) Protein buffer **and in erythrocytes, hemoglobin buffer.**

Bicarbonate buffer

It is the principal buffer in extracullar fluids such as the blood plasma. It comprises bicarbonte (HCO_3^-) and carbonic acid (H_2CO_3) as the base and acid members respectively, the bicarbonate buffer neutralizes stronger dietary and metabolic acids (HA), changing them to the corresponding weak conjugate bases (A^-); as a result of which there is a simultaneous increase in H_2CO_3 Stronger bases (B) get also changed to the corresponding weak conjugate acids (BW) with a concomitant rise in HCO_3^-.

$$HA + HCO_3^- \rightleftharpoons A^- + H_2CO_3$$
$$B + H_2CO_3 \rightleftharpoons BH^+ + HCO_3^-$$

Whenever the bicarbonate buffer neutralizes any acid or base, the replacement of one of the members of the buffer pair by the other member changes the buffer ratio and consequently the blood pH but the buffer ratio is immediately restored by altering either the respiratory elimination of H_2CO_3 as CO_2 or the urinary elimination of HCO_3^-.

The plasma HCO_3^- content is called the alkali reserve because of its outstanding role in buffering acids entering the blood.

The bicarbonate buffer has far less importance inside the cell because cells contain much lower amounts of HCO_3^-. The [HCO_3^-]/[H_2CO_3] ratio is as low as 11-13 in the cells having a HCO_3^- concentration like 15-18 mM.

Phosphate buffer : It is next to the

bicarbonate buffer in importance in the extracellular fluids other than blood. It is also of primary importance in most cells other than RBCs. In the blood plasma, its concentration is only about 8% of that of the bicarbonate buffer, therefore, its buffering capacity is far lower than the bicarbonate in the plasma.

The phosphate buffer contains dibasic phosphate and monobasic phosphate as the base and acid members respectively. It has a pK of about 6.8 for the dissociation $H_2PO_4^- \rightleftharpoons H^+ + HPO_4^{--}$ which means it is more effective in the pH range of 5.8-7.8, therefore, at the pH of blood i.e. 7.4., it operates relatively close to its pK and consequently has got a high buffering capacity. Plasma normally has a $[HCO_3^-]/[H_2CO_3]$ ratio of 4. The Henderson- Hasselbalch equation indicates that this buffer ratio corresponds to the pH of blood i.e. 7.4.

or pH = pK_a + log $\dfrac{[HPO_4^{--}]}{[H_2PO_4]}$

or pH = 6.8 + log 4 = 7.4

The phosphate buffer has a far higher concentration in intracellular fluids than in extracellular fluids. Moreover, the pH of intracellular fluids (6.0 - 6.9) is closer to the pK of the phosphate buffer which means that the phosphate buffer has much higher buffering capacity inside the cells. Similar reasons make the phosphate buffer considerably effective in the urine inside the renal distal tubules and collecting ducts.

When HPO_4^{--} buffers any acid (including some H_2CO_3). $H_2PO_4^-$ gets protected and the $[HPO_4^{--}]/[H_2PO_4^-]$ratio tends to change. The ratio can be restored by the renal eliminiation of $H_2PO_4^-$, but not by respiratory adjustment.

Protein buffers

These are of considerable importance in the plasma and the intracellular fluids, but are too low in concentration in lymph; interstitial fluids and cerebrospinal fluids. Many of the proteins in the plasma are acidic proteins with acidic isoelectric pHs. Therefore, at the pH of blood i.e. 7.4 these exist as anions to serve as conjugate bases (Pr^-) and may accept H^+ ions to form the corresponding conjugate acids (HPr). Protein buffers may even buffer some H_2CO_3 in the blood.

$$H_2CO_3 + Pr^- \rightleftharpoons HCO_3^- + HPr$$

Hemoglobin buffer

Particularly due to reversible changes in the buffering capacity of hemoglobin on oxygenation and deoxygenation, it plays the major role in buffering CO_2 inside erythrocytes. Deoxyhemoglobin is a weaker acid (pK_a 8.18) and consequently pessesses a much higher capacity than oxyhemoglobin (pK_a 6.62) for accepting H^+ and buffering CO_2. On entering the RBCs in tissue capillaries, CO_2 combines with H_2O to form H_2CO_3 under the action of carbonic anhydrase (Fig 5.1). H_2CO_3 remains 95% dissociated into H^+ and HCO_3^- at the blood pH of 7.4 and consequently needs immediate buffering. Side by side, oxyhemoglobin (HbO_2^- or $HHbO_2$) has lost O_2 to form deoxyhemoglobin (Hb^- or HHb) but while $HHbO_2$ remains about 85% ionized as HbO_2^- at pH 7.4, 85% of Hb^- remains as undissociated HHb by accepting H^+ from the ionization of H_2CO_3. Thus, Hb^- buffers H_2CO_3 in RBCs.

$$HbO_2^- \rightleftharpoons Hb^- + O_2$$
$$Hb^- + H_2CO_3 \rightleftharpoons HHb + HCO_3^-$$

Acidosis and alkalosis

Acidosis: it is a fall in the $[HCO_3^-]/[H_2CO_3]$ ratio of blood below 20, threatening to lower the pH of blood. Hypoventilation (e.g. in asthma, respriratory paralysis or lobar pneumonia) causes retention of CO_2 and raises the PCO_2 and H_2CO_3 of blood with little change in HCO_3. This tends to lower the $[HCO_3^-]/[H_2CO_3]$ ratio and consequently the ratios of all other buffer pairs as well as the blood pH (respiratory acidosis). **Excessive loss of bases such as in diabetic ketosis, severe diarrhoea and nephritic acidosis lowers the plasma HCO_3^-** concentration with little change in H_2CO_3 concentration, thus lowering their ratio **(metabolic acidosis).**

Alkalosis: It is a rise in the $[HCO_3^-]/[H_2CO_3]$ ratio of blood above 20, tending to raise the pH of blood. **Pulmonary hyperventilation as happens in fever, mountain sickness, hysterical overbreathing, voluntary hyperpnea (abnormal increase in depth and rate of respiration)** etc. removes excess CO_2 from the blood and lowers the H_2CO_3 content of blood with little change in HCO_3^-. This tends to raise the $[HCO_3^-]/[H_2CO_3]$ ratio and consequently the ratios of all other buffer pairs as well as the blood pH **(respiratory alkalosis).** Violent vomiting, pyloric stenosis or high intake of bases or alkaline substances like $NaHCO_3$ may raise the plasma HCO_3^- with little change in H_2CO_3, thereby raising their ratio **(metabolic alkalosis).**

In both the acidosis and alkalosis, the body tries to restore the normal $[HCO_3^-]/[H_2CO_3]$ ratio by changing the pulmonary elimination of CO_2 and / or the urinary elimination of HCO_3^-. **If it succeeds to restore the normal buffer ratio, the acidosis or alkalosis is said to be compensated. If the buffer ratio fails to return to normal, the acidosis or alkalosis is said to be uncompensated.**

Role of lungs in the regulation of pH

Lungs serve to normalize the $[HCO_3^-]/[H_2CO_3]$ ratio and the pH of blood by changing the rate of respiratory elimination of CO_2 from the blood. A rise in alveolar ventilation lowers the alveolar Pco_2 and consequently increases the diffusion of CO_2 to the alveolar air from the dissolved state in blood. As the concentration of HCO_3^- is in equilibrium with that of dissolved CO_2 in the blood, hyperventilation increases the $[HCO_3^-]/[H_2CO_3]$ ratio simultaneously with a fall in the CO_2 concentration, Thus, a doubling of ventilation may raise the pH of blood by 0.4. Hypoventilation, on the contrary, increases the concentration of dissolved CO_2 in blood as a result of which ratio of buffer gets lowered. Thus, a fall in alveolar ventilation to 1/4th the normal value may lower the blood pH by 0.46. the pulmonary ventilation is adjusted according to the pH of the blood. For instance, a fall in blood pH to 7.1 raises the alveolar ventilation to almost 2.5 times the normal value while arise in blood pH to 7.6 reduces the ventilation to almost half the normal value. Thus, acidosis and alkalosis may produce hyperventilation and hypoventilation of the lungs respectively and these in turn respectively raise and lower the $[HCO_3^-]/[H_2CO_3]$ ratio to normal by respectively washing off and retaining more CO_2. Pulmonary hypoventilation however, has got limited significance in compensating for metabolic alkalosis because hypoventilation not only retains CO_2 to lower the $[HCO_3^-]/[H_2CO_3]$ ratio but also simultaneously curtails the O_2 supply-an undesirable effect. The role of lungs in the functioning of hemoglobin buffers through the oxygenation of hemoglobin is much.

Role of Kidneys in the regulation of pH

Kidneys normally eliminate around 50 mEq of non volatile acids in 24 hours and conserve bases by minimizing their urinary elimination. The pH of the glomerular filtrate is almost 7.4 as it enters the proximal tubule but the pH of the filtrate falls to about 6.9 in the proximal tubule, then to about 6 – 6.5 in the distal tubule and ultimately to about 4.5-4.7 in the collecting ducts. The urinary pH is maintained by a cooperation between the urinary buffer and the renal ion-exchange mechanism. Major urinary buffers consist of bicarbonate and phosphate buffers which come into the urine by filtration from glomeruli. As the filtrate proceeds along the tubules, the ratio between the base member and the acid member of each urinary buffer falls progressively with a consequent fall in the urinary pH.

In the renal ion-exchange mechanism, some urinary Na^+ ions are actively, reabsorbed by the tubule cells and in exchange, an equivalent amount of H^+ ions is secreted into the tubular filtrate of the total amount *of* H^+ secreted by the tubules, nearly 85% is secreted by the proximal tubules and the remaining 15% by the distal tubules and the collecting ducts. The H^+ ions arise mainly from the ionization of H_2CO_3 formed from CO_2 and H_2O by the action of enzyme carbonic anhydrase in the tubule cells.

$$H_2O + CO_2 \rightleftharpoons H_2CO_3 \rightleftharpoons H^+ + HCO_3^-$$

While the H^+ ion is secreted in the urine, the HCO_3^- formed simultaneously is returned to blood alongwith the reabsorbed Na^+ ions.

Although most of the urinary H^+ ions are secreted in the proximal tubules, the H^+ concentration in the proximal tubular lumen does not exceed 3.2 times that in the extracellular fluid.

The serection of H^+ continues in exchange of reabsorbed Na^+ even in the collecting ducts till the urinary pH declines to about 4.5. At this stage, the H^+ concentration in the tubular filtrate attains a maximum level of about 3.16×10^{-5} mol litre^{-1}. H^+ ions cannot be secreted any more against such a high concentration

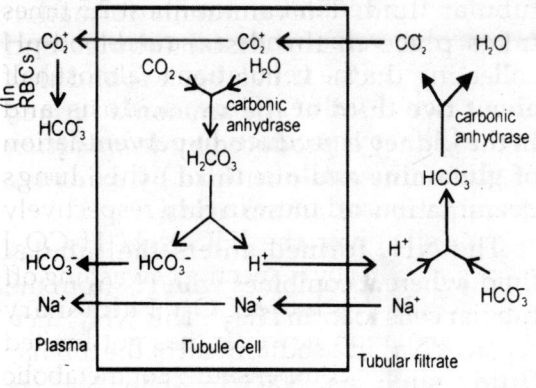

Fig. 5.1 : Buffering of H^+ ions by HCO_3^- ions in the renal tubules

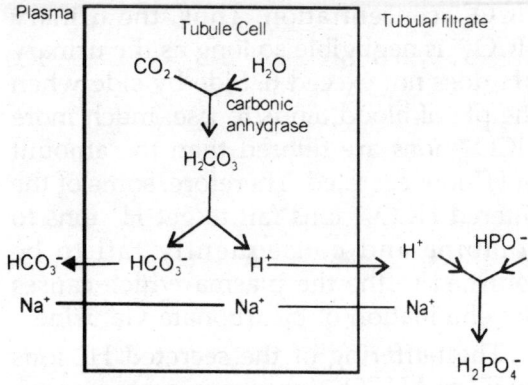

Fig. 5.2 : Buffering of H^+ by HPO_4^{--} in the renal tubules

gradient between the filtrate and the blood. This explains why the urinary pH never falls below pH 4.5. The buffering of the secreted H^+ ions is therefore, esential for containing their secretion in the urine which is carried out in the tubular filtrate in the following four ways:

(a) Buffering by bicarbonate

The proximal tubule is the site for about 80-90% of HCO_3^- mediated buffering of H^+ ions depending upon the rate of renal flow, blood Pco_2 and the HCO_3^- concentration of the ECF. The H_2CO_3 formed in the process gets immediately cleaved into H_2O and CO_2 in the proximal tubular lumen by *carbonic anhydrase* enzyme of the luminal plasma membrane of the proximal tubule cells. (Fig. 5.1). This CO_2 diffuses very readily into the proximal tubule cells and then ro the blood. In RBCs, enzyme carbonic anhydrase converts this CO_2 into H_2CO_3 which dissociates to give fresh HCO_3^- ions. Thus, the HCO_3^- ions which were filtered out in the glomerular filtrate are restored in the plasma.

Thus, whenever H^+ ions are secreted in excess due to a fall in the blood pH, almost all the filtered HCO_3^- ions change into H_2CO_3 by combining with H^+ and are then returned to plasma as CO_2 to restore its HCO_3^- concentration. Thus, the urinary HCO_3^- is negligible so long as the urinary pH does not exceed 6: Side by side when the pH of blood tends to rise, much more HCO_3^- ions are filtered than the amount of H^+ ions secreted. Therefore, some of the filtered HCO_3^- ions fail to get H^+ ions to combine and consequently fail to be returned to the the plasma which causes the elimination of bicarbonate via urine.

The buffering of the secreted H^+ ions by filtered HCO_3^- ion serves two pruposes:

(i) it does not allow the pH to fall below 6.9 in the proximal tubule and consequently allows more H^+ ions to be eliminated by tubule cells into the urine.

(ii) It helps to reabsorb the filtered HCO_3^- and to restore it in the blood.

(b) Buffering by phosphate buffer

Some secreted H^+ ions are buffered by the phosphate buffer, especially in the distal tubules. HPO_4^{--} filtered into the glomerular filtrate, accepts the secreted H^+ to form $H_2PO_4^-$ (Fig. 5.2) which changes the $[HPO_4^-]/[H_2PO_4^-]$ ratio from 4 in the Bowman's capsule to 0.02 - 0.05 in the final urine; the lower this ratio, the more acidic is the urine. But unlike H_2CO_3, $H_2PO_4^-$ is eliminated in the urine carrying some Na^+ ions with it and consequently causes some urinary loss of Na^+ ions. Moreover, the concentration of HPO_4^- is far less than that of HCO_3^- in the plasma and consequently in the glomerular filtrate also, therefore, the total buffering power of urinary phosphate buffer is far less than that of the bicarbonate buffer.

(c) Buffering by ammonia: Renal tubular cells form ammonia from a precursor in renal arterial blood and secrete it into tubular fluid. This ammonia formation takes place in the distal tubules and collecting ducts. **It has been found that about two third of the ammonia formed in the kidney is produced by *deamidation* of glutamine and one third by oxidative deamination of amino acids.**

The NH_3 formed enters the tubular fluid, where it combines with H^+ from the tubular cells to form NH_4^-. This NH_4^- then replaces Na^+ in a sodium salt of the tubular fluid, such as Na^+Cl^-. The Na^+ is reabsorbed by the H^+–Na exchange mechanism and reenters the plasma as

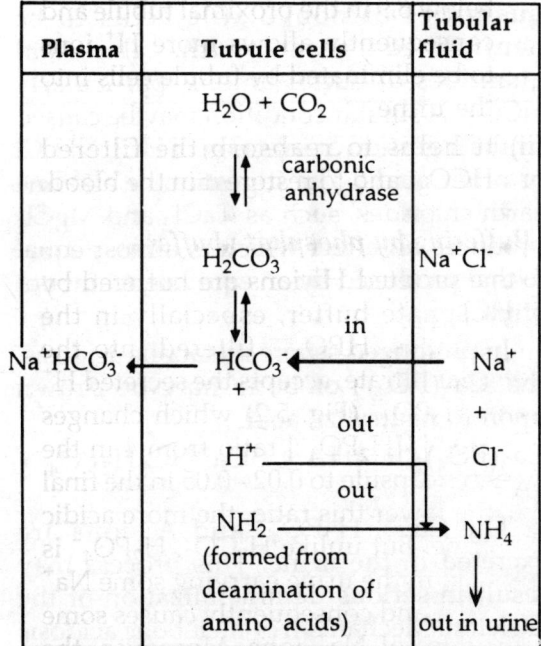

Plasma	Tubule cells	Tubular fluid
	$H_2O + CO_2$	
	$\updownarrow$ carbonic anhydrase	
	H_2CO_3	Na^+Cl^-
	$\updownarrow$ in	
$Na^+HCO_3^- \longleftarrow$	$HCO_3^- \longleftarrow$	Na^+
	$+$	$+$
	out	
	H^+	Cl^-
	out	
	NH_2 (formed from deamination of amino acids)	NH_4
		out in urine

Fig. 5.3: Buffering of H^+ by ammonia in renal tubules

$Na^+HCO_3^-$. The NH_4 is excreted in the urine as NH_4Cl (Fig. 5.3). In this way production of ammonia helps in regulating acid-base balance. Acidosis and dehydration may result from the failure of the ammonia secreting mechanisms of the kidneys, as in the syndromes of **Fanconi** and of **lower nephron nephrosis.**

It is also clear that the kidneys play a major role in controlling the electrolyte and acid base balance of the body which is achieved principally through the $H^+ - Na^+$ exchange mechanism, NH_3 formation and the kidney threshold for bicarbonate. The chief cation concerned in the regulation of electrolyte concentration and acid-base balance is Na^+.

(d) Eliminatioin of free acids

Elimination of free acids also helps in the regulation of acid-base balance of the body.

Some H^+ ions are accepted by strong conjugate bases such as lactate, acetoacetate, urate and oxalate anions, replacing the Na^+ reabsorbed from their salts as a result of which free weak acids such as lactic acid, acetoacetic acid and uric acid are formed. These may be excerted without any base because they have poor ionizability and their elimination changes the urinary pH to some extent. For example, 50% of acetoacetate is eliminated as free acid in the urine during ketosis.

Disturbances in Acid-Base balance

Disturbances in acid-base balance can be broadly classified into two headings:

1. **Acidosis** ⟶ **Respiratory acidosis**
   ⟶ **Metabolic acidosis**

2. **Alkalosis** ⟶ **Respiratory alkalosis**
   ⟶ **Metabolic alkalosis**

Respiratory acidosis: It is caused by CO_2 retention (CO_2 excess). In this type, the ionic shifts between extracellular and intracellular compartments are reversed to those in respiratory alkalosis, with W and K^+ entering the cells and Na^+ passing from the cells into extracellular fluid. The shift *of* H^+ into the cells leaves HCO_3^- in the extracellular fluid to raise the pH,

$$H_2CO_3 \rightleftharpoons HCO_3^- + H^+$$

into cells

and the H^+ is taken up by intracellular buffers. The kidneys *compensate* by increased excretion of H^+ and of NH_4^+ with anions such as Cl^-, and by decreased excretion of Na^+ and K^+ (NH_4^+ is substituted for these).

Such condition occurs in **pneumonia, asthama, etc.**

Metabolic Acidosis: Metabolic type of acidosis refers to decreases in total buffer anions, chiefly HCO_3^- and is not related to respiratory changes in blood CO_2,

In this type, the main three effects encountered are:

(i) a decrease in the alkali reserve HCO_3^-

(ii) a decrease in the total CO_2 of the blood and

(iii) a lowered pH of blood.

The lowered pH stimulates respiration to blow off CO_2 in an attempt to bring the ratio HCO_3^-/H_2CO_3 and the pH to normal. Also, the kidneys excrete a more acid urine and more ammonia to conserve HCO_3^-. If the condition is mild and the pH is within normal range, it is referred to as *'compensated metabolic acidosis'* and if the pH is below the normal range, the condition is known *as" uncompensated metabolic acidosis'*

In Metabolic acidosis the ionic shifts between extracellular and intracellular fluids are reversed. The movement of H^+ (and K^+) from extracellular fluid into the cells in exchange for Na^+ leaves HCO_3^- in the extracellular fluid, to help raise the pH. The H^+ entering the cells is taken up by the intracellular buffer systems. The kidneys increase excretion of H^+ and NH_4^+ and decrease excretion of Na^+, K^+ and HCO_3^-. Respiration is stimulated to increase excretion of CO_2. Each of these processes helps compensate the acidosis.

$$H_2CO_3 \rightleftharpoons HCO_3^- + H^+$$

into cells

Examples of metabolic acidosis are observed in uncontrolled diabetes with ketosis and nephritic acidosis when the quantities of nonvolatile acids to be neutralized react with abnormal quantities of buffer anions, particularly HCO_3^-. A similar condition may be caused by the ingestion or injection of HCl, NH_4Cl or other acids, The ingestion of alkaline earth chlorides, such as $CaCl_2$ and $MgCl_2$ produces an effect which is almost equal to that produced by an equivalent amount of HCl.

In prolonged severe metabolic acidosis, the $Ca_3(PO_4)_2$ of bone may be drawn upon to neutralize acid.

$$Ca_3(PO_4)_2 + 4HA \rightarrow 3Ca^{++} + 2H_2PO_4^- + 4A^-$$

The Ca^{++}, $H_2PO_4^-$ and A^- ions are excreted in the urine. This process may result in serious demineralization of the skeleton. Mechanism of metabolic acidosis may be understood easily by figure 5.4.

Respiratory alkalosis: It is caused by excessive CO_2 excretion (CO_2 deficit). This is referred to the increases in total buffer anions, chiefly HCO_3^- which is not related to respiratory changes in the CO_2 of blood.

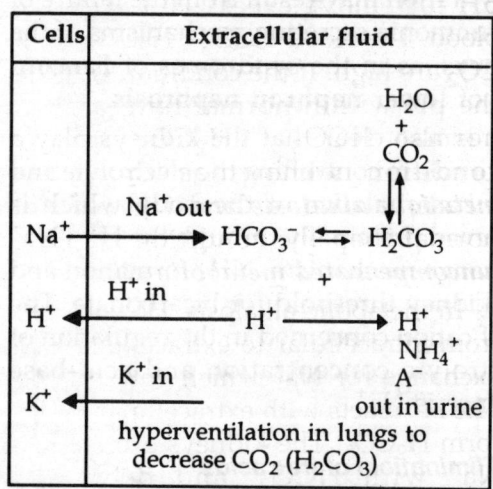

Fig. 5.4: Metabolic acidosis, pH of extracellular fluid increased by ionic shifts

In this type, due to hyperventilation H^+ and K^+ pass from intracellular to extracellular fluid in exchange for Na^+, which enters the cells. The H^+ reacts with HCO_3^- to form H_2CO_3 to compensate the alkalosis. The kidneys excrete less H^+ and NH_4^+ and more HCO_3^- alongwith Na^+ and K^+.

In respiratory alkalosis, with decreased pCO_2 and H_2CO_3 in the tubular cells, H^+ excretion is decreased and K^+ and HCO_3^- excretions are increased.

Such condition occurs in **hepatic coma.**

Metabolic alkalosis: Metabolic type of alkalosis refers to the increases :,n total buffer anions, mainly HCO_3^- and is not related to respiratory changes in blood CO_2.

Metabolic alkalosis may be caused by the ingestion or injection of $NaHCO_3$ or other basic substances or of substances such as sodium lactate and sodium citrate which give $NaHCO_3$ when metabolized. As the pH rises, the respiration is depressed to retain CO_2 and lower the pH and the kidneys excrete urine at a higher pH to remove excess HCO_3^- from the blood. The blood HCO_3^-, H_2CO_3 and total CO_2 are high. If the condition is mild and the pH within normal ranges due to a normal HCO_3^- / H_2CO_3 ratio, the condition is known as *'Compensated metabolic alkalosis'* and if the pH is above normal then the condition is called as *'uncompensated metabolic alkalosis '.*

In metabolic alkalosis, H^+ and K^+ shift from intracellular to extracellular fluid in exchange for Na^+ which enters the cells. The H^+ reacts with extracellular HCO_3^- to form H_2CO_3. The kidneys excrete K^+ and Na^+ with HCO_3^- and decrease the excretion of NH_4^+. Respiration is decreased

to retain CO_2 (H_2CO_3). Each of these processes helps in compensating the alkalosis.

Conditions of alkalosis are seldom treated by the administration of acids, though occasionally NH_4Cl solution are used, the ammonia being converted to neutral urea in the liver with the release of HCl, which reacts with body buffers. The administration of isotortic NaCl solution dilutes the extracellular HCO_3^- to improve the alkalosis and expands the extracellular fluid volume. Often in such cases as the alkalosis of vomiting there is K^+ depletion, and this deficit must be corrected by administering potassium before the kidneys can compensate the alkalosis by excreting bicarbonate and retaining Cl^-.

Such condition may occur in **Cushing's Syndrome.**

The mechanism of metabolic alkalosis may be easily understood by studying the Figure 5.5.

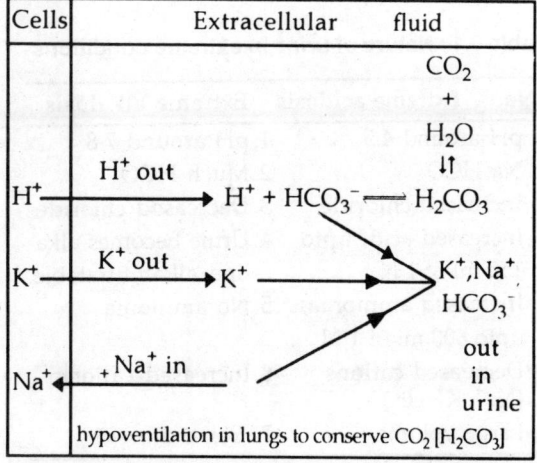

Fig. 5.5: Metabolic alkalosis. pH of extracellular fluid decreased by ionic shifts

Alkaline Tide

It has been found that shortly after a meal, the alveolar CO_2 gets increased, the pH of urine rises, the plasma bicarbonate rises and the chloride falls. This so-called alkaline tide after a meal is due to the formation of gastric HCl to increase pH. The condition is very mild and disappears after the gastric HCl is neutralized in the intestine to from NaCl, which is absorbed into the blood and reestablishes the status quo. The alkaline tide gets more pronounced after meals that stimulates much gastric secretion, such as heavy protein meals. It may be greatly diminished or disappear in conditions of achlorhydria in which little gastric HCl is secreted. This may be true after meals consisting chiefly of fat and carbohydrate.

Nature of Urine in Extreme Conditions

The nature of the urine excreted in extreme conditions of acidosis and alkalosis is of considerable interest. The main relevant characteristics are as follows (Table 5.1):

Table 5.1 : Nature of urine in extreme conditions

SNo.	Extreme acidosis	Extreme alkalosis
1.	pH around 4.5	pH around 7.8
2.	Na HCO_3^-	Much HCO_3^-
3.	Increased chloride	Decreased chloride
4.	Increased acid, upto 150 ml of 1 N	Urine becomes alkaline, alkali titratable.
5.	Increased ammonia, upto 600 ml of 1 N	No ammonia
6.	Decreased cations (Na^+, K^+. etc.)	Increased cations
7.	Large volume	Some diuresis

VARIATIONS OF PLASMA ELECTROLYTES IN PATHOLOGICAL STATES

Table 5.2 shows the variations of plasma electrolytes in various pathological states. The cation variations chiefly involve Na^+.

Table 5.2: Cations and Anions of plasma in various pathological states compared to those of normal plasma. (values are in milli equivalents per litre of water)

Condition	Cations, total	Anions			
		HCO_3^-	Cl^-	Keto-acids	other anions
Normal	155	27	103		25
Diabetic ketosis (acidosis)	142	5	80	24	33
Fasting ketosis (acidosis)	155	I5	101	13	26
Diarrhoea	148	11	100		37
Addison's disease	126	22	73		31
Nephrosis	150	20	113		17
Chronic nephritis	157	21	101		35
Chronic nephritis (terminal)	146	6	87		53
Pyloric obstruction (vomiting)	146	59	42		45
Duodenal obstruction (vomiting)	150	43	48	32	27
Habitual vomiting	155	33	96		27

Ratio of H_2CO_3 versus HCO_3^- in different states

Following Table 5.3 gives an idea of pH and $H_2CO_3^-/HCO_3^-$ ratio in different states:

Table 5.3 :To show pH and $H_2CO_3^-/HCO_3^-$ ratio in different states

State	pH	$H_2CO_3^-/HCO_3^-$
Normal	6-6.5	1:20
Respiratory acidosis	↓	< 1:20
Respiratory alkalosis	↑	> 1:20
Metabolic acidosis	↓	< 1:20
Metabolic alkalosis	↑	> 1:20

CHAPTER 6

BIOCHEMISTRY OF CANCER
(MALIGNANT NEOPLASM)
(A relative Autonomous Growth of Tissue, causing great panic in humans)

> Who is not scared of the name 'cancer'? May be there a person per thousand who is not scared. By its name only, one loses its hunger and thinks himself/herself closer to 'God'. There are several causes known so far for the onset of this disease; its permanent cure especially when the metastasis has taken place, is not yet known. If it is detected in the first stage, then victory may be got by various kinds of treatment. Its incidence is on increase side somehow. Certain hospitals meant exclusively for the treatment of 'cancer' are coming up annually in big cities which itself indicates the rising trend of this disease in our society.
>
> On the other hand, scientists are also busy day and night in bringing out its permanent solution which should be cheaper and trouble free as well.

One of the key differences between the cancer cells and the normal cells is the *inability* of *cancer cells* to stop dividing. Why does it so happen, is not yet clear? Focus of the scientific community of the globe is to find out the cause of the same and the permanent cure of the same for the betterment of mankind. Scientists around the world are working seriously day and night in this field for more than four decades and have yet to reach the depth of the same.

Cancerous cells are characterized by three main properties:

(i) **Unrestricted growth;**

(ii) **Invasion on local tissues; and**

(iii) **Spread or metastasis to other parts of the body**

Cells of benign tumors have also been found to show unrestricted growth but do not invade local tissue or spread to other parts of the body.

Biochemical tests for the detection of cancer

Several biochemical tests are on date

Cancer is supposed to be the second largest killer after the cardiovascular diseases throughout the globe.

Breast cancer is the leader, followed by the cancer of the prostate, lung, colon-rectum and the bladder.

No age is immune. Victims may be children, young ones or older people. It's an expensive disease. Its victims may die within a month or months or may even remain alive for years together with the help of treatment and proper care.

helpful in the management of patients with cancer. Many cancers are found to be associated with the abnormal production of enzymes, proteins and hormones, which can be easily estimated in serum or plasma. These molecules are called as *"tumor markers"*. Measurement of some tumor markers is now a days an integral part of the management of some types of cancer (Table 6.1).

Electrophoresis and detailed salt fractionation are the other valuable biochemical techniques which have revealed a number of interesting variations in the size of the globulin fraction in certain diseases including some types of cancers. Examples of electrophoretic patterns have been exhibited in Fig. 6.1. A small to moderate increase in α_1 and α_2-globulins is seen in some cases of cancer. A fall in the mean concentration of the γ-globulins has been reported in lymphatic leukaemia in contrast to an increase in myelogenous and monocytic leukaemias. The albumin tends to fall in all cases.

Varied patterns are obtained in multiple myeloma. The most characteristic and peculiar observation is the presence of the

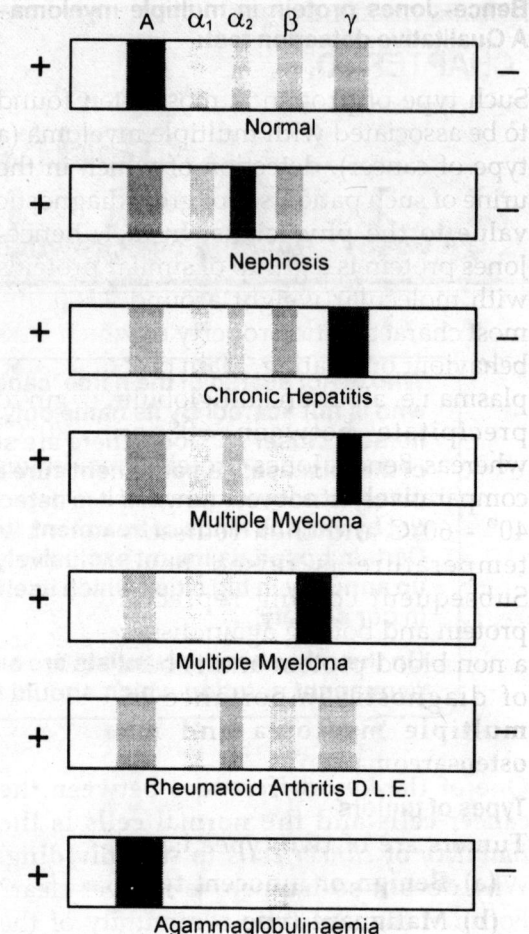

Fig. 6.1 : Electrophoretic patterns in different disorders

band of abnormal protein which has been termed as the M protein. It occurs as an intense, narrow band most often found with the γ-globulins, then in diminishing frequency between the γ and β-globulins, with the β, and very rarely between the β and α_2. There is often dissociation between the presence of the M protein in the serum and Bence-Jones protein in the urine; only occasionally both are seen in the same patient.

Table 6.1: Some clinically useful tumor markers

Sl. No.	Marker	Associated cancer
1.	Carcinoembryonic antigen (CEA)	Colon, lung, breast, pancreas
2.	Human chorionic gonadotropin (HCG)	Trophoblast, germ cell
3.	Alpha-fetoprotein (AFP)	Liver, germ cell
4.	Calcitonin (CT)	Thyroid (medullary carcinoma)
5.	Prostatic acid phosphatase (PAP)	Prostate

Bence–Jones protein in multiple myeloma– A Qualitative detection test:

Such type of protein is most often found to be associated with multiple myeloma (a type of cancer), detection of which in the urine of such patients is of great diagnostic value to the physicians. In fact, Bence-Jones protein is a group of similar proteins with molecular weight around 2,500; the most characteristic property of which is its behaviour on heating. Main proteins of the plasma i.e. albumin and globulin begin to precipitate between 60° and 70°C; whereas Bence- Jones protein precipitates comparatively at a lower range i.e. between 40° - 60°C and then redissolves as the temperature is raised beyond 60°C. Subsequent cooling reprecipitates the protein and boiling again dissolves it. It is a non blood protein and is believed to be of diagnostic importance in cases of **multiple myeloma and myelogenic osteosarcoma too.**

Types of tumors

Tumors are of two types i.e.

(a) **Benign or innocent type,** and

(b) **Malignant type**

Benign tumors are the growths which although may continue to grow slowly over long periods but remain restricted in area. They do not spread to the other parts of the body. They have little or no tendency of recurrence after surgical removal. The danger of benign tumors is limited to their effects of pressure and obstruction.

Contrarily, a malignant tumor to which the most common term of today i.e. *cancer* has been given is one whose growth is unrestricted and which has a tendency to infiltrate the neighbouring tissues of the body. As a result of transmission of such cells i.e. malignant cells via the blood or lymphatic system, even the farthest portions of the body may be easily victimized. Portions of a tumor which have taken root in distant part(s) of the body are *commonly referred to as metastases,* and a tumor resulting from such a process is termed as a *metastatic tumor.*

Two main classes of the malignant tumors are the:

(a) **Carcinomas, and**

(b) **Sarcomas**

Carcinoma is a tumor which arises from epithelial tissues whether pavement or glandular, while *sarcoma* is the one which originates from the connective and allied structures of mesenchymal origin including muscles also. Either name may be modified by a *prefix* to designate the particular tissue from which the tumor is derived. Cancer is not confined to any particular site/place of the body. It may develop in any organ or tissue of the body; however, common sites are liver, breast, uterus, uterine cervix, bone marrow, vagina in young women, colon, scrotum, skin, blood, etc.

CARCINOGENESIS

Cancer is not a single entity with a single etiology. Today, many *carcinogens* are on the list which can produce cancer in the humans. These carcinogens may either be *exogenous* or *endogenous* in nature. *Co-carcinogens* are the substances which have got the capability to activate/induce the carcinogen. **Methylcholanthrene for instance can cause carcinoma of the skin at a very high concentration but if croton oil is mixed with it, then it can cause skin cancer even at a very low concentration. In this case, croton oil acts as a cocarcinogen, hence termed as a cocarcinogen.** The known **carcinogens** (agents that are responsible for the causation of cancers) may be arbitrarily placed in the following four groups:

(i) **Chemical compounds,**

(ii) **Endocrine factors,**

(iii) **Oncogenic viruses,** and

(iv) **Ionizing radiations.**

Rous, Peyton (U.S.A.) **a Physician** was awarded Nobel Prize in Medicine in 1966 for his discovery of tumour inducing viruses.

Chemical compounds

A wide variety of chemical compounds are carcinogenic in nature (Table 6.2) the structure of some of them are given below.

Table 6.2: Chemicals recognised as carcinogens in humans and experimental animals

Sl No.	Carcinogens	Target organs/ tissues affected
1.	Benzidine	urinary bladder
2.	2-naphthylamine	urinary bladder
3.	4-nitrobiphenyl	urinary bladder
4.	4-aminobiphenyl	urinary bladder
5.	Nickel compounds	lungs and nasal sinuses
6.	Asbestos	lungs and pleura
7.	Cigarette's smoke	lungs and other tissues
8.	Chromium compounds	lungs
9.	Soot, tar, mineral oils	skin and lungs
10.	Betel nut	buccal mucosa

The induction of cancer by chemicals was first discovered more than two centuries ago in man. **Hill for the first time had reported nasal cancer in snuff users,** whereas, **scientist Pott** had **reported high incidence of scrotal cancer in chimney sweepers. Carcinogenesis may be caused by both, inorganic and organic chemicals.**

Inorganic carcinogens are rare as compared to organic carcinogens. Cancers particularly involving lungs have been observed in persons working in the factories of nickel, chromium, cadmium and beryllium. Inhalation of asbestos has also been found to cause *asbestosis* and *cancer of lungs;* these diseases are more prevalent in the workers of asbestos factories.

Amongst the **organic carcinogens,** the common ones include methylcholanthrene, benzpyrene, benzidine, 2-naphthylamine, 2-acetaminofluorene, N-methyl-4-aminoazobenzene etc., the structures of which are as given over here (Fig 6.2).

The most important compounds are of the polycyclic hydrocarbon group. A second group is of the 'azo-compounds;. Cancer of skin is very common in the persons working with *tar* because it is a highly complex substance containing many carcinogenic agents. One of the active compounds that has been isolated from *tar* is **benzpyrene.**

A large number of the fungal infected foods·have been found to be potent carcinogens. The carcinogenic substances present in such foods are called *"natural carcinogens"* (Fig 6.2). Many of them are responsible for the causation of cancer particularly in the tropical areas with low standard of living and low socio-economic status. Contamination of the foods by *Aspergillus flavus* results in the accumulation of toxic and carcinogenic compound (aflatoxin-B) in the food. The suspicion that some of the **aflatoxins** are carcinogens in man is based upon the observation that **aflatoxin B_1 and C_1 have been found to be potent carcinogens causing liver cancer** in a wide variety of

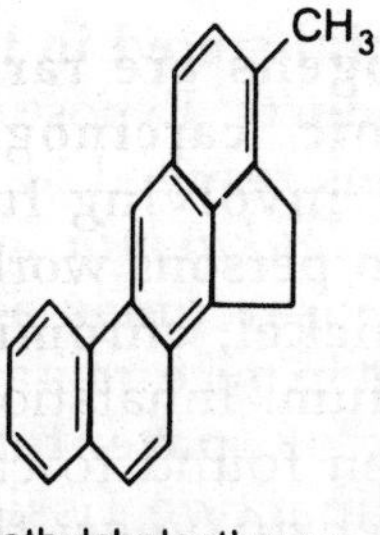

Methylcholanthrene
(extremely potent)

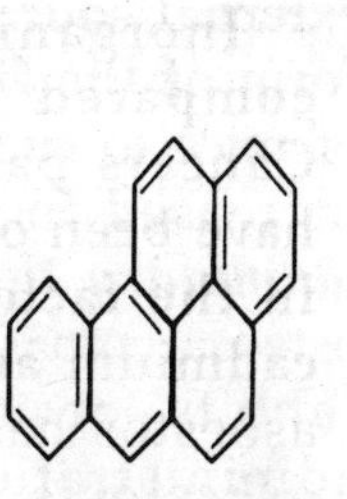

3 - 4 - Benzpyrene
(Source - Tar)

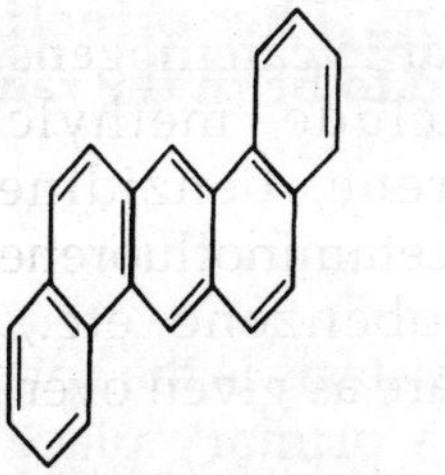

1,2,5,6 - Dibenzan-
thracene

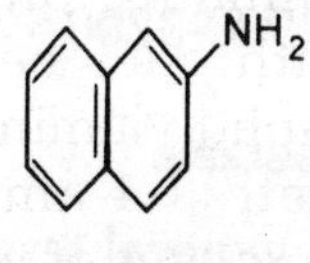

2 - Naphthylamine

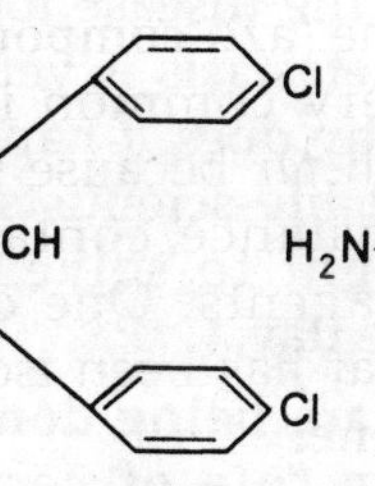

CCl₃CH

D.D.T.

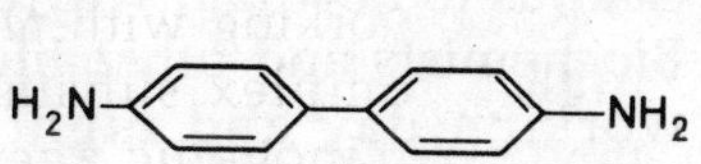

Benzidine

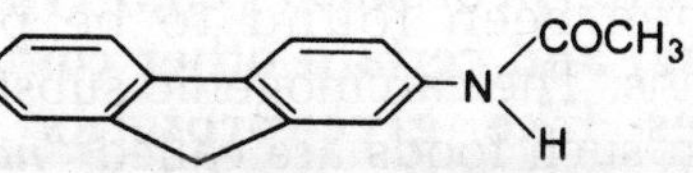

2 - Acetaminofluorene

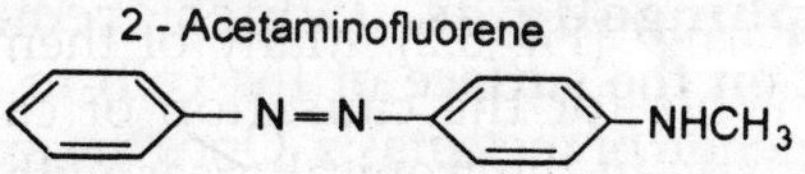

N - Methyl - 4 - aminoazobenzene

Fig 6.2 : Structures of some chemical carcinogens

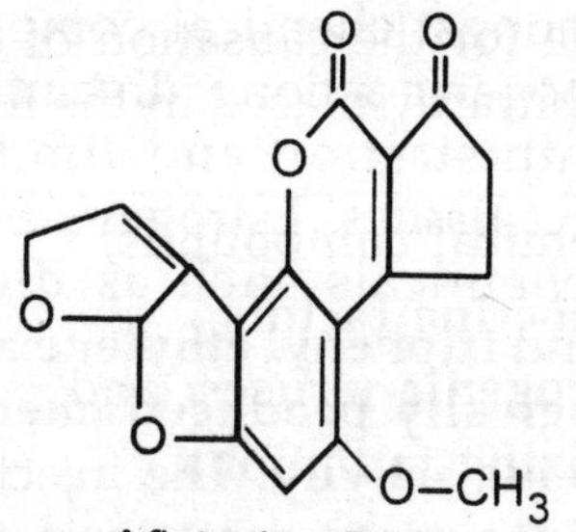

Aflatoxin - B₁
(source - Aspergillus flavus)

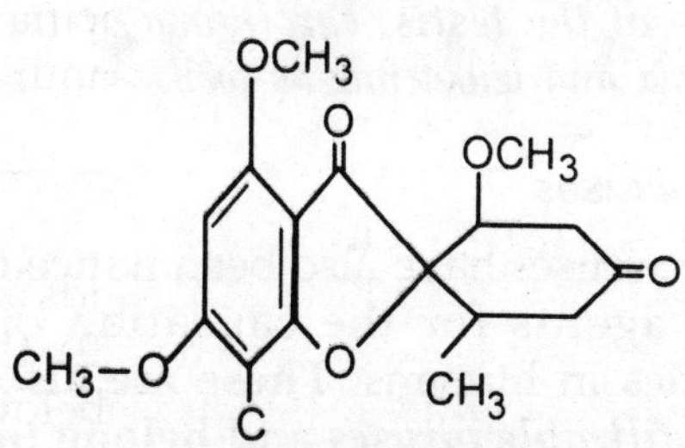

Griseofulvin
(source - Penicillium griseofulvum)

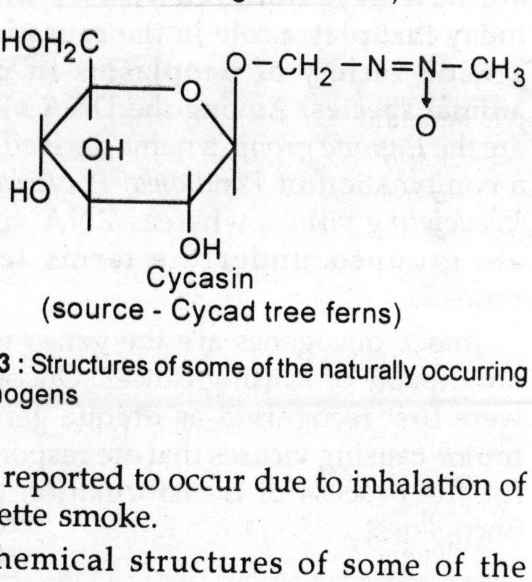

Cycasin
(source - Cycad tree ferns)

Fig 6.3 : Structures of some of the naturally occurring carcinogens

been reported to occur due to inhalation of cigarette smoke.

Chemical structures of some of the important naturally occurring carcinogens are as mentioned in the last of this chapter.

Endocrine factors

It has been established that many hormones are responsible for the onset of cancers. Examples include estrogens and androgens for premenopausal breast and prostatic carcinoma, respectively. Estro-

animals. Secondly, high incidence of carcinoma has been noticed in the parts of the world where fungal contaminated food is carelessly consumed. An increasing number of chemical carcinogens has been found in certain green plants and fungi (Fig. 6.3). Widespread carcinogenic exposure has gens are amongst chemical compounds whose carcinogenic action is **distant.** to the site of administration and limited to specific target tissues. **Estrogens include synthetic** chemicals such as **diethyl-stilbestrol** and **triphenyl ethylene as well as physiologically produced chemicals with estrogenic activity.** The injection of estrogens into mice may lead to the appearance of *pituitary adenoma, interstitial cell tumors of the testis, carcinoma of the uterine cervix and leukaemia as well.*

Oncogenic viruses

Oncogenic viruses have also been noticed to be the agents for the causation of malignancies in humans. **These are also known as** *filtrable viruses* **and belong to both DNA and RNA virus groups. There are now over hundred viruses known today that play a role in the causation of a wide variety of neoplasms in many animal species.** Among the DNA viruses are the *Papova group,* a name derived from a combination of *Papilloma, Polyoma* and *Vacuolating viruses* whereas RNA viruses are grouped under the terms *leuko-viruses.*

Infact, oncogenes are the genes which are capable of causing cancer. Oncogenes were first recognised as unique genes of tumor-causing viruses that are responsible for the process of transformation (viral oncogenes).

Ionizing Radiations

The fact that the ionizing radiations are carcinogenic was shown within ten years of their discovery by the tragic occurrence of skin carcinoma in the physicians and other workers who exposed themselves to the new rays. **Ionizing radiations are carcinogenic whether delivered from external sources or admini-stered in the form of the fission products.** Exposures of mice to such radiations resulted in an increased incidence of *leukaemia* **and** *mammary tumors.* Fibrosarcomas and osteosarcomas developed in mice, rats and rabbits at the sites of **parenteral** administration of radioactive fission products of **plutonium. Likewise, ultraviolet rays are also responsible for the cancers of skin. The effective wavelength was found to be in the range of 2900-3200Å.**

Metastasis

In a general term, metastasis is the spread of cancer cells from a primary place of origin to other tissues where they grow as secondary tumors, and it is the major problem presented by the disease today. The biochemistry of metastasis is yet not clear as to how and why does it happen. Biochemists and other life-scientists are working day and night to solve this burning problem of the day.

Many studies also are being done to uncover the possible role of certain enzymes like proteases (e.g., type 4-collagenase) and certain other complex substances like glycoproteins and glycosphingolipids (which remain present on the surface of the cell) in the phenomenon of metastasis. Once the exact biochemistry of metastasis is known, only then the accurate and effective anticancer therapy shall come forward.

Metabolism of Cancer Cells

Cancer cells have an unique type of metabolism. Although, they possess all the enzymes required for most of the central pathways of intermediary metabolism; cancer cells of nearly all types exhibit an anomaly in the integration of the glycolytic pathway and the tricarboxylic acid cycle. Remarkable thing is that the rate of oxygen consumption of cancerous cells is somewhat less than the normal cells. Malignant cells tend to utilize anywhere from 5 to 10 times as much glucose as normal cells and convert most of it to lactic acid, even though they have nearly normal rate of respiration. Several malignant tumors have been found to have high levels of glycolytic enzymes and the necessary cofactors (phosphate and nicotinamide adenine dinucleotide) and are able to withstand considerable period of oxygen deprivation due to either failure of blood flow (ischaemia) or due to failure of blood oxygenation (anoxia). Malignant tumors and embryonic cells exhibit high rate of anaerobic glycolysis. Rapidly growing tumors resemble embryonic cells in another respect. Each type of cells has a high rate of DNA synthesis whereas the synthesis of less essential products is depressed. The very structure of the malignant cell resembles that of the embryonic cell as regards the disposition of certain cell surface proteins; the difference being that in an embryonic cell, the genes which are responsible for its biochemical characteristics are under specific control and become modulated as the embryo develops whereas; in a malignant cell, the capacity to exercise that control is lost.

Malignant tissue is comparatively more deficient in *cytochrome* C than the *cytochrome oxidase* and that, it is the concentration of the former which is the rate limiting factor for the chemical reaction.

The pH of the growing tumors in *situ* was measured and found to be distinctly lower than that of the normal tissues i.e.

about 7.0 as compared to 7.4. The pH of the tumor cells was found to drop still lower to as low as 6.3 after the administration of glucose either subcutaneously or intraperitoneally without any signs of systemic acidosis which indicates that the drop in pH is confined to the tumors only. This is a strong evidence in favour of higher *in vivo* glycolysis of tumors. Since glycolysis involves the production of lactic acid as an end-product which is relatively a strong organic acid and easily available in sufficient quantity to lower down tissue pH.

The most striking change among the individual enzyme systems of cancerous cells is the decline in the content of various enzymes involved in aerobic oxidation such as *cytochrome oxidase, succinic acid dehydrogenase,* and *D-amino acid oxidase.* The activity of enzymes involved in the metabolism of nucleic acids and the proteins continues to be high in most of the cancers; examples of such enzymes are the *nucleases, arginase,* certain *peptidases, xanthine oxidase* and *β-glucuronidase.* Enzyme hyaluronidase is found to be absent in the cancerous cells. Hepatoma cells in rats are characterized by very low catalase activity as compared to the normal liver cells. In the mouse, hepatoma cells also exhibit decrease in *catalase* concentration but this is not as marked as in the rat. Furthermore, the *catalase* deficiency in hepatomas varies with the strain of the rat.

The double stranded DNA may then be integrated with the host cell DNA and when *turned on* may transcribe viral RNA molecules. Every oncogenic RNA virus tested so far contains *reverse transcriptase* activity. *Reverse transcriptase* has been found to be present in the particles present in human milk with a familial history of *breast cancer. Visna virus* which is the cause of a progressive neurological disease of sheep that leads to paralysis and death has also been shown to contain the enzyme *reverse transcriptase.*

Cancerous cells exhibit the following salient features:

1. **Low (↓) levels of enzymes, i.e.,**
   (a) Cytochrome oxidase,
   (b) Succinic dehydrogenase

The formation of *thymidylic acid* has been found to be specially higher in the patients of *leukaemia* (blood cancer). The activity of *dihydrofolate reductase* required for thymidylic acid formation is also found to be elevated in white blood cells of such patients whereas in the normal individuals, its concentration is found to be very low.

The plasma of most of the patients suffering from *multiple myeloma shows considerably raised levels of cryoglobulins.*

In tumor virology, excitement has also aroused by the discovery of the enzyme *RNA-dependent-DNA-polymerase.* It is now suggested that the transformation of the host cells by RNA tumor viruses might depend on the activity of the *reverse transcriptase.* This enzyme may be essential for viral replication and cell transformation. The enzyme might be possibly working in the following manner in two steps sequence during reverse transcription.

Viral - RNA

↓

RNA - DNA hybrid

↓

Double stranded DNA

(c) D-amino acid oxidase, etc.

2. **Raised (↑) levels of enzymes, i.e.,**
   (a) Nucleases,
   (b) Arginase,
   (c) Xanthine oxidase
   (d) β-glucuronidase
   (e) Certain peptidases,
   (f) Glycolytic enzymes, etc.

3. **Enzyme hyaluronidase is found to be totally absent in cancerous cells.**

4. Rate of oxygen consumption of cancerous cells is somewhat less than the normal cells.

5. **Malignant cells utilise 5-10 times more glucose than the normal cells and convert most of it to lactic acid.**

6. **Several malignant tumours have been found to have high levels of glycolytic enzymes and the necessary cofactors (phosphate and nicotinamide dinucleotide.**

7. **Role of aldoreductases in such cells is of considerable importance.**

Cancer therapy

The development of effective cancer therapy is a major focus of biomedical research. As a result of fundamental and applied research, certain previously lethal malignancies have become curable now a days.

True cancer therapy involves the people from the following three sub-specialities, namely the role of:

(i) The surgeon
(ii) The radiation oncologist and the
(iii) The medical oncologist

Antitumor agents (chemotherapeutic agents)

Special emphasis is being laid down these days to find out the ways of preventing the growth and development of tumors. It has been found that the use of nucleotide biosynthetic inhibitors prevents the growth of such cells and arrests the pathological development to a certain extent. In the past four decades, over 75 such agents having antitumor property have been identified and out of them more than 40 drugs have become commercially available. Some of the important types of antitumor agents are as given below:

(a) **Alkylating agents,**

(b) **Nucleic acids inhibitors,**

(c) **Plant alkaloids,**

(d) **Anti-tumor antibiotics,**

(e) **Hormonal agents,** and

(f) **Immunotherapy**

(a) Alkylating agents

Commonly used alkylating agents are **mephalan, cyclophosphamide, busulphan, etc.** These agents act on such cells in all the phases of cell cycle but the proliferating cells are more vulnerable to their effects. Busulphan has a greater effect on *granulopoiesis* and *myelogenous leukaemia;* whereas mephalan and cyclophosphamide are the most effective agents for the treatment of myeloma. Cyclophosphamide is the only alkylating agent which can produce and maintain complete remissions in *acute leukaemia.*

(b) Nucleic acids inhibitors

Inhibitors of nucleic acids biosynthesis behave as antitumor agents. Such inhibitors are of great significance as they are responsible for establishing the interdependence of DNA synthesis, RNA synthesis and protein synthesis. Those currently in use are 6-mercaptopurine, 5-fluorodeoxyuridine, 6-thioguanine, 5-fluorouracil, aminopterin, amethopterin, etc (Fig. 6.4). Mechanism of action of some of these is as follows:

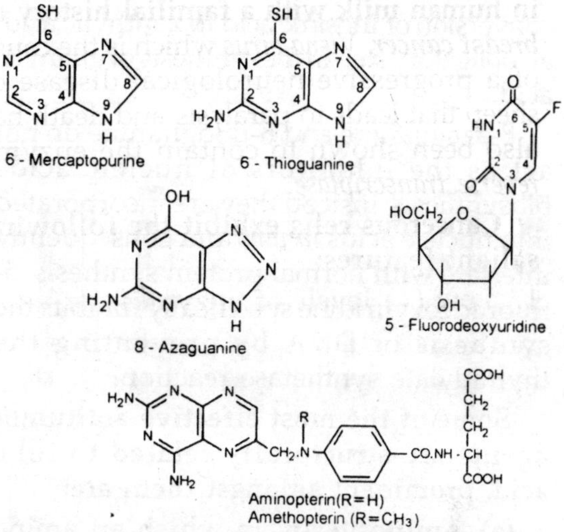

Fig. 6.4 : Structures of some of the nucleotide inhibitors having antitumor properties

The best known and one of the clinically most useful inhibitor is *6-mercaptopurine* which is supposed to be the potent inhibitor of both the steps involved in the conversion of inosinic acid to adenylic acid. Consequently, this compound causes an inhibition in the synthesis of adenylic acid, vis-a-vis nucleic acids biosynthesis. In addition, 6-mercaptopurine also inhibits the

---

ALKYLATING AGENTS

1. Cyclophosphamide,
2. Mephalan,
3. Busulphan, etc.

NUCLEIC ACIDS INHIBITORS

1. 6 - Mercaptopurine,
2. 8 - Azaguanine,
3. 6 - Thioguanine,
4. 5 - Fluorodeoxyuridine,
5. 5 - Fluorouracil,
6. Aminopterin,
7. Amethopterin, etc.

conversion of inosinic acid to xanthylic acid, an obligatory step in the synthesis of guanylic acid.

8-azaguanine and 6-thioguanine do not act as the inhibitors of nucleic acids biosynthesis; instead they are incorporated into nucleic acids *in vivo* and consequently interfere with normal protein synthesis. 5-fluorodeoxyuridine specifically inhibits the synthesis of DNA by preventing the thymidylate synthetase reaction.

Some of the most effective antitumor agents are structurally related to folic acid, prominent amongst them are:

(a) **Aminopterin,** in which an amino group replaces the 4-hydroxyl group of folic acid, and

(b) **Amethopterin,** which is N^{10}– methyl-aminopterin. At two stages in the biosynthesis of purines and at one stage in the biosynthesis of pyrimidines, **'one carbon' transfer reactions occur for which folic acid derivatives are required as coenzymes.** Aminopterin and amethopterin prevent the reduction of dihydrofolic acid to tetrahydrofolic acid (THFA), the active coenzyme required for the synthesis of nucleic acids.

(c) *Plant alkaloids:* Alkaloids namely vincristine and vinblastine are derived from periwinkle plants. They are cell cycle specific and produce metaphase arrest in dividing cells.

(d) *Anti-tumor antibiotics:* Important anti-tumor antibiotics in clinical use include azaserine, DON (6-diazo-5-oxo-L-norleucine), actinomycin-D, mitomycin C, mithramycin, adriamycin, bleomycin, phleomycin, etc. (Fig. 6.5). Mechanism of action of

some of these is as follows:

Antibiotics azaserine and DON

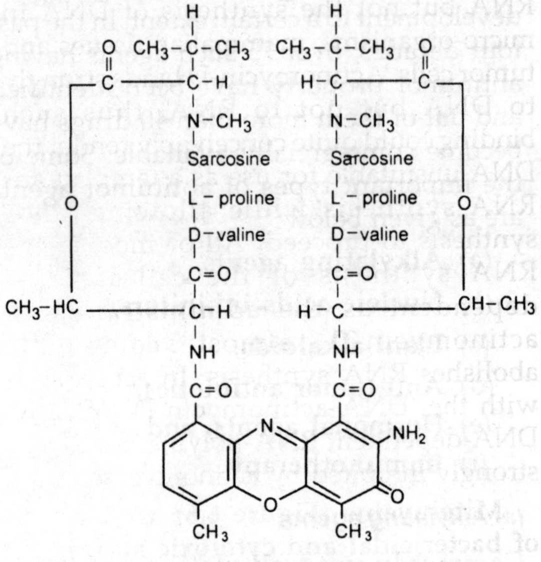

Fig. 6.5 : Structures of some of the antitumor antibiotics

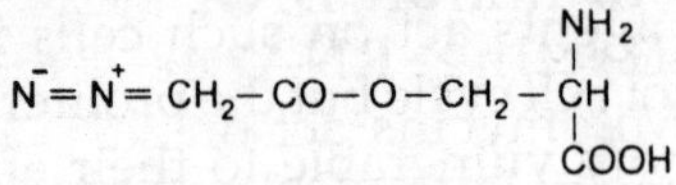

derived from *streptomyces* are structurally related to glutamine. These antibiotics have a property to inhibit to varying extents the aminations in which glutamine serves as the amino group donor. Since, several such aminations are involved in the biosynthesis of nucleic acids precursors, azaserine and DON are ought to inhibit the biosynthesis of nucleic acids. Of the various glutamine dependent aminations, the one involved in the conversion of formylglycinamide ribonucleotide to the corresponding amidine is most sensitive to inhibition by these glutamine analogues.

Actinomycin-D, like azaserine and

DON, is an antibiotic, isolated from streptomyces. *In vivo*, actionomycin-D at low concentration inhibits the synthesis of RNA but not the synthesis of DNA in micro-organisms, mammalian tissues and tumor cells. Actinomycin-D binds strongly to DNA but not to RNA, thus such binding could quite conceivably render the DNA unsuitable for use as a template for RNA synthesis while allowing DNA synthesis to proceed. All or most of the RNA synthesis of the cell is DNA dependent as the administration of actinomycin-D almost completely abolishes RNA synthesis. In accordance with the 'DNA actinomycin-D' concept, DNA-dependent RNA-polymerase is very strongly inhibited by actinomycin-D.

Mitomycins (Figure 6.6) are a group of bactericidal and cytotoxic antibiotics prepared from *streptomycetes* **and have a property to inhibit DNA synthesis without affecting RNA or protein synthesis.** Mitomycins act on the DNA-priming capacity in the DNA polymerase reaction, but not in the DNA primed RNA

Plant alkaloids

1. Vincristine,
2. Vinblastine

Anti-tumor antibiotics

1. Azaserine,
2. DON,
3. Actinomycin-D,
4. Mitomycin C,
5. Mithramycin,
6. Adriamycin,
7. Bleomycin,
8. Phleomycin, etc.

Hormonal agents

1. Estrogens,
2. Androgens,
3. Progestins,
4. Thyroxine,
5. Adrenal corticosteroids, etc.

polymerase reaction. Mechanism involves inhibition by forming covalent cross linkages of the complementary strands of DNA. They act as alkylating agents, attacking either the guanine or cytosine residues, or both. It is probable that a preliminary reduction of the quinone is required for its activity.

Phleomycin antibiotic inhibits DNA synthesis but not RNA or protein synthesis. In vitro, it inhibits the enzyme DNA polymerase by binding the DNA primer, showing preference for adenine-thymine pairs. It also inhibits enzyme *exonuclease I*, which normally has got a tendency to degrade single stranded DNA, starting from the 3'-hydroxyl end, releasing deoxynucleoside -5'-monophosphates.

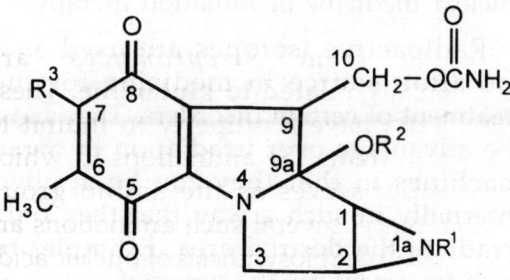

Fig 6.6 : Structures of

a. Mitomycin A where R^1=H, R^2=CH$_3$, R^3=H$_3$CO,

b. Mitomycin B where R^1=CH$_3$,R^2=H, R^3=H$_3$CO,

c. Mitomycin C where R^1=H,R^2=CH$_3$, R^3=NH$_2$

(e) *Hormonal agents:* **Major diseases responsive to hormonal therapy are carcinoma of the breast, prostate, uterine endometrium and thyroid.** Estrogens, androgens, progestins and thyroxine have been therapeutically used in certain types of cancers. Adrenal corticosteroids are unique in the form of hormonal treatment because they are also active against nonendocrine related tumors such as lymphomas and leukaemia.

Huggins, Charles Brenton (Canada/ U.S.A.) **a Surgeon was awarded Nobel Prize in Medicine in 1966 for his discoveries concerning hormonal treatment of prostatic cancer.** He for the first time demonstrated that the injection of a synthetic female sex hormone causes the disappearance of tumours in the prostate glands of males. He established the feasibility of hormonal therapy in the control of cancer. **He was a surgeon.**

(f) *Immunotherapy:* Since the host's immunologic system may be involved in the control of malignant processes, immunologic approaches to cancer are under active investigations.

Radiation therapy

Radiation therapy, like surgery, is a local modality used in the treatment of cancer. This type of therapy for most solid tumours involves the administration of ionising radiation in the form of x-rays or gamma rays to a tumour site. The term x-ray denotes high-energy electromagnetic radiation (4 to 25 MeV) produced by electron-level transitions within the atom.

X-rays are generated by instruments such as linear accelerators. **Gamma rays are also high energy radiation but are produced by radioactive isotope decay, typically from Cobalt-60, Cesium-137 or Radium-226.**

Although, there is no difference in the physical characteristics or biologic effects of x-rays and gamma rays, linear accelerators are more widely used and produce a more focussed beam with a smaller penumbra. Mega voltage x-rays are commonly used to irradiate internal, deep-seated lesions, since high-energy penetrating beams deliver a less intense superficial dose and spare the skin.

Radiation therapy is known to be mutagenic, carcinogenic and teratogenic and is associated with an increased risk of developing both secondary leukaemias and solid tumours.

Radionuclides

For decades, radionuclides have been used systematically to treat malignant disorders. They are administered by specialists in nuclear medicine or radiation therapy.

Radioactive isotopes are used as a radiation source in medicine for the treatment of certain disorders. They have the advantage over irradiation by x-ray machines in that they can be applied internally in such a way that they only irradiate the desired area. Examples of such treatment are the usage of :

(A) **Radioactive iodine (^{131}I) in the treatment of :**
   (i) Hyperthyroidism
   (ii) Certain cancers of the thyroid
   (iii) Certain cardiac diseases, e.g., intractable angina pectoris, congestive failure, and

Stages of Cancer	
Ist stage (generally ignored by the victim)	: Chances of cure are very good if detected in the begining
IInd stage	: Chances of cure are almost 60%
IIIrd stage	: Chances of cure are almost 20%
IVth stage	: Chances of cure are nil

(iv) Certain pulmonary diseases.

(B) **P^{32}-labelled sodium phosphate for the treatment of polycythemia vera and leukaemia.** ^{32}P concentrates in bone marrow and irradiates the dividing parent cells of the red and white cell lines.

Strontium-89 (^{89}Sr) is used for the treatment of bony metastases.

Diet

No specific diet or food factor or combination of food factors have so far been found to be carcinogenic. **There is some reason to think, however, that excessive caloric intake may be correlated with a somewhat increased incidence of cancer.** Scientist Strong points out that man and domestic animals are more prone to cancer than are the wild animals and suggests that one possible explanation for this is that man and domestic animals have a tendency to eat more than their counterparts i.e., wild animals.

Mutagens and antimutagens in foods

Early in 20th century, a **Dutch Botanist Hugo De Vries** noted sudden, heritable unusual changes in an otherwise fairly uniform population of a certain species of plant, for which he used the word **'mutation'**. These changes were found to take place during cell division. Substances

- Radioisotopes have been used as a radiation source for many purposes in Science and Industry.
- Industrial radiography is a prominent example where ^{192}Ir, ^{137}Cs and ^{60}Co are used for the inspection of steel products fabricated by welding. Defects permit penetration of the gamma rays and can be recorded on film.
- Radioisotopes are being used to produce luminescence. Alpha and beta sources are mixed with phosphorus to produce luminous signs and dials. Tritium has been of particular value in this use because of its weak beta emission and long half- life.
- Radioactive isotopes are being used for radiopasteurization and radiosterilization of foods. Radiopasteurization may extend the refrigerator shelf life of perishable foods. Generally food sterilisation requires 2 to 5 million rads. This amount of radiation plus suitable packaging will keep some foods sterile at room temperature for months. **Fifty to one hundred thousand rep will permit storage of apples for over one year.**

which can cause mutation are known as 'mutagens'. Risk of cancer is greater on exposure to these mutagens. There has been increasing awareness that exposure to environmental pollution due to indiscriminate use of a wide range of chemicals in agriculture and industrial pollutants can lead to genetic damage. The study of this science is known as genetic toxicology.

Mutagens in foods

Food is a complex commodity on which humans depend for their existence. Wyander (1975) estimated that 50% of cancer deaths in women and 30% in men are due to toxicants and natural chemicals present in our foods. Doll (1981) had estimated that 35% of cancer deaths are due to food toxicants. Hence, it is very important to evaluate the hazards caused by various environmental agents and to eliminate them.

Chemical components of foods get altered prior to ingestion, by processing like cooking or by storage or by the addition of certain food additives. The major components of foods which are known as mutagens are indicated below in Table 6.3.

Cereals, pulses, vegetables and fruits are amongst the several natural foods which are rich in a number of chemical compounds like flavonoids, alkaloids and furans. Some of these compounds are known mutagens. Lot of pesticides are used as post harvest preservatives of food commodities e.g., grapes are sprayed with suitable pesticide from being attacked by pests. Pesticides include herbicides, fungicides, etc. **These substances are toxic at certain levels and the suitable cleaning procedures should be followed before using such foods.** Similarly, materials used for packaging foods like milk, oil, etc., can also react with the material if they are acidic or the package material can pass out slowly into the food and contaminate it. Nitroso compounds and polycyclic aromatic hydrocarbons can be formed in foods by heating, smoking, curing the meat with nitrates and similar processes where high temperature is required to facilitate oxidation in free air. These processes like heating, boiling, deep fat frying, smoking, broiling, curing, irradiation of foods and solvent extraction of oils are the normal processes where these changes can take place resulting in the formation of mutagens.

We use lot of food additives like food colours in jams, marmalades, squashes, ice creams, and sweets for aesthetic reasons. There are some permitted food additives which have been tested for their safety. Some of the food colours in small quantities can also be mutagenic. Food flavours are also used similarly in food and more in paediatric drugs. Preservatives are used to prevent fungal growth and bacterial attack in the above food preparations. Artificial sweeteners like saccharin are used in many of the above preparations. Antioxidants are used in many preparations to prevent oxidation at high

Table 6.3: Classes of mutagens in foods

Natural food constituent	Food contaminants	Food additives	Mutagens generated by food processing	Mutagens generated by storage of food
Flavonoids	Pesticides	Food colours	Products of heating	Malonaldehyde
Furans	Package materials, solvents	Food flavours, preservatives, sweetners	Smoking, broiling (cooking on coal), curing	Mycotoxins, fumigation products
Alkaloids	Nitroso compounds, polycyclic aromatic hydrocarbons	Antioxidants, miscellaneous food additives	Irradiation, solvent extraction	

> Epidemiological studies have shown that vegetarians have lower risk of cancer than the non-vegetarians because of the fact that green coloured raw vegetables possess antimutagens and anticarcinogens in abundance which include methylated flavonoids, aromatic isothiocyanates, coumarins, plant sterols, protease inhibitors, ascorbic acid, tocopherols, retinols, etc. Scientist Wattenberg bas suggested that these compounds can certainly reduce the risk of cancer.
>
> Food processing involves high temperature, oxidation, polymerization and production of nitrosamines, polycyclic aromatic hydrocarbons, etc, which are injurious to health, therefore, as far as possible, **intake of processed foods should be discouraged.**

temperatures. The type of these chemical **"additives"** and the level of their usage have to be chosen with great care. Due to improper storage conditions, certain types of fungus can grow upon many cereals, oil seeds, and other food materials. The fungal metabolites are quite toxic and they can cause health hazards if they enter the food chain. Therefore, great care has to be taken to avoid these compounds in foods beyond their permitted limits.

Although, many carcinogens have been identified in the diet, only naturally occurring contaminants have been casually associated with cancer in humans. It has been clearly demonstrated that carcinogenic N-nitroso compounds may be formed within the body from non-carcinogenic precursors present in the diet.

Antimutagens in foods

Food contains some chemical components which have neither any nutritional property nor any role in the normal metabolic processes. These components are generally removed in the process of refining. Such compounds generally are fibres, polyphenols (which impart colour), saponins, lectins, tannins, coumarins, amines, flavonoids and anthocyanins. Recent studies revealed that most of these compounds have some beneficial effects like reducing blood cholesterol and triglycerides and other useful properties like antidiabetic, antifertility, anticarcinogenic, antiallergic, antimutagenic effects. **Wattenberg (1983) reported that foods contain large number of anticarcinogens and antimutagens, i.e., these compounds counteract the effect of carcinogens. The compounds are polyphenols, aromatic isoth-iocyanates, methylated flavonoids, coumarins, plant sterols, selenium salts, protease inhibitors, ascorbic acid, tocopherols and retinols which are known to inhibit cancer formation.**

Prevention of Cancer by Vegetarianism

Cancer, as everyone knows is the most dreadful disease of the day, the name of which causes so much panic in one's mind that it cannot be described in words.

Now, the scientists have reached the conclusion that special phytochemicals present in the vegetables/ fruits/spices, etc. have got the capability to prevent cancers which means we must understand the meaning of vegetarianism and must follow in one's life. It appears that **'Nature'** has already made certain arrangement to fight/prevent cancer, the follow-up of which is not being done satisfactorily by majority of us. Following Table 6.4 gives an account of anticancerous sources, phytochemical present in them etc.

Table 6.4 : Showing anticancerous sources, phytochemicals present etc.

Sl No.	Fruit/vegetable/ spices	Phytoche- mical present	Biochemical basis of action	Comments
1.	(i) Citrus fruits like orange, lemon, amla, malta, kino, etc. are rich in vitamin C, folate and fibres.	Limonin	Limonin increases the level of natural enzymes by increasing their synthe- sis which have got the capability to disintegrate the cancer causing substa- nces and then eliminates them from body.	(i) Various organs are protected from cancer.
	(ii) Cardamom and aniseed (saunf)	Limonin		(ii) Are also antic- ancerous
2.	Grapes (black grapes are richer in phenolics than the green).	(i) Allomic acid (ii) Flavonoids (especially phenolics)	Inhibit the enzymes which may otherwise help the biochemical reactions causing cancer.	(i) Various organs are protected (ii) In the countries where grapes- wine is used in abundance for e.g., France, incidence of heart ailments is less.
3.	Apple, strawberry, plum (Ber)	(i) Antioxidants (ii) Phenols (iii) Reveratol	–	(i) Various organs are protected. (ii) **Raveratol has got the property to control the level of bad cholesterol (LDL- cholesterol) as well in blood.**
4.	Watermelon	Carotenoids, especially cantalop	–	(i) Various organs are protected (ii) It also contains an anticoagulant named 'adenosine which protects from heart ailm- ents.
5.	Tomato, papaya, carrot, strawberry, apricot, etc.	(i) Vitamin 'C' (ii) Lycopene	Prevents biochemical changes of DNA of the cell.	Protects from the cancers of pros- tate glands, lungs, stomach, etc.
6.	Chillies	Capsenin	Checks the possible growth of gene by creating interruption which may be caused by the cancerous agents present in the smoke of cigarettes.	(i) Protects from the lung cancer (ii) **More bitter the chillies-more is the capsenin in them.**
7.	Garlic and onion	Alicin	(i) Increases the synthe- sis of enzymes which have got the capability	(i) Protects from the cancer of oesophagus

(Contd.)

		to disintegrate the cancerous substances (ii) Gives more energy to immune cells	(ii) Regular intake of garlic also protects from the cancer of anus as per the latest findings published in the American Journal of Clinical Nutrition. (iii) Regular intake of garlic also controls the level of cholesterol in blood. (iv) Garlic also contains antibiotics.
8.	Cauliflower, cabbage, radish, mustard	Indole-3-carbinol	Increases the synthesis of enzymes responsible for degrading cancerous substances	Protects from the cancer of stomach, lung and breasts
9.	Carrots	β-carotene		(i) Protects from the cancer of lungs, stomach (ii) Also lowers down the level of cholesterol in blood
10.	Soyabean, groundnut and germinating alfa-alfa	Genistin	Interrupts the blood supply to the cancerous cells.	(i) Estrogen hormone found in the females induces the cancerous cells whereas genistin protects from the cancer of breast and ovaries
11.	Spinach, fenugreek, green leaves of mustard, chaurai	(i) Leutein (ii) Geoxanthine		Protects from loss of eyesight and blindness as well
12.	Tea leaves (especially green leaves)	Polyphenols	(i) Antioxidant property (ii) Controls the multiplication of cancerous cells. (iii) Eliminates cancerous substances from the body	Protects from the cancer of oesophagus.

As we know, mutation mechanism is responsible for cancer, as a result of which several genes get altered unexpectedly without knowing the automatic changes in their DNA sequence.

Scientist Francis Barani (Weyl Medical College, Cornell University, U.S.A.) has prepared such a wonderful sensitive device which can recognise very easily and promptly the 'fast mutations' (cell division). This device can also predict that which type of mutation will give birth to cancer.

CHAPTER 7

EICOSANOIDS

(PROSTAGLANDINS, THROMBOXANES AND LEUKOTRIENES)

> We are C_{20} fatty acids derivatives having complicated structures and play numerous very important roles in the body like we help in controlling (i) blood pressure (ii) secretion of gastric HCl, (iii) inflammation (anti inflammatory agents), etc.

Arachidonic acid and some other C_{20} fatty acids with methylene-interrupted bonds give rise to eicosanoids which are physiologically and pharmacologically very active compounds and are known as **prostaglandins (PG), thromboxanes (TX),** and **leukotrienes (LT).**

Arachidonic acid which is usually derived from the 2nd position of phospholipids in the plasma membrane, as a result of phospholipase A_2 activity, is the substrate for the biosynthesis of the PG_2, TX_2, and LT_4 compounds. The pathway for the synthesis of prostaglandins and thromboxanes is known as a 'cyclooxygenase pathway' whereas the pathway for the synthesis of leukotrienes is known as a 'Lipooxygenase pathway' as shown in Figure 7.1.

The figure indicates various stimulants as well as inhibitors. **It also indicates as to why steroids, which inhibit total eicosanoids production, are better anti-** **inflammatory agents than aspirin like drugs which inhibit only the cyclooxygenase pathway.**

PROSTAGLANDINS (PG)

Prostaglandins may be defined as the compounds which are fatty acid derivatives with hormones like activities. They are in fact, unsaturated cyclic hydroxy fatty acids with a five membered ring in a 20 carbon skeleton. This group of hormone like substances was first of all detected in seminal fluid of man and other species, hence the name given as prostaglandins.

Prostaglandins are a group of naturally occurring substances having in common a structure which is based on prostanoic acid which contains 20 carbon atoms.

Sixteen naturally occurring prostaglandins have been described (Table 7.1), but only seven along with two

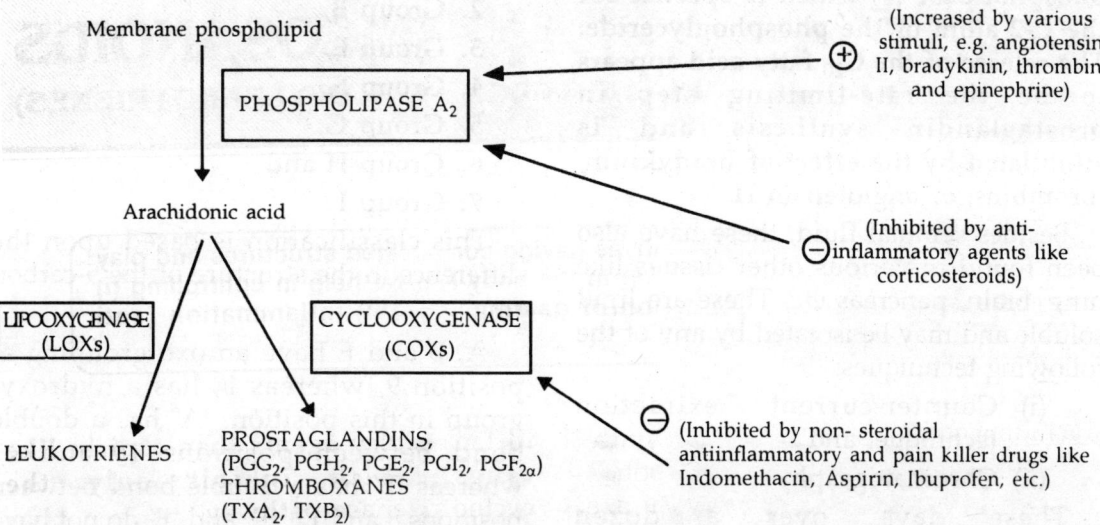

Prostanoic acid

Membrane phospholipid

PHOSPHOLIPASE A_2

(Increased by various stimuli, e.g. angiotensin II, bradykinin, thrombin, and epinephrine) ⊕

(Inhibited by anti-inflammatory agents like corticosteroids) ⊖

Arachidonic acid

LIPOOXYGENASE (LOXs)

CYCLOOXYGENASE (COXs)

(Inhibited by non-steroidal antiinflammatory and pain killer drugs like Indomethacin, Aspirin, Ibuprofen, etc.) ⊖

LEUKOTRIENES

PROSTAGLANDINS, (PGG_2, PGH_2, PGE_2, PGI_2, $PGF_{2\alpha}$) THROMBOXANES (TXA_2, TXB_2)

Fig. 7.1 : Conversion of archidonic acid to prostaglandins and thromboxanes via cyclooxygenase pathway and leukotrienes via lipooxygenase pathway

Although PGs appear **hormone like in action but they are different from** hormones in atleast two respects; they are synthesized at the site of action and made in almost all the tissues. **Linoleic acid** ($C_{18}:2^{9,12}$) is the precursor of two of the three 20- carbon fatty acids that form PGs; linolenic acid ($C_{18}:3^{9,12,15}$) is the other precursor. **Both these fatty acids are considered essential because they can not be synthesized in the body and therefore must be taken through diet.** The three C_{20} fatty acids subsequently formed are $C_{20}:3^{5,8,11}$ (eicosatrienoic acid), $C_{20}:4^{5,8,11,14}$ (eicosatetraenoic acid or **arachidonic acid),** and $C_{20}:5^{5,8,11,14,17}$ (eicosapentaenoic acid). These fatty acids form the PG_1, PG_2 and PG_3 series respectively.

Once formed, prostaglandins exert very short-lived effects and are catabolized rapidly (their half-life being expressed in seconds). Inactivation of prostaglandin appears to be mediated by two enzymes,

Table 7.1: Naturally occurring Prostaglandins

Primary PG	Other PG
PGE_1	PGA_1
$PGF_{1\alpha}$	PGA_2
PGE_2	19 α- OH PGA_1*
$PGF_{2\alpha}$	19 α- OH PGA_2**
PGG_2	PGB_1
PGH_2	PGB_2
PGI_2	19 α- OH PGB_2
Thromboxane A_2	PGE_3
Thromboxane B_2	$PGF_{3\alpha}$

* hydroxy-prostaglandin A,** hydroxy-prostaglandin B

thromboxanes are found commonly throughout the body. These are termed as the **primary prostaglandins.**

15α-hydroxy-prostaglandin dehydrogenase and Δ^{13}- prostaglandin reductase. **Prostaglandins are not stored; instead the precursor C_{20} fatty acids are present in tissues attached to the C-2 of phosphoglycerides. When needed, the C_{20} precursor is hydrolyzed by phospholipase A_2 which is specific for the C-2 atom of the phosphoglyceride. The release of the C_{20} fatty acid appears to be the rate-limiting step in prostaglandin synthesis and is stimulated by the effect of bradykinin, thrombins, or angiotensin II.**

Besides seminal fluid, these have also been found in various other tissues like lung, brain, pancreas etc. These are lipid soluble and may be isolated by any of the following techniques:

(i) Counter-current extraction technique, and

(ii) Chromatography

These days, over a dozen prostaglandins have been isolated from seminal plasma and sheep vesicular glands. They can be synthesized (Fig. 7.2) by the seminal vesicle from polyunsaturated fatty acids like arachidonic acid, linolenic acid, etc.

For convenience, they have been put into atleast seven categories, viz:

1. **Group A,**
2. **Group B,**
3. **Group E,**
4. **Group F,**
5. **Group G,**
6. **Group H and**
7. **Group I**

This classification is based upon the difference in the structure of the 5-carbon ring.

A, B and E have an oxo-grouping at position 9, whereas F, has a hydroxyl group in this position. 'A' has a double bond between positions 10 and 11 whereas 'B' has a double bond between positions 8 and 12. 'E' and 'F' do not have a double bond in the ring but possess a hydroxyl group at position 11. It has been

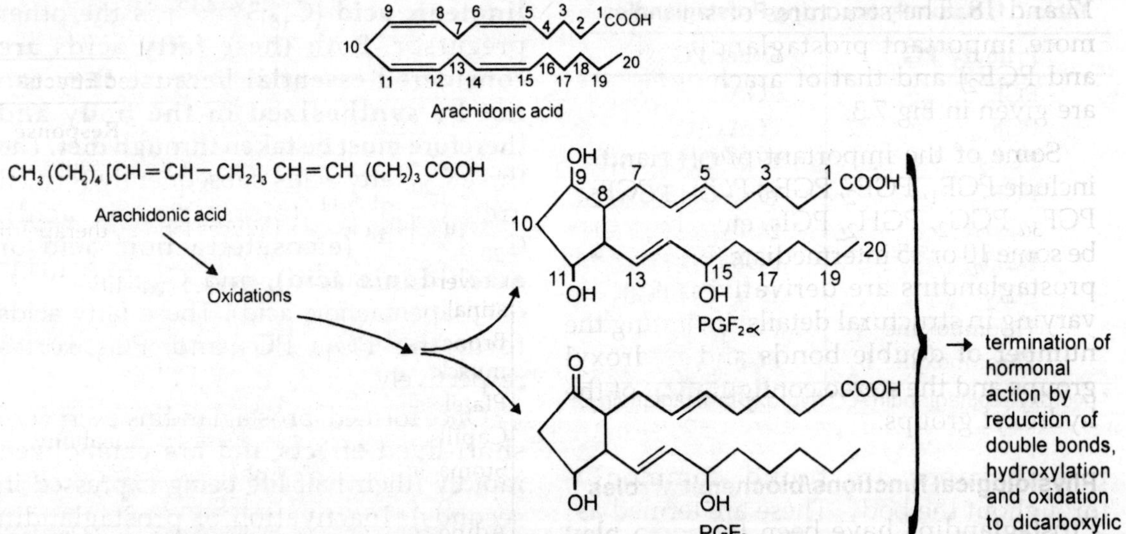

Arachidonic acid

$$CH_3 (CH_2)_4 [CH = CH - CH_2]_3 CH = CH (CH_2)_3 COOH$$

PGF$_{2\alpha}$

PGE$_2$

→ termination of hormonal action by reduction of double bonds, hydroxylation and oxidation to dicarboxylic acids

Fig. 7.2 : Biosynthesis of prostaglandins.

Bergstrom, Sune K (Sweden), a Chemist; Samuelsson, Bengt (Sweden), a Chemist and Van, Sir John R (UK), a Chemist were jointly awarded Nobel Prize in Medicine in 1982 for their discoveries concerning the biosynthesis, metabolism, etc of prostaglandins (PGF_2, PGF_{2a}, PGD_2, etc.), thromboxane A_2 prostacyclin and the leukotrienes and related biologically active substances. All are potent chemical transmitters of intercellular and intracellular signals that mediate a diversity of **physiological** and **pathological** functions. They all are formed from oxygenation of arachidonic acid, a 20 - carbon polyunsaturated fatty acid.

studied that all the active prostaglandins have got at least one double bond between positions 13 and 14; even some have two double bonds, the second being between positions 5 and 6 and finally some are found to have three double bonds; the additional bond being between positions 17 and 18. The structures of some of the more important prostaglandins ($PGF_{2\alpha}$ and PGE_2) and that of arachidonic acid are given in Fig 7.3.

Some of the important prostaglandins include PGE_1, PGE_2, PGE_3, $PGF_{1\alpha}$, $PGF_{2\alpha}$, $PGF_{3\alpha}$ PGG_2, PGH_2, PGI_2, etc. There may be some 10 or 15 intermediate forms. Other prostaglandins are derivatives of PGE_1, varying in structural details, including the number of double bonds and hydroxyl groups and the stereo configuration of the hydroxyl groups.

Physiological functions/biochemical roles

Prostaglandins have been found to play following important roles in the human body (Table 7.2):

(i) They exert profound effects in facilitating fertilization of the ovum by causing uterine and cervical movements that help in the movement of the spermatozoa from the vagina into the cervix and uterus. In this way, they are believed to stimulate the smooth muscle of the uterus, particularly at the time of ovulation.

(ii) They help in controlling blood pressure.

(iii) Infertility in males has been found to be associated with low levels of seminal prostaglandins in some cases; whereas high levels of the same have been noticed in the amniotic fluid of those women who have a tendency of premature abortion.

(iv) Prostaglandins are believed to inhibit lipolysis in adipose tissue, possibly by inhibiting the conversion of ATP to cyclic

Table 7.2 : Prostaglandin-Mediated Effects	
Site of Action	**Physiological Response**
Arterial smooth muscle	Alters blood pressure
Uterine muscle	Induces labour, therapeutic abortion
Lower gastrointestinal tract	Increases motility
Bronchial smooth muscle	Induces bronchospasm
Platelets	Increases coagulability
Capillaries	Increases permeability
Stomach	Enhances gastric acid secretion
Adipose tissue	Inhibits triglyceride lipolysis

AMP. Prostaglandins, thus, have the opposite effect of epinephrine, norepinephrine, glucagon and ACTH on the release of fatty acids from adipose tissue.

(v) **They also appear to control the secretion of gastric hydrochloric acid, the excess of which may otherwise cause gastric ulcers.**

(vi) They antagonize the action of catecholamines, in general.

(vii) They are also being extensively used as **abortificants** in some countries as they have got a tendency to induce abortions. The use of PGE_2 and $PGE_{2\alpha}$ are under extensive clinical trials in countries like Sweden, U.K., U.S., Uganda, etc., that is to say they help preventing conceptions.

(viii) Their exact role in human reproduction is still uncertain.

(ix) They give relief in **asthma** and **nasal congestion.**

(ix) **They help in controlling the** **inflammation.**

THROMBOXANES

These are synthesized in platelets and when released are responsible for vasoconstriction and platelet aggregation. They are of different types like TXA and TXB etc. Structures of some important thromboxanes are as given in Fig. 7.3.

LEUKOTRIENES

These are arachidonic acid metabolites. When these are conjugated to glutathione, then they are termed as peptidoleukotrienes. These are abbreviated as LT, thus LTC_3 denotes leukotriene C_3. These are of various types like LTA, LTB, LTC, LTD etc. Structure of LTB_4 is as shown in Fig. 7.4.

Functions/Importance

(i) They are responsible for the causation of **vascular permeability.**

(ii) They are also responsible for the attraction and activation of leukocytes.

(iii) They appear to be important

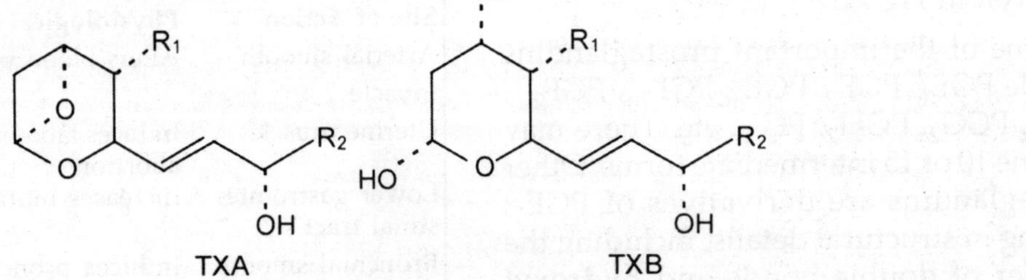

Fig 7.3: Structures of thromboxanes (TXA & TXB)

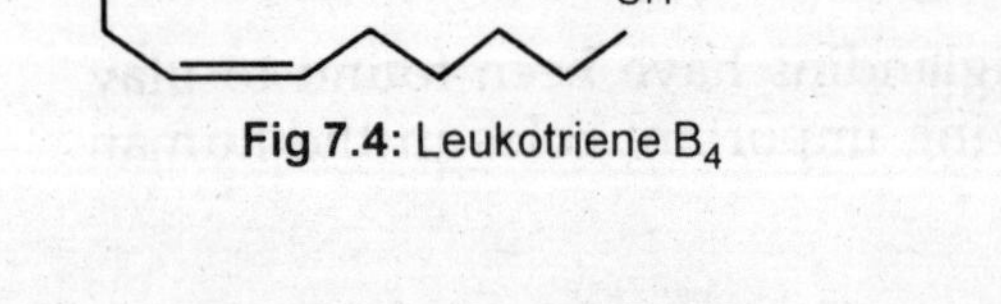

Fig 7.4: Leukotriene B_4

regulators in many diseases which involve inflammation or

immediate hypersensitivity reactions, such as asthma.

Nonsteroidal anti-inflammatory drugs (NSAIDs), such as aspirin, ibuprofen, and indomethacin, inhibit the COXs, thereby decreasing prostaglandins synthesis. **Two isoforms of COX are known as COX-1 and COX-2. COX-1 level is in general rather constant in cells, whereas COX-2 is synthesized in response of inflammation. Certain drugs that inhibit both COXs have nephrotoxic and ulcerogenic side effects.** Therefore, new NSAIDs are being tested to inhibit preferentially COX-2 to reduce side effects while maintaining the desirable anti-inflammatory therapy.

Prostaglandin I_2, or prostacyclin, is derived from arachidonic acid in the vascular endothelium. It has a powerful vasodilatory action, especially on the coronary arteries, and also is responsible for inhibiting platelet aggregation.

Thromboxane A_2 is synthesized from arachidonic acid but also is produced by platelets. It has the opposite effect of prostacylin; that is, it stimulates the contraction of arterial smooth muscle and enhances platelet aggregation. It has a very short half-life, about 30 seconds, and is converted rapidly to its inactive metabolite thromboxane B_2. The thromboxanes are slightly different from the other prostaglandins in that they contain six sided rings of five carbon atoms and one oxygen atom (Figure 7.4). Table 7.2 lists some of the reported functions of the various prostaglandins. With the increasing knowledge of the physiological role of the prostaglandins, discrete disorders of prostaglandin metabolism are likely to be discovered, and prostaglandins, prostaglandin analogues, or prostaglandin antagonists are likely to be used in clinical practice.

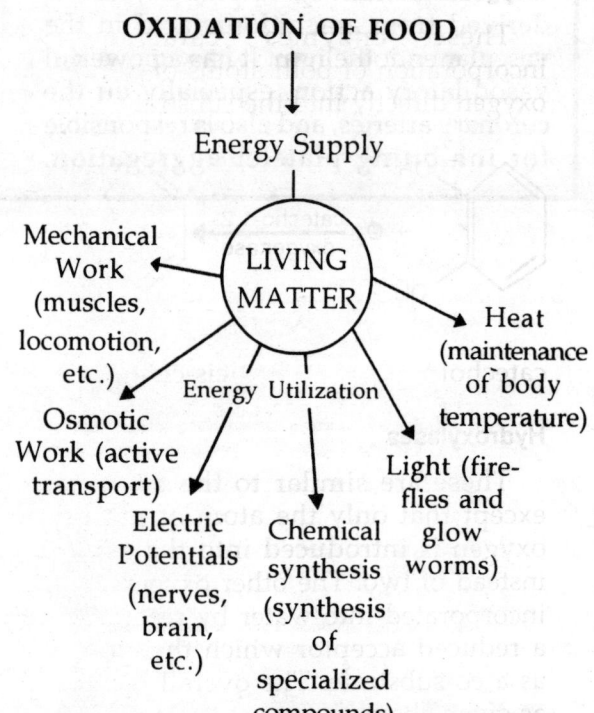

CHAPTER 8

BIOENERGETICS/BIOLOGICAL OXIDATIONS

> We are the chemical reactions of paramount importance to the living matter where we supply energy for various types of works like mechanical work (muscles, locomotion, etc.), osmotic work, electric potentials, chemical synthesis, light, heat maintenance, etc.

THE OXIDOREDUCTASE

Living organisms require continuous nonstop supply of energy to carry out different types of functions of living matter (Fig. 8.1). In most of the cases, the energy is obtained by the oxidation of metabolites which are formed from the digestion of food. There are three ways by which such oxidations can take place. All the ways are basically the same and involve the loss of electrons from the compound being oxidized (Fig. 8.2).

The enzymes responsible for biological oxidation are classified in group 1, the oxidoreductases. Trivial names are still used for enzymes in this group which are as considered below in brief:

Oxygenases and Hydroxylases

A few metabolites are oxidized by the direct addition of molecular oxygen, but this is the exception rather than the rule

OXIDATION OF FOOD

Energy Supply

Mechanical Work (muscles, locomotion, etc.)

LIVING MATTER

Energy Utilization

Osmotic Work (active transport)

Electric Potentials (nerves, brain, etc.)

Chemical synthesis (synthesis of specialized compounds)

Heat (maintenance of body temperature)

Light (fire-flies and glow worms)

Fig. 8.1: Energy turnover in living organisms

Addition of Oxygen

$$CH_3CHO + \tfrac{1}{2}O_2 \longrightarrow CH_3COOH$$

acetaldehyde   acetic acid

Removal of Hydrogen

$$\begin{array}{ccc}
CH(OH).COOH & & CO.COOH \\
| & \longrightarrow & | \qquad +2H \\
CH_2COOH & & CH_2COOH \\
\text{malic acid} & & \text{oxaloacetic acid}
\end{array}$$

(H to acceptor)

Removal of Electrons

Cytochrome (Fe^{++})

↓

Cytochrome (Fe^{+++}) + Electron (to acceptor)

Fig. 8.2 Methods of Biological Oxidation

for biological oxidations.

Oxygenases

These enzymes catalyse the incorporation of both atoms of molecular oxygen directly into the substrate.

catechol   cis-cis-muconate

Hydroxylases

These are similar to the oxygenases except that only the atom of molecular oxygen is introduced into the substrate instead of two. The other oxygen atom is incorporated into water by reaction with a reduced acceptor which therefore acts as a co-substrate. The overall reaction is as given above:

aniline + NADPH + H$^+$ + O$_2$

aryl-4-hydroxylase

p- hydroxyaniline + NADP$^+$ + H$_2$O

Dehydrogenases and Oxidases

Nearly all biological oxidations take place by the removal of hydrogen from the substrate. Hydrogen atoms are removed from a metabolite (AH$_2$) and passed on to an acceptor (B).

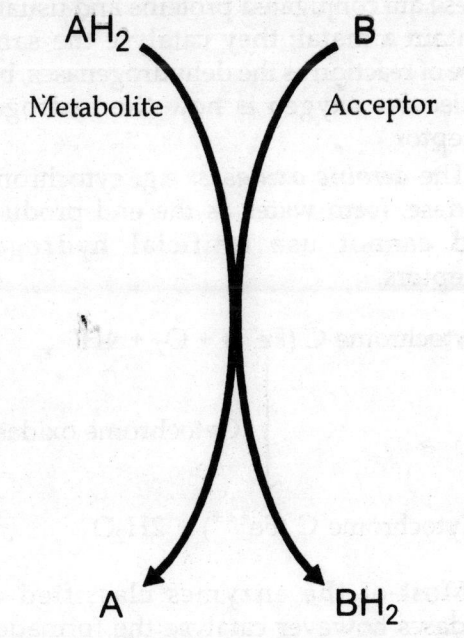

AH$_2$ B

Metabolite   Acceptor

A   BH$_2$

Oxidized metabolite   Reduced acceptor

Dehydrogenases

If the acceptor is not molecular oxygen, then the enzymes are known as **dehydrogenases**. For the purpose of studying a dehydrogenase catalysed reaction in the laboratory, artificial hydrogen acceptors can be used instead of the 'natural' coenzymes of the cell.

$CH_3CH (OH) CH_2COOH + NAD^+$
D-3 hydroxybutyrate

$\updownarrow$ 3-hydroxybutyrate dehydrogenase

$CH_3CO.CH_2COOH + NADH + H^+$
acetoacetate

Oxidases

These are conjugated proteins and usually contain a metal; they catalyse the same type of reaction as the dehydrogenases, but molecular oxygen is now the hydrogen acceptor.

The *aerobic oxidases:* e.g. cytochrome oxidase, form water as the end product. and cannot use artificial hydrogen acceptors.

$4 \text{ cytochrome C (Fe}^{++}) + O_2 + 4H^+$

$\downarrow$ Cytochrome oxidase

$4 \text{ Cytochrome C (Fe}^{+++}) + 2H_2O$

Most of the enzymes classified as oxidases however catalyse the formation of hydrogen peroxide and *not* water. These oxidases are also known as *aerobic dehydrogenases* which can utilize artificial

$RCH_2NH_2 + H_2O + O_2$
primary amine

$\downarrow$ Monoamine oxidase

$R.CHO + NH_3 + H_2O_2$
aldehyde

hydrogen acceptors instead of molecular oxygen. Monoamine oxidase, for instance, catalyses the oxidation of a number of primary, secondary and tertiary amines.

Reductases

Oxidative reactions involving the removal of electrons but *not* hydrogen ions *from* the substrate are catalysed by enzymes which are known as **reductases**. Some plants and micro-organisms are known *to* contain an enzyme which catalyses the reduction of nitrate.

$-NO_3^- + NADH + H^+$

$\updownarrow$ Nitrate reductase

$-NO_2^- + NAD^+ + H_2O$

Catalase and peroxidase

Hydrogen peroxide formed by the catalytic action of the **aerobic dehydrogenases** is highly toxic to living cells but does not accumulate due to the rapid action of catalase or a peroxidase. Catalase is found in both the animals and the plants, whereas peroxidases are found in plants only.

$$2H_2O_2 \xrightarrow{\text{Catalase}} 2H_2O + O_2$$

$$\underset{\text{donor}}{AH_2} + \underset{\text{peroxide}}{H_2O_2} \xrightarrow{\text{Peroxidase}} 2H_2O + \underset{\text{oxidized donor}}{\bar{A}}$$

ELECTRON TRANSPORT CHAIN (RESPIRATORY CHAIN)

Components of the Chain
Pyridine nucleotides

Dehydrogenase enzymes cannot catalyse the removal of hydrogen from a substrate unless low molecular weight cofactors are also present to act as hydrogen acceptors. The compounds that are most frequently found as coenzymes for dehydrogenases are the two pyridine nucleotides, nicotinamide adenine dinucleotide (NAD) and nicotinamide adenine dinucleotide phosphate (NADP); both are freely soluble. These have a typical nucleotide type of structure, as given below:

Nicotinamide—D—ribofuranose-phosphate
|
Adenine—D—riboturanose-phosphate

Nicotinamide adenine dinucleotide (NAD)

The nicotinamide part of the molecule is only involved in the reaction, therefore, the structure can be simplified to ;

$$NAD^+ \text{ or } NADP^+$$ —CONH$_2$

N$^+$
|
R

Nicotinamide

where R represents the rest of the molecule. Work with isotopes has revealed that the hydrogen atoms from the substrate

HC—C-CONH$_2$ + 2H $\rightleftharpoons$ HC—C-CONH$_2$ + H$^+$

NAD$^+$
(oxidized form)

NADH
(reduced form)

add on the 1 and 4 positions of the nicotinamide ring but, at neutral pH, the hydrogen at position 1 dissociates as an hydrogen ion.

This reaction is usually abbreviated as :

$$NAD + 2H \rightleftharpoons NADH_2$$

or

$$NAD^+ + 2H \rightleftharpoons NADH + H^+$$

Flavoproteins

Another major group of reversible hydrogen acceptors are the flavoproteins, which consist of a protein moiety and a prosthetic group containing riboflavin. These compounds are often called nucleotides although the sugar component linked to the isoalloxazine ring is present as the alcohol ribitol and not the sugar ribose, and the link between base and 'sugar' is not glycosidic. The two flavin prosthetic groups are flavin mononucleotide (FMN) and flavin adenine dinucleotide (FAD).

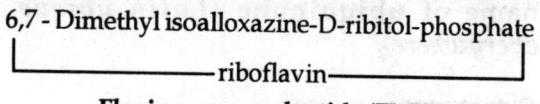

6,7 - Dimethyl isoalloxazine-D-ribitol-phosphate
|_____riboflavin_____|

Flavin mononucleotide (FMN)

6,7 - Dimethyl-isoalloxazine- D-ribitol-phosphate
|
Adenine-D-ribose-phosphate

Flavin adenine dinucleotide (FAD)

The hydrogen atoms react with the isoalloxazine part of the molecule so that the prosthetic groups, can be conveniently represented as shown below where R is the rest of the molecule.

Coenzyme Q

An important part of the chain of compounds involved in cellular respiration

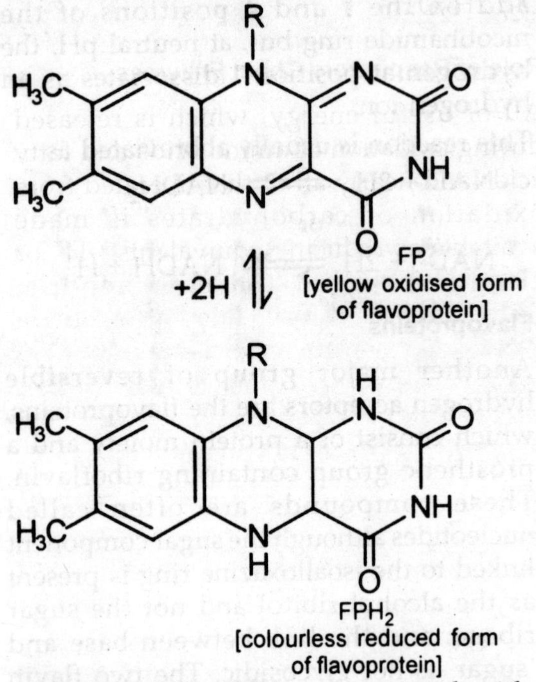

FP
[yellow oxidised form
of flavoprotein]

+2H

FPH$_2$
[colourless reduced form
of flavoprotein]

is coenzyme Q, which is associated with the lipoprotein part of the mitochondria. Coenzyme Q is found widely in living materials and has therefore been given the name of **ubiquinone** (*Latin ubique, everywhere*).

Cytochromes

The word cytochrome means cellular pigment, and the name is derived from the

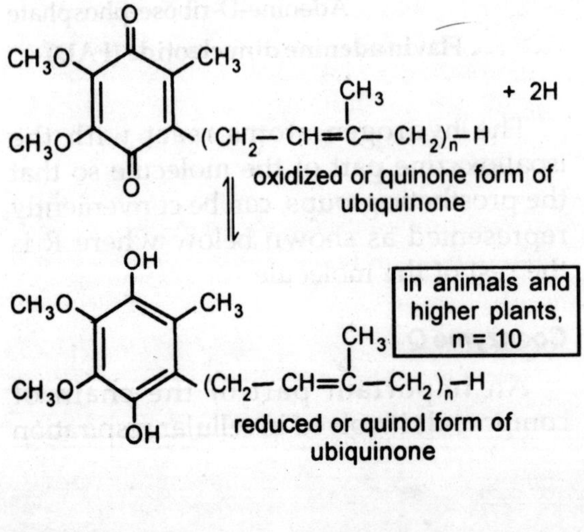

oxidized or quinone form of ubiquinone

in animals and higher plants, n = 10

reduced or quinol form of ubiquinone

fact that all living cells exhibit characteristic absorption bands in the visible region of the spectrum due to these iron porphyrin compounds. The cytochromes are redox catalysts of major importance in cellular respiration. Unlike the compounds previously considered, they act by reversibly donating and accepting electrons, not hydrogen atoms. Electrons are transported by the haem iron which undergoes a change of valency in the process.

Cytochrome (Fe^{+++}) + e $\rightleftharpoons$ Cytochrome (Fe^{++})
Oxidized form   Electron   Reduced form

Cytochromes were first discovered by McMunn in 1886, then rediscovered by Keilin in 1925. On the basis of spectroscopic data, Keilin demonstrated the existence of three cytochromes designated a, b and c and later cytochrome d was also discovered. Classification of a cytochrome into one of these 4 groups is on the basis of the absorption spectra of the haem prosthetic group and certain chemical properties.

In the mitochondria, cytochromes act together as a coordinated system for electron transfer. Most cytochromes are intimately associated with the membranes and are extremely difficult to isolate. Cytochrome c, a low molecular weight protein (12,000) with one atom of iron per molecule, is the only cytochrome which is readily soluble.

The Function of the Chain

Formation of water

In the mitochondria, above compounds, i.e, pyridine nucleotides, flavoproteins, coenzyme Q (ubiquinone) and cytochromes act together as an integrated chain during biological oxidations. This sequence of redox compounds is known as the electron transport chain or respiratory chain. Reducing equivalents from most metabolites are transferred to NAD, pass down the chain and finally react with molecular oxygen to form water (Fig. 8.3). The first part of the chain involves the transfer of a pair of hydrogen atoms, while the cytochromes transfer only a single electron.

Water is probably formed from H^+ discharged at the CoQ-Cyt b step and OH^- arising from the reaction of molecular oxygen with cytochrome a_3.

$$CoQ.2H + 2Cyt.b^{+++} \rightarrow 2\,Cyt.b^{++} + 2H^+ + CoQ$$
$$\downarrow$$
$$2H_2O$$
$$\uparrow$$
$$2Cyt.a_3^{++} + \tfrac{1}{2}O_2 + HOH \rightarrow 2Cyt.a_3^{+++} + 2OH^-$$

Arrangement of components of the chain

The major components of the respiratory chain are arranged sequentially in order of increasing redox potentials (Table 8.1).

Hydrogen or electron flows through the chain in a *step-wise manner from the more electro-negative components to the more electro-positive oxygen* through a redox span of 1.1 volts from NAD/NADH to

Table 8.1: Some redox potentials in oxidation systems

System	Eo' volts
H^+/N_2	- 0.42
$NAD^+/NADH$	- 0.32
Flavoprotein-old yellow enzyme, ox/red	- 0.12
Cytochrome b; Fe^{+++}/Fe^{++}	+ 0.08
Ubiquinone; ox/red	+ 0.10
Cytochrome c; Fe^{+++}/Fe^{++}	+ 0.22
Cytochrome a; Fe^{+++}/Fe^{++}	+ 0.29
Oxygen/Water	+ 0.82

$O_2/2H_2O$.

Role of Respiratory Chain Enzymes

All of useful energy, which is released during oxidation of amino acids and fatty acids and nearly all of that liberated from oxidation of carbohydrates is made available as reducing equivalents ($-H^+$ or electrons) within the mitochondria. **Mitochondria are well known to contain various key enzymes which are important for the energy production (as shown ahead in 1st Box). These enzymes perform various important functions such as :**

(i) **collection and transport of reducing equivalents,**

(ii) **trapping the liberated free energy as high energy phosphates, and**

(iii) **production of most of reducing equivalents in earlier stages i.e. β-oxidation and citric acid cycle (TCA Cycle).**

OXIDATIVE PHOSPHORYLATION

Introduction

At first sight, the chain appears to be a rather complicated way of producing water, but this sequence of carriers has a more important function than that.

The transfer of hydrogen from a substrate (AH_2) to NAD generally involves a relatively small change in free energy:

$$AH_2 + NAD^+ \rightleftharpoons A + NADH + H^+$$
$$\Delta G \text{ small}$$

The oxidation of reduced coenzyme by molecular oxygen however releases a large amount of energy:

$$NADH + H^+ + \tfrac{1}{2}O_2 \rightleftharpoons NAD^+ + H_2O$$
$$\Delta G = -52 \text{ kcal}$$

The release of this energy does not take

place in one step, as suggested by the overall equation, but in a series of different stages. This is the difference between stepping out of a first floor window to reach the ground and going down the stairs; the overall energy change is the same in both cases, but using the stairs is less traumatic and also more reversible. In the electron transport chain, the energy is not only released in different steps but at certain points is converted into a form which can be used by cell. **Adenosine triphosphate (ATP) is the** *'energy currency'* **of the cell** and the formation of 1 mol from ADP and inorganic phosphate (P_i) requires 7.5 kcal.

$$ADP + Pi \rightarrow ATP + H_2O$$

$$\Delta G = + 7.5 \text{ kcal}$$

At certain points in the chain, enough energy is available to form ATP and 3 molecules of this compound are believed to be formed for each pair of hydrogen atoms oxidized. The means whereby this is accomplished are, to say the least, obscure but some form of **'coupling'** exists between oxidation and the phosphorylation of ADP. In the case of dehydrogenases with NAD as coenzyme, 3 molecules of phosphate (P) are incorporated into ATP for each atom of oxygen (O) utilized, so that a P/O ratio of 3 is obtained. Some substrates such as succinate and fatty acyl CoA react directly with flavoproteins and therefore bypass the step involving NAD; in these cases, a P/O ratio of 2 is found (Fig. 8.3).

Definition

The oxidation of a substrate with accompanying phosphorylation of ADP to ATP is known as oxidative *phosphorylation.* This process takes place in mitochondria as the enzymes concerned with **"Citric acid cycle"** are located in the

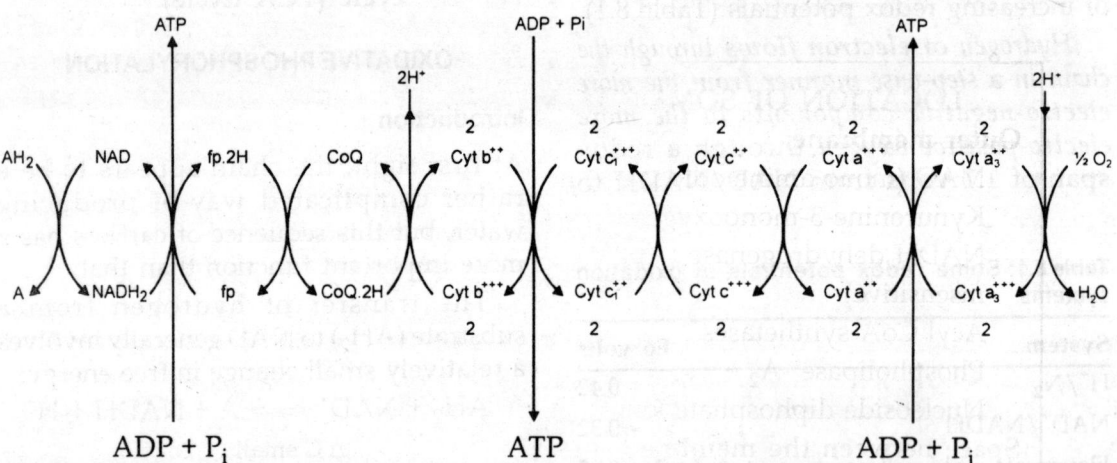

AH$_2$ = most substrates
ATP = adenosine triphosphate
NAD = nicotinamide adenine dinucleotide
ADP = adenosine diphosphate

fp = flavoproteins
Pi = inorganic phosphate
Cyt = cytochromes

Fig. 8.3 : The electron transport chain

space between the cristae and the enzymes concerned with **"electron transport"** (Fig 8.3) are arranged in an appropriate pattern in cristae themselves.

Biomedical Importance

Oxidative phosphorylation is fundamental to all *aspects of cellular life* in *aerobic organisms since it is their main source of useful energy.* It enables aerobic organisms to capture a far greater proportion of available free energy of respiratory substrates compared with anaerobic organisms. **A number of inherited defects of mitochondria which invade the components of respiratory chain and oxidative phosphorylation are responsible for several disorders in men like myopathy, encephalopathy and often lactacidosis too.**

Agents affecting Oxidative Phosphorylation

There are various chemical agents which affect the oxidative phosphorylation. Broadly, they are divided into three categories:-

1. **Uncoupling agents**
2. **Inhibitors**
3. **Ionophores**

Uncoupling agents

These agents allow electron-transport to continue but prevent the phosphorylation of ADP to ATP, that is, they uncouple energy yielding from the energy conserving reactions. The very first uncoupling agent to be described by W.F. Loomis and F. Lipmann in 1948 was 2-4 Dinitrophenol (DNP).

Inhibitors

These agents prevent both stimulation of oxygen consumption by ADP and phosphorylation of ADP to ATP. The *antibiotic oligomycin*, whose action for the first time was described by H.A. Lardy and his colleagues, *is the prototype of this class.*

LOCATION OF SOME ENZYMES IN RAT LIVER MITOCHONDRIA

Outer membrane
    MAO (mono amine odidase)
    Kynurenine-3-monooxygenase
    NADH dehydrogenase (Antimycin insensitive)
    Acyl CoA synthetases
    Phospholipase A_2
    Nucleoside diphosphate kinase

Space between the membranes
    Adenylate kinase

Inner membrane
    NADH dehydrogenase (Antimycin sensitive)
    Iron-sulphur proteins

Cytochrome b, c, c_1 and a a_3
F_1 ATPase
Succinate dehydrogenase
D-β Hydroxybutyrate dehydrogenase
Carnitine acyl transferase

Matrix
    Citrate synthetase
    Isocitrate dehydrogenase
    Fumarase
    Malate dehydrogemse
    Glutamate dehydrogenase
    Asparate transaminase
    Fatty acyl-CoA oxidation enzyme

TYPES OF AGENTS AFFECTING OXIDATIVE PHOSPHORYLATION

Uncoupling agents

2, 4-Dinitrophenol

Dicumarol

Carbonylcyanide phenylhydrazone

Salicylanilides

Arsenate

Inhibitors of ATP formation

Oligomycin

Rutamycin

Aurovertin

Triethyltin

Ionophores (Carriers of cations)

Valinomycin

Gramicidin

Nonactin

Nigericin

Ionophores

These agents cause breakdown of high energy intermediate state only if certain monovalent cations are present. The *prototype of this group is the antibiotic Valinomycin* which requires K^+ for its inhibitory effect, other agents include *Nigericin* and *Nonactin.*

Mechanism of Oxidative Phosphorylation

(Formation of ATP by Oxidative Phosphorylation)

Despite all the complexities of (a) glycolysis, (b) citric acid cycle, (c) dehydrogenation and (d) decarboxylation, only small amounts of ATP (two ATP molecules in glycolysis and another two ATP molecules in the citric acid cycle) are formed during all these processes. Instead 90 per cent of the total ATP formed by glucose metabolism is formed during subsequent oxidation of the hydrogen atoms that are released during these earlier stages of glucose degradation. Truly speaking, the main function of all these earlier stages is to make the hydrogen of the glucose molecule in forms that can be utilized for oxidation.

Oxidation of hydrogen is completed by a series of enzymatically catalyzed reactions in the mitochondria which (a) split each hydrogen atom into a hydrogen ion and an electron i.e., $H \rightarrow H^+ + e^-$, and (b) use the electrons finally to change the dissolved oxygen of the fluids into hydroxyl ions, i.e.

$O_2 \longrightarrow OH^-$. Then the hydrogen and hydroxyl ions combine with each other to form water i.e., $H^+ + OH^- \longrightarrow H_2O$. During the sequence of oxidative reactions, large amount of energy is released to form ATP. Formation of ATP in this way is called *'oxidative phosphorylation'.* This occurs exclusively in the mitochondria by a highly specialized process called the *'chemiosmotic mechanism.*

In all there are three hypotheses regarding the mechanism of oxidative phosphorylation:

(i) **Chemical coupling hypothesis**

(ii) **Conformational coupling hypothesis**

(iii) **Chemiosmotic hypothesis**

Chemical Coupling Hypothesis

It proposes that electron transport is coupled to ATP synthesis by a sequence of consecutive reactions in which a high energy covalent intermediate is formed by electron transport and subsequently is cleaved and donates its energy to generate ATP.

Conformational Coupling Hypothesis

It postulates that the transfer of electrons along the respiratory chain causes a conformational change in protein components of inner membrane to yield a high-energy form. The conformational change so produced is transmitted to the F_0F_1 ATPase molecule, causing it to become energized. Relaxation of the energized F_0F_1 ATPase to its normal conformation has proposed to provide energy for the synthesis of ATP and its release from the enzyme.

Chemiosmotic Hypothesis

It was for the first time proposed by the *British Biochemist* named *Peter Mitchell*, which postulates that 'electron transport' pumps H^+ form the matrix across the inner mitochondrial membrane to the outer aqueous phase, thus generating a H^+ gradient across the inner membrane. The osmotic energy inherent in its gradient was postulated to drive the energy requiring synthesis of ATP.

This mechanism mainly involves the following three important stages:

   (i) **Ionization of Hydrogen,**

   (ii) **Electron Transport Chain, and**

   (iii) **Formation of Water**

The first step in the oxidative phosphorylation in the mitochondria is to ionize the hydrogen atoms that are removed from the food substrates. These hydrogen atoms are removed in pairs; one immediately becomes a hydrogen ion, H^+, and the other combines with NAD^+ to produce NADH. The upper portion of Figure 8.4 reveals the subsequent fate of the NADH and H^+. The initial effect is to release the other hydrogen atom bound with NAD to form another hydrogen ion, H^+; this process also re-forms NAD^+ that will be reused again and again.

Now, the electrons that are removed from the hydrogen atoms to cause the ionization immediately enter an *electron transport chain* (ETC) which is an integral part of the inner membrane of the mitochondria. This transport chain (Fig. 8.4) consists of a series of electron acceptors which can be reversibly reduced or oxidized by accepting or giving up electrons. The important members of this ETC include flavoprotein, several iron sulfide proteins, ubiquinone and the cytochromes B, C_1, C, A and A_3. Each electron gets shuttled from one of these acceptors to the next until it finally reaches cytochrome A_3, **which is called** *cytochrome oxidase* because it is capable, by giving up two electrons, of causing elemental oxygen to combine with hydrogen ions to form water.

Figures 8.3 and 8.4 illustrate transport of electrons through the electron chain and then ultimate use of these electrons by *cytochrome oxidase* to cause the formation of water molecules. During the transport of these electrons through the electron transport chain, energy is released which is later on used for the generation of ATP.

Pumping of Hydrogen ions into the outer chamber of the mitochondrion is caused by the Electron Transport Chain. **As the electrons pass through the ETC,** large amount of energy is released which is eventually used to pump hydrogen ions from the inner

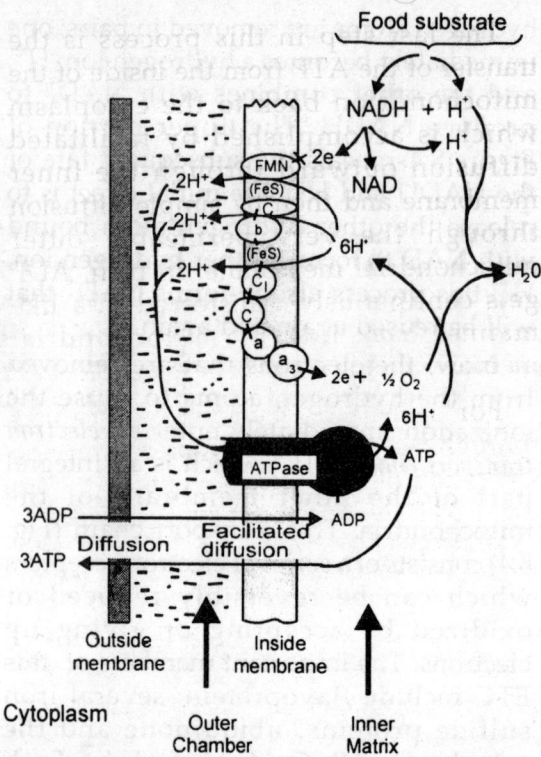

Fig. 8.4: The chemiosmotic theory of oxidative phosphorylation for the generation of large amount of ATP.

Central role of transmembrane gradient of H^+ in providing energy for different cell activities :

ΔH^+ membrane gradient

- **ATP synthesis**
- **Transport of Ca^{++}**
- **Transport of PO_4**
- **Transport of ADP and ATP**
- **Heat**
- **Rotation of bacteria flagella**

matrix of the mitochondrion into the outer chamber between the inner and outer mitochondrial membranes. This creates a high concentration of hydrogen ions in this chamber; besides, it also creates a strong negative electrical potential in the inner matrix.

Generation of ATP

The next step in the oxidative phosphorylation is to convert ADP into ATP, which occurs in the large protein molecule that protrudes all the way through the inner mitochondrial

---

SUBSTRATE LEVEL PHOSPHORYLATION

In addition to oxidative phosphorylation, some ATP is produced in direct association within the individual steps of certain metabolic pathways. The process of transfer of a phosphate group from a very high energy phophate donor to ADP is called **substrate level phosphorylation,** To cite few examples;

(i) The enzyme phosphoglycerate kinase acts on 1, 3-diphosphoglyceric acid resulting in the synthesis of ATP and formation of 3-phosphoglyceric acid **(step of glycolysis)**. This step is a good example of **substrate level** phosphorylation; since ATP is synthesized from the substrate without the involvement of electron transport chain. Phosphoglycerate kinase reaction is reversible, a rare example among the kinase reactions.

(ii) The enzyme pyruvate kinase catalyses the transfer of high energy phosphate from phosphoenolpyruvate to ADP, leading to the formation of ATP **(step of glycolysis)**. This step is another example of **substrate level phosphorylation. This reaction is irreversible.**

membrane and projects with a knob like head into the inner matrix. This protein molecule is known as ATPase (Fig 8.4), which is also called as ATP synthetase. It is believed that the high concentration of hydrogen ions in the outer chamber and the large electrical potential difference across the inner membrane are responsible for the flow of hydrogen ions into the mitrochondrial matrix through the substance of the ATPase molecule. In doing so, energy derived from the hydrogen ion flow is utilized by the ATPase to convert ADP into ATP in the presence of inorganic phosphate (Pi), thus forming an additional high energy phosphate bond.

The last step in this process is the transfer of the ATP from the inside of the mitochondrion back to the cytoplasm which is accomplished by facilitated diffusion outward through the inner membrane and then by simple diffusion through the very permeable outer mitochondrial membrane. In turn, ADP gets continuously transferred in a like manner back into the mitochondrial matrix for continuous conversion into ATP

For each two electrons which pass through the entire ETC (representing the ionization of two hydrogen atoms), upto three ATP molecules get synthesized.

Plasma

CHAPTER 9

VASCULAR SYSTEM (CHEMISTRY OF BLOOD)

I play ever very important functions in humans and animals; out of the
numerous important functions, the first important is to supply the nutrients
to the cells and the second one is to remove the endproducts of metabolism.
Whereas, the third main function is to transport hormones between tissues
and organs.

Donation of mine saves lives. I can so far be replaced by myself only, that's
why it is said that donation of mine is the ever greatest donation. Scientists
have so far not been able to synthesize me as such but are still trying hard
for the same. The day I am synthesized commercially shall be a breakthrough
revolutionary day in 'science'.

Vascular system by and large means the
blood, its chemistry, functions, etc.

Sugars, amino acids, fats, vitamins and
hormones are transported by the fluid part
of blood i.e. *plasma*. Some end-products of
metabolism, such as H_2O, CO_2 and urea
are also transported by plasma. Oxygen
and some CO_2 are transported by the *red
cells*.

In addition to plasma and red cells,
blood contains white cells and platelets
(Table 9.1). The function of *white cells* is
predominantly that of protecting the body
against *infection* which means the
neutralization and elimination of viruses,
bacteria and other microbes.

The function of platelets is to prevent
accidental loss of blood. By initiating the

clotting of blood at sites of damage to the
vascular system and thus 'sealing' the
injury, platelets prevent blood supply. In
this way, continuous supply of blood is
maintained to all organs, especially brain
and heart. A disruption of the blood supply
by mechanical stoppage or by excessive loss
rapidly leads to organ failure and death.

Table 9.1 : Constituents of blood

Constituent	Amount present
Plasma volume	55-60% by
Cells	40-45% by volume
Red	$4-7 \times 10^{12}$ cells/l
White	$4-11 \times 10^9$ cells/l
Platelets (thrombocytes)	$1-4 \times 10^{11}$ cells/l

Plasma

Constituents

Plasma is defined as the fluid part of the blood which is obtained by removing red cells, white cells and platelets; this is obtained by centrifuging whole blood in the presence of anticoagulants such as citrate or heparin. Plasma is found to account for half the volume of blood, whereas the cellular part makes up the other half. The **total volume of blood in a 70 kg man is nearly** *six litres;* **in addition there is some** *twelve litres* **of interistial fluid, with another 30 litres of fluid within cells. In other words, nearly 70 per cent of the body is water.**

The main constituents of plasma are proteins, lipids, carbohydrates, low molecular weight compounds and ions. A typical distribution is shown in Table 9.2.

If the blood is a allowed to coagulate before it is centrifuged, one of the components of plasma, namely fibrinogen is removed. In this case the supernatant fluid; i.e., **fibrinogen-free plasma is termed as** *serum.*

Proteins and lipids: The predominant protein in plasma is *albumin* (molecular weight 65,000). **If its concentration falls, as in protein malnutrition and certain types of renal failure, then water gets retained in the interistitial fluid as a result of which edema develops.**

Albumin is the main carrier of free fatty acids in plasma. The free fatty acids pass across the blood vessels and the cell plasma membrane while albumin remains in the blood stream. **Analbumin-like molecule,** present at much lower concentration has a specific site for the fat soluble vitamin A.

Some of the globulins have binding sites for steroid hormones and other lipids. The majority of **triglyceride and cholesterol is transported in the form of** *lipoprotein complexes.* **These are actually vesicles made up of a membrane containing** α - **and** β - **globulins surrounding a mixture of triglyceride and cholesterol.** Depending upon the relative amounts of triglyceride and cholesterol compared to protein, the vesicles are known as very low density lipoproteins (VLDL), low density lipoproteins (LDL), and high density lipoproteins (HDL).

After a fatty meal the plasma concentration of triglycerides rises.

Table 9.2 : Constituents of plasma

Constituent	Amount present
Protein	69-85 g/l of which
	61 % is albumin
	9% is α - globulins
	11 % is β - globulins
	14% is γ - globulins
	4% is fibrinogen
Fat	3.5-8.5 g/l of which approx.
	30% is cholesterol
	30% is phospholipid
	30% is triglyceride
Inorganic ions	~ 6g/l of which approx.
	140 meq/l is Na^+
	4 meq/l is K^+
	2.5 meq/l is Ca^{++}
	1 meq/l is Mg^{2+}
	100 meq/l is Cl^-
	27 meq/l is HCO_3^-
	2 meq/l is phosphate
Carbohydrate	~ 0.8 g/l of which most is glucose
Urea	~ 0.3 g/l
Amino acids	~ 0.2 g/l of which alanine, glutamine, lysine, glycine, proline and valine are the predominant one.
Ketone bodies	~ 0.02-0.2 g/l

Triglyceride is initially in the form of chylomicrons, absorbed into the lymphatic system and released into the blood stream by way of the thoracic duct. **Triglyceride is broken to free fatty acids and glycerol by the enzyme 'clearing factor lipase'** which remains present on the outside of certain cells. The enzyme is called the **'clearing factor lipase' as it clears the blood of its milky appearance caused by the presence of triglyceride.** Production of this enzyme is stimulated by heparin.

The values refer to a normal adult. A value of $< 4 \times 10^{12}$ red cells/l is referred to as **anemia;** a value of $< 4 \times 10^9$ white cells/l is referred to as **leucopenia;** and a value of $<1 \times 10^{11}$ platelets/l is referred to as thrombopenia.

These values refer to a normal adult but may vary cosiderably after meals. There are in addition other low molecular-weight components, ions, vitamins, proteins, hormones, enzymes etc.

The enzyme facilitates the uptake of some of the free fatty acids into adipose cells and muscle. The rest of the free fatty acids become bound to albumin. In the liver, such free fatty acids are reconstituted into triglyceides and then these in association with phospholipid and protein are released in the form of VLDL. Triglyceride is again degraded to free fatty acids by clearing factor lipase of adipose cells, muscle and other tissues such as heart and kidney cortex. Most of the free fatty acids are taken up into cells. The triglyceride depleted VLDL is now LDL, carrying mainly cholesterol. Cholesterol is not utilized so effectively and much of it remains in the blood stream. Exactly, how the circulatioin of cholesterol in LDL or HDL is controlled is not clear.

The major outcome of the processes described above is to store triglyceride in adipose tissue; at the same time some of the free fatty acids are oxidized by muscle, heart, and other tissues. **During starvation, triglyceride of adipose tissue is broken down to free fatty acids, which are utilized by muscle and other tissues either directly or indirectly often conversion to ketone bodies by the liver.**

Globulins play other roles. **The γ-globulins, or immunoglobulins, act as antibodies to neutralize foreign antigens:**

Whereas other globulins, such as prothrombin and various clotting factors, are together with fibrinogen involved in the coagulation of blood. The coagulation of blood is closely associated with the function of platelets. Several other globulins, some with as yet undefined functions, exist. A very minor globulin, for example, specifically binds thyroxine (thyroxin binding protein) and is responsible for its transport in the blood. Most of the proteins, with the exception of immunoglobulins, are mostly synthesized in the liver. Plasma contains circulating proteins and peptide hormones in very low concentration which are synthesized in respective endocrine organs. Plasma also contains several enzymes which are synthesized invarious tissues. These enzymes if found in abnormal concentration in blood are indicative of damage of the cells of origin as shown in Table 9.3.

Low molecular weight components and ions

Low molecular weight components present in plasma comprise of water soluble and fat-soluble molecules. The fat soluble molecules include cholesterol, steroid hormones, fat-soluble vitamins and other lipids which are protein-bound and are transported, partly in the form of vesicles.

Table 9.3 : Elevation of serum enzymes in various diseases

Sl. No.	Enzyme	Cellular origin	Disease
1.	Most; some transaminases upto 10-200 folds	Liver	Acute hepatitis
2.	Transaminases upto 2-8 folds	Liver	Chronic hepatitis,
3.	Alkaline phosphatase	Liver	Obstructive jaundice
4.	Creatine kinase, aldolase, aspartate transaminase and LDH (type 1 + 2) upto 2-10 folds	Heart	Myocardial infarction
5.	Creatine kinase, aldolase, aspartate transaminase, and LDH (type 5) upto 3 - 6 folds	Muscle	Muscular disease (e.g., muscle injury, muscular dystrophy)

The water soluble molecules include glucose and other sugars, amino acids, glycerol, ketone bodies, urea and vitamins; some water-soluble molecules for instance certain vitamins and hormones are also transported in a protein-bound form. Following a meal, amino acids and sugar are absorbed by the intestine and their concentration in blood-stream rises. They are then utilised for storage, energy porduction and biosynthesis of important substances by liver, muscle and other tissues. The deamination of amino acids by liver results in the formation of urea which is excreted by the kidneys. During starvation/fast, the level of nutrients returns to normal or a little below. Glucose is obtained by glycogen breakdown (glycogenolysis) and gluconeogenesis. Amino acids are obtained by an excess of protein breakdown, over protein synthesis. At the same time, the output of liver ketone bodies, formed from free fatty acids derived from adipose tissue triglyceride,

increases. *Ketone bodies are a major energy source for muscle, heart and other tissues.*

Carbon dioxide, derived from cells as the end product of sugar, amino acid and fat metabolism, is transported largely as bicarbonate ion. The equilibrium position is rapidly reached by participation of the enzyme carbonic anhydrase present in RBCs. Main functioin of carbonic anhydrase may be easily understood by the following equation:

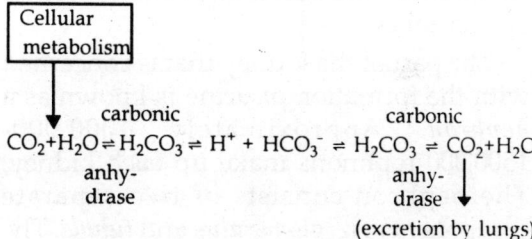

$$CO_2 + H_2O \rightleftharpoons H_2CO_3 \rightleftharpoons H^+ + HCO_3^- \rightleftharpoons H_2CO_3 \rightleftharpoons CO_2 + H_2O$$

(excretion by lungs)

Red blood cells are freely permeable to CO_2. Transient lowering of pH (acidosis) due to excessive production of CO_2 or other cause is avoided by the buffering capacity of plasma proteins. In addition, the kidneys do also control plasma pH.

The concentration of the major inorganic ions in the blood stream is like that of bicarbonate, linked to the metabolism of cell. Failure to absorb Na^+ and K^+ across the epithelial cells of intestine or renal tubules, or failure of the Na^+ pump to maintain ionic asymmetry in other cells, leads to an imbalance of plasma Na^+ and K^+. Ca^{2+} levels are controlled by the action of two hormones i.e., (i) **calcitonin,** which stimulates Ca^{2+} removal by deposition as calcium phosphate in bone, that is to say that it is responsible for lowering the level of serum calcium, and (ii) **parathormone** which has the reverse effect i.e. it is responsible for elevating the serum calcium level with a concomitant decrease in the plasma Pi, reflecting an increase in urinary phosphate (**phosphaturia**). Besides these two hormones, vitamin D also helps a lot in controlling blood calcium level as it stimulates Ca^{2+} absorption by the small intensine. Vitamin D also increases reabsorption of Ca^{2+} from bone.

Excretion of Waste products

The main function of the kidneys, two organs, each weighing approximately 150g, is the formation of *urine*. **Another function of the kidneys is the secretion of** *hormones*.

The part of the kidney that is concerned with the formation of urine is known as a *nephron*. Approximately 1000,000-1500,000 rephnons make up each kidney. The nephron consists of two separate components viz; *glomerulus* and *tubule*. The function of *glomerulus* is to filter the blood and thus to retain cells, proteins and other high moelcular weight substances. The function of the *tubule* is to *reabsorb* most of water, ions, sugars and amino acids that are present in the glomerular filtrate, back into the blood stream. What is afterwards left is a concentrated solution of urea, uric acid, creatinine and other-excretory products which are passed via collecting duct to the bladder.

The absorptive capacity of the tubule is enormous. Out of some 160-180 litres of fluid that may pass through the glomerulus in one day, only approximately 1-5 litres is excreted. The rest, about 99 per cent of the glomerular filtrate is reabsorbed. This is achieved largely as a result of the increased osmotic pressure of the protein-rich fluid leaving the glomerulus, which flows through blood-vessels. **Additional water is reabsorbed by active transport, linked to the Na^+ pump and controlled by the antidiuretic hormone (ADH or vasopressin).** Moreover, the anatomical arrangement of the tubules is such that a counter-current system of absorption is set up, which serves to absorb more water. Failure to synthesize and to secrete ADH (from the posterior **pituitary** gland) results in diuresis which means the production of too watery a urine. **This is a characteristic of the type of diabetes known as diabetes insipidus.**

As in the case of water, much of the sugar, amino acids and ions are reabsorbed by active transport. The Na^+ *pump* is the main driving force. It is situated within the epithelial tubule cells, so as to pump Na^+ from cell into the bloodstream. In order to reabsorb something like 1.4 kg of NaCl per day, the pump utilizes most of the ATP generated by oxidative phosphorylation within the kidney. **The hormone aldosterone potentiates the reabsorption of Na^+ from the glomerular filtrate but not of K^+.** Moreover, as Na^+ is secreted from the tubule cell into the bloodstream, it exchanges with K^+. As a result, almost as much Na^+ as water is reabsorbed (98-99 percent) whereas only some 90% of K^+ is reabsorbed. In other words, urine is relatively richer in K^+ than is plasma.

Urine provides a useful diagnostic system for many diseases affecting metabolism. **Diseases resulting from lack of a particular degradative enzyme, such** as *phenylketonuria* or *galactosaemia*, etc. **are characterized by the presence of** *phenylpyruvate or galactose* in the urine.

Maintenance of the pH of plasma

The kidney performs a second role, which is related to its function as an excretory organ. Its role is in the maintenance of plasma pH near neutrality. Basal metabolism releases H^+ (Fig. 9.1) due to:

(a) the ionization of CO_2 produced by respiration

(b) the ionization of acids such as lactic acid and ketogenesis respectively, and

(c) the ionization of H_2SO_4 produced by the oxidation of cysteine and methionine.

H⁺ producing processes

(a) Oxidation of nutrients CO_2 (in all tissues)

$$CO_2 + H_2O \rightleftharpoons H_2CO_3$$
$$H_2CO_3 \rightleftharpoons HCO_3^- + H^+$$

(b) glycolysis →lactic acid (skeletal muscle, red cells, other tissues)

$$CH_3CH(OH)COOH \rightleftharpoons CH_3CH(OH)COO^- + H^+$$

Ketogenesis $\longrightarrow$ ketone bodies (liver)

$$CH_3COCH_2COOH \rightleftharpoons CH_3COCH_2COO^- + H^+$$

acetoacetic acid

$$CH_3CH\,(OH)CH_2COOH$$

β hydroxybutyric acid

$$CH_3CH(OH)CH_2COO + H^+$$

(c) Oxidation of sulphur-containing amino acids (liver and other tissues)

cysteine $\longrightarrow$

$\longrightarrow$ $H_2S \rightarrow \rightarrow H_2SO_4$

methionine $\longrightarrow$

$$H_2SO_4 \rightarrow SO_4^{2-} + 2H^+$$

H⁺ removing processes

(d) amino acids → keto acids $+NH_3$ (liver and other tissues)

$$NH_3 + H^+ \rightleftharpoons NH_4^+$$

Fig. 9.1: Control of plasma pH

The kidney achieves the maintenance

of plasma pH near 7.4 by excreting a slightly *acidic urine* (normal pH range between 5.3 and 7.0) with an average of 6.0.

The kidney is able to control the rate at which Na^+ bicarbonate, phosphate and other anions are reabsorbed. It is therefore able to control the pH of plasma; decreased reabsorption of bicarbonate, for instance leads to a fall in plasma pH; increased reabsorption has the opposite effect. **The kidney is also able to control the action of glutaminase; i.e., the rate** at which ammonia is produced (Fig. 9.2). This too controls the pH of plasma: a fall in plasma pH is corrected by increased activity of glutaminase, whereas a rise in plasma pH is corrected by a decrease of glutaminase activity. Damage to the renal tubule and failure to secrete ammonia therefore has a direct effect upon the maintenance of plasma pH and leads to an acidosis (and excessive loss of Na^+).

Kidneys do regulate acid-base balance by the formation of ammonia. Renal tubular cells form **ammonia** from a precursor in renal arterial blood and secrete it into tubular fluid. This ammonia formation takes place in the distal tubules and collecting ducts. **It has been found that about two thirds of the ammonia formed in the kidneys is produced by deamidation of glutamine and one third by oxidative deamination of amino acids as shown below (Fig 9.2).**

The NH_3 formed enters the tubular fluid, where it combines with H^+ from the tubular fluid to form NH_4^+. This NH_4^+ then replaces Na^+ in a sodium salt of the tubular fluid, such as Na^+Cl^-. The Na^+ is reabsorbed by the H^+-Na^+ exchange mechanism and reenters the plasma as $Na^+HCO_3^-$. The NH_4^+ is excreted in the urine as NH_4Cl.

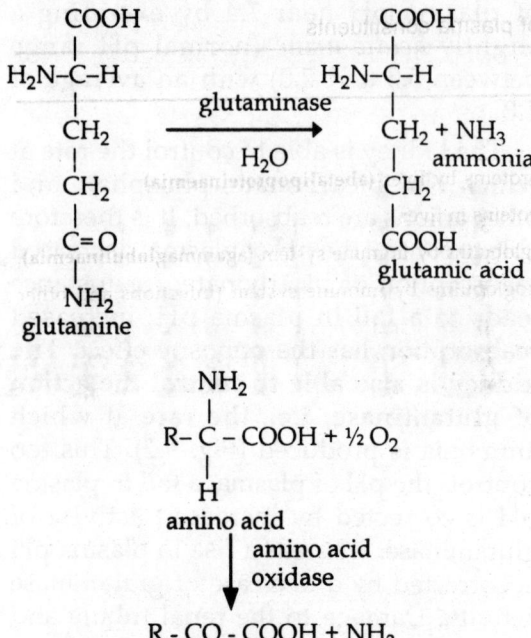

Fig. 9.2 : Production of ammonia in kidneys

Diseases

An abnormal concentration of plasma constituents generally reflects either a nutritional deficiency, or an impairement in the function of organs such as liver or the endocrine glands (Table 9.4). Liver diseases affect the levels of plasma protein such as albumin, α- and β–globulins; hormones. In each case the levels may either be found to be increased or decreased.

Changes in plasma proteins affect those substances that are transported by them, for example in abetalipoproteinaemia, a lowered concentration of the proteins responsible for transporting triglycerides and cholesterol results in an altered deposition of fat. Conversely; an increase of β - lipoproteins can result in an increaesed level of cholesterol (cholesterolaemia) and triglyceride in plasma, which may be a contributing factor to the development of atherosclerosis. **Atherosclerosis is caused due to the deposition of lipid 'plaques' containing cholesterol, triglyceride and proteins in the wall of blood-vessels. Such plaques tend to form a** *clot* **(thrombus) with platelets and red blood cells. Thrombi present a danger and they may detach and block a vessel in the heart (leading to angina pectoris and myocardial infarction, that is, coronary thrombosis) or the brain (leading to a cerebral infarct, i.e. stroke).**

Diseases of the kidney have two effects:

(i) failure to retain substances such as amino acids, proteins, sugars, water and ions.

(ii) failure to excrete substances such as urea, creatinine and other waste products.

The first consequence is generally not so serious as the second.

In acute nephritis, on the other hand, the glomerulus is often affected (perhaps by an autoimmune reaction) and ceases to function. No fluid is filtered with the result that all the toxic components of the blood are retained and accumulate. Besides, there is also retention of water, leading to oedema. Such defects of glomerular filtration are the most common forms of renal diseases.

Other diseases of the kidney are those that reflect an endocrine imbalane, such as an insufficiency or excess of vasopressin (ADH), or aldosterone. A malfunctioning kidney is also *a common site for the start of bacterial infections;* **blockage due to precipitation of calcium oxalate or other material (renal calculi) is often the cause.**

Red blood cells

The main function of red blood cells

Table 9.4 : Abnormal levels of plasma constituents

Constituent	Alteration	Cause
Albumin; proteins in general	Decrease	Kwashiorkor, liver disease
β- lipoproteins	Decrease	Defective synthesis of β-lipoproteins by liver (**abetalipoproteinaemia**)
	Increase	Increased synthesis of β-lipoproteins in liver
γ - globulins	Decrease	Defective synthesis of immunoglobulins by immune system (**agammaglobulinaemia**).
	Increase	Incerased synthesis of immunoglobulins by immune system (infections and other causes)
Fibrinogen	Decrease	Defective synthesis of fibrinogen by liver (**afibrinogenaemia**).
Cholesterol	Increase	Hyperlipidaemia, cholesterolaemia
Triglyceride	Increase	Hyperlipidaemia
Glucose	Increase	Diabetes mellitus
Urea, creatinine	Increase	Renal disease, e.g. acute nephritis
Na^+	Decrease	Lack of aldosterone (**Addison's disease**); excessive loss from gastrointestinal tract (e.g., vomiting).
	Increase	Excess of aldosterone (**certain adrenal tumors**); **excessive water loss.**
K^+	Decrease	Excessive loss from gastrointestinal tract (e.g. vomiting) or from kidney.
	Increase	Addison's disease
Ca^{2+}	Decrease	Hypoparathyroidism
	Increase	Excessive vitamin D intake; excessive bone destruction; hyperparathyroidism
Insulin	Decrease	Diabetes mellitus
	Increase	Hypoglycemic coma
Thyroxine	Decrease	Endemic goitre; primary hypothyroidism (myxoedema)
	Increase	Thyrotoxicosis
Oestrogens	↓	Female hypogonadism (**failure of sexual development in females; amenorrhea**)
Androgens	↓	Male hypogonadism (**failure of sexual development in males**)
Mineralocorticoids	↑	Aldosteronoma (Conn's syndrome) - cause is due to tumor of adrenal cortex
Glucocorticoids	↑	Cushing's syndrome (due to tumor of adrenal cortex)
Vitamin A	↓	Xerophthalmia, nightblindness, etc.
Thiamine (B_1)	↓	Beriberi
Riboflavin (B_2)	↓	Various skin lesions
Pyridoxin (B_6)	↓	Various skin lesions
Cobalamin (B_{12})	↓	Pernicious anaemia
Niacin	↓	Pellagra
Folic acid	↓	Anaemia (**macrocytic** and **megaloblastic**)
Biotin	↓	Various skin lesions
Ascorbic acid (Vit. C)	↓	Scurvy
Calciferol (Vit. D)	↓	Rickets (children), Osteomalacia (adults)
Phylloquinone (Vit. K)	↓	Tendency of haemorrhage

(erythrocytes) is to *carry oxygen* **from the lungs to the other organs of the body.** At the same time, red cells accelerate the removal of CO_2 from the tissues back to the lungs. The constituents and metabolism of RBCs reflect these two functions. Blood-flow through tissues is designed so that incoming blood (containing oxygen) is kept separate from outgoing blood (containing CO_2). This is achieved by having separate networks of incoming (arterial) and outgoing (venous) blood within tissues. Within tissues the blood vessels become progressively smaller, until they are some 5- 10 µm in diameter. Such capillaries then form a network of ingoing (arterial) and outgoing (venous) vessels for the supply and removal of nutrients from cells.

Constituents

The chief constituent of RBCs is *haemoglobin.* **It is the compound that transports oxygen and about 15% of the** CO_2 **in blood.** Hemoglobin accounts for some 90% of the dry weight of RBCs. The remainder, which is largely plasma membrane (red cells have no nucleus, mitochondria, endoplasmic reticulum or other internal membrane system) consists of other proteins, glycoproteins, phospholipids, cholesterol, inorganic ions (Na^+, K^+, Mg^{2+}, Cl^-, etc.) and low molecular weight compounds such as sugar phosphates and other metabolic intermediates.

Hemoglobin : It is a protein made up of 4 subunits. In adult hemoglobin, the subunits are two α - chains and two β-chains ($\alpha_2 \beta_2$). Each subunit, called globin contains a haem group. The essential component of the hemoglobin is the iron atom in each of the 4 haem groups. Of the six coordinate valency of the iron, only one is linked to globin; four remain linked to the pyrrole groups of haem; and the last is free to bind oxygen, CO or other ligand. **CO binds 500 times more tightly than oxygen (to yield an inactive hemoglobin -CO complex),** which explains its greater toxicity.

The binding of *oxygen* by hemoglobin is characterized by *cooperativity* between the four haem groups. That is to say, the affinity of anyone haem groups for oxygen gets affected by the presence of an oxygen molecule on one of the other haem groups. As a result, a plot of the amout of oxygen bound against the concentration of oxygen is sigmoidal (Fig. 9.3).

In contrast, the binding of oxygen to a haem group that is present as a single chain only, as is the case for the muscle protein myoglobin, is characterized by the more useful rectangular hyperbola.

The physiological advantage of cooperativity in oxygen binding by

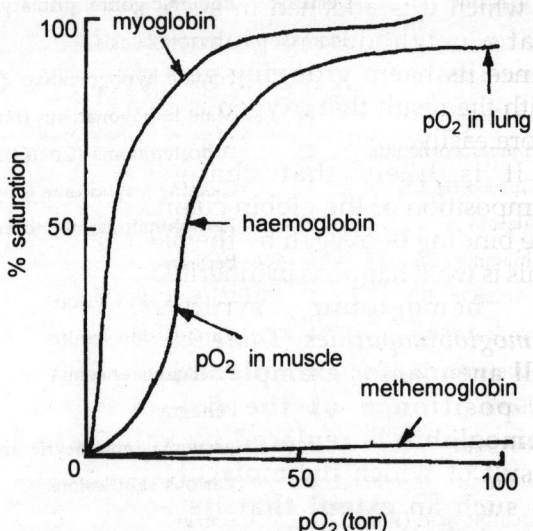

Fig. 9.3 : Binding of oxygen to hemoglobin (the binding of oxygen to hemoglobin is characterized by a S-shaped curve, indicative of co-operativity between the 4 subunits).

hemoglobin is as follows. In the lungs, where oxygen tension is high, hemoglobin is fully saturated with oxygen. As it passes through the arterial system to the tissues, the oxygen tension, and hence the amount of oxygen bound, drops; at this point myoglobin (which also remains present in tissues other than muscle) has a relatively greater affinity for oxygen than hemoglobin (Fig. 9.3), thus facilitating transfer. Once this has occurred, hemoglobin tends to bind CO_2 (at free amino groups of globin, not at the iron atom of haem), and the hemoglobin -CO_2 is carried by the venous system to the lungs. Many other factors, such as the concentration of chloride, affect the transport of CO_2.

The mechanism whereby in hemoglobin the affinity of one haem group for oxygen is modulated by the presence or absence of oxygen or another haem group is due to the quaternary structure of hemoglobin. Athough the four haem groups are not in direct contact, the binding of oxygen by one haem group distorts the globin chain to which it is attached in such a manner that a neighbouring globin chain and hence its haem grouping gets distorted, with the result that oxygen is able to bind more easily.

It is likely that changes in the composition of the globin chain can affect the binding of oxygen by the haem group. This is what happens in inherited disorders of hemoglobin synthesis, the *hemoglobinopathies (Table 9.5)*. In sickle cell anemia, for example, the glutamate at position 6 of the β - chain of hemoglobin is replaced by valine as a result of which the molecule is altered to such an extent that its solubility, especially in the mono-oxygenated state gets reduced to the point of precipitation.

As a result, the red cells are distorted in a characteristic **'sickling' manner.** The anemia results from the fact that sickled cells are unable to bind oxygen normally; moreover the cells are recognized as **'foreign' or 'aged' by the spleen and hence degraded** faster than the normal.

Many other types of hemoglobinopathy have now been recognized. *Anemia* and *muscular fatigue* due to the failure of proper oxygenation are common symptoms. In each case, the hemoglobin has an abnormal electrophoretic mobility, generally due to the replacement of a particular amino acid in one of the two globin chains (Table 9.5). In some instances, entire globin chain is found to be missing. This could be due to a **'nonsense'** mutation, so that m-RNA that is untranslatable into protein is produced.

Metabolism of RBCs

The human red cell has no nucleus, mitochondria, endoplasmic reticulum or other organelle. It therefore cannot synthesize DNA, RNA, protein, phospholipid, or carbohydrate, nor can it obtain ATP by oxidative phosphorylation. Its **major metabolic transformation is the breakdown of glucose to lactate by the pathway of** *glycolysis.* **Glucose is therefore the major metabolic fuel required by red cells. The ATP that is generated is used primarily to drive the Na^+ pump. Its main function in red cells is to maintain a high internal K^+ concentration (conducive to glycolysis) and to prevent excessive entry of water.**

In addition to being broken down to lactate by glycolysis, glucose is oxidized to CO_2 and H_2O by the pentose phosphate shunt.

Table 9.5 : Some hemoglobinopathies*

Sl. No.	Disorder	Type of Hb	Subunits	Abnormality	Result	Clinical manifestation
Change in gene structure						
1.	Sickle cell disease	HbS	αα ββ	Glu → Val at position 6 of β chain	Decreased sol. of Hb; sickling	Hemolytic anemia
Change in gene expression						
1.	α - thalassaemia	HbH	ββββ	Defective synthesis of α chains	Insol. Hb; decreased red cell survival	Mild anemia
2.	β - thalassaemia	HbF**	αα γγ	Failure to switch from synthesis of γ - chains to β - chains at birth	Abnormal O_2 affinity	Anemia

* over 400 types are known today
** Normal Hb prior to birth

Formation and destruction of RBCs

Red cells have a life span of 120-130 days. This means that approximately 2 x 10^{11} red cells, or 1 per cent of the total red cell population is formed (and destroyed) every day.

Since a red cell contains some 3 x 10^8 molecules of hemoglobin, the rate of synthesis is 6 x 10^{19} molecules or about 8 grams of hemoglobin per day; this corresponds to about 5 percent of the total weight of proteins turned over per day. **During pregnancy, the demand for hemoglobin synthesis is increased, as a result of which an extra intake of iron is required in this state.**

The formation of red cells takes place in the bone marrow. The precursor cells are known as erythroblasts and contain nucleus, mitochondria and endoplasmic reticulum. Hemoglobin begins to be synthesized at this stage. As the erythroblast matures, it loses its nucleus to become a reticulocyte (Fig. 9.4). This contains sufficient of the hemoglobin m-RNA synthesized in the erythroblast to continue hamoglobin synthesis. The pathway for the synthesis of hemoglobin is outlined in Fig. 9.5. Failure to absorb sufficient dietary iron prevents hemoglobin synthesis and leads to anemia. **Anemia also results from failure to absorb sufficient vitamin B_{12} or folic acid, both of which are required for the rapid DNA synthesis that accompanies the formation and proliferation of erythroblasts.**

In foetal development, during which a blood-supply is initiated long before the establishment of bones, synthesis of hemoglobin takes place in the liver. The type of hemoglobin that is synthesized differs from adult hemolgobin in having two γ chains instead of two β chains. The resultant hemoglobin is known as foetal hemoglobin (HbF). In **β-thalassaemia,** foetal hemoglobin synthesis continues into

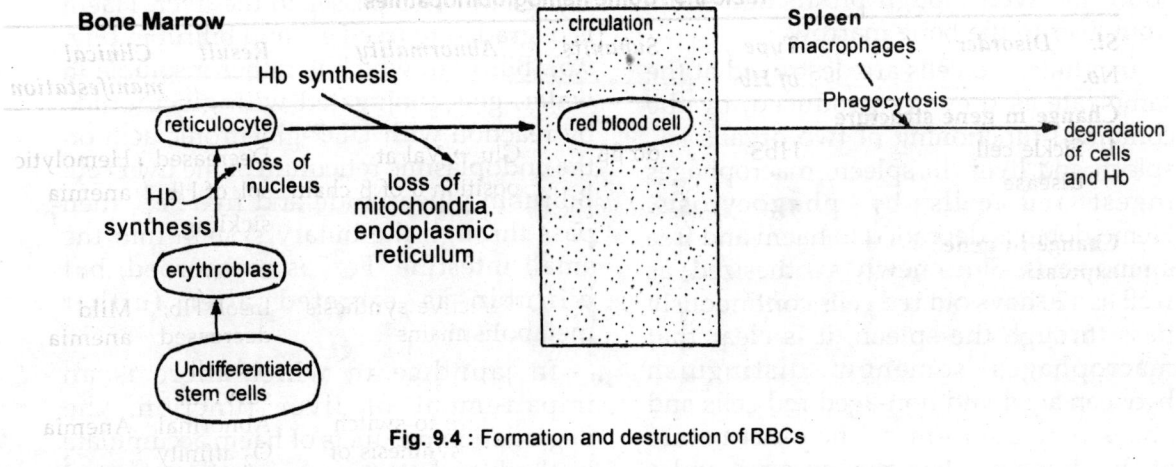

Fig. 9.4 : Formation and destruction of RBCs

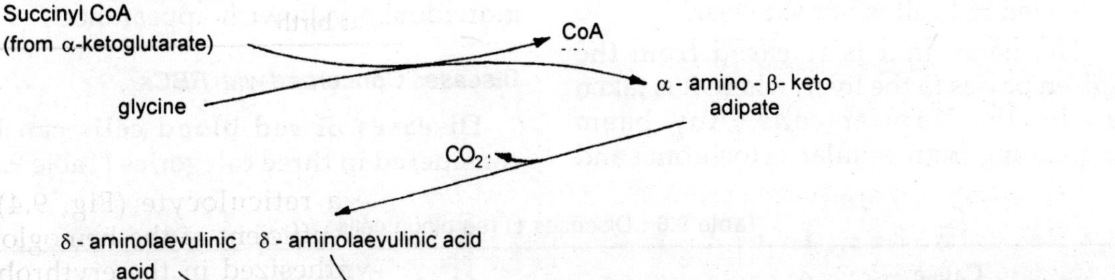

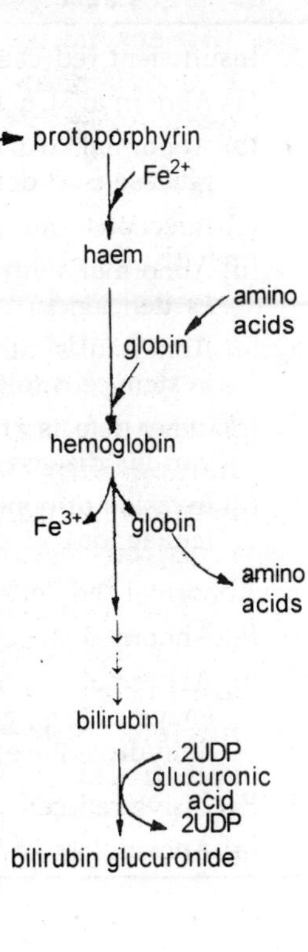

Fig. 9.5 : Biosynthesis and degradation of hemoglobin {Synthesis of Hb takes place in the erythroblasts and reticulocytes, whereas synthesis of haem takes place in most of the cells, since it is the precursor of cytochromes and of myoglobin, as well as of Hb too. Degradation of Hb begins in the spleen and is continued in the liver, the product (bilirubin glucuronide) is secreted in the bile}.

adult life, even though production shifts from liver to the bone marrow.

In adults, red cells are destroyed at the same rate as they are produced, by the combined functioning of two organs i.e., spleen and liver. In spleen, macrophages ingest red cells by phagocytosis. Hemoglobin is degraded to haem and free amino acids. Since newly synthesized, as well as 120 days old red cells continuously pass through the spleen, it is clear that macrophages somehow distinguish between aged and non-aged red cells and attack only the former. The exact nature of the difference between an aged and a non-aged red cell is not yet clear.

The haem that is released from the spleen passes to the liver, where it is taken up by the Kupffer cells. Any haem originating from cellular cytochrome and myoglobin also passes to the liver. Haem is degraded to free Fe^{2+} and bilirubin (Fig. 9.5). Bilirubin which is rather insoluble in water, gets conjugated with glucuronide by reaction with UDP-glucuronic acid on the endoplasmic reticulum of the liver cell. Bilirubin glucuronide and free Fe^{2+} then pass through the biliary system into the small intestine. Fe^{2+} is reabsorbed, but bilirubin is excreted after further metabolism.

In jaundice in which there is an impairement of liver function, the degradation products of haem accumulate in the blood-stream, giving the affected individual a yellowish appearance.

Diseases Concerned with RBCs

Diseases of red blood cells can be considered in three categories (Table 9.6),

Table 9.6 : Diseases of red blood cells

Cause	Result
1. Insufficient red cells: anaemia	
(a) Abnormal structure of Hb	Increased loss of red cells due to haemolysis
(b) Abnormal structure of enzymes (e.g., glucose-6- P-dehydrogenase)	- do -
(c) Infections, immune disorders, etc.	- do -
(d) Abnormal synthesis of haemoglobin (e.g., Fe deficiency)	Decreased production of red cells
(e) Abnormal synthesis of nucleic acids in stem cells (e.g. B_{12} or folate deficiency)	" "
(g) Other defects of erythropoiesis (e.g., various diseases, protein deficiency)	" "
(g) Invasion of bone marrow (e.g., leukaemia)	" "
2. Abnormal red cells	
(a) Abnormal structure of Hb	Abnormal O_2 transport by red cells
(b) Abnormal structure of enzymes (e.g., glucose -6- P dehydrogenase)	Abnormal metabolism of red cells
3. Excessive red cells: polycythaemia	
(a) Anoxia; loss of blood	Increased production of red cells; generally only temporary

i.e.,

(i) production of insufficient red cells (anaemia)

(ii) production of faulty red cells, and

(iii) production of an excess of red cells

Category (i) is by far the most common, the cause of which may be nutritional due to less intake of iron, folic acid and vitamin B_{12}; the cause may also be infections as in malaria or infectious mononucleosis or it may be due to a diseased bone marrow.

Category (ii) includes the haemoglobinopathies and other hereditary disorders such as G-6-P-DH deficiency. These disorders may themselves lead to anaemia.

Category (iii) known as polycythaemia, is much less serious than category (i). It occurs in situations in which an excessive demand for RBCs has arisen for example: loss of blood, anoxia, etc. Only where excessive production fails to return to normal, does polycythaemia become a hazard.

Anaemia is by far the most common disorder of red blood cells; some 20 per cent of hospital admissions are due to anaemia.

White blood cells (Leucocytes)

Leucocytes or white cells of mammalian blood differ structurally from the erythrocytes in many ways, such as being larger in size, containing at least a single nucleus and possessing ameboid movement. They are typical animal cells and therefore contain the following substances which are customarily present in such cells for e.g., protein, fats, glycogen, purines, enzymes, phosphatides, cholesterol, inorganic salts and water. Compound proteins make up the chief part of the protein quota of leucocytes, the nucleoproteins predominating. Powerful proteotytic and glycolytic enzymes also remain present. It is claimed that the granular leucocytes originate in the bone marrow, whereas the nongranular leucocytes (lymphocytes) have a lymphatic origin (lymphglands or lymphoid tissue). **The normal number of leucocytes in human blood varies between 5,000 and 10,000 per cmm.** The ratio between the leucocytes and erythrocytes is about 1 :350 to 500.

A leucocytosis is said to exist when the leucocytes count gets increased above normal limits. **Leucocytosis may be divided into two general classes, viz; the *physiological* and *pathological*, the examples of physiological state are pregnancy, parturition (process of giving birth to a child), digestion, excessive physical exercise, etc. and those of pathological state include inflammations, infections,** post hemorrhagic, toxic, malignancy etc.

Leucocytosis is also found to be associated with such emotional states as fear, rage (a state of violent anger), or apprehension.

The function of leucocytes is to combat and prevent infection.

When the total leucocyte count is decreased than the normal which is rare, the condition is known as *leucopenia*.

In certain types of cancer affecting the bone marrow or other site of white cell production, the number of white cells gets increased, a disease known as *leukaemia* according to which cells proliferate the most. Leukaemias are defined as granulocytic, lymphocytic and so forth. Unlike nonleukaemic cells, leukaemic cells divide *indiscriminately* and invade other tissues to form malignant growths.

PLATELETS: **The main function of platelets or thrombocytes, which are the smallest cells in the body is to promote the** *coagulation* **of blood.** This is achieved by the release of certain factors from platelets that activate a series of enzymes present in plasma, which results in the formation of a *fibrin clot.*

Mechanism of Blood coagulation

This is very complex and not completely understood. The key and final step of blood coagulation involves the trapping of red blood cells in a network of strands composed of the *protein fibrin.* Fibrin is produced from a soluble precursor protein present in plasma called fibrinogen.

Its mechanism in brief may be understood as in (Fig. 9.6).

Failure (due to hereditary or nutritional causes) to coagulate blood when necessary, leads to diseases such as *haemophilia* **in which one of the clotting factors is either found completely missing or defective with the result that** *thrombin* **formation is retarted.** Afflicted persons are therefore at risk of extensive internal or external bleeding (e.g. when an injury is sustained).

Certainly, excessive coagulation may lead to coronary or cerebral thrombosis.

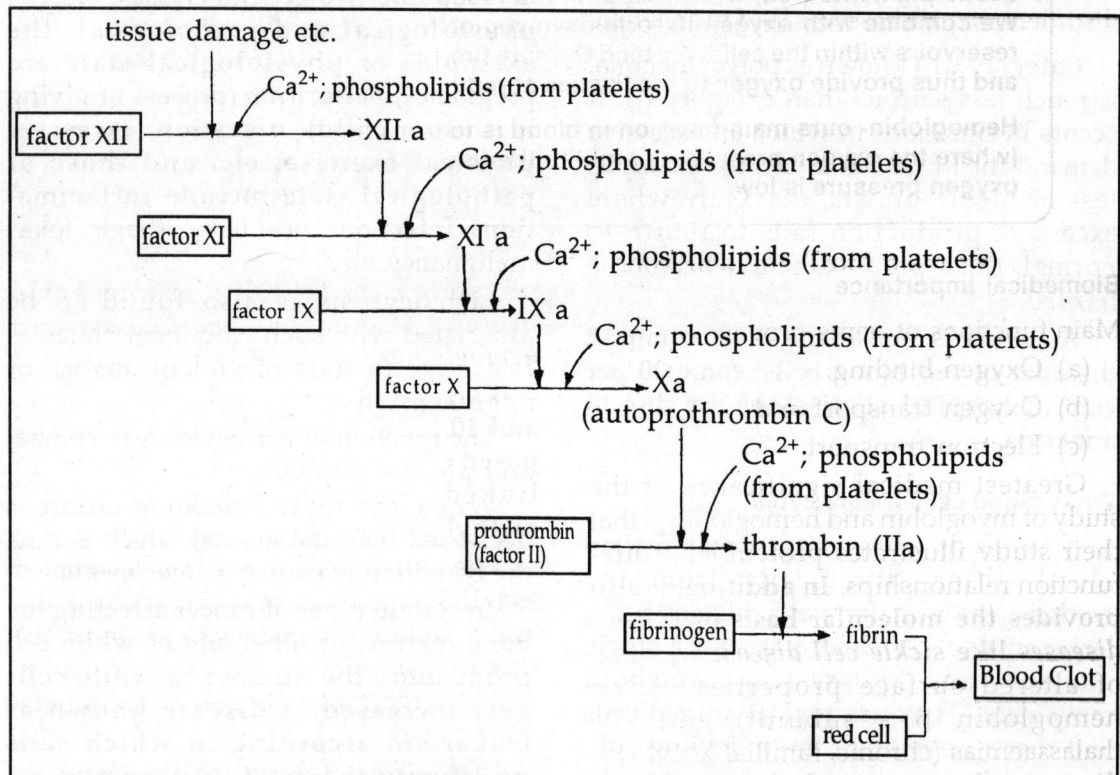

Fig. 9.6: Blood Coagulation (factors XIIa, XIa, IXa, Xa and thrombin are proteolytic enzymes. Like chymotrypsin, each is derived from an inactive precursor; also like chymotrypsin, their action involves acylation of a serine residue at the active site. The factors are all plasma proteins; their concentration in the blood stream reflects the fact that each acts catalytically for the next step (i.e., the concentration of XII < XI < IX, etc.). Note that other factors, in addition to Ca^{2+} and phospholipids, are invovled at various stages.

CHAPTER 10

MYOGLOBINS AND HEMOGLOBIN

Myoglobins- we are small proteins having M.W. of about 17,000 and consist of a single globin peptide chain combined with heme. We are intracellular tissue pigments (red) which occur in red muscle fibres of the vertebrates. We combine with oxygen to form oxymyoglobins; which serve as oxygen reservoirs within the cells. We bind O_2 more firmly than does the hemoglobin and thus provide oxygen to the tissues at reduced tension.

Hemoglobin- ours main function in blood is to transport O_2 from the lungs (where the oxygen pressure is high) to the tissues for utilization where the oxygen pressure is low.

Biomedical importance

Main functions of heme proteins are in :

(a) Oxygen binding,

(b) Oxygen transport and

(c) Electron transport

Greatest medical significance of the study of myoglobin and hemoglobin is that their study illustrates protein structure-function relationships. **In addition, it also provides the molecular basis of** *genetic diseases* like *sickle cell disease* (a result of altered surface properties of the hemoglobin β - subunit) and the thalassaemias (chronic, familial hemolytic disease characterized by defective synthesis of hemoglobin).

Cyanide and carbon monoxide finish the life because they disrupt the

physiological fuctions of the heme proteins i.e., *cytochrome oxidase* and *hemoglobin,* respectively.

Porphins : Porphins [Figures 10.1 (a) and 10.1 (b)] are cyclic compounds composed of four *pyrrole rings* which remain linked to each other by-CH -, methylidyne bridges.

The four pyrrole rings are designated as I, II, III and IV and the bridges as α, β, γ and δ. Different substituent groups on the rings are labelled as 1,2,3,4,.5,6,7, and 8. In short the molecule may, however be represented as:

Porphyrins: Substituted porphins are known as porphyrins.

Porphyrins are of two types, i.e.

(i) Type I and (ii) Type III

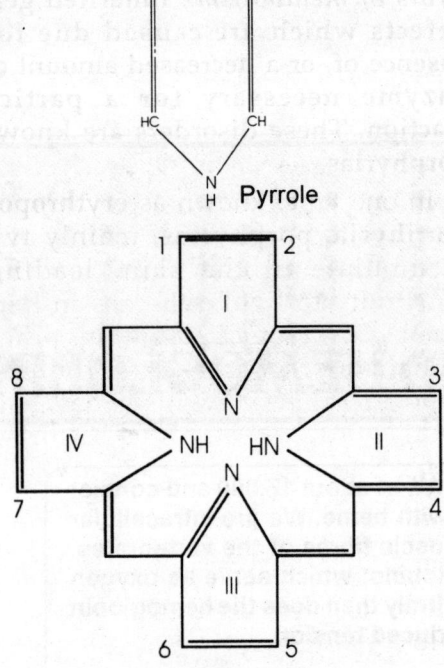

Fig. 10.1 (a) : Porphin

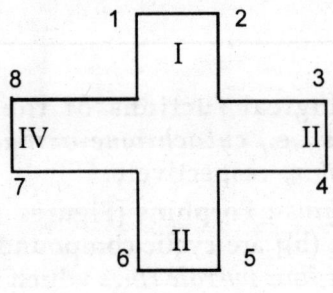

Fig. 10.1 (b)

Type I porphyrin consists of completely symmetrical arrangements of substituents, whereas Type III Porphyrins consist of assymetrical arrangements of substituents. In nature both types of porphyrins namely I and III are found, out of which type III is more abundant. Some of the important porphyrins are as shown in Table 10.1:

Table 10.1: To show different types of porphyrins

Sl. No.	Porphyrins	Nature of the substituents at the following positions			
		1,2	3,4	5,6	7, 8
1.	Mesoporphyrin	ME	ME	MP	PM
2.	Uroporphyrin	AP	AP	AP	PA
3.	Coproporphyrin	MP	MP	MP	PM
4.	Protoporphyrin	MV	MV	MP	PM

Where: M = - CH$_3$ (methyl group)

V = - CH = CH$_2$ (vinyl group)

P = - CH$_2$ -CH$_2$ - COOH (propionic acid)

A = - CH$_2$ -COOH (acetic acid)

E = - C$_2$H$_5$ - (ethyl group)

In reactions which follow, four molecules of porphobilinogen are joined to form a pophyrin ring.

By decarboxylation of the acetic acid side chain and decarboxylation and desaturation of the propionic acid side chain, these groups are altered producing methyl and vinyl groups, resulting finally in protoporphyrin IX (Fig 10.2).

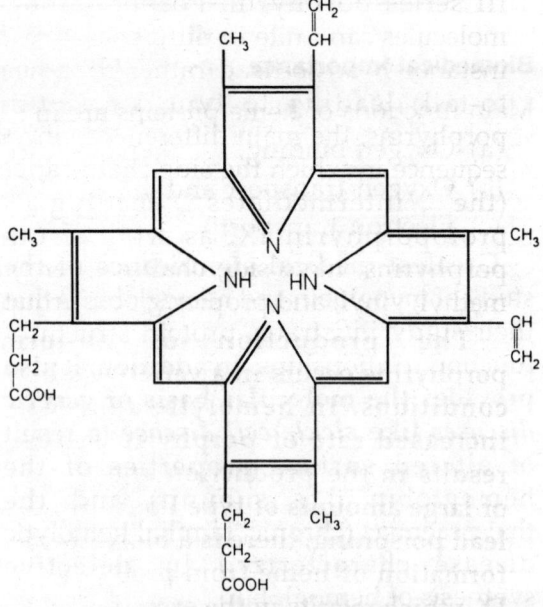

Fig. 10.2 : Protoporphyrin IX

Porphyrins contribute the prosthetic group of many important biological substances, including hemoglobin, the cytochromes, peroxidases, catalase, etc. **It has been studied that porphyrin of hemoglobin is synthesized from glycine and succinyl CoA.** The complete synthesis of protoporphyrin IX, the porphyrin of hemoglobin, is complex and some of the details have yet to be discovered. However, the synthetic route is as shown below which takes place in two stages.

(1) Succinyl CoA+glycine→5 - Aminolevu-
        linic acid
(2) 5-Aminolevulinic acid→Porphobilinogen
        (2 moles)

Incorporation of Fe^{++} into this compound produces heme.

Protoporphyrin IX is known as a type III series porphyrin. Porphobilinogen molecules can unite in different ways (for instance head-to-head rather than head-to-tail) leading to type I and other porphyrins, the main difference being the sequence in which the side chains appear (the intermediates leading to protoporphyrin IX, as well as other porphyrins, have side chains other than methyl, vinyl, and propionic acid groups).

The production of abnormal porphyrins occurs in a variety of disease conditions. In hemolytic anemias, an increased rate of porphyrin synthesis results in the production and excretion of large amounts of type I porphyrins. In lead poisoning, there is a blocking of the formation of heme from protoporphyrin IX, which results in the excretion of Type III porphyrins. Porphyrin metabolism is also affected by a number of '*inborn

***errors of metabolism'*, inherited genetic defects which are caused due to the absence of, or a decreased amount of an enzyme necessary for a particular reaction. These disorders are known as porphyrias.**

In one type, known as **erythropoietic porphyria,** porphyrins, mainly type I, accumulate in the skin, leading to sensitivity to light; whereas in **hepatic porphyrias,** Type III porphyrins primarily and their precursors are produced in abnormal amount which may lead to neurological and intestinal disturbances **(acute porphyria),** or sensitivity to light, or both.

Hemoglobin and Related Substances

The heme proteins, to which hemoglobin belongs, constitute one of the most important classes of biological substances. Among the heme proteins are found the respiratory proteins of animals such as the haemoglobins, myoglobins, erythrocruorins, etc.; cellular oxidation catalysts of both animals and plants, such as the cytochromes, cytochrome oxidase and peroxidase; and catalase, which catalyze the decomposition of H_2O_2 in both the animals and the plants.

The heme proteins are formed by conjugation of proteins with heme, an iron-porphyrin compound, which serves as the prosthetic group.

The red colour material of blood is because of hemoglobin which remains present in RBCs.

RBCs have a life-span of about 120 days after which they are broken down and the hemoglobin is degraded by the liver, spleen, bone marrow and reticuloendothelial cells forming bile pigments, mainly bilirubin and biliverdin. A considerable

---

Functions of Hemoglobin

1. In the transport of oxygen from the lungs to the tissues and in the transport of CO_2 from tissues to the lungs.
2. As buffers: The buffering action of hemoglobin is due to the amino acid *histidine* which remains present in the globin part of hemoglobin. Histidine comprises 8% of the total amino-acid make up of the globin.

---

number of pigments are produced which are found not only in the bile but also in plasma, urine, and feces.

Hemoglobin belongs to the class of conjugation proteins where heme is the prosthetic group and globin, the protein part.

Hemoglobin = Heme + Globin

Carbon Monoxide Poisoning

Poisoning by carbon monoxide is very fatal because of the fact of greater affinity of hemoglobin for CO than for oxygen **(about 200 times greater).** The products formed are carboxyhemoglobin and oxyhemoglobin respectively as shown below:

$$HbO_2 + CO \rightleftharpoons HbCO + O_2$$

$$Hemoglobin + O_2 \rightleftharpoons Oxyhemoglobin$$

If air is breathed containing CO in one two-hundredth the concentration of oxygen, equal amounts of carboxyhemoglobin and oxyhemoglobin will be formed which means a concentration of about 0.1 per cent of CO in the air breathed will lead to 50 per cent of the hemoglobin being present as carboxyhemoglobin and will eventually produce marked symptoms within about an hour. With 0.2 per cent concentration in the air death may occur within a few hours.

In a person with a normal blood count, symptoms may start to appear when there is about 20 per cent saturation of the Hb with CO. There may be a feeling of lassitude (heaviness) with headache. Above this point, symptoms steadily worsen, the headache becomes more severe, with increasing feeling of fatigue and muscular weakness, giddiness, fainting and shoutness of breath which are very marked at 50 percent saturation. Unconsciousness occurs between 50-70%, with death following soon if exposure to the gas continues. **Death follows quickly when 80% saturation gets reached.**

Methemoglobin: It is a hemoglobin derivative in which iron remains present in the ferric state hence it is also called *ferrihemoglobin.* It is formed by the oxidation of hemoglobin and oxyhemoglobin, for example, by the action of potassium ferricyanide. Methemoglobin is dark brown in colour.

Conversion of ferrous to ferric iron in hemoglobin destroys its property to combine with oxygen, therefore no transport of oxygen takes place, vis-a-vis methemoglobin has got no capacity to transport oxygen.

Normally, the conversion of hemoglobin to methemoglobin occurs in the blood but reducing substances present in red blood cells tend to prevent the deposition of any appreciable amount of methemoglobin which is not a good substance for the human system.

Methemoglobin is usually detected by means of its characteristic absorption spectrum. It does not combine with either oxygen or CO but does form a coloured cyanide derivative. There is found little or no hemoglobin in the normal blood.

Appearance of methemoglobinemia is noticed in certain diseases and after the administration of certain chemicals like nitrites and aniline derivatives such as the drug sulphanilamide. Methemoglobin is not toxic but its presence in blood simply means a proportional reduction in the oxygen-carrying capacity of the blood. **Symptoms of methemoglobinemia are cyanosis (blue skin) and dyspnea (difficulty in breathing).**

When hemoglobin comes in contact with certain oxidizing agents, either in vitro or in vivo, methemoglobin in formed which is a brown pigment; it differs from hemoglobin and oxyhemoglobin in that the iron is in the ferric form, i.e., methemoglobin is a combination of heme, or ferriprotoporphyrin, and globin.

The clinical induction of a moderately severe methemoglobinemia has been proposed as an aid in the treatement of *cyanide poisoning*, since methemoglobin combines with cyanide and may thus prevent the latter i.e., cyanide from reacting with enzymes in the tissues.

Hemoglobin Variants
Hemoglobin A₁

HbA$_1$ contains two α - chains and two β_2- chains. HbA$_1$constitutes over 98% of the total hemoglobin of the normal adult hemoglobin and is designated as α_2A β_2A or more simply as $\alpha_2\beta_2$.

Hemoglobin A₂

HbA$_2$ contains two α_2 - chains and two δ_2 - chains. Hb A$_2$ constitutes about 3% of the total hemoglobin in the normal adult and is designated as $\alpha_2\delta_2$.

Hemoglobin F

This is found in high proportion (upto 90 percent) in the new born, falling gradually within the first two years of life to reach 1 per cent of the total hemoglobin. This persits throughout adult life during which amounts in excess of 1 per cent are treated as abnormal. In this type polypeptide chains are designated as α and γ chains.

This type of hemoglobin is designated as HbF and is represented as $\alpha_2\gamma_2$. It contains two α - chains and two γ- chains.

Hemoglobin S (Sickle cell Hemoglobin)

HbS contains two α- and two β - chains in which *glutamic* acid at 6th position from the N-terminal end of the β - chain is replaced by *valine*. This type of hemoglobin is also called sickle hemoglobin due to the fact that the RBCs assume the shape of sickle cell on deoxygenation.

Presence of such type of Hb was for the first time detected by scientist Pauling et al in 1949 in RBCs in sickle cell anaemia cases.

Hemoglobin C : In 1951 hemoglobin C was found in some **Negros** in which *glutamic acid* at the 6th position from the **N-terminal end of the β - chain is replaced by *lysine*.**

Besides the above variants, today more than 100 Hb variants are knwon out of which some like hemoglobin D, E, G, Hb Barts, H, I, M, O, etc. are important.

Metabolism of Hemoglobin

Hemoglobin is synthesized in our system from the :

(i) **Protein and**
(ii) **Iron present in the diet**

Glycine and other amino acids are of

In short, hemoglobin variants may be represented as given in Table 10.2.

Table 10.2: To show different types of hemoglobin variants

	Chains	
HbA$_1$	2 α	2 β
HbA$_2$	2 α	2 δ
HbF	2 α	2 γ
HbS	2 α	2 β glu → val at position 6th from N-terminal end

obvious importance in this connection for both globin and nitrogen in the **porphyrin ring.** Inorganic iron, which is contributed by both the body pool of this importnat element and the diet, cannot be directly converted to heme. The synthesis of the protoporphyrin has been shown to occur from acetate and glycine fragemnts and the inclusion of iron is catalysed by utilization of iron-bearing protein i.e., *siderophyllin* in which copper appears to play an important role. The complete mechanism of the synthesis of heme has not yet been known.

In the embryo, the liver is an important source of erythrocyte production and during maturation, this process passes to the bone marrow. Destruction of RBCs has been traced to liver and the spleen where hemoglobin gets split into porphyrin and protein portions. The iron is removed and the remaining protoporphyrin like material gets converted to a number of pigments which are finally eliminated through bile.

Anemia, the lack of sufficient hemoglobin for the transport of oxygen, can be caused by a number of pathological conditions. These vary from reduced hemoglobin formation due to nutritional lack of iron, lack of a factor required for absorption of iron (as in pernicious anemia), loss of hemoglobin due to errors in metabolism or due to the presence of toxic substances as in **uremia.** Thus, we find that the cycle of production and degradation of hemoglobin gets controlled by a number of factors ranging from dietary to hereditary.

Biosynthesis and degradation of hemoglobin may be understood by the following schematic diagram (Fig. 10.3).

Synthesis of hemoglobin takes place in erythrocytes and reticulocytes; (synthesis of haem takes place in mast cells, since it is the precursor of cytochromes, myoglobin and as well as of Hb). Degradation of Hb begins in the spleen and is continued in the liver. The product i.e. the bilirubin glucuronide is secreted in the bile.

Diseases of RBCs

Diseases of red blood cells can be considered in the following three categories:

(i) production of insufficient red cells (anemia)

(ii) production of faulty red cells, and

(iii) production of an excess of red cells (polycythemia)

Category (i): It is by far the most common: The cause may be nutritional, as in iron, folate, or vitamin B$_{12}$ deficiency. It may also be infectious, as in malaria or infectious mononucleosis or it may be due to a diseased bone marrow.

Category (ii): It includes hemoglobinopathies and other hereditary disorders such as G-6-P-DH deficiency.

Category (iii): It's known as

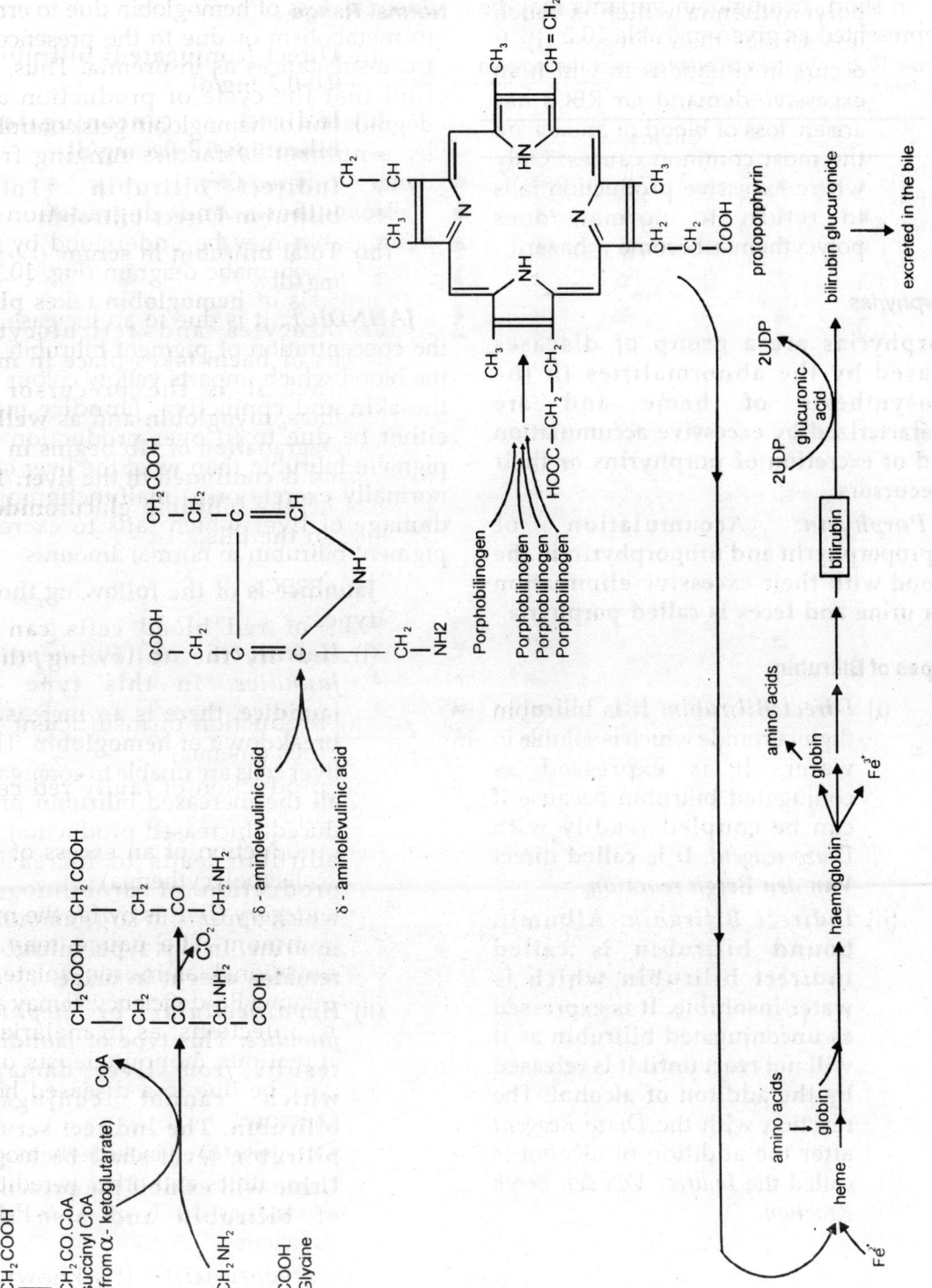

Fig. 10.3 : Biosynthesis and degradation of hemoglobin i.e. metabolism of Hb

polychythemia which is much less serious than category (i). It occurs in situations in which an excessive demand *for* RBCs has arisen: loss of blood or anoxia are the most common causes. Only where excessive production fails to return to normal, does polycythemia become a hazard.

Porphyrias

Porphyrias are a group of diseases caused by the abnormalities in the biosynthesis of heme and are characterized by excessive accumulation and or excretion of porphyrins or their precursors.

Porphyria: **Accumulation of coproporphyrin and uroporphyrin in the blood with their excessive elimination via urine and feces is called porphyria.**

Types of Bilirubin

(i) *Direct Bilirubin:* It is bilirubin diglucuronide which is soluble in water. It is expressed as conjugated bilirubin because it can be coupled readily with *Diazo reagent.* **It is called direct** *Van den Bergh reaction.*

(ii) *Indirect Bilirubin:* Albumin bound bilirubin is called indirect bilirubin which is water-insoluble. It is expressed as unconjugated bilirubin as it will not react until it is released by the additon of alcohol. The reaction with the *Diazo Reagent* after the addition of alcohol is called the *Indirect Van den Bergh Reaction.*

Normal Range

(i) **Direct (conjugated) bilirubin:** *0.0-0.2* **mg/dl**

(ii) **Indirect (unconjugated) bilirubin:** *0.2-0.8* **mg/dl.**

Indirect bilirubin =Total bilirubin-Direct bilirubin

(iii) **Total bilirubin in serum:** *0.2-1.0* mg/dl

JAUNDICE: It is due to an increase in the concentration of pigment bilirubin in the blood which imparts yellow colour to the skin and conjuctiva. Jaundice may either be due to (i) over production of pigment bilirubin than what the liver can normally excrete or(ii) malfunctioning/ damage of liver which fails to excrete pigment bilirubin in normal amounts.

Jaundice is of the following three types:

(i) *Hemolytic or Pre-hepatic jaundice:* **In this type of jaundice, there is an increased breakdown of hemoglobin.** The liver cells are unable to conjugate all the increased bilirubin produced. Increased production of bilirubin leads to increased production of urobilinogen which appears in large **amounts in urine. In this type, bilirubin remains absent in urine.**

(ii) *Hepatocellular or hepatic jaundice:* **This type of jaundice results** *from* **liver damage which cannot conjugate bilirubin. The indirect serum bilirubin level shall be high. Urine will exhibit the presence of bilirubin and also the** increased amount of urobilinogen. Stool is light in colour.

(iii) *Obstructive or post-hepatic jaundice:* This type of jaundice as the name itself indicates, results from the obstruction in common bile duct. As a result of obstruction, bilirubin does not pass into the intestine, therefore no urobilinogen is found in the urine. Direct serum bilirubin level will be high and urine will exhibit the presence of bilirubin. Moreover, the colour of stool shall be *clay-coloured*

Raised levels of bilirubin and its fractions may be understood by the following table 10.3.

Table 10.3 : To show raised levels of bilirubin and its fractions in different diseases

Sl.No.	High in
(A) Total Bilirubin	Obstructive jaundice, hemolytic *(prehepatic)jaundice,* neonatal jaundice and hepatitis.
(B) Direct Bilirubin	Acute or chronic hepatitis, biliary tract obstruction (cholangiolar, *hepatic,* or common ducts); Dubin Johnson and Rotor's syndromes, toxic reactions to many drugs, chemicals, toxins, etc.
(C) Indirect Bilirubin	-do- i.e., as mentioned in (B) and in hemolytic *(prehepatic)* diseases or reactions and absence or deficiency of enzyme glucuronyl transferase as in Gilbert's disease and Crigler-Najjar syndrome.

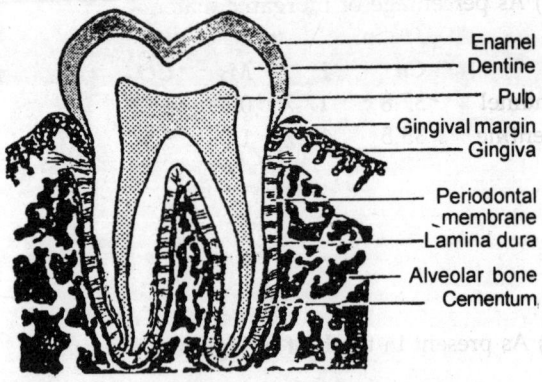

CHAPTER **11**

CHEMICAL COMPOSITION OF TEETH

> Without us life is unenjoyable and of almost no meaning. We are 32 in number. We, the humans (and the animals) are alive by and large for good quality delicious food and we earn day and night only for the same. Ours care from the very begining is must; if we get damaged partially or wholly, then we make the life miserable and painful. Our functions are numerous. Humans thought that we are made up of only Ca and P but the fact is that we are made up of nearly 30 elements.
>
> For ours good care, we wish that you do brushing twice i.e., morning and evening.

Inorganic Composition of Enamel and Dentine

The composition of enamel and dentine differ very much. The separation of the cementum from the dentine is less important because these two tissues have a similar composition and side by side the proportion of cementum present in the normal tooth is too small.

The anatomical relations of the dental tissues are shown in Fig. 11.1.

The approximate composition of human enamel and dentine which is very complicated has been expressed in different ways as shown in Table 11.1.

MINOR INORGANIC CONSTITUENTS OF ENAMEL AND DENTINE

One of the most important findings on the lesser constituents of the enamel and

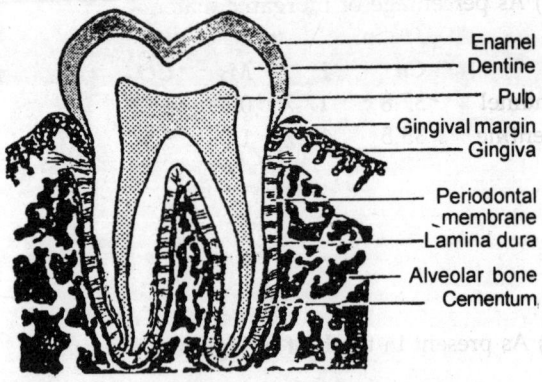

Fig. 11.1 : The relations of the main dental tissues.

Labels: Enamel, Dentine, Pulp, Gingival margin, Gingiva, Periodontal membrane, Lamina dura, Alveolar bone, Cementum

dentine is that their distribution throughout these tissues is not uniform. These ions can be classified into following three groups, namely:

(a) higher concentration on the surface of enamel than within (F,

Table 11.1 : The approximate composition of human enamel and dentine expressed in different ways

	Ca	P	Mg	CO_2	Organic matter	Comments
(1) As percentage of dry weight						
Enamel	36	17	0.4	2.5	1.3	(a) Tooth material heated to about 105°C till weight constant. Some water removed but 'bound' water retained.
Dentine	27	13	0.9	3.3	20	

(b) The large differences between the figures for enamel and dentine are due to the larger organic and water contents of dentine.

(c) More analytical figures are available for this material than for others; these results can be regarded as being more fully established than are those below.

(d) Variations between results of different workers are too great to justify the calculation of accurate averages.

	Ca	P	Mg	CO_2	Organic matter	
(2) As percentage of ash						
Enamel	38	18	0.4	none	none	(a) Tooth material heated strongly - all water-removed organic matter destroyed and CO_2 driven off from carbonates.
Dentine	38	18	1.2	none	none	

(b) Note that in this material, the only major difference is in the magnesium content.

	Ca	P	Mg	CO_2	Organic matter	
(3) As percentage of inorganic material						
Enamel	37.8	17.7	0.4	2.5	none	(a) Tooth material boiled with 3 percent KOH in ethylene glycol which removes organic matter and water but leaves carbonates intact.
Dentine	35.5	16.7	1.0	3.9	none	

(b) In detine, the figures given are those actually found, but they are lower than would be expected probably because some Ca and P are dissolved by the reagent.

	Ca	P	Mg	CO_2	Organic matter	
(4) As present in tooth of living animal (calculated)						
Enamel	35	16.5	0.4	2.5	1.3	
Dentine	24	11.5	0.9	3.0	18	

Note that the second column of figures refers to P, and not PO_4, and that CO_3, is present in the tooth which is usually expressed as CO_2. This explains why the figures do not add up to 100 per cent.

Actual analysis of fresh tooth, material is technically difficult. These approximate figures are calculated from those given in

(1) above assuming:

    (i) that enamel contians 4 per cent of water,

    (ii) that dentine contains 10 per cent of water.

Pb, Zn, Fe, Sb);

(b) lower concentration on surface than within (Na, Mg, CO).

(c) distribution approximately uniform (Sr, Cu, Al, K).

Ions which readily become attached to the apatite crystals tend to build up in those parts of the tooth which are exposed for the longest time to the body fluids, i.e., outer enamel, which is bathed in tissue fluid after calcification and before eruption and in saliva, food and drinks after eruption. The outer cementum and inner dentine are also in contact with tissue fluid throughout life and tend to concentrate trace elements in the same way as outer enamel.

Most trace elements are present throughout the bulk of the tooth in concentrations ranging from a few parts per million to less than 0.01 p.p.m, although in certain places, such as the outer enamel surface, the concentration may be much higher. Only *strontium fluoride* and *zinc reach or exceed concentrations of 100 pp.m. throughtout the tooth.*

SODIUM: Estimates of the amount of sodium in enamel and dentine vary widely but there is general agreement that enamel contains a higher proportion (about 0.7 per cent of enamal ash) than dentine (about 0.3 percentof dentine ash). **The sodium concentration of enamel is higher than that of any other tissue in the body.**

POTASSIUM: The concentration is probably less than 0.1 per cent of the ash.

CHLORIDE: The concentration of chloride in enamel (between 0.2 per cent and 0.3 per cent of dry weight) appears to be higher than that in dentine but a smaller proportion of it is water soluble.

CARBONATE: It's usually referred to as either *bicarbonate* or simply CO_2 adsorbed as such.

The carbonate content of enamel has been found to be lower on the outermost surface and to rise steadily towards the amelodentinal junction. There is a tendency for the carbonate on the outer layer to fall with increasing age.

TRACE ELEMENTS

The presence of about 20 elements has been detected by *spectrographic* study of enamel and dentine. The following elements have been detected spectrographically in most or an of the teeth studied:

Ag, Al, Ba, Cu, Fe, Mg, Ni, Pb, Si, Sr, Ti, V, and Zn. The following elements have been found in some samples but are not always detectable by spectroscopy, namely:

Teeth represent complex calcified structures in which calcification is differentiated in three distinct anatomical regions, i.e.,

(i) enamel,

(ii) dentine and

(iii) cementum

Dentine is the major tooth component; into it extends the pulp cavity containing the blood vessels and nerves.

The dentine is covered with a layer of cementum in the root and a layer of enamel in the exposed part of the tooth. Enamel is the most highly calcified and also the hardest tissue of the body. Dentine is softer than enamel but harder than bone and shows an intermediate degree of calcification.

(a) Cr

(b) K

(c) Li

(d) Mn, and

(e) Sn

Fluorine cannot always be detected by spectrographic means, probabely owing to its loss from the sample by volatilization at the high temperatures used in this method.

Not much is known till date about the significance of most of these elements in teeth. A few points of interest about some of the trace elements in teeth shall now be discussed.

FLUORIDE: The fluoride content of teeth has received a good deal of attention since the discovery of the relation between the intake of fluoride and the incidence of caries. It is quite clear that the fluoride content of enamel and dentine depends upon the amount of fluoride ingested in food and drinking water (also tea), mainly during calcification of teeth. The concentration of fluoride in dentine is between two and three times higher than the enamel. It has been analysed that the deciduous teeth contain a lower concentration than do permanent teeth. It is now known that much of the fluoride enters the enamel during calcification.

The concentration of fluoride on the extreme outer surface of the enamel has been found to be up to 10 times higher than that of the enamel as a whole. This is true even in areas where fluoride is found to be absent from the tap water. **Presumably, the fluoride enters the body via food and drink (especially via tea which contains about 1 p. p.m and has become very popular as a cheaper beverage in almost all the countries of the world.**

The main change with age is an increased depth of the fluoride rich-layer rather than in the concentration. The fluoride of dentine rises with age. The fluoride rich layer also occurs in deciduous teeth but the concentrations are lower than the permanent teeth.

SELENIUM: In some geographical areas, incidence of caries is found to be related to a high urinary excretion of selenium. Why does it happen, is not yet clear?

IRON: The presence of iron in human teeth has been established, but the exact concentration is not clear and its importance has not also been established so far. The yellow pigment of rodents' incisors is an iron containing compound.

LEAD: It has been found that the concentration of lead in human teeth increases with age upto early adulthood and then remains constant. It is found in **the concentration between 30 and 90 p.p.m. in moist dentine and enamel.**

COPPER: An average of approximately 20 p.p.m. of copper has been detected spectroscopically in enamel and about half of this concentration by activation analysis. It is randomly distributed and is not correlated with solubility, hypoplasia or caries.

ZINC: Zinc is found to have a distribution similar to that of fluoride, i.e., high (up to 2000 p.p.m.) on the outer surface of enamel decreasing to about 10-20 per cent of this figure at the amelodentinal junction. The level in coronal dentine is highest on the pulpal surface but in the root both the cemental and pulpal surface levels are higher than that of the inner dentine. The zinc concentration of teeth varies in different geographical areas.

Chemistry and Physiology of Collagen

> Collagen (Fig. 11.2) is the main protein constituent of most connective tissues and is the most prevalent single organic substance in the higher animals, *since it makes up about one-third of body protein.*
>
> Collagen in the form of microscopical fibres is widely distributed and is found in areolar tissue, tendons, ligaments and the connective tissue capsules of most organs. It also remains present in the matrix of bone, dentine, cementum and cartilage but in these tissues the fibres are so fine and tightly packed that histologically their matrix appears homogeneous when stained by routine methods, although special methods like electron micrographs reveal their fibrous pattern.

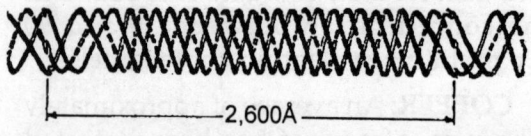

|← ——————— 2,600Å ——————— →|

Fig.11.2: A diagram of the arrangements of the three peptide chains in the collagen molecule. Two of the chains are identical but the third is different. The 2600 Å banding is believed to be inherent in the peptide chain and the periodicity at 640 Å appears because the chains are 'quarter staggered'.

There is evidence that zinc may exchange with calcium. It also binds with proteins in the body fluids and is consequently less readily available than fluoride for uptake by the tissues.

THE ORGANIC MATTER OF TEETH

It has been found that specimens of collagen from different organs show only very slight differences in constitution. After collagen has been hydrolysed, the product (known as hydrolysate) contains 18 amino acids. The approximate percentage of which is as given in Table 11.2 and the relative proportions of the amino acids in collagen are as given in Fig 11.3.

Collagen belongs to the group of fibrous proteins, its molecule being made up of long chains of amino acids (two chains are alike but the third one differs in amino acid composition) coiled together (Fig.11.2) and linked by hydrogen bonds.. **When collagen is heated with boiling water, it is converted into gelatin,** probably because the three chains become separated. These molecules polymerize very readily and this has made molecular weight determinations uncertain; figures between 340,000 and 10 millions have been quoted. The figure of 340,000 probably represents the basic unit of

Table 11.2 : Approxiamte percentage of amino acids in collagen

Sl. No.	Amino acid	Percentage
I.	glycine	nearly 26%
2.	proline	nearly 15%
3.	alanine	nearly 14%
4.	hydroxyproline	nearly 13%
5.	glutamic acid	nearly 8%
6.	arginine	nearly 5%
7.	aspartic acid	nearly 5%
8.	serine	nearly 3%
9.	leucine	nearly 2%
10.	valine	nearly 2%
II.	lysine	nearly 2%
12.	threonine	nearly 1%
13.	phenylalanine	nearly 1%
1.	isoleucine	nearly 1%
15.	hydroxylysine	nearly 0.7%
16.	methionine	nearly 0.5%
17.	histidine	nearly 0.5%
18.	tyrosine	nearly 0.3%

DENTINE COLLAGEN

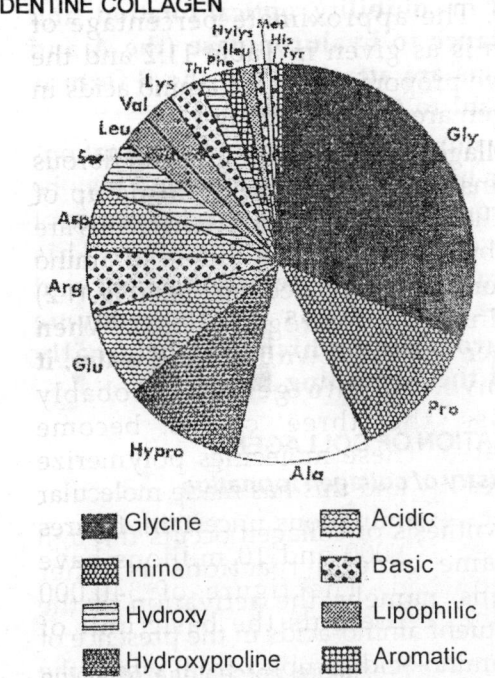

Glycine — Acidic

Imino — Basic

Hydroxy — Lipophilic

Hydroxyproline — Aromatic

Fig. 11.3 : The relative proportions of the amino-acids in collagen,

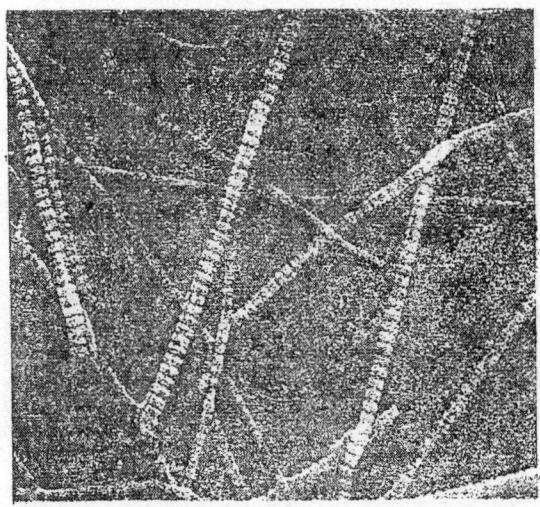

Fig. 11.4 : An electron micrograph of collagen fibres from a human tendon

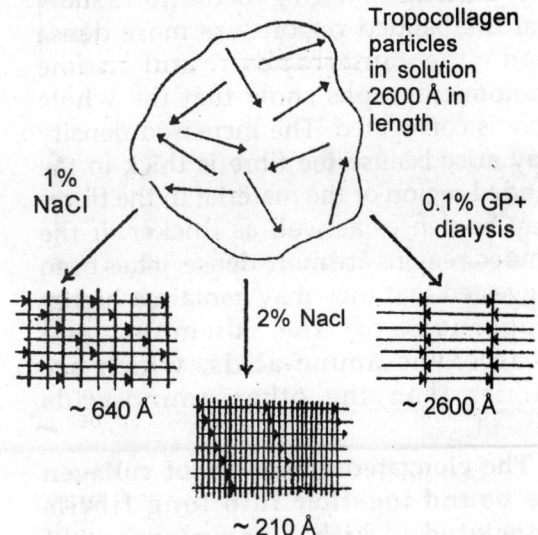

Fig. 11.5 : Diagram to illustrate how tropocollagen fibrils precipitated by different reagents may be arranged in different ways to give the various types of banding seen with the electron microscope. The 640 Å banding, as observed on collagen *in vivo*, is shown on the left and is made by a 'quarter stagger' of the molecules which possess a banding of approximately 2600 Å.

tropocollagen, a molecule with dimensions approximately 14 x 2800 Å which readily polymerizes to form collagen.

The electron microscope shows that collagen fibres have highly characteristic regular striations at intervals of 640 Å (Fig. 11.4). Their significance has been explained by the following observations illustrated in Fig. 11.5.

Collagen dissolves in dilute acids and if certain substances are added to the solution, the collagen is precipitated as fibres which also show the banding, whilst the distances between the bandings depend on the substance used to form the precipitate. With 1 per cent NaCl as the precipitating agent; the bands correspond with the 640Å of natural collagen. With 2 per cent NaCl, however, the bands are only about 210Å apart whereas with 0.1 per cent of a particular glycoprotein followed by dialysis they vary between 2600 and

3000 Å (FLS or 'fibrous long spacing' type). These finding are interpreted as follows: the smallest units of collagen have a banding of 2600 Å but in the natural form they are lying parallel (see Fig. 11.5) and the individual molecules are staggered about a quarter of their length and so the bands of adjacent fibres are 640 Å apart (a 'quarter stagger'); the 210 Å bands are staggered one twelth of their length whereas in the FLS type the bandings are all in the same place. Chondroitin sulphate is another substance which precipitates the fibres and as this substance is invariably associated with collagen in tissues, it may perhaps be concerned with the formation of the fibres *in vivo*.

Densitometer tracings of the fibres show that the banded regions are more dense than the interbands, and some photomicrographs show that the whole fibre is corrugated. The increased density may arise beause the fibre is thick in the banded region or the material in the fibres may be denser as well as thicker. If the banded regions are more dense, it has been suggested that they may contain a higher proportion of the diamino and dicarboxylic amino-acids, which are bulkier than the other amino-acids present.

The elongated molecules of collagen are bound together into long fibrils associated with complexes of mucopolysaccharides and non-collagenous proteins. There are two main kinds of mucopolysaccharides in connective tissues: (1) hyaluronic acid (a polymer of equimolecular parts of N-acetyl glucosamine and glucuronic acid) and (2) chondroitin sulphate (a polymer of N-acetyl galactosamine sulphate and glucuronic acid) of which three types are known (described as A, B and C), which differ in solubility, optical rotation and resistance to hyaluronidase (the A and C forms are attacked, but the B form is resistant to the enzyme).

Hyaluronic acid is found in situations where lubrication is required and may be the ground susbtance in which bundles of collagen fibres are embedded. This substance can be depolymerized and made less viscous by the enzyme hyaluronidase which was originally called the 'spreading factor.'

FORMATION OF COLLAGEN
Chemistry of collagen formation

The synthesis of collagen occurs through the same general reactions as other proteins, namely, the activation of the constituent amino-acids in the presence of ATP amino-acid complex from which the amino-acid is transferred into the peptide chain of the protein being synthesized. Some more specialized reactions appear to be involved during collagen synthesis.

Ascorbic acid and alkaline phosphatase play role in collagen formation

In severe ascorbic acid deficiency in guinea pigs, collagen formation does not occur although fibroblasts survive and may even proliferate although they have an abnormal appearance. It has further been seen that much more collagen is formed in areas receiving ascorbic acid.

Collagen formation is accompanied by the presence of high concentration of alkaline phosphatase in the fibroblasts and on the fibre itself. In scurvy, neither alkaline phosphatase nor collagen appear, suggesting that collagen synthesis requries the action of phosphatase and that ascorbic acid is related to the presence of the enzyme. It has been suggested that this enzyme is in some way connected with the synthesis of other fibrous proteins: for example, the keratin of hair.

Hormones and Collagen formation

Glucocorticoids of the adrenal cortex (eg. cortisone) have a marked action in inhibiting collagen formation, thus interfering with wound healing and the repair of the fractured bones. Adrenocorticotrophic hormone, which causes the release of glucocorticoids, has a similar action.

Mineralocorticoids (such as deoxycorticosterone) on the other hand, stimulate fibroblasts and favour collagen formation.

Organic Matter of Dentine

Dentine contains roughtly 19.66 per cent organic matter as shown in Table 11.3.

Table 11.3 : Organic constituents of dentine (approximate percentage on dry weight basis).

Collagen	18
Citrate	0.9
Chondroitin sulphate	0.2
Other proteins	0.2
Lipid	0.36

Organic Matter of Enamel

The approximate composition of the organic matter of enamel is summarized in Table 11.4.

Table 11.4 : Organic Constituents of enamel (percentage on dry weight basis).

Insoluble proteins	0.25
Soluble proteins	0.25
Lipid	0.6
Citrate	0.1

Enamel has been found to contain 0.6 per cent of lipid, mostly unidentified which also includes some phosphatide and cholesterol.

Enamel contains proteins as described above. Most proteins contain about 16% of nitrogen.

Citrate is found at the lower average concentration of 0.1 %; it is higher on the surface and near the amelodentinal junction than in the middle of the enamel.

Lactate is also found in human enamel with a distribution similar to that of citrate but at a lower concentration.

CHAPTER 12

BIOCHEMISTRY OF SALIVA

I am a natural lubricant secreted by mouth and my composition is not so easy as you think; besides so many organic and inorganic constituents, I do also contain so many enzymes which help in digestion. I get secreted in higher quantity when I come across any flavoured, good looking, good smelled food. Higher the flavour- higher mine secretion. If I am higher in quantity, I help in swallow process and digestion.

Composition of Saliva

Saliva (Table 12.1) is produced by three pairs of large glands and the smaller glands of the oral mucosa (labial, lingual, buccal and palatal), whose secretions differ in composition and whose relative contribution to the mixed saliva present in the mouth varies with conditions. Since little is known about the factors which decide the relative secretion rates of each source, this variable is difficult to control.

The composition of the saliva produced from any one gland varies with the rate of flow which itself varies with the type and intensity of stimulus used for obtaining the sample. Consequently the composition of saliva may vary with the changes in the stimulus.

Saliva varies greatly in different individuals and in the same individual under different circumstances. An approximate composition of mixed human

saliva is as given in Table 12.1.

Organic Constituents

The total protein content of human saliva averages about 0.3% but may vary widely.

Mucoids: One of the main proteins in saliva is what is often called *'mucin'*. This name implies to a definite single substance but, as it is a somewhat ill-defined mixture, the term 'mucoid' has come into general use, indicating a class of substance (within the wider group of mucoproteins) rather than one substance. Mucoids contain carbohydrate derivatives, such as hexosamine in their molecules and it has been proposed by scientist Meyer that the term be confined to those proteins which contain more than 4% hexosamine. Many proteins contain small proportions of hexosamine (e.g., serum globulins) and the term *'glycoprotein'* has been suggested for those

Table 12.1 : Data on the approximate composition of mixed human saliva

Substance	Unstimulated saliva (mg/100 ml)		Stimulated saliva (mg/100 ml)		Comments
	Average	Range	Average	Range	
Total solids	no data	-	530	410-720	Usually expressed as
Total ash	no data	-	250	170-350	0.53% and 0.25%
Organic Constituents					
Total Protein	similar to stimulated?		280	180-420	No separate figure available for mucoid but most of the protein exists in this form
Amino-acids	no data	-	4	no data	
Lysozyme	no data	-	10	?	
Urea	20	?	13	?	
Ammonia	?	?	7	1-12	
Uric acid	?	?	3 (approx.)	1-21	Presumably stimulated but not clearly stated. Over 4.0 mg abnormal.
Creatinine	up to 1	?	no data		
Cholesterol	7.9	2.5-50	no data		
Glucose	-	-	1.0	0.5-3.0	Many published figures probably too high because reducing substances other than glucose included.
Citrate	-	-	1	0.2-2.0	
Lactate	-	-	?	1-5	
Vitamins (µg/ml)					
Aneurin HCl	0.7		no data		
Riboflavin	5.0		no data		
Nicotinic Acid	3.0		no data		
Pyridoxine HCl	60.0		0.6	0.1-1.7	No Explanation of wide differences between these figures
Folic Acid	0.01		2.4	0.3-7.5	
Pantothenic Acid	8.0		-	-	
Biotin	0.08		-	-	
Vitamin K	1.5		-	-	
Inorganic Constituents (mg/100ml)					
Sodium	30	15-60	60	29-111	
Potassium	80	53-125	80 (same)	53-125 (same)	
Thiocyanate	13	3-27	?	?	
Calcium	5.8	2.2-11.3			

Table 12.1 : Data on the approximate composition of mixed human saliva

Substance	Unstimulated saliva (mg/100 ml)		Stimulated saliva (mg/100 ml)		Comments
	Average	Range	Average	Range	
Phosphate (P)	16.8	6.1-71			When estimations are made on saliva secreted by paraffin wax stimulation, then Ca and phosphate concentrations are found to be lower than in the unstimulated saliva.
Magnesium	1.0	0.76-1.3	no data	no data	
Chloride	50	?	50	?	
CO_2 (vols. %)	15		150		
Bromide	no data	no data	?	0.1-0.7	Usually expressed as part per million. (1 p.p.m. = 0.1 mg/100ml)
Iodide	no data	no data	?	0.35-0.24	
Fluoride	no data	no data	?	0.01-0.02	
Copper	no data	no data	0.025	0.010-0.047	

'No data' means that no figures appear to have been published? indicates that although figures are available but they are uncertain or cannot be averaged. This table is not intended to be a complete record of all salivary constituents, but it does show (l) the wide range of substances which saliva is already known to contain, and (2) the gaps in present knowledge.

which have less than 4%. All these terms are still often used rather loosely, however. **The most important property of mucoid is the sliminess of the solution which** *makes saliva an excellent lubricant.* **Saliva mucoid is only slighty soluble in water,** is insoluble in weak acids and may be precipitated from saliva by dilute acetic acid or alcohol but redissolves in the form of sodium salt in NaOH.

Mucoids from mixed human saliva contain an average of :

(i) 10-11 % of nitrogen and

(ii) approximately twenty percent of mucopolysaccharides made up of 6- 7% hexosamine, 8-10% hexose, 3% fucose (a methyl pentose), 1-2% sialic acid.

Silaic acid (which is also called N-acetyl neuraminic acid or NANA) is an acetylated form of one of the neuraminic acids which can be regarded as the condensation products of an amino sugar (usually mannosamine) and pyruvic acid.

The proportion of sialic acid in mucoid from human saliva is much lower than in that from animal saliva, which may contain upto 20%.

Other protein Constituents: By electrophoresis of saliva, presence of many additional proteins has been established **which include mucoids, minute concentration of** *albumins* **and globulins, lysozyme, amylase and other enzymes.** Immunological tests have confirmed that atleast 6 salivary proteins are serum proteins but have also established that some distinctive salivary proteins are present.

Other nitrogenous Constituents

18 amino acids have been detected in whole saliva: of these 9 have been found consistently and 9 are found sometimes. The concentration of most of the individual amino-acids was less than 0.3 mg%. An unusual aminoacid-porbably γ - amino-butyric acid (GABA) has been detected in whole saliva.

Peptides remain present in saliva and there is evidence that they, and perhaps some amino acids act as cofactors in the metabolism of salivary bacteria.

Urea, creatinine, uric acid and ammonia are also found in saliva but their significance, if any, is not properly known.

Glucose: Sugars in free form are found only in traces in fasting saliva (0.5-1.0 mg %). Figures based upon the reducing power of saliva suggest much higher levels (upto 30 mg %) but it is now known that most of these reducing substances are not sugar.

Much higher concentrations of sugar are found in the saliva after eating carbohydrate.

Other Organic Constituents

Citrate: It has been found in saliva in concentrations ranging from 0.2 to 2.0 mg %. Since citrate is a chelate of calcium, which means that it forms a complex ion even at the normal salivary pH; **it has been suggested that high salivary citrate might be a factor concerned in a clinical condition known as *'dental erosion'* in which the enamel becomes dissolved without the usual symptoms of dental caries.**

Lactate: It is found in very variable quantities since it is one of the main products of bacterial degradation of carbohydrates by salivary bacteria. After a meal, 10 fold increases in concentration upto 50 mg% have been found.

Agglutinogens : The agglutinogens A, B and O, which are soluble polysaccharides, are found in the saliva of about 80% of the people ('secretors') whose cells contain them and have been isolated in yields of about 3 mg %.

Vitamins: Vitamins like thiamine, riboflavim, niacin, pyridoxine, folic acid, pantothenic acid, biotin and vitamin K are also found in saliva.

Apoerythein : Saliva is also stated to contain *apoerythein* **a substance related to the** 'intrinsic factor' concerned in the utilization of vitamin B_{12}.

Lipids: Chromatography has revealed the presence of many lipids, including cholesterol and cholesterol esters, fatty acids, glycerides, and phospholipids in saliva but all of them are found in very low concentration.

Corticosteroids: These are also found in saliva but in vary low concentration than the blood.

Enzymes of saliva : Salivary amylase is found in sufficient quantity but it is not the only enzyme found in saliva. **Besides salivary amylase other found in saliva include:**

  (i) **acid phosphatase**
 (ii) **esterases**
(iii) **choline esterase**
 (iv) **lipase**
  (v) **aldolase**
 (vi) **lysozyme**
(vii) **β- glucuronidase**
(viii) **succinic dehydroganase**
 (ix) **peroxidase**
  (x) **carbonic anhydrase, etc.**

Some of the enzymes play important role in various processes.

Inorganic Constituetns

Calcium and phosphorus: **Because of their possible connections with dental caries the calcium and phosphorus concentrations in saliva** have been studied and thoroughly investigated by several workers. Extensive study was carried out by the scientists **Becks and Wainwright** who have given the following Table 12.2.

Phosphorus of saliva remains present in several forms. About 90% phosphorus of saliva remains present in inorganic form. Traces of many organic phosphorus compounds are also found for e.g. phosphorylated carbohydrate compounds such as hexose phosphates, phospholipids, nucleoproteins and nucleic acids. It has been further studied that upto 10% of the inorganic phosphate remains present as pyrophosphate.

The concentrations of calcium and inorganic phosphate in saliva are, even more than the blood.

Other inorganic constituents

The following ions remain presnet in saliva in readily detectable amounts: sodium, potassium, magnesium, chloride, sulphate and thiocyanate.

Minute traces of fluoride, iodide, bromide, nitrite and copper have also been recorded.

The average concentration of thiocyanate is about 13 mg% with a wide range (3 to 27 mg %).

The fluoride content of saliva is of interest in connection with the important effect of fluoride in reducing dental caries. The concentration found by chemical methods is about 0.1 to 0.2 p.p.m. but recent results with the fluoride electrode suggest much lower figures i.e., between 0.01 and 0.05 p.p.m. (mostly in ionic form with very little bound). Experiments indicate a slight rise after drinking water.

Hydrogen ion concentration

pH of unstimulated saliva ranges from 5.6 to 7.6 with an average of 6. 7 5. No sex differences are found as regards pH.

The cells of saliva : Microscopical examination of saliva shows that epithetial cells (buccal squames) are always present in addition to leucocytes, mostly polymorphs.

The gases dissolved in saliva: Like all body fluids, saliva contains oxygen, nitrogen and CO_2 in solution. The oxygen and nitrogen centents are stated to be between 0.18 and 0.25 volumes per cent and about 0.9 volumes per cent respectivety.

Unstimulated saliva contains 10-20 volumes percent of CO_2 and vigorously stimulated saliva upto 150   volumes per cent.

Saliva contains the enzyme *carbonic anhydrase* **which catalyses the reaction:**

$$CO_2 + H_2O \rightleftharpoons H_2CO_3$$

Bicarbonate is the main buffering system of saliva.

Effect of diet on the composition of saliva

Nearly 120 years ago, several workers had

Table 12.2 : Effect of rate of flow on Ca and inorganic P contents of unstimulated saliva

	Av. rate of flow (ml/hr)	Av. conc. of Ca (mg%)	Av. amount of Ca (mg/hr)	Av. conc. of P (mg%)	Av. Amount of P (mg/hr)
Slow secretors	13.4	5.99	0.80	17.0	2.21
Rapid secretors	39.6	5.66	2.26	11.8	4.42

reported that the consumption of diets high in carbohydrates is followed by a rise in the amylase content of saliva and this was later on confirmed in different studies carried out by different scientists at different places.

The first group normally ate a predominantly carbohydrate diet, the second group ate a protein rich diet. The second group had an average of 1/10th of the activity of salivary amylase found in the first group.

Effect of fatigue: If the salivary glands are stimulated vigorously for an hour or so, the volume of saliva secreted per minute shows little tendency to fall, but some of the solid constituents (e.g., γ - globulins) do decrease whereas others (e.g. urea) may maintain their concentration for as long as 3 hours. The fall in organic constituents probably arises from the exhaustion of reserve material in the cells whereas the fall in inorganic constituents is probably caused by fatigue making it more difficult for the cells to transfer substances from the blood to the saliva.

Effect of hormones

It has been shown in man that the injection of adrenocorticotrophic hormone and cortisone causes a lowering of salivary sodium but little change in salivary potassium. Effects of other hormones on saliva have not yet been established.

Physical Properties of Saliva

- The specific gravity of saliva varies between 1.000 to 1.010 and increases with increasing rate of flow.
- The osmotic pressure is between half and three - quarters that of blood but sublingual saliva has

got approximately the same osmotic pressure as blood.

- Saliva is a viscous fluid and also shows the property of' *spinbarkest*, i.e. the ability to be drawn out into long elastic threads. On standing for an hour or so even at room temperature, the viscosity of mixed saliva falls.

The relative viscosities of the three main secretions after acetic-acid stimulation are found to be :

(a) Parotid   :   1.5
(b) Submaxillary :   3.4
(c) Sublingual   :   13.4

- The buffering power (that is, the power to resist changes of pH when acid or alkali are added) of saliva varies at different pH values because different systems of buffers are effective over different parts of the pH range. Salivary buffers consist of bicarbonates and phosphates
- Saliva contains a complex mixture of substances with reducing properties which have been mistakenly assumed in the past to be glucose. These include carbohydrates split off from mucoids, proteins, nitrites and some unidentified substances of low molecular weight.
- The total volume of saliva amounts to between 1.0 and 1.5 litres a day.

Control of the Secretion of Saliva

Saliva seems to be unique among the digestive juices in that its secretion is controlled exclusively by nerves. No hormone has been discovered which

controls specifically its rate of flow.

The salivary glands receive a double nerve supply (1) from the parasympathetic (a branch of the facial nerve to the sublingual and submaxillary and a branch of the glossopharyngeal to the parotid), and (2) from the sympathetic (fibres arising between the first and fourth thorasic segments and relaying in the superior sympathetic ganglion).

Secreting Cell of a salivary gland **(The nature of the secretory process).**

Electron micrographs have made it possible to picture the main sequence of events during the process of secretion.

The basal side of the glandular and duct cells have been found to be elaborately infolded thus giving the appearance of presenting an increased surface area-even upto 60 fold-which presumably facilitates the uptake of water and dissolved substances from the tissue fluid. Mitochondria are sometimes but not always, closely associated with the infoldings.

The endoplasmic reticulum is concerned with the synthesis of proteins including the enzymes and mucoids of saliva which are released as microsomes. When ^{14}C amino acids are injected, the microsomes contain labelled amylase within 5-10 minutes. It is probable that the newly synthesized protein molecules are transported to the golgi apparatus which converts them into the secretion granules very well as may be seen by the light microscope.

The number of granules increases after various procedures such as injection of pilocarpine or adrenaline which are known to increase secretion.

In the parotid gland (as in the pancreas) synthesis of amylase appears to be independent of nerve control and is regulated by a chemical equilibrium so that when stores are depleted after secretion, more synthesis occurs. In the suubmandibular, and sublingual glands, however, synthesis is increased by pilocarpine or by eating (which causes nerve stimulation) and is prevented by atropine. **These observations strongly suggest that in these glands synthesis is under nervous control.**

Several types of extrusion mechanism have been described from electron micrographs of various secreting cells; the one most frequently seen in the salivary glands is as follows. In the cytoplasm a secretion granule forms, the outer membrane of which approaches and fuses with the microvilli of the inner secreting surface of the cell. The membrane then ruptures allowing the contents of the granule to escape. The wall of the secretion granule then straightens out and becomes a new part of the cell wall (Fig. 12.1).

The structure of the 'secretary capillaries' between the serous cells (Fig. 12.2) has been clarified in the human submandibular gland. They have many microvilli projecting into them (unlike the inner surface of the cells on which microvilli were found to be rather spares) and this is presumably the route by which some of the products reach the lumen.

Movement of the secretion along the ducts may be encouraged by the branched myoepithelial cells (basket cells) whose cytopalsm contains fibres similar to those of smooth muscle. These cells are state to be widely distributed in the acini and ducts of the salivary glands (Fig. 12.3).

Functions of Saliva

Saliva has many functions and although, not essential for the maintenance of life,

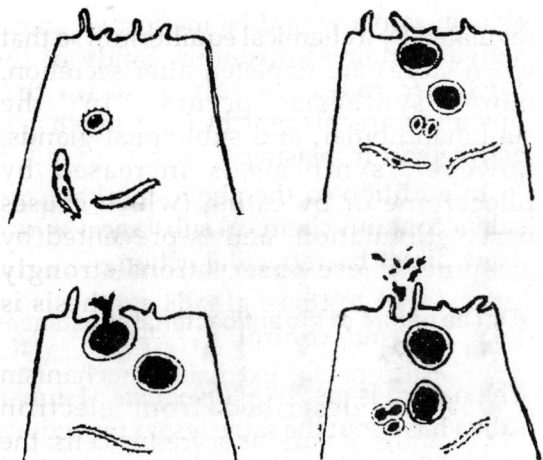

Fig. 12.1 : Successive stages in one method of extrusion of secretion granules observed in the salivary glands.

it makes important and varied contribution to the efficient working and protection of the body.

(A) **Digestive Functions:** The only important digestive enzyme in the saliva is ptyalin or salivary amylase. This enzyme digests starch provided it has been previously cooked. The significance of the cooking of starch is that heat breaks up starch granules, after which their contents form a colloidal suspension which can be attacked by the enzyme.

Amylases are of 2 types referred to as

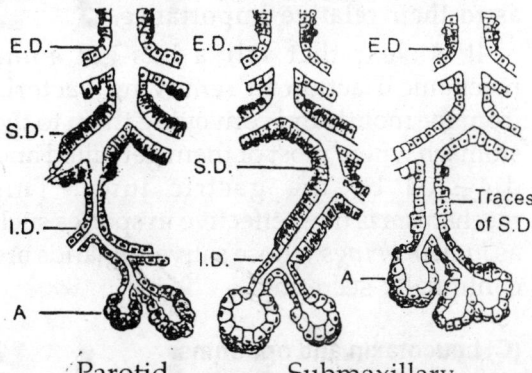

Fig. 12.3: The distribution of the salivary ducts in the various salivary glands

E.D.- excretory duct, S.D.-striated duct,
I.D. - intercalated duct (absent from sublingual),
A-alveolus containing serous cells (in the parotid)
or serous and mucous cells (submandibular).

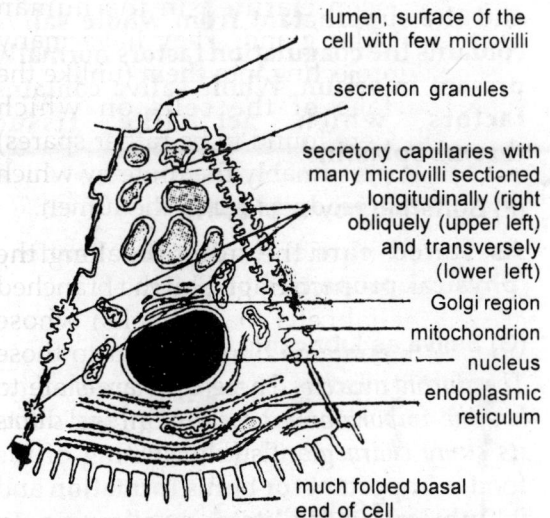

lumen, surface of the cell with few microvilli
secretion granules
secretory capillaries with many microvilli sectioned longitudinally (right obliquely (upper left) and transversely (lower left)
Golgi region
mitochondrion
nucleus
endoplasmic reticulum
much folded basal end of cell

Fig. 12.2 : Diagram of a secreting cell of a salivary gland based upon electron microscope studies.

α - and β amylases. α- amylase breaks down the starch molecule simulataneously at many places into a large number of dextrin molecules which are then more slowly attacked, chiefly forming maltose.

Contrarily, β amylases are found in plants and attack starch molecules by breaking off maltose units one at a time, thus gradually reducing the size of the starch molecule.

Three stages in the process of amylase digestion can be recognized by means of iodine reaction:

Starch→ Soluble→ erythrodextrin→ achrodextrin→ maltose
 starch

Blue with iodine	Blue with iodine	Red with iodine	No colour with iodine	Reduces Fehling's solution

(B) The Antibacterial function of Saliva

It is often stated that although bacteria are always present, wounds in the mouth heal rapidly and rarely become infected.

Many antibacterial actions of saliva have been observed but opinions differ as to their relative importance.

It is clear that saliva has got some mechanical action in removing bacteria from the mouth and conveying them to the stomach where most of them get killed and digested by the gastric juice. This mechanism is most effective in species such as *human beings* whose salivary glands are continually secreting.

(C) Leucotaxin and opsonins

Two properties of saliva have been described which, although not fully established, may be related to its antibacterial power. It has been shown, firstly, that saliva increases capillary *permeability* and secondly, that it possesses *chemotactic activity* towards leucocytes (i.e. the power of attracting leucocytes, by a mechanism not yet understood). **Both these properties remain present in a polypeptide isolated in a crystalline form from inflammatory exudates and are called as 'leucotaxin'.**

It is well known that leucocytes thoroughly washed free of plasma and suspended in saline do not phagocytose bacteria but if a trace of plasma is added, phagocytosis readily occurs. **The substances in plasma which make bacteria more *'palatable'* to leucocytes are called *'opsonins'*.** Similarly, the phagocytic cells in saliva would be ineffective unless saliva contained opsonins. Study of the *'opsomic index'* of saliva shows that opsonins are present but are much less active than in plasma.

In addition to the above mechanisms, saliva contains chemical substances which exert direct bacteriocidal action.

(D) The nature of the antibacterial substances in Saliva

The nature is just like *'lysozyme'*. Human saliva has about the same lysozyme activity as blood. Lysozyme is an enzyme which has got the capability to disintegrate certain complex polysaccharides present in some bacteria and thus causes their death. If these polysaccharides are absent from certain species of bacteria, then they are not destroyed by lysozyme.

(E) Saliva and blood coagulation

When freshly shed blood is diluted with saliva, its clotting time is reduced. **It has been studied that saliva from all the three glands as well as both the sediment and the supernatant from whole saliva contains the coagulation factors normally present in serum. Whole saliva contains factors which act like tissue thromboplastins.**

(F) Buffering power of saliva

As stated earlier under the heading 'physical properties of Saliva':

(G) Saliva as lubricant

The mucoid which is the main protein of saliva, has the important property of giving saliva its slimy character. The moistening of the food is important **for bolus formation** and its lubrication facilitates swallowing. **In man the lubrication of the mouth is necessary for clear speech.** The accurate positioning of the tongue in relation to the teeth becomes difficult when the mouth is dry. The lubricating function of saliva is perhaps best appreciated when salivary flow gets inhibited during nervousness or embarrassment. Under these special circumstances, the swallowing of dry food or clear speaking in public becomes very difficult.

(H) Saliva and Taste

The sensation of taste is produced only by substances in solution. Some foods such as fruits, contain such a high proportion of water that probably all the substances which have a taste and already in solution and their taste may be perceived as soon as they are released by mastication. Other foods, biscuits for example, contain relatively little water and before their taste becoems apparent, saliva must dissolve out the flavoured constituents. By this means, saliva not only makes eating more pleasurable but may assist in the detection of unwholesome contaminants of food.

(I) Saliva as a route of Excretion

Saliva is a route by which certain substances are excreted. Saliva can only be an effective route of excretion for substances that are either destroyed or rendered insoluble during their passing through the gut after swallowing. **Thiocyanate is one of the normal constituents of saliva which has been regarded as an excretion.**

It is undoubtedly true that mercury and lead are present in traces in saliva of people suffering from poisoning by these metals but both. are known to be absorbed by the intestine.

Among the symptoms of severe mercury poisoning are an unpleasant metallic taste and an increased flow of saliva. The amount of excretion through saliva would seem to be insignificant compared with that via the kidneys. The stated presence of glucose in the saliva of diabetics and salivary urea in kidney diseases are often considered to be *excretions.*

The viruses responsible for such diseases like *hydrophobia, poliomyelitis, saliva (in minute quantity),* mumps, etc. remain present in the saliva of infected individuals and would therefore be swallowed. Since the viruses are proteins, they would at least in some cases, be destroyed by the digestive mechanisms of the gut.

Incidentally, the saliva of sufferers from these virus diseases is a potential source of infection for others.

(J) Saliva and the Iodine Metabolism

Saliva contains iodide in the concentrations between 20 and 100 times that of the plasma. It has been suggested that the glands deiodinate thyroxine and diiodotyrosine, secreting the released iodine (in the form of iodide), which, after swallowing and absorption from the gastroi testinal tract, becomes available for use by the thyroid.

The Effect of Desalivation on other Organs

A fall in body weight and especially in the weight of adrenals, testis, ovary and uterus has been reported by various scientists following the removal of the salivary glands in the rat. The effects on the testis and adrenals and the fall in body weight were probably caused by the reduced food consumption which occurs in the absence of saliva.

CHAPTER 13

DIGESTION AND ABSORPTION

We (digestion & absorption) two are the most important aspects for any living organism, especially for the animals. If we do not work simultaneously in a satisfactory way, then we make the life of any millionaire very miserable and shocking. We are always very friendly to any human (animal) system but we advise them not to consume food in bulk and too frequently at short intervals as various enzymes and other factors bringing out these processes are afterall also in limited amount and secreted in small amount. Afterall we also want some rest. We shall take care of you and your system provided you too behave in the same way.

Introduction

The alimentary tract extends from the mouth to the anus (Fig. 13.1) which remains in contact to the external environment at both ends, which can be sealed only partially. **Main functions of the tract are** *digestion* **and** *absorption* **of food, as well as excretion of the residues as stool.** These functions are carried out in different compartments like mouth, stomach, small intestines (comprising of duodenum, jejunum and ileum) and colon (large intestine). The tract terminates in the sigmoid and the rectum.

All movements and secretions are controlled by nerve impulses. An involuntary wave like contraction of muscles lining the walls of the tract (peristaltic movement) facilitates the passage of the food. The mucus present in the mucosal lining of the epithelial cells acts

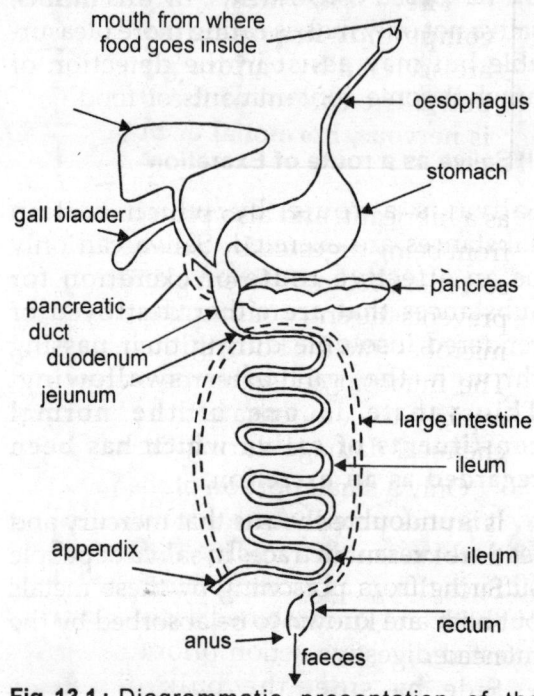

Fig. 13.1 : Diagrammatic presentation of the Alimentary tract

Labels: mouth from where food goes inside; oesophagus; stomach; gall bladder; pancreas; pancreatic duct; duodenum; jejunum; large intestine; ileum; appendix; ileum; anus; faeces; rectum

A number of factors assist the digestive processes. Cooking of food produces several changes. It softens certain tissues, breaks the cellulose covering around starch granules allowing better access to digestive enzymes, partially hydrolyzes some food components, brings about coagulation of liquid proteins of eggs and other foods and also improves the flavour of some, which may result in increased flow of saliva and gastric juice.

Marsication greatly increases the surface area of food for better contact with the digestive juices. The most important factor in digestion, is of course, the action of the enzymes and other specific components of the digestive juices.

The enzymes and other compounds important in digestion are secreted by various glands of the body. The control of these secretions is nervous, hormonal or both.

as a lubricant, and also protects these cells from being digested by the enzymes of the secretions from different glands. It further prevents the entry of infectious viruses and microbes into the body through these cells. The mucosal cells are regenerated very rapidly to compensate the physical and chemical damage during their function.

Only a small portion of the food we eat is in the proper form for absorption into the blood or the lymph system of the body. Such things as water, uncombined mineral salts, and uncombined vitamins may not need digestive action prior to absorption. Side by side, the bulk of our food undergoes many chemical changes before the resulting molecules can be absorbed.

The proteins and protein split products must be hydrolyzed to amino acids; the polysaccharides and the oligosaccharides to hexose sugars and the lipids to fatty acids and glycerol, in part at least. Other lipids are also hydrolyzed to smaller product molecules.

Digestion of Carbohydrates

Carbohydrates being used most by human beings in food consist of polysaccharides i.e. starch (vegetables, grains, cereals, pulses etc.) and glycogen (animal sources like liver, muscles etc.). To a lesser extent are the disaccharides i.e., lactose of milk and sucrose of molasses and the ordinary sugar. Other related compounds less commonly present are lactic acid, alcohol, pectins etc.

The digestive process involves the enzymatic hydrolysis of the poly and disaccharides to the simplest constituent units i.e., monosaccharides, consisting mainly of glucose with small amount of fructose and galactose. First of all ptyalin (an (α- amylase) secreted from the parotid glands in the mouth, hydrolyzes starch to maltose mainly with few other smaller polymers of glucose containing 3-9 units (e.g., maltotriose, dextrin). The action of ptyalin continues in the fundus of the stomach till the food is mixed with the gastric secretion producing a low pH at which ptyalin gets inactivated. However, this appears to cause at the most 30% digestion of starch. When the food passes into the duodenum and the upper jejunum, the pH gets raised by the bicarbonate in the pancreatic secretion. **Virtually, whole of the starch gets hydrolysed to maltose and other polymers in about 30 minutes by the action of pancreatic amylase which remains present in the pancreatic** secretion. **At this site, glycogen is also hydrolysed to smaller fragments due to the splitting of (α -1$\rightarrow$ 4 linkages for which this amylase is specific.**

Lactose $\xrightarrow{\text{(lactase)}}$ glucose + galactose

Maltose $\xrightarrow{\text{(maltase)}}$ glucose + glucose

Sucrose $\xrightarrow{\text{(sucrase)}}$ glucose + fructose

Dextrin $\xrightarrow{\text{(dextrinase)}}$ glucose (several molecules)

Further digestion of maltose and other disaccharides as well as of small polymers of glucose takes place in the epithelial cells lining the intestinal lumen.Enzymes i.e., lactase, maltase, sucrase and dextrinase are found to be located in the membrane of the microvilli brush border and the sugars are hydrolysed as soon as they come in contact with these membranes.

In this way, the final product of the digestion of carbohydrates is almost wholly glucose with little fructose and galactose and are absorbed immediately after formation.

Another polysaccharide i.e., cellulose remains abundantly present in the vegetable food; but the enzyme necessary for its-breakdown remains absent in humans, therefore, it's excreted as such in stool. Cellulose is a polymer of β - glucose; herbiborous animals i.e., cattles do possess the corresponding enzyme i.e., cellulase, therefore, they can digest it.

Absorption of Carbohydrates

Be it known that glucose is the most abundant monosaccharide available after digestion of carbohydrates; however, there may be found small amounts of other

monosaccharides viz., fructose, galactose and perhaps mannose also. Some amount of the disaccharides, i.e., sucrose and maltose may also remain unhydrolysed. All these are absorbed easily through the intestinal mucosa. Glucose and galactose are also absorbed by the same process. The latest theroy is that these carbohydrates are not absorbed by simple diffusion, but by the *sodium ion dependant transport mechanism* requiring special carrier protein. This is well established in case of glucose and galactose, whereas, other carbohydrates may have a facilitated diffusion mechanism with special carrier proteins. The disaccharides are hydrolysed into the monosaccharides by specific enzymes inside the eptithelial cells and it is only the monosaccharides that are passed ito the portal blood.

Fructose is absrobed much more slowly than glucose and galactose. It does not require any extra energy and more Na^+ ions. Some of it may be converted to glucose during absorption. Mannose and pentoses are absorbed even more slowly than fructose.

Digestion of Lipids

The most abundant fat in the human diet is triglycerides or neutral fats with smaller proportion of some phospholipids and cholesterol (mainly in the form of esters).

Fats are digested due to hydrohysis by the action of enzyme *lipase* into fatty acids plus glycerol; **in case of cholesterol ester, it is fatty acid + steroid.**

Gastric lipase digests small amount of fat in the stomach which is mostly tributyrin (butter fat). Most of the fat is digested in the intestines by pancreatic lipase which remains present in bulk in the pancreatic secretion. There is some enteric lipase also secreted in the intestine, the role of which is not important.

The enzyme lipase is soluble in water but its substrates, the lipids are water-insoluble. So lipase can attack on a lipid only at the water-oil interface. This is facilitated by emulsification of lipids by bile suuplied form the liver, it is present in the aqueous medium of the intestinal lumen. Bile contains bile salts and phospholipids (mostly lecithin). These are in ionised form with negatively charged organic part and positively charged sodium ions. The organic ion behaves as an amphipathic lipid and its polar part is soluble in water. The nonpolar part is soluble in fat and is dissolved in the surface layer of the dietary fat globule, while the polar part remains outward dissolved in the aqueous medium (Fig. 13.2) which lowers the surface tension, and the fat globule becomes liable to easy fragmentation by the mechanical agitation of the peristaltic movement of the intestine. **As a result, an emulsion is formed by the dispersion of the minute fat globules in the aqueous medium, thus increasing the surface area of the fat by nearly 1000 fold.**

The attack of lipase, therefore gets immediately increased though it is not in a common solvent with its substrate. The action of pancreatic *co-lipase* and phospholipase A_2 (both are released from their precursor by the action of enzyme trypsin) in the presence of Ca^{2+} ions facilitates the firm binding of the enzyme pancreatic lipase to the substrate at the water-oil interface. In this way, by the action of pancreatic lipase ester bond in the α - positions of a neutral fat i.e., a triglyceride are rapidly hydrolysed firstly forming one molecule each of α–β- diglyceride and a fatty acid and finally one molecule each of β- monoglyceride and a fatty acid as shown below in Fig. 13.3. Now by the action of yet another enzyme known as *intestinal isomerase* β - monoglyceride is converted to α - monoglyceride which in turn by the action of enzyme *intestinal lipase* in the presence of water molecule in finally broken down to yield one molecule each of glycerol and a fatty acid (Fig. 13.3).

Products so formed are capable of blocking the digestion of more fat globules but as they are removed quickly in the micelles formed by the bile salts, the digestion of more fat continues. These micelles are spherical globules (Fig. 13.2), 3-4 nm in diameter, composed of 20-40 molecules of bile salt. The sterol nucleus of the bile salt is fat soluble whereas the polar group is water soluble. The sterol nuclei aggregate together, forming a small fat globule in the middle of the micelle while the polar groups projecting outward cover the surface of the micelle, whole of which is kept in solution in the aqueous medium due to the negative charge on the polar part.

Bile salt micelles do also have a tendency to transport the monoglycerides and fatty acids engulfed in them to the brush borders of the epithelial cells and then the bile salts return to the chyme to be reused.

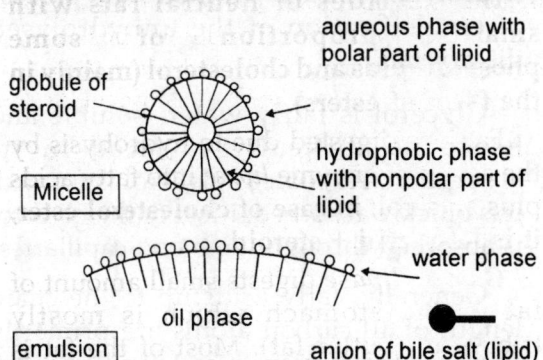

Fig. 13.2: Emulsification and micelle formation by bile acids

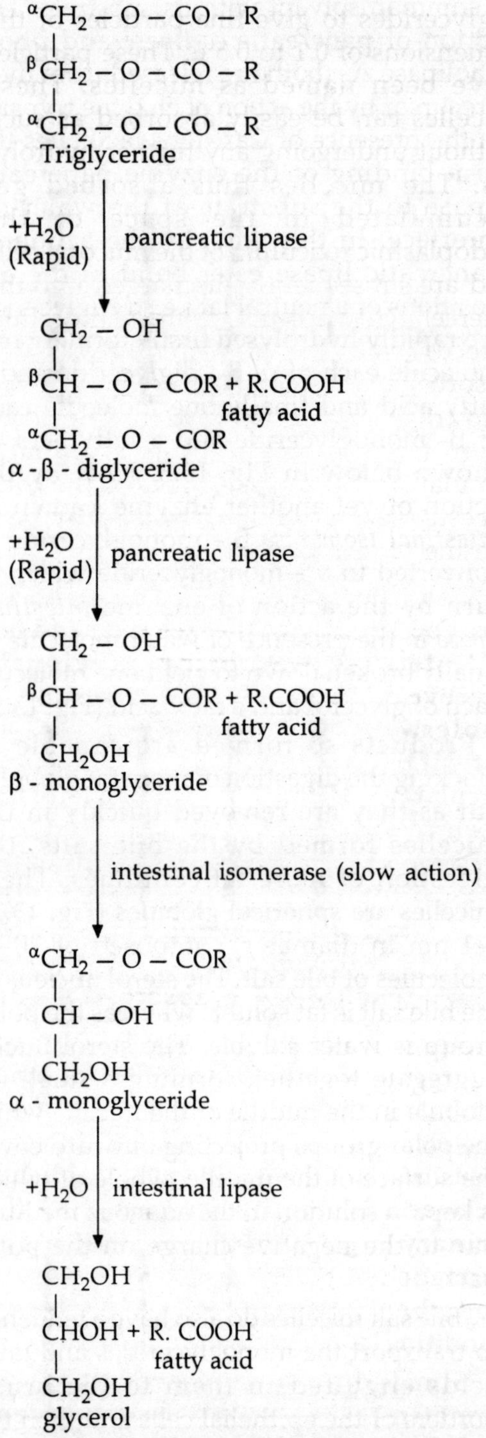

$$^\alpha CH_2 - O - CO - R$$
$$|$$
$$^\beta CH_2 - O - CO - R$$
$$|$$
$$^\alpha CH_2 - O - CO - R$$

Triglyceride

$$\downarrow \quad \begin{array}{l} +H_2O \\ \text{(Rapid)} \end{array} \Big| \text{ pancreatic lipase}$$

$$CH_2 - OH$$
$$|$$
$$^\beta CH - O - COR + R.COOH$$
$$| \qquad\qquad\qquad \text{fatty acid}$$
$$^\alpha CH_2 - O - COR$$

α - β - diglyceride

$$\downarrow \quad \begin{array}{l} +H_2O \\ \text{(Rapid)} \end{array} \Big| \text{ pancreatic lipase}$$

$$CH_2 - OH$$
$$|$$
$$^\beta CH - O - COR + R.COOH$$
$$| \qquad\qquad\qquad \text{fatty acid}$$
$$CH_2OH$$

β - monoglyceride

$$\downarrow \quad \text{intestinal isomerase (slow action)}$$

$$^\alpha CH_2 - O - COR$$
$$|$$
$$CH - OH$$
$$|$$
$$CH_2OH$$

α - monoglyceride

$$\downarrow \quad +H_2O \Big| \text{ intestinal lipase}$$

$$CH_2OH$$
$$|$$
$$CHOH + R. COOH$$
$$| \qquad\qquad \text{fatty acid}$$
$$CH_2OH$$

glycerol

Fig. 13.3 : Hydrolysis of triglycerides

The lipase present in the epithelial cells slowly hydrolyses the monoglyceride but not completely. Free fatty acids and unhydrolysed monoglycerides are absorbed. Fig. 13.3 represents the scheme of hydrolyis.

Phospholipase A$_2$ has got a tendency to hydrolyse ester bond of phospholipids at β - position forming free fatty acid and a lysophospholipid. Cholesterol esterase enzyme which is found in pancreas hydrolyses cholesterol esters yielding free fatty acid and free cholesterol. These digested products are also 'ferried' to the brush border by the bile salt micelle.

Absorption of Lipids

Lipids are mostly absorbed in the duodenum and the jejunum. Lipids are hydrolysed yielding a mixture of glycerol, diglycerides, monoglycerides and free fatty acids. Dietary lipids are never digested completely in the alimentary canal. Hydrolysis of the trigycerides to diglycerides and β - monoglycerides occurs easily but hydrolysis of the β - monoglycerides is relatively very difficult. The mixture of these intermediary hydrolytic products promotes the process of emulsification of the unhydrolysed dietary fats.

Glycerol is fairly water- soluble and hence no difficulty is faced in its absorption. As soon as glycerol is formed, it is quickly absorbed. Most of the glycerol is absorbed through the blood capillaries.

Generally, fatty acids up to the chain length of 10 carbon atoms are primarily absorbed through the blood capillaries but fatty acids of higher chain length are primarily absorbed through the lymphatic route. The low molecular weight fatty acids are absorbed without much difficulty but the complexity goes on increasing as the molecular wieght of the fatty acids goes on increasing. This is due to the fact that low M.W. fatty acids are relatively hydrophilic whereas the high M. W. fatty acids are hydrophobic. The hydrophobic fatty acids can not be absorbed till these are brought into some soluble form. This is brought about by the formation of *fatty acid-bile salt complexes* which are more soluble and can be absorbed without much difficulty. Fatty acids ean also be absorbed in combination of the steroids by forming more soluble esters. The fatty acid present in the β monoglycerides is hydrolysed within the mucosal cells by a *distinct lipase* which is found in these cells.

The short chain fatty acids (upto 10 carbon atoms) are transported directly into the blood stream in the free form and get bound to the plasma albumin. These fatty acids comprise nonesterified fatty acid (NEFA) fraction. The fate of the longer chain fatty acids is different. These are converted into triglycerides by intermediate formation of the phosphatidic acids and then carried away by the lymphatic system to the venous blood. The triglyceride thus synthesized in the mucosal cells are transported into the lymphatic circulation in two forms, namely, chylomicrons and *invisible fatty particulates*. An enzyme **lipoprotein lipase** present in the blood stream is responsibie for splitting of the complexes of chylomicrons and thus removes milky appearance of blood. Previously, the name **clearing factor** was given to this enzyme.

The undigested fat is finely emulsified by the intestinal movement in the presence of bile salts, monoglycerides and diglycerides to give fine particles of the dimensions of 0.1 to 0.5 μ. These particles have been named as micelles. These micelles can be easily absorbed as such without undergoing any further hydrolysis. The micelles thus absorbed get accumulated in the space of the endoplasmic reticulum of the mucosal cells and are subsequently discharged into the intercellular space and corium of the villus. The diglycerides and monoglycerides absorbed in this manner are resynthesized into triglycerides. These triglycerides are then transported by the lymphatic circulation. Thus, about 95% of the total ingested lipids may be absorbed by both the mechanisms.

Cholesterol has been shown to be absorbed mostly in the free state and not as esters as was being previously believed. However, absorption of cholesterol is followed by its re-esterification in the lymphatic circulation. Absorption of cholesterol has been reported to be facilitated by the presence of unsaturated fatty acids in the intestine. Bile salts are necessary for the absorption of cholesterol. Plant sterols are not absorbed. Out of the different sterols, cholesterol is absorbed mostly easily.

Absorption of different types of lipids gets markedly lowered in states like *biliary-obstruction* and *liver dysfunction*. **In some cases, an abnormal link gets established between lymphatic system and the urinary tract which results in the formation of milky urine and loss of the absorbed fats through urine. Such a condition is known as** *chyluria.*

Similarly, a connection might sometimes be established between lymphatic system and the pleural space

as a result of which fats may pass into the pleural fluid giving it a milky appearance. Such a condition is cIinicalIy known as chylothorax.

Digestion of Proteins

Before understanding the digestion of proteins, it's important to know, what proteins are. These are large polypetide molecules coiled by weaker bonds in their tertiary structure. The digestion of proteins involves step by step breakdown of these polypeptides by enzymatic hydrolysis into their constituent units, i.e., amino acid molecules which are then absorbed in the blood stream. The breaking of a peptide bond by a specific enzyme in general is as shown below:

$$- NH - CO - \xrightarrow[+H_2O]{enzyme} -NH_2 + HOOC -$$

Digestion involves the following protocol/ procedures:

1. Heat and hydrochloric acid denature proteins which expose hidden peptide bonds, hence help in digestion.

2. Proteolytic (protein breaking) enzymes are secreted in the gut as inactive zymogens. Acid or another enzyme converts them into active form as shown below:

Pepsinogen $\xrightarrow{H^+}$ Pepsin

Trypsinogen $\xrightarrow{Enterokinase}$ Trypsin

Procarboxypeptidase $\xrightarrow{Trypsin}$ Carboxypeptidase

3. Protein is first of all acted upon by endopeptidases and then by exopeptidases. The action of former produces polypeptides and peptides and the action of later i.e., exopeptidases produces amino acids

and the remaining protein molecule.

4. Proteolytic enzymes are found in various juices which are secreted by stomach, pancreas and intestine, they are as follows.

(a) Gastric juice :

 (i) Pepsin : Acts on protein and forms proteoses and peptones. It acts on peptide bonds formed by aspartic acid, glutamic acid and aromatic amino acids (phenylalanine and tyrosine).

Proteins
$\downarrow$ Pepsin
Proteoses + Peptones

 (ii) Renin : It is found in infants and acts on caseinogen to form calcium paracaseinate.

Caseinogen
$\downarrow$ Renin
Calcium Paracaseinate

(b) Pancreatic juice :

 (i) Trypsin : It acts upon proteins, proteoses and peptones to form polypeptides, dipeptides and peptides. This enzyme acts on peptide bonds formed by basic amino acids i.e., arginine and lysine.

Proteins + Proteoses + Peptones
$\downarrow$ Trypsin
Polypeptides + Dipeptides + Peptides

 (ii) Chymotrypsin : This acts upon proteins, proteoses, peptones and peptides. It acts upon peptide bonds of polar amino acids, i.e., phenylal-anine, tyrosine, tryptophan,

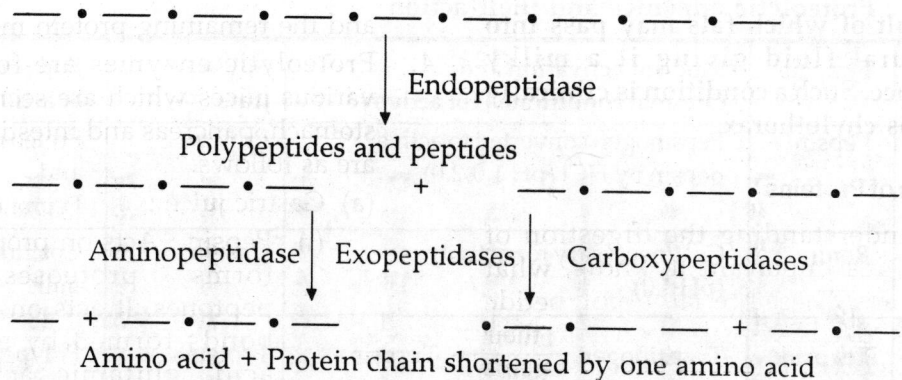

Endopeptidase

Polypeptides and peptides

Aminopeptidase | Exopeptidases | Carboxypeptidases

Amino acid + Protein chain shortened by one amino acid

leucine and methionine.

(iii) Carboxypeptidase : It acts on polypeptides at carboxyterminal to form lower peptides and free amino acids.

(c) Intestinal juice :

(i) Aminopeptidase : It acts upon polypeptides at amino terminals to form lower peptides and free amino acids

(ii) Dipeptidases : These act upon dipeptides to yield amino acids

In this way, by the combined action of these enzymes, protein is completely hydrolyzed to its constituent units i.e. amino acids, and some dipeptides and tripeptides.

Details of various proteolytic enzymes found in the gut and their action is as has been described in Table 1.

Absorption of Proteins :

Proteins are rarely absorbed in the intact form except in the cases of foetal and newborns. These are absorbed in the form of amino acids through the blood route. Almost negligible amount may also be absorbed through the lymphatic route. Amino acids obtained during the process of digestion do not accumulate in the intestine indicating that these are absorbed very rapidly.

This phenomeon can be well understood by considering the following points :

1. As amino acids are water soluble, their absorption takes place by portal venous system. The fasting amino nitrogen level in blood is from 4-6 mg% which gets raised by 2-4 mg% after meals.

2. All amino acids are absorbed by passive diffusion but the active transport process is more important. Absorption is a carrier mediated, energy requiring process. It is having a co-transport of Na^{++}

At least four different transport systems are there for different groups of amino acids which are as follows :

i) For acidic amino acids

ii) For basic amino acids

iii) For neutral amino acids, and

iv) For imino acids and glycine

The general scheme of Na^+ dependent

Table - 1 : Proteolytic enzymes and their action

Source	Enzyme	Mode of activation and Optimal condition(s) for activity	Substrate	End product(s) of action
Stomach	Pepsin	Pepsinogen converted to active pepsin by HCl (pH 1.0-2.0)	Protein	Proteoses and Peptones
	Renin	Ca^{++} necessary for activity (pH 4.0)	Casein	Coagulates milk
Pancreas	Trypsin	Trypsinogen $\xrightarrow{\text{Entero-kinase}}$ Trypsin Enterokinase of intestine (pH 5.2 to 6.0) Autocatalytic at pH 7.9	Proteins Proteoses Peptones	Polypeptides and Dipeptides
	Chymo-trypsin	Chymotryp-sinogen $\xrightarrow[\text{pH 8.0}]{\text{Trypsin}}$ Chymo-trypsin	Proteins Proteoses Peptones	Polypeptides and Dipeptides
	Carboxy-peptidase	Procarboxypeptidase $\downarrow$ Trypsin Active enzyme	Polypeptides with free carboxyl groups	Lower peptides and free amino acids
Small Intestine	Amino-peptidase		Polypeptides with free amino groups	Lower peptides and free amino acids
	Dipepti-dase		Dipeptides	Amino acids

secondary active transport is as shown below in Figure 13.4.

There are common sites for the absorption, therefore competition occurs.

3. Some di- and tripeptides are also absorbed by intestinal mucosa. These are digested by intramucosal hydrolases.

4. For 2 - 3 days, intestinal mucosa of new borns absorb proteins and polypeptides which enables the child to acquire passive immunity by absorption of immunoglobulins present in colostrum and milk.

5. Sometimes proteins in small amount may be absorbed by pinocytosis by adults which may cause allergic reaction i.e., allergy in an individual.

Small amounts of proteins may remain undigested which are absorbed by **pinocytosis**. Although, their amounts may be insignificant from nutritional point of view, such proteins may act as antigen to form antibody. **However an excess may lead to allergy.** In the new borns, the proteins may not be digested completely; the immunoglobulin, IgA from mothers's milk is absorbed as such which contributes

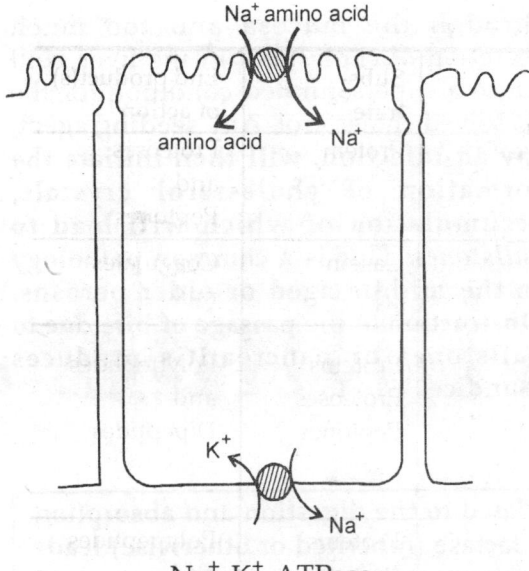

Na⁺ amino acid

amino acid   Na⁺

K^+

Na^+

$Na^+ \, K^+$ ATPase

Fig.- 13.4 : Na⁺ dependent active transport of amino acids.

to the immunity in the child.

Disorders of the Alimentary tract

Derangement in the function of the organs concerned with the alimentary system is associated with various disease conditions as mentioned below:

(A) Stomach disorders

The alteration in the normal secretion of the gastric juice is reflected primarily in the concentration of HCl in the stomach. There may be *hyperchlorhydria* (increased concentration of HCl) or *hypochlorhydria* (decreased concentration of HCl). **In hyperchlorhydria, the acid together with pepsin released from pepsinogen, may attack the very cells of their origin exposing the wall of stomach. Contact of acid with this may produce** *ulcer*, **accompanied with pain and other discomforts.**

The final result of continued hyperchlorhydria is the development of peptic ulcer, that may further be aggravated by the reduced secretion of alkaline fluid from the pancreas and/or inability of the layer of mucus to protect the wall of that part of the duodenum from the action of gastric acid in the chyme. **Peptic ulcer is a common ailment especially amongst malnourished and undernourished people.**

Hypochlorhydria evidently leads to digestive insufficiency. **There may even be** *achlorhydria* **(absence of HCl) and** *achyla* **when associated with the absence of enzymes and the intrinsic factor secreted in the stomach. Pernicious anemia presents the latter condition. Carcinoma of stomach has hypochlorhydria or even achlorhydria.**

(B) Pancreatic disorders

Disorder in the external secretion of the pancreas may cause a wide range of digestive disorders since the enzymes necessary for the hydrolysis of carbohydrates, lipids and proteins are all originated from the pancreas. The reduction in the acidity of the chyme from the stomach is also due to the bicarbonate secreted by the pancreas. **The important internal secretions of the pancreas are** *insulin* **and** *glucagon.* In pancreatitis, benign or malignant, there may be found excessive secretion of enzymes amylase and lipase and also elevated levels of the same in blood. One may also find elevated urinary levels of these enzymes.

(C) Bile disorders

Liver is the site of formation of bile which excretes bile acids, bilirubin, cholesterol, etc., besides being the most important factor in the emulsification of fats in the small intestine. Any disorder in the liver affecting the bile formation will certainly disturb the above functions. Cholesterol is insoluble in water, but is solubilized in bile due to the presence of phospholipids an bile acids, water content also having an important role. Alteration in the proportion of these substances in bile may reduce the solubility of cholesterol. This, as well as too much concentration of bile in the gall bladder by excessive absorption of ions and water through the mucosa and too much secretion of cholesterol in the liver, will cause a supersaturated condition for the dissolved cholesterol. **Any seeding agent, say an infection, will then initiate the formation of cholesterol crystals, accumulation of which will lead to** *gallstones*. **This is a common pathology in the middle aged or older perosns. Obstruction to the passage of bile due to gallstones or pancreatitis produces jaundice.**

(D) Disorders in the small intestine

A large number of clinical conditions are related to the digestion and absorption in the small intestine. Deficiency of *enzyme* lactase (inherited or otherwise) leads to the accumulation of lastose *(milk intolerance)* with abdominal cramps and diarrhea. Similar condition may also take place from the deficiency of enzymes sucrase and maltase. Hereditary defect in the carrier protein may cause reduced absorption of glucose and galactose. Under certain conditions, a few proteins or small polypeptides (for instance wheat gluten or its fraction) get absorbed and produce their antibodies in the system which may produce *coeliac disease)* in children and a similar one in adults *(non-tropical sprue)*. Anemia results from reduced absorption of iron, folic acid, and vitamin B_{12}. *Protein deficiency syndrome* is the result of malabsorption of amino-acids; *tetany* may take place with the malabsorption of Ca^{2+}, Mg^{2+} and vitamin D. *Steatorrhea* (excess fat in the feces) is mostly the result of unabsorbed fat and fat soluble vitamins. Deficiency of vitamin K (lack of production and/or absorption) contributes to *bleeding* diseases/disorders.

Hormonal control of digestion:

Mechanical pressure of food against the stomach wall initiates endocrine (hormonal) control, the gastric phase of digestion. Food stretches the pylorus, and it secretes **gastrin** into the circulation. This has no particular effect until the secretion has returned to the parietal cells of the cardiac area of the stomach. Digestive juices and HCl are secreted in response to the hormone. The presence of HCl itself serves as a feed back mechanism to inhibit gastric secretion. HCl and the hormone **enterogastrone** act to inhibit the secretion of gastric juices. When fats enter the intestine, duodenal glands release enterogastrone into the circulation and in this way partly digested food present in the intestine gradually shows gastric activity.

The presence of th HCl and fat in the duodenum also triggers the release of a second intestinal hormone, cholecystokinin, which stimulates the gallbladder to release bile. In this way, a bile sample is promptly added to the intestinal content in response to the fat which requires it for digestion.

Two very important hormones control the secretory action of pancreas. The presence of acid chyme in the intestine stimulates the duodenal mucosa to secrete secretin ; the products of carbohydrate digestion stimulate the duodenal mucosa

to secrete **pancreozymin.** Both hormones stimulate the pancreas to secrete its digestive enzymes and alkaline salts.

Two other digestive hormones are concerned with the action of duodenum itself. Chyme in the upper intestine stimulates the release of **enterokinin (duocrinin),** which releases enzymes at several points in the small intestine. A second duodenal hormone, **villikinin** stimulates the motility of the absorptive villi.

CHAPTER 14

VITAMINS

Do not worry. We are found in abundance in eatables whether vegetarian or non-vegetarian and we are required by the body in small quantity only but mind it, ignorance of ours is very dangerous and causes several deficiency disorders. Side by side, excess intake of ours also causes hypervitaminosis which is also not good. We are of so great value that ours coenzymic forms like TPP, FMN, FAD, NAD, NADP etc., make the basis of innumerable biochemical reactions of the system. You can judge our importance that ours discovery led many scientists to win Nobel Prize.

In addition to oxygen, water, carbohydrates, lipids, proteins and inorganic salts, a number of organic compounds are also necessary for the life, growth and health of animals including man. These compounds are known as the accessory dietary factors or vitamins and are required only in very small amount.

Vitamins are defined as organic compounds, occurring in natural food either as such or as utilisable precursors which are required in small quantity for:

(i) normal growth
(ii) maintenance of various metabolic processes of the body, and
(iii) reproduction.

They differ from other organic foodstuffs in that they do not enter into the tissue structure and do not undergo degradation for the purpose of providing energy. The absence of these results in deficiency diseases.

Most of the vitamins are supplied by the diet. Majority of the vitamins which is synthesized in the intestines belongs to the vitamin-B group.

Vitamins which are synthesized by the intestinal flora include:

(a) Thiamine i.e. B_1
(b) Riboflavin i.e. B_2 (G)
(c) Niacin i.e. B_3
(d) Pantothenic acid, B_5
(e) Pyridoxine i.e. B_6
(f) Biotin, i.e. H (B_7)
(g) Folic acid i.e. B_9, and
(h) Vitamin K

Vitamins
↓

Fat soluble vitamins
(A, D, E & K)

Water soluble vitamins
(vitamin C and all vitamins of B complex group,
i.e., B_1, B_2, B_3, B_5, B_6, Biotin, B_9, B_{12}, etc)

Most of the vitamins form the integral part of the coenzymes as shown below (Table 14.1):

Table 14.1 : Vitamins as coenzymes

Vitamin	Active form(s)	Functions performed
Thiamine	Thiamine pyrophosphate i.e. TPP	Transfer of aldehyde group
Riboflavin	(i) Flavin mononucleotide, i.e. FMN	Transfer of hydrogen group
	(ii) Flavin adenine dinucleotide, i.e. FAD	Transfer of hydrogen group
Nicotinamide	(i) Nicotinamide adenine dinucleotide. i.e. NAD	Transfer of hydrogen
	(ii) Nicotinamide adenine dinucleotide phosphate, i.e. NADP	Transfer of hydrogen
Pyridoxine	Pyridoxal phosphate, i.e. PP	Transfer of amino group
Biotin	Biocytin	Transfer of carboxyl group i.e. CO_2 fixing
Pantothenic acid	Coenzyme A	Transfer of acyl group
Folic acid	Tetrahydrofolic acid i.e., Folacin	Transfer of methyl, methylene, formyl or formimino groups
Cyanocobalamine	Cobamides	Transfer of alkyl group
Lipoic acid	Lipoyl lysine	Transfer of acyl group

But the entire requirement of these vitamins is not met by the endogenous synthesis.

Vitamins, on the basis of solubility, have been divided into two categories as shown below:

Vitamin A

This is also called as Retinol, or Growth-promoting vitamin or Anti-infective vitamin or Anti-xerophthalmic vitamin.

History : Scientist Mc Collum is generally credited for the discovery of this vitamin.

Chemistry: Vitamin A occurs in two forms i.e., vitamin A_1 and vitamin A_2. The structure of vitamin A_1 is as shown below:

Vitamin A_2 contains one more double bond in the ring. It is a dehydro vitamin A_1 formed by the loss of two hydrogen atoms in the body. **Vitamin A_1 is more potent, whereas A_2 is only 40% active in comparison to A_1.**

Certain carotenes called provitamins A are converted in to vitamin A in the body. β-carotene gives rise to two molecules of vitamin A whereas α-and γ-carotenes give rise to one molecule each of vitamin A.

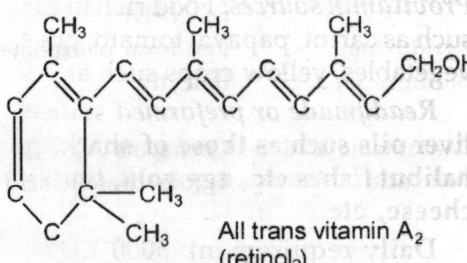

β-Carotene

A ring   B ring

B ring in α- carotene
shift in double bond

B ring in
γ - carotene
open ring

All trans vitamin A$_1$
(retinol$_1$)

All trans vitamin A$_2$
(retinol$_2$)

Functions

1. The most important function of vitamin A is in the visual cycle (Fig 14.1), also known as rhodopsin cycle.

2. In the maintenance of proper health of epithelial tissue.

3. In the stability and integrity of cellular and subcellular membranes.

4. It's necessary for the synthesis of mucopolysaccharides as it helps in the incorporation of sulphur in chondroitin sulphates.

5. It is also involved in the metabolism of nucleic acids.

6. **It is also involved in the**

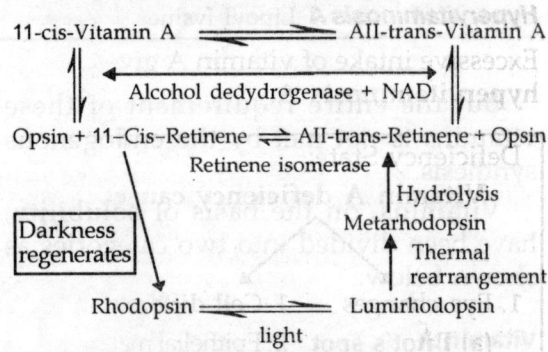

11-cis-Vitamin A ⇌ All-trans-Vitamin A

Alcohol dedydrogenase + NAD

Opsin + 11–Cis–Retinene ⇌ All-trans-Retinene + Opsin

Retinene isomerase

Hydrolysis

Metarhodopsin

Darkness regenerates

Thermal rearrangement

Rhodopsin ⇌ Lumirhodopsin

Darkness regenerates

light

Fig. 14.1 : Vitamin A Visual Cycle

electron transport chain and in oxidative phosphorylation.

Deficiency Diseases:

1. It's   deficiency   causes

nightblindness i.e. **nyctalopia**.

2. It's deficiency causes **xeroderma** in adults.

3. It's deficiency causes poor dark adaptation, **xerosis, growth failure, keratomalacia** and even **death in children**.

4. It's deficiency affects growth.

5. It's deficiency affects the **development of tooth**.

6. It's deficiency affects the development of bones.

7. It's deficiency lowers down the **resistance against infections**.

Sources

Provitamin sources: Food rich in carotenes such as carrot, papaya, tomato, green leafy vegetables, yellow crops such as corn, etc.

Readymade or preformed sources: **Fish liver oils such as those of shark, cod and halibut fishes etc., egg yolk, butter, meat, cheese, etc.**

Daily requirement: 5000 I.U.

Hypervitaminosis A

Excessive intake of vitamin A gives rise to **hypervitaminosis A.**

Deficiency State:

Vitamin A deficiency causes

1. Eye changes
   (a) **Bitot's spot**
   (b) Corneal ulcer
   (c) Keratomalacia
2. Blindness

1. Cell differentiation
2. Epithelial metaplasia
3. Keratin debris leading to **stones in kidneys**
4. **Cancer**

Vitamin D

The term vitamin D does not refer to a single dietary factor but to a number of chemically related compounds, all of which have a tendency to prevent or cure *rickets.* The two most important antirachitic substances in this respect are:

(i) **Vitamin D_2 also known as ergocalciferol**

(ii) **Vitamin D_3 also known as cholecalciferol**

(i)
$$\text{Cholesterol}$$
$$\downarrow$$
$$\text{7-dehydrocholesterol (skin)}$$
$$\downarrow \text{ Irradiation by uv light}$$
$$\text{Cholecalciferol i.e. VitD}_3$$

(ii)
$$\text{Ergosterol}$$
$$\downarrow \text{ Irradiation by uv light}$$
$$\text{Pre-ergocalciferol}$$
$$\downarrow$$
$$\text{Ergocalciferol i.e. Vit D}_2$$

Chemistry: There is no vitamin D_1 but vitamins D_2 and D_3 are of great importance to human beings. **Vitamin D_4 is activated 22-dehydroergosterol;** whereas **vitamin D_5 is activated 7-dehydrositosterol.**

The immediate precursor of D_3 is 7-dehydrocholesterol which is found in skin and sebum and the agent promoting the change is ultraviolet light as shown above. If the skin is exposed sufficiently to direct sun light then sufficient vitamin will be formed; its intake in food is unnecessary then.

Vitamin D_2 differs from vitamin D_3 with respect to a double bond which remains additionally present in the side chain at position 20 and 21.

Regulation of Vitamin D

It's regulation is monitored through the action of parathyroid hormone on the renal cells and not through direct feedback by plasma Ca^{++} or calcitonin.

Owing to the regulatory action of the parathyroid gland, serum Ca level in rickets is rarely low; instead inorganic phosphate level usually gets lowered.

Functions

1. It increases the absorption of calcium and phosphorus from the intestine.
2. It promotes the deposition of minerals mainly Ca and P in the bones.
3. It is required for normal growth in mammals.
4. It has got a specific function on kidney tubular reabsorption of calcium and phosphorus, thus inhibits their excretion via urine.

Deficiency diseases

It's deficiency gives rise to *rickets* in infants and *osteomalacia* in adults.

Daily requirement

(a) **Infants** : 400 IU/day
(b) **Children** : 400 IU/day
(c) **Pregnancy and lactation** : 400 IU/day
(d) **Adults** : 100 IU/day; apparently no need of this vitamin.

Hypervitaminosis: Serious overdosage is *toxic* which may cause calcificatin of the renal tubules. Several deaths, mostly of children from vitamin D overdosage have been reported in last few years in several countries.

Sources: Naturally occurring foods have practically no vitamin D activity. However, the best sources are:

(i) Fish liver oils, and
(ii) Margarine (imitation butter).

Vitamin E
(Antisterility Vitamin, Fertility factor)

Today, at least seven compounds with vitamin E activity are known to occur in a variety of plant and animal tissues which are called as 'tocopherols'.

Chemistry: There are, eight naturally occurring tocopherol derivatives known. There are six toco-derivatives and rest two are tocotrienol derivatives, as follows:

α-tocopherol (alpha)
β-tocopherol (beta)
γ- tocopherol(gamma)
ζ_2–tocopherol (zeta$_2$) } toco-derivatives
η-tocopherol (eta)
δ-tocopherol (delta)

ε-tocopherol (epsilon)] tocotrienol
ζ_1-tocopherol (zeta$_1$) } derivatives

α-**Tocopherol is biologically more potent than any other form,** the structure of which is as shown below:

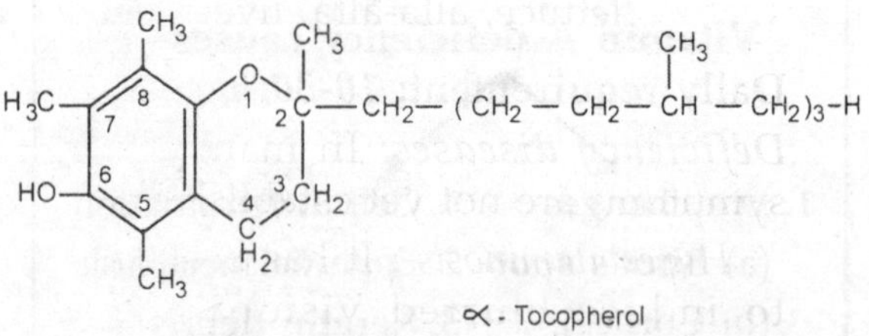

$\propto$ - Tocopherol
(5,7, 8-Trimethyltocol)

Functions:

1. Tocopherols act as powerful antioxidants to prevent many

undesirable oxidations in the body out of which some important ones are:

(i) **They act as scavanger of free radicals like OH radical, superoxide anion, free halogen radicals, etc;** in this way they prevent their peroxidative effects on unsaturated lipids present in membranes, and thus are responsible for stabilizing the membranes.

(ii) They help preserving the integrities of membrane-bound organelles and thereby prevent muscular dystrophy, hepatic necrosis or increased erythrocyte fragility.

(iii) They help maintaining the translocation of phosphate ions into mitochondria; **in this way they increase the rate of oxidative phosphorylation.**

(iv) They help protecting selenide at the active sites of membrane scleroproteins against the harmful effects of free radicals.

2. They prevent rancidity.

Sources: Wheat germ oil, corn oil, cottonseed oil, safflower oil, lettuce, alfa-alfa, liver, etc.

Daily requirement: *10-30 mg.*

Deficiency diseases: In man, deficiency symptoms are not yet established.

Hypervitaminosis : It has been reported to induce blurred vision, headache, dizziness, fatigue, acne, vasodilation, gastrointestinal symptoms, prolonged clotting time and rise in the levels of cholesterol and fats in the blood.

Vitamin K
(Coagulation factor)

There are several compounds that exhibit vitamin K activity; two important ones are:

(i) **Vitamin K_1 and**

(ii) **Vitamin K_2**

Both are naphthoquinone derivatives. Vitamin K_1 is phylloquinone and is chemically known as 2-methyl-3-phytyl-l, 4-naphthoquinone.

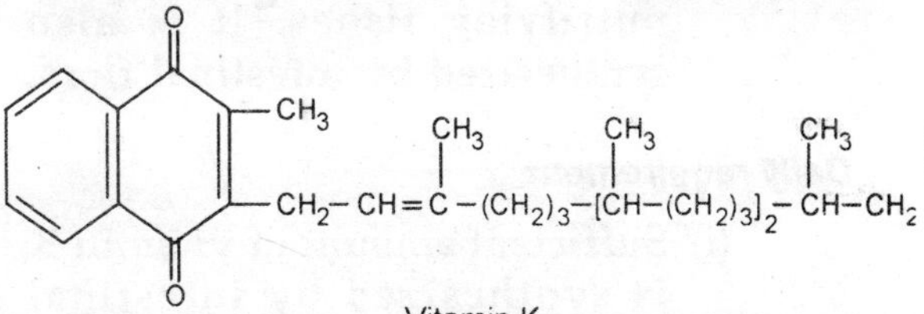

Vitamin K_1

(2 - methyl - 3 - phytyl - 1, 4 - naphthoquinone)

The original K_2 contains two *farnesyl* units in the side chain at position 3 whcih is equivalent to 6 isoprene units or 30 carbon atoms. Other K_2 molecules contain 7 and 9 isoprene units respectively in the side chain.

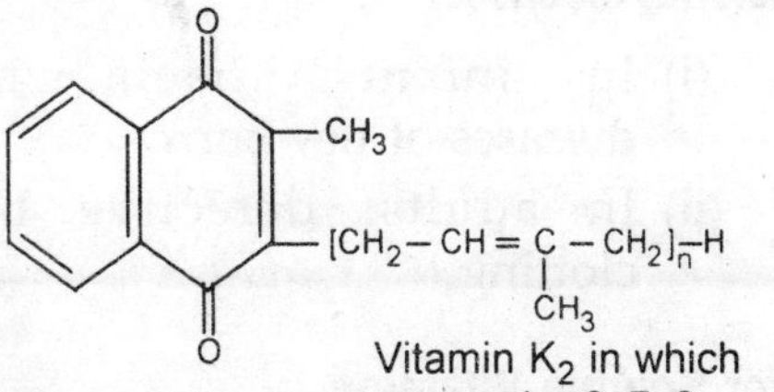

Vitamin K_2 in which
n can be 6, 7, 9,

Functions

1. In the production of **prothrombin.**

2. **In the manufacture and preservation of other blood clotting factors like proconvertin, Christian factor and Stuart factor.**

3. It is involved in the **mitochondrial electron transport and oxidative phosphorylation.**

Vitamin K Antagonist: *Dicumarol*

Sources

(i) Vitamin K_1 is found in green leafy vegetables such as alpha-alpha, spinach, cabbage, etc.

(ii) Vitamin K_2 remains present in putrifying fishes. **It is also synthesized by intestinal flora.**

Daily requirement

(i) **Sufficient amount of vitamin K is synthesized by intestinal bacteria** and also one gets sufficient amount through regular diet.

(ii) A minimal amount of 2 mg for adults has been established in the form of menadione which is given intravenously.

Deficiency diseases

(i) In infants: haemorrhagic diseases of newborn.

(ii) In adults: defective blood clotting.

Water Soluble Vitamins

Water soluble vitamins include vitamin C and members of vitamin B complex.

Vitamin C

(Ascorbic acid, Antiscorbutic Vitamin)

Chemistry

Vitamin C is soluble in water. It is a very strong reducing agent and is easily oxidized by air to dehydroascorbic acid.

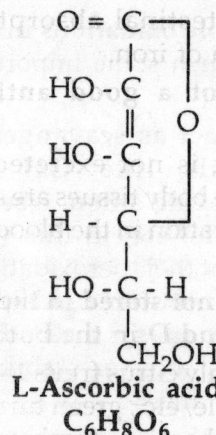

L-Ascorbic acid
$C_6H_8O_6$

Both forms are biologically active.

It melts at 190-192 °C and is stable for years in crystalline form. Its taste is sour. It is insoluble in most organic solvents.

Synthesis: **Vitamin C is not synthesized in men due to the absence of enzyme L-gulonooxidase and its entire requirement is met by the diet.**

Functions

1. In the formation of normal collagen, an intracellular cementing substance.

2. In the formation of hydroxyproline from proline.

3. In the formation of hydroxyllysine from lysine.

4. Participates in the synthesis of steroid hormones both in adrenal cortex and corpus luteum.

5. Participates as cofactor in the following reactions:

   (a) In phenylalanine metabolism: p-hydroxyphenylpyruvic acid → homogentisic acid

   (b) Dopamine → Norepinephrine

   (c) Folic acid → Folinic acid.

6. In the intestinal absorption and utilization of iron.

7. **It has got a good antioxidant property.**

Excretion: It is not excreted by the kidneys until the body tissues are saturated and the concentration in the blood exceeds a certain level.

Storage: **It is not stored in the body as are vitamin A and D in the body fat.**

Sources: Mainly citrus fruits like lemon, orange, pineapple, etc., green turnip, fresh cabbage, strawberries, fresh tomatoes, fresh potatoes and other fresh vegetables.

Deficiency diseases

1. It causes **scurvy** which is manifested in the form of:

   (i) weakness

   (ii) loosening of teeth and shrinkage of gums

   (iii) weakening of blood vessels

   (iv) failure of wounds to heal

   (v) failure of fractures to heal

   (vi) swollen and painful joints

2. Causes inpaired collagen formation

3. Causes inadequate synthesis of osteoid.

Daily requirement: **60-100 mg depending upon the age, size and associated stressful conditions.**

Large doses should be avoided: In large doses vitamin C predisposes *urinary tract stones,* may be responsible for aspirin-induced gastric erosions, unnecessarily increases intestinal absorption of iron and may lead to *iron overload* and other side-effects.

Vitamin B Complex Group

The members of this group are:
1. Thiamine **(B_1)**
2. Riboflavin **(B_2)** or **(G)**
3. Niacin **(B_3)**
4. Choline **(B_4)**
5. Pantothenic acid **(B_5)**
6. Pyridoxine **(B_6)**
7. Biotin **(B_7)**
8. Folic acid **(B_9)**
9. Cyanocobalamine **(B_{12})**
10. Para Amino Benzoic acid **(PABA)**
11. Inositol
12. Lipoic acid

Thiamine (B_1)

(Antineuritic vitamin, anti beriberi factor, aneurin)

Chemistry: Its structure consists of a pyrimidine and a thiazole ring system joined by a methylene bridge as shown below:

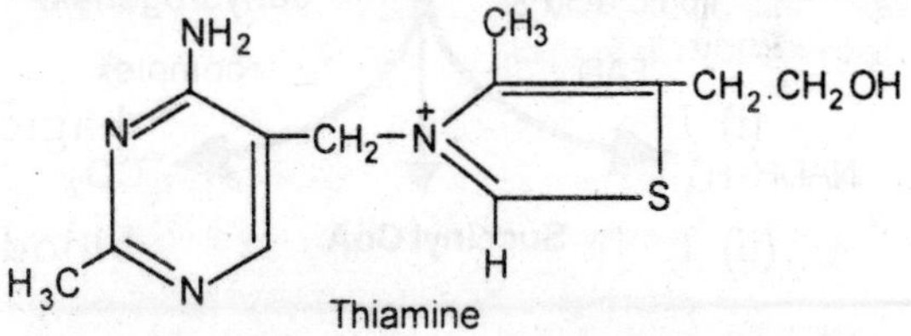

Thiamine

Thiamine is largely found in the cells in the form of its coenzyme form, i.e., thiamine pyrophosphate (TPP), also known as cocarboxylase. TPP is the coenzyme or prosthetic group of the enzyme decarboxylase.

Functions: **TPP participates mainly as a coenzyme in the carbohydrate metabolism:**

(a) **In oxidative decarboxylation of α-keto acids:** Puruvic acid and α-ketoglutaric acid which are intermediates in the carbohydrate metabolism **(glycolysis and TCA cycle)** are oxidatively decarboxylated to acetyl CoA and succinyl CoA respectively as shown below:

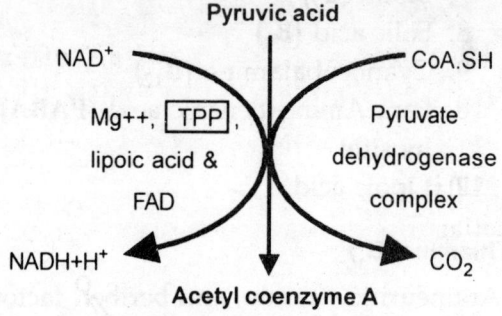

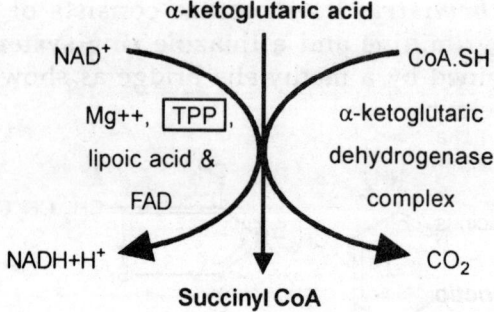

(b) In transketolation reaction: An intermediate step in HMP shunt where TPP plays role as shown below:

$$D-xylulose-5-P + D-Ribose-5-P$$

$$\downarrow \text{Transketolase}, \boxed{TPP}, Mg^{++}$$

$$D-sedoheptulose-7-P+D-glyceraldehyde-3-P$$

(c) In yeast, TPP acts as a coenzyme for nonoxidative decarboxylation of α-keto acids, i.e., pyruvate to CO_2 and acetaldehyde.

Deficiency diseases: 1. **In humans its deficiency causes 'beriberi' which is of three following types:**

(i) *Dry or neuritic beriberi:* In this type, pain, paralysis and wasting of limb muscles, enlarged heart, inflammation of ophthalmic nerve leading to blindness etc. may take place.

(ii) *Wet or edematous beriberi:* **Extensive edema in the extremities and the heart takes place.**

(iii) *Wernicke-Korsakoff syndrome:* **It's characterized by lesions and hemorrhages near the third cerebral ventricle, paralysis of eye movements, depression, insomnia, disorientation, extreme anxiety, mental confusions, severe loss of memory, etc.**

2. In birds and animals, its deficiency causes polyneuritis.

Sources: Dry peas, beans, soyabeans, bran, rice polishings, whole wheat flour, nuts, yeast, seeds, oranges, pork chops, fat ham, etc.

Daily requirement: **Nearly 1 mg (333 I.U.).**

Riboflavin

(Vitamin B_2 or G, Lactoflavin)

Chemistry: It is a derivative of isoalloxazine i.e., dimethylisoalloxazine attached to ribityl group as shown below:

B_2 is thermolabile, destroyed in alkaline medium, active in acidic medium. Its aqueous solution imparts a yellow-green

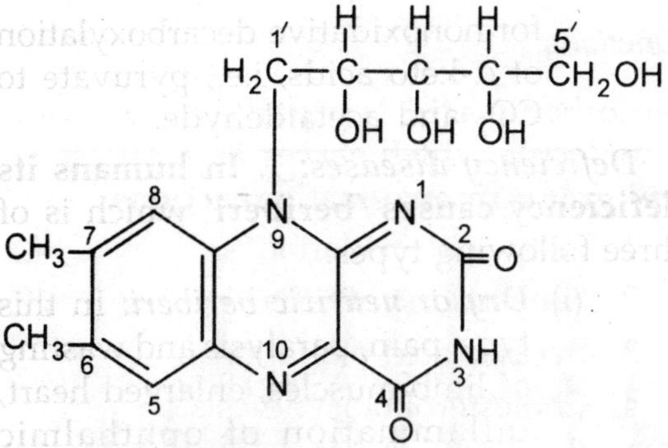

Riboflavin

(6,7 - dimethyl - 9 - (D - 1' - ribityl) - isoalloxazine)

fluorescence.

Functions

1. Riboflavin remains present as such in retina where it plays a part in light adaptation.
2. **It exists as components of two most important coenzymes called flavin mononucleotide (FMN) and flavin adenine dinucleotide (FAD) which act as coenzymes or prosthetic groups of many flavoprotein enzymes.**

Examples of flavoprotein enzymes containing FMN and FAD as prosthetic group are:

Containing FMN

(a) Warburg yellow enzyme
(b) L-amino acid oxidase
(c) Cytochrome C-reductase

Containing FAD

(a) D-amino acid oxidase
(b) Xanthine oxidase
(c) Acyl CoA dehydrogenase
(d) Succinic dehydrogenase
(e) Glycine oxidase

Sources: Liver, kidney, eggs, cheese, peanuts, milk, ham, soyabean flour, white bread, dry peas, dry beans, etc.

Daily requirement; 1.0 - 2.0 mg

Deficiency diseases; Important deficiency symptoms are:

(a) Glossitis (inflammation of the tongue).
(b) Cheilosis or fissuring at the corners of the mouth and the lips.
(c) **Seborrheic dermatitis, often manifested by the shark like apearance of the skin.**

Niacin (B₃)

(Pellagra preventing factor)

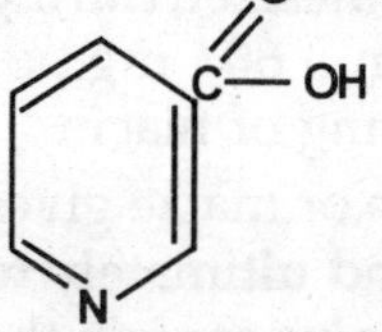

Niacin
(nicotinic acid)

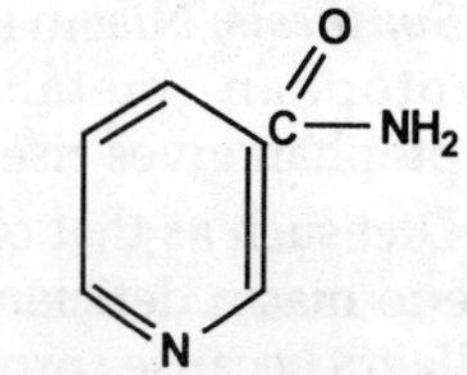

Niacinamide
(nicotinic acid amide)

Niacin is a pyridine derivative.

Functions

Nicotinamide is a component of nicotinamide adenine dinucleotide (NAD), also known as DPN or CO I and nicotinamide adenine dinucleotide phosphate (NADP), also known as TPN or CO II which act as coenzymes for many anaerobic dehydrogenases by accepting hydride ions during oxidation of their substrates, i.e., these act with a large group of hydrogen transport enzymes.

Enzymes requiring NAD or NADH as coenzymes are:

(a) Glyceraldehyde-3-P-dehydrogenase

(b) Malic dehydrogenase

(c) Lactic dehydrogenase

Enzymes requiring NADP or NADPH as coenzymes are:

(a) Isocitrate dehydrogenase

(b) Glucose- 6-PO_4 dehydrogenase

(c) Aldolase reductase

Sources: Liver, kidney, heart, lean meat and some fish flesh are outstanding sources. Plant sources include peanuts, wheat germ, dried legumes, yeasts etc.

Deficiency diseases: **Its deficiency in man gives rise to pellagra which is characterized by 3 D's i.e. (a) Dermatitis (b) Diarrhoea and (c) Dementia and black tongue in dogs.**

Synthesis; Niacin is synthesized during tryptophan metabolism. 60 mg of tryptophan gives rise to 1 mg of niacin.

Diet such as that of corn or maize gives rise to niacin deficiency and ultimately to pellagra because corn or maize contain the **protein *zein* which is deficient in tryptophan.** Corn or maize form the major dietary sources of rural population of **Rajasthan, a part of U.P. and M.P. and other states.**

Daily requirement: **19 mg.**

Pantothenic Acid (B₅)

(Filtrate factor, Chick antidermatitis factor)

Chemistry: It is a condensation product of β-alanine and a hydroxyl-and methyl substituted butyric acid.

$$
\begin{array}{ccccccccc}
H_2 & CH_3 & OH & O & & H & H_2 & H_2 & \\
| & | & | & \| & & | & | & | & \\
C & - C & - C & - C & - & N & - C & - C & - COOH \\
| & | & | & & & & & & \\
OH & CH_3 & H & & & & & & \\
\end{array}
$$

Pantoic acid   β-alanine

Pantothenic acid (Pantoyl-β-alanine)

Functions

Pantothenic acid is a part of coenzyme A molecule which serves as a carrier of acyl group in enzymatic reactions.

1. Fatty acid oxidation

2. Fatty acid synthesis

3. Pyruvic acid oxidation

4. Cholesterol biosynthesis

5. In acyl carrier proteins

6. Biological acetylations, etc.

Sources: Liver, kidney, egg yolk, peas, peanuts, tea, rice bran, barley, sweet potatoes, etc.

Deficiency diseases: Since this vitamin is synthesized in abundance in man by the intestinal flora, hence, symptoms of its deficiency are rarely met which may include *meuromotor disorders*, **cardiovascular instability, gastrointestinal distress, susceptibility to infections and mental depression.**

Daily requirement: **10 mg.**

Pyridoxine (B₆)

(Antichrodynia factor)

Chemistry: Vitamin B_6 refers to a group of substances namely pyridoxine, pyridoxal and pyridoxamine which possess similar biological activity. Their structures are as given below:

Biosynthesis: **A limited amount of pyridoxine can be synthesized by the bacterial flora of the gut.**

Functions

1. Pyridoxine exists in the form of *pyridoxal phosphate* in the cells and functions as a coenzyme for a variety of chemical reactions of amino acids and protein metabolism.

2. **The enzymes which require**

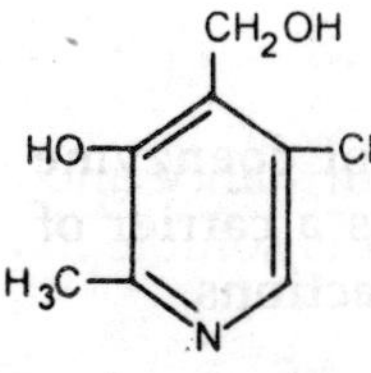

Pyridoxine

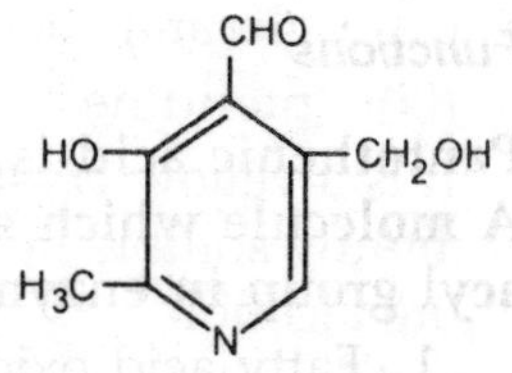

Pyridoxal

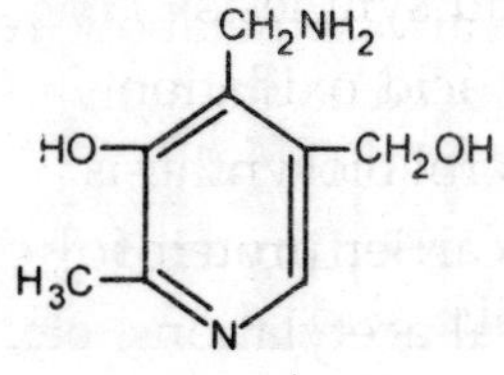

Pyridoxamine

pyridoxal phosphate (PP) as a coenzyme are:

(a) **Amino acid decarboxylases,** examples:

 (i) **Histidine → Histamine**

 (ii) **Tyrosine → Tyramine**

 (iii) **Glutamic acid**

   ↓

   γ-amino butyric acid (GABA)

(b) Transaminases, i.e., **GOT (AST)** and **GPT (ALT)**.

(c) Enzymes involved in tryptophan metabolism e.g., **tryptophanase which converts tryptophan to indole, pyruvate and ammonia.**

(d) Cystathionase which converts cystathionine to serine and homocysteine.

3. It is also believed to facilitate the transport of some amino acids across the cell membrane.

Deficiency diseases: Dermatitis, glossitis, cheilosis and in infants and children diarrhoea, anaemia, peripheral neuropathy, etc.

Secondary deficiency states maybe produced by long term use of a variety of drugs such as isoniazid.

Alcoholism may also lead to its deficiency.

Hypervitaminosis: Severe neuropathy has been described in patients taking megadoses of pyridoxine in the ill-founded belief that it is 'body building' or a remedy for the premenstrual syndrome.

Antagoist : Isonicotinic acid hydrazide is a potent antagonist of B_6

Sources : Vegetables, fruits, grains, meats and other food stuffs. Synthesized by the intestinal flora.

Daily requirement: 2-2.5 mg

Biotin (Vitamin H)

Chemistry: It is acyclic compound containing two rings, i.e., acyclic ureid and the other a reduced thiophene ring. A valeric acid side chain remains attached to the reduced thiophene ring. Its structure is as shown below:

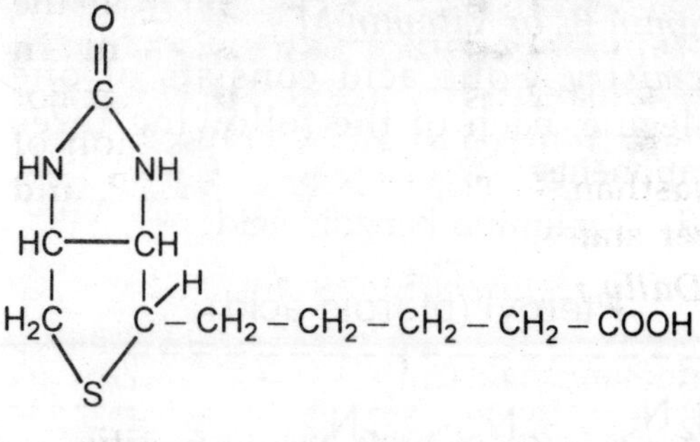

Biotin

Functions

Its main role is in carbon-dioxide fixation reactions. Reactions where biotin is involved include:

1. Acetyl CoA → Malonyl CoA (fatty acid synthesis)

2. CO_2 + NH_3 → Carbamoyl phosphate (urea cycle)

3. Pyruvic acid → Oxaloacetic acid

(gluconeogenesis)

4. Propionyl CoA → D-methyl malonyl CoA

5. In purine ring synthesis, i.e., the C-6 position in purine ring skeleton.

Deficiency states: **Intake of raw egg white induces the deficiency of biotin because it contains a protein 'avidin' which tightly binds biotin and thus prevents its absorption from the intestines and leads to** (i) **depression,** (ii) **nausea,** (iii) **easy fatigue,** (iv) **incoordination,** (v) **movements,** (vi) **dermatitis, etc.**

Sources: Liver, kidney, peas, yeast, cauliflower, egg yolk, milk, etc.

For man and other animals, synthesis by bacteria in the intestinal tract is an important source.

Daily requirement; 150-300 μg.

Folic Acid (pteroyl glutamic acid)

Vitamin B₉ or Vitamin M

Chemistry: Folic acid consists of one molecule, each of the following three components :

(i)   p-amino benzoic acid

(ii)   glutamic acid, and

(iii) pteridine

It is a yellow crystalline substance and is slightly soluble in water. It is soluble in dilute alcohol.

Before folic acid can function as coenzymes in various metabolic reactions, it must be reduced to its active form i.e. tetrahydrofolic acid (FH_4)

Folic acid → dihydrofolic acid →tetrahydrofolic acid

Folic acid coenzymes collectively are known as *folacin.*

Functions

1. **Folic acid coenzymes are involved in the transfer and incorporation of single carbon moiety. One carbon moieties are :**

(i) Formyl group and formate group i.e.,—CHO and

(ii) Hydroxy methyl group, i.e.,— CH_2OH

(iii) Methyl group, i.e.,—CH_3

(iv) Formimino group, i.e.—CH=NH

All of these are interconvertible.

Pteroyl (pteroic acid)

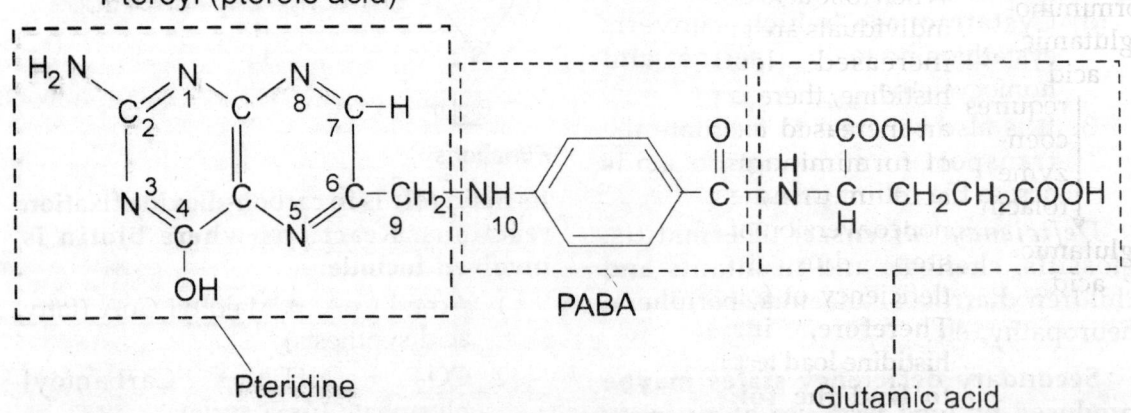

Folic acid, pteroylglutamic acid (PGA)

$$CH_2OH \rightarrow CHO \rightarrow COOH$$

Sources of one carbon moieties are:

   (i) α– carbon of glycine gives rise to-CHO group

  (ii) Histidine gives rise to-CH=NH group

 (iii) Biotin gives rise to-CH_3 group

 (iv) β- carbon of serine gives rise to-CHO group

  (v) Choline gives rise to-CH_3 group via betaine (choline as such cannot give rise to methyl group).

Utilisation of one carbon moiety

   (i) Conversion of ethanolamine to choline

  (ii) Conversion of glycine to serine

 (iii) Conversion of norepinephrine to epinephrine

 (iv) Conversion of guanidoacetic acid to creatine

  (v) In the formation of formimino-glutamate

 (vi) Histidine synthesis

 (vii) Purine and pyrimidine synthesis

(viii) Methionine-homocysteine reactions, i.e., methyl synthesis.

Folic acid antagonists are :

   (i) **Aminopterin**

  (ii) **Amethopterin**

These are used to some extent in the treatment of cancers in medicine.

Deficiency states :

   (i) **Folic acid deficiency occurs most commonly among pregnant women because of their increased need for this nutrient.**

  (ii) **Its deficiency causes macrocytic and megaloblastic type of anemia, i.e., reduced ability to produce RBCs.**

 (iii) It causes *sprue syndrome*

 (iv) It causes **diarrhoea, gastrointestinal lesions, etc.**

It is synthesized in sufficient amount by the intestinal bacteria unless their growth is inhibited by the intake of sulfonamide drugs and antibiotics.

Sources: Green leafy vegetables, fruits and yeast.

Daily requirement:

Adult man/woman	:	0.1 mg
Lactating woman	:	0.15 mg
Pregnant woman	:	0.3 mg

FIGLU excretion test (Formiminoglutamic acid excretion test)

This is a diagnostic test for the detection of folic acid deficiency.

About the Test:

Histidine
↓
formimino-glutamic acid
↓ requires coenzyme folacin
glutamic acid

In the histidine metabolism, the conversion of N-formiminoglutamic acid to glutamic acid is a folic acid dependent step. When folic acid deficient individuals are given an increased load of histidine, there is found an increased excretion of formiminoglutamic acid in urine due to nonconversion of above step due to the deficiency of folic acid. **Therefore, increased histidine load test is used to find the folic acid deficiency.**

Vitamin B$_{12}$
or
Cyanocobalamine/Cobalamine
(Anti pernicious factor, Castle's extrinsic factor)

Antipernicious anaemia factor from liver extract was isolated in 1948 by Rickes and coworkers and by Smith. This factor is known as 'animal protein factor' and has got the capability to cure pernicious anaemia and is now termed as vitamin B$_{12}$. It is to found in animal tissues in the form of a conjugate with a polypeptide.

Chemistry: **Vitamin B$_{12}$ (Fig 14.2) is a dark red compound. It is made up of two components:**

The centrally located larger component is known as *Corrin ring system* which

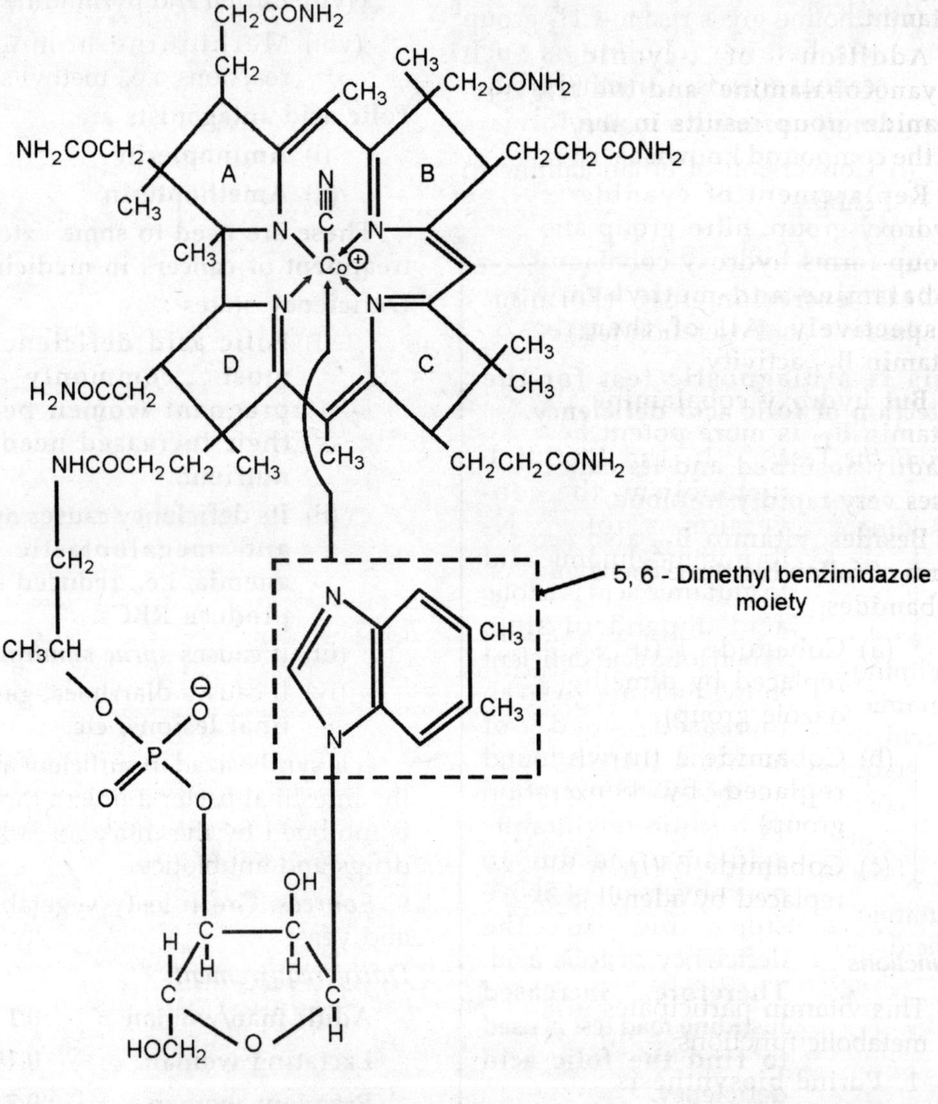

Fig. 14.2 : Vitamin B$_{12}$, C$_{63}$H$_{88}$N$_{14}$O$_{14}$PCo

contains 4 pyrrole rings. Cobalt remains coordinated to the four nitrogen of the pyrrole rings.

The second comparatively smaller component is a ribonucleotide called as 5,6 dimethyl benzimidazole riboside which remains connected to the central cobalt atom at one end and to the ribose moiety at the other end. Presence of **'cobalt'** **imparts dark red/pink colour to this vitamin.**

Addition of cyanide forms 'Cyanocobalamine' and the removal of cyanide group results in the formation of the compound known as 'cobalamine'.

Replacement of cyanide group by hydroxy group, nitro group and methyl group forms hydroxy cobalamine, nitro cobalamine and methyl cobalamine respectively. All of them have got vitamin B_{12} activity.

But hydroxy cobalamine also called vitamin B_{12} is more potent because it's readily absorbed and its concentration rises very rapidly in blood.

Besides, vitamin B_{12} also acts in the form of following three coenzymes, called cobamides.

    (a) Cobamide 1 (in which CN-is replaced by dimethyl benzimidazole group).

    (b) Cobamide 2 (in which CN-is replaced by benzimidazole group)

    (c) Cobamide 3 (in which CN-is replaced by adenyl group).

Functions

This vitamin participates in a number of metabolic functions:

1. **Purine biosynthesis**
2. **Synthesis of labelled methyl** group.
3. **It plays an important role in the stimulation of protein synthesis.**
4. In the conversion of carbohydrate to lipid.

Deficiency diseases

1. **Its deficiency gives rise to pernicious anaemia which is not simply the result of vitamin B_{12} deficiency in the diet but is caused due to lack of specific glycoprotein (so called intrinsic factor) in the gastric juice. Intrinsic factor with a factor present in the food (extrinsic factor) forms a system responsible for the proper maturation of RBCs. People with pernicious anaemia do not make this protien, hence pernicious anaemia is a genetic defect of the stomach.**

2. **Achlorhydria** (No HCl in gastric juice).

3. **Neurological degeneration, and**

4. **Glossitis.**

Sources:

    (i) Liver, kidney, meat, fish, oysters, egg yolk, etc. **Animal proteins are the sole source of this vitamin but it remains absent in plant sources.**

    (ii) **Microorganisms present in the intestinal tract have got the capability to synthesize vitamin B_{12}.**

Daily requirement :

    (a) Adult man/woman.   : 1 µg
    (b) Pregnant/lactating woman : 1.5 µg
    (c) Infants and children   : 0.2-1 µg

Antivitamins

Antivitamins are those substances which possess structural similarity to certain vitamins but behave antagonistically to these vitamins when incorporated into the body, thereby, preventing the normal functions of these vitamins. Examples of vitamins with their antivitamins are:

	Vitamin		*Antivitamin/Antagonist*
(i)	Thiamine	:	Pyrithiamine
(ii)	Ribioflavin	:	Isoflavin
(iii)	Pyridoxine	:	Isonicotinic acid hydrazide (INH)
(iv)	Folic acid	:	Aminopterin, Amethopterin
(v)	Vitamin K	:	Dicumarol.

CHAPTER 15

METABOLISM OF CARBOHYDRATES

We have a beautiful scene in intermediary metabolism. We include very important anabolic and catabolic pathways. Our anabolic pathways include glycogenesis (synthesis of glycogen) and gluconeogenesis (synthesis of glucose or glycogen); whereas catabolic ones include glycogenolysis, glycolysis, TCA cycle and the pentose phosphate pathway. Ours catabolic routes have a tendency to liberate energy which is used for various purposes in the human body whereas ours anabolic routes have a tendency to synthesize glycogen/glucose and then store it so that the same may be utilized in odd situations.

We include in ourselves the only hypoglycaemic hormone i.e., insulin, the deficiency of which leads to a very fierceful disease of carbohydrate metabolism called as Diabetes Mellitus.

The major function of carbohydrate metabolism is to provide energy for various metabolic processes of the body. In this role, carbohydrates are utilised by the cells mainly in the form of glucose. Carbohydrates have the advantage of being cheap, easily digestible and rapidly metabolizable.

Carbohydrates' metabolism is basically the metabolism of glucose and substances related to it.

The sugar of the blood is glucose. The digestion of carbohydrates such as starch, sucrose and lactose produces glucose, fructose and galactose respectively which pass into the blood circulation. Conversion of fructose and galactose into glucose occurs in the liver.

Carbohydrates supply nearly 2/3 energy requirement of the body.

HEMOLYTIC ANEMIAS

The importance of carbohydrate and energy metabolism for the survival of the erythrocyte is emphasized by several inborn errors of metabolism that lead to hemolysis and anemia. In type VII glycogen-storage disease, e.g., phosphofructokinase enzyme of the erythrocytes is partly deficient, which results in reduced efficiency of ATP production and mild hemolytic symptoms.

A more severe disorder is associated with another recessively inherited condition, *pyruvate-kinase deficiency*, in which the enzyme in the erythrocytes is specifically decreased. Since glycolysis is blocked before the last energy-producing step, there can be no net ATP generation from glucose catabolism. The affected cells also accumulate increased amounts of 2, 3-diphosphoglycerate, but they cannot use the latter for ATP production because of the kinase deficit. The resulting lack of cellular energy sources causes an impaired maintenance of internal composition and

---

The black groups are very sensitive to antimalarial drugs such as primaquine and this condition is often termed *primaquine sensitivity*. The Mediterranean groups show similar sensitivity to such drugs and may also react to the *fava bean*, which has thus led to the term *favism* to designate this disorder. In both cases, the, individuals are without symptoms until they are exposed to the causative agents, which trigger a severe hemolytic anemia that may be fatal. **These agents promote the oxidation of erythrocytic glutathione.** In the absence of glucose-6phosphate dehydrogenase, the cells are unable to provide the increased NADPH required to restore the oxidized glutathione to the - SH form. The failure to sustain reduced glutathione is associated with the appearance of deposits of denatured hemoglobin *(Heinz bodies)*, and the resulting deformations of the cell membrane single out the defective erythrocytes for destruction in the sinusoids of the spleen, thereby producing the acute hemolytic episode.

---

disruption of membrane integrity. Deformation and other alterations in surface properties lead to the recognition by the spleen of such cells as abnormal, and they are consequently removed and destroyed by the reticuloendothelial system. Other similarly severe hemolytic anemias have been described with inherited lesions of the erythrocytic enzymes of the glycolytic pathway (triose-phosphate isomerase, glucose-phosphate isomerase, phosphoglycerate kinase and hexokinase), but these conditions seem to be very rare.

The significance of pentose-phosphate pathway for the ability of the erythrocyte to withstand external stresses is demonstrated by a group of common, drug-induced, hemolytic anemias that are characterized by glucose-6-phosphate dehydrogenase deficiency. The diseases are transmitted as sex-linked recessive traits and are found most frequently among black people who are inhabitants of the Mediterranean area.

Carbohydrate Metabolism

The major anabolic route open for carbohydrates in the human body is *glycogenesis* in which genesis of glycogen (biosynthesis of the polysaccharide glycogen) takes place whereas the catabolic routes are many, e.g. (i) *glycogenolysis* (ii) *glycolysis* (iii) *citric acid cycle*, and (iv) *pentose phosphate* **pathway**. These routes of catabolism liberate energy which is used for various purposes in the human body. **Side by side, certain noncarbohydrate substances lead to the biosynthesis of glucose and glycogen; this process is referred to as *gluconeogenesis* or neoglucogenesis.** We will take up these pathways one by one.

GLYCOGENESIS

(Genesis i.e. synthesis of glycogen)
This process is an anabolic process which requires energy expenditure both from ATP and uridine triphosphate (UTP). This process may be referred to as the genesis (synthesis) of glycogen from glucose or other sugars. Glycogen is synthesized in practically all the tissues of the body but the major sites are:

(a) Liver, and

(b) Muscles

Glycogenesis starts with glucose. In the very first reaction glucose gets phosphorylated to form glucose-6-phosphate in the presence of ATP; this reaction is catalyzed by glucokinase. Thus, it may be seen that glucose-6-phosphate so formed occupies a key position as a common intermediate in carbohydrate metabolic pathways: it may be converted reversibly to pyruvate by glycolysis or gluconeogenesis; it may be converted to pentoses or to CO_2 irreversibly by the pentose phosphate pathway; and it may be converted reversibly to glycogen also.

In the next step, mutation of the phosphate group of glucose-6-phosphate from position 6 to the position 1 takes place in the presence of a cofactor glucose-1, 6-diphosphate; this reaction is catalysed by the enzyme phosphoglucomutase. In the next reaction, glucose-1-phosphate reacts with uridine triphosphate (UTP) to form active nucleotide i.e. uridine diphosphate glucose in the presence of an enzyme UDPG pyrophosphorylase; in this process, two terminal phosphates are removed from UTP as inorganic pyrophosphate,. while the remaining UMP portion gets joined by a pyrophosphate bridge to glucose-1-phosphate to form UDP-glucose.

The next reaction is catalyzed by the enzyme glycogen synthetase, in this reaction, the C_1 of the activated glucose of UDPG forms a glycosidic bond with the C_4 of a terminal glucose residue of glycogen, liberating uridine diphosphate (UDP) with the formation of unnatural glycogen i.e. straight chain; a pre-existing glycogen or "primer" must be present to initiate this reaction (Fig 15.1).

Mechanism of Branching

The addition of a glucose residue to the pre-existing glycogen chain or "primer" occurs at the nonreducing outer end of the molecule so that branches of the glycogen become elongated as successive -1 → 4-linkages occur, **as a result of which a 'tree' like molecule of glycogen gets synthesized.** When the chain acquires a length of minimum of 11 glucose residues, a second enzyme called a branching enzyme (amylo-[1 → 4] → [1 → 6]-transglucosidase) transfers a part of the -1 → 4- chain (minimum length of 6 glucose residues) to a neighbouring chain to form α -1 → 6-linkage, thus a branch point is established in the molecule. The branches grow by further additions of -1 → 4-glucosyl units and further branching. This highly branched structure serves two major purposes in the cell:

(a) firstly, it provides numerous ends for glucose molecules to be attached or removed rapidly;

(b) secondly, it forms a dense and compact storage particle in the cell.

In this way, natural molecule of glycogen with α-1, 6 linkages i.e. branches is synthesized.

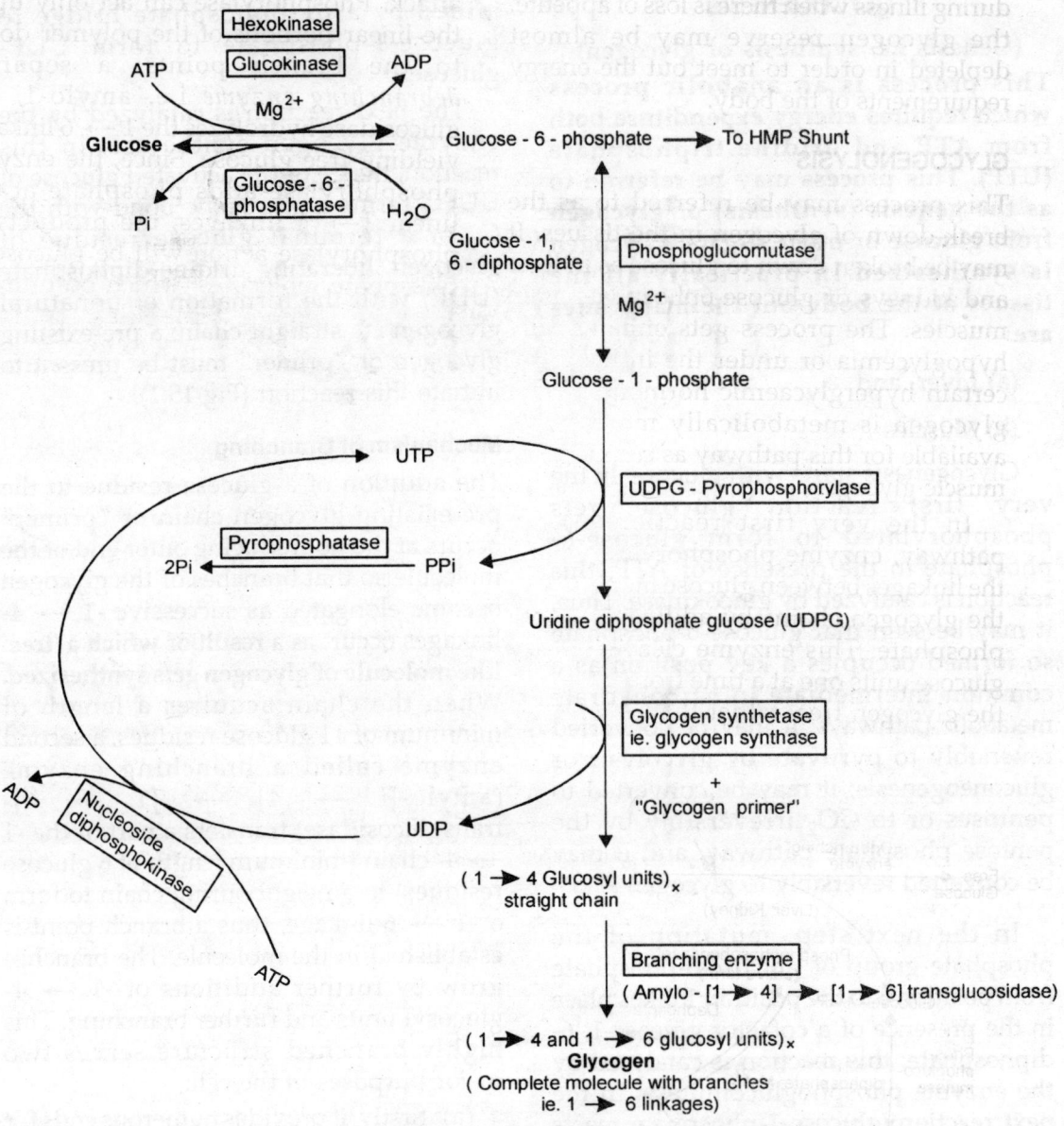

Figure 15.1 : Pathway of Glycogenesis

Significance of the pathway

Significance of this pathway lies in the fact that it acts as a source of sugar, both for the blood that nourishes other tissues and for the needs of the liver itself especially when one is starved or sick. **Glycogen** in fact, is a **reservoir** of energy. After a heavy intake of carbohydrates, as much as one tenth of the liver mass may consist of this storage form of glucose, whereas in starvation or during illness when there is loss of appetite, the glycogen reserve may be almost depleted in order to meet out the energy requirements of the body.

GLYCOGENOLYSIS

This process may be referred to as the break-down of glycogen in the tissues. It may be broken down to glucose as in liver and kidneys or glucose-6phosphate as in muscles. The process gets enhanced by hypoglycemia or under the influence of certain hyperglycaemic hormones. Liver glycogen is metabolically more easily available for this pathway as compared to muscle glycogen.

In the very first reaction of this pathway, enzyme phosphorylase breaks the linkages between glucose monomers of the glycogen chains by adding inorganic phosphate. This enzyme cleaves off the glucose units one at a time from the tips of the glycogen tree, rather than by random

attack. Phosphorylase can act only upon the linear portions of the polymer down to the branch points; a separate *debranching enzyme* i.e. amylo-1, 6 - glucosidase hydrolyzes the 1 → 6 linkage, yielding free glucose. Since, the enzyme phosphorylase adds phosphate at the linear 1→ 4 linkages, the products of phosphorylase action will be glucose-1-phosphate molecules, which outnumber the free glucose molecules from the debranching process by a ratio of roughly 10:1.

In the next reaction (Fig 15.2), in the liver/kidney tissues, glucose -1-phosphate molecule is converted to glucose 6-phosphate by the action of enzyme phosphoglucomutase in the presence of coenzyme glucose-1, 6-diphosphate; this reaction being reversible. Now, in the third and last reaction of this pathway, glucose-6-phosphate is acted upon by the enzyme glucose-6-phosphatase, as a result of which glucose is formed along with the

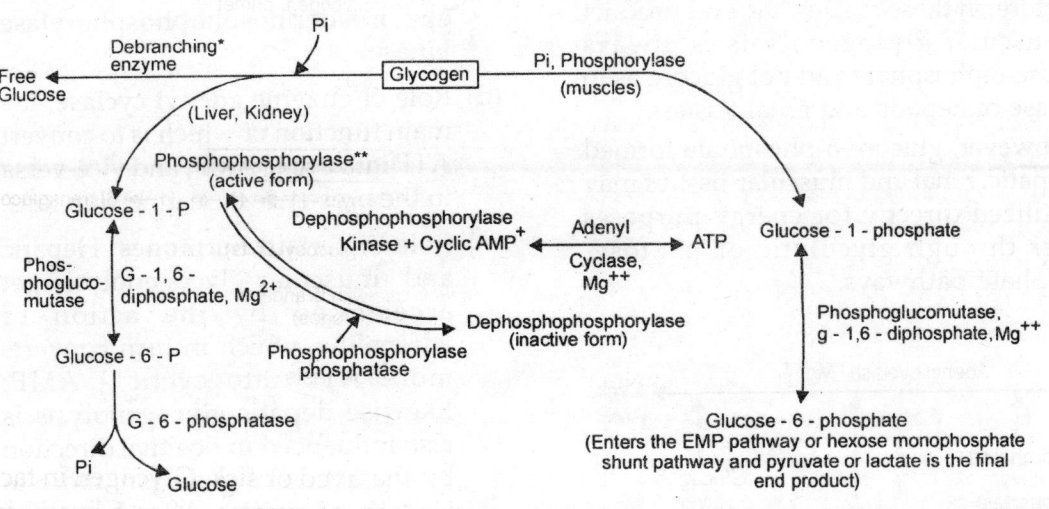

Figure 15.2 : Mechanism of glycogenolysis in liver, kidney and muscles

---

Glycogenolysis = Glycogen + Lysis

The breakdown of liver glycogen occurs in response to the accelerated requirements for glucose by the hepatic tissue itself or by other parts of the body.

End product of this pathway in liver and kidney tissues is glucose whereas glucose-6-phosphate in the muscles.

It's an energy liberating process. There are several factors like various enzymes, cyclic AMP, various hormones etc. which regulate this pathway.

Its rate gets increased in starvation, sickness, less carbohydrate consumption and other states.

---

liberation of inorganic phosphate. Glucose, so obtained is freely diffusible through the blood stream.

Be it known, that muscles lack the enzyme glucose-6-phoshatase (Fig 15.2), therefore, in these tissues, the end product of muscular glycogenolysis is always glucose-6-phosphate and not glucose as in the case of hepatic and renal tissues.

However, glucose-6-phosphate formed in hepatic, renal and muscular tissues may be utilized directly for energy purposes either through glycolytic or pentose-phosphate pathways.

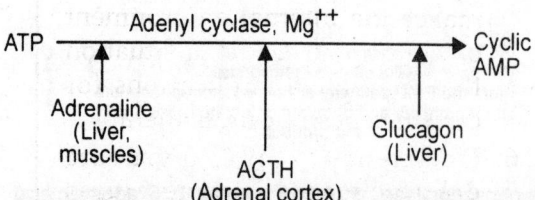

Regulatory factors of Glycogenolysis

There are several regulatory factors which play vital role in the regulation of this pathway, namely:

(a) **Active phosphorylase or phosphophos phorylase** is the *rate-limiting* enzyme of glycogenolysis: Inactive dephospho-phosphorylase is converted to its active form i.e; phosphophosphorylase by the action of enzyme dephospho-phosphorylase kinase (Fig 12.3).

(b) **There is yet another enzyme phos-phophosphorylase phosphatase** which may convert phosphopho-sphorylase into dephospho-phosphorylase. In this way the above named phosphatase enzyme has got a regulatory effect. If the rate of this pathway is to be decreased, then the activity of this phosphatase becomes more and vice-versa.

(c) Role of **cyclic AMP,** the presence of which is must for the activity of enzyme dephosphophosphorylase kinase.

(d) Role of enzyme **adenyl cyclase**, the main function of which is to convert ATP into cyclic AMP, and vice-versa in the pres-ence of magnesium ions.

(e) Role of certain **hormones:** Hepatic and muscular glycogenolysis get accelerated by the action of adrenaline, which in turn converts more ATP into cyclic - AMP; likewise hepatic glycogenolysis is also influenced in positive direction by the action of glucagon; more to say, in adrenal cortex, hormone ACTH plays the same role (Fig 15.2).

Insulin appears to suppress glucose-6-phosp-hatase activity, thereby reducing glycogenolysis. Contrarily, starvation, less carbohydrate consumption, glucocorticoids, thyroid hormones and glucagon may stimulate glycogenolysis by enhancing the activity of enzyme glucose-6-phosphatase.

Significance

It lies in the fact that this pathway is very important and essential as well from the point of view of giving energy to various tissues of the body, especially in starvation, sickness, carbohydrate deprivation and other similar conditions.

Sutherland (USA), a Physician was awarded Nobel Prize in Medicine in 1971 for his discoveries concerning the mechanism of the action of hormones. He was awarded Nobel Prize for isolation of cyclic AMP in 1952 and demonstrated its involvement in numerous metabolic processes which occur in animals.

GLYCOLYSIS
OR
EMBDEN MEYERHOF parnas PATHWAY
(emp pathway)

There is a minimum requirement of glucose in all the tissues of the body but some tissues *like brain and erythrocytes require it in a good concentration*. It is the major pathway for the utilization of glucose which operates in all the cells. **It is a unique pathway because it can operate under aerobic and as well as anaerobic conditions.**

GLYCOLYTIC PATHWAY

This is **a very important pathway from** several points and may be referred to as **the breakdown of glucose or glycogen to produce pyruvate or lactate. This operates in almost all the tissues of the body but liver and muscles are the main sites. Various enzymes involved in this pathway are found in the extramitochondrial soluble fraction of the cell, the cytosol.**

Glucose units derived from dietary carbohy-drates or from glucose synthesized in the liver, enter cells as free

Biomedical Importance

1. **It is the main pathway for the oxidation of glucose.**
2. It is also the main pathway for the metabolism of fructose and galactose, which one consumes daily in moderate quantity via diet.
3. It provides ATP
4. **A small number of diseases occur in which enzymes of glycolysis (e.g., puruvate kinase) are deficient in activity; such conditions are mainly manifested as hemolytic anemias.**
5. In fast growing cancerous cells, this pathway proceeds at a much higher rate resulting into more production of pyruvate. This in turn results in excessive production of lactate, which makes the internal environment of the tumour acidic, a situation that may have implications for certain types of cancer therapy.
6. **Deficiency of pyruvate dehydrogenase enzyme causes lactic acidosis.**

glucose. In the very first reaction of this pathway glucose molecule gets phosphorylated with ATP by an enzyme called hexokinase to yield glucose-6-phosphate (Fig. 15.3) in the presence of Mg^{++} ions. **Several hereditary disorders of hexokinase deficiency are known today, the reason being that it exists in different isoenzymic forms. In each case, the main symptom of enzymic deficiency is anemia.** Another glucose phosphorylating enzyme exists in liver which is called as glucokinase; this has got greater specificity for glucose than the hexokinase.

The very first reaction i.e. the conversion of glucose to g-6-P is irreversible but can be reversed by another enzyme glucose-6-phosphatase which remains present in liver and kidney tissues. Muscles do not contain glucose-6-phosphatase hence the formation of glucose from g-6-phosphate is not possible in such tissues. Side by side, glucosyl units obtained from glycogen in the presence of inorganic phosphate may also be converted to glucose-1-phosphate by the action of phosphorylase; these units do not require ATP for activation. G-1- P may then be converted to G-6-P by the action of phosphoglucomutase in the presence of cofactor glucose-1,6 diphosphate and Mg^{++} ions.

Glucose-6-phosphate forms the active substrate of glycolysis, which is now isomerized to form fructose -6-P in the presence of enzyme phosphohexose-isomerase. At this juncture fructose can also enter into glycolytic pathway by forming fructose-6-P; this reaction being catalysed by an unspecific hexokinase in the presence of ATP and Mg^{++} ions. In the next reaction, fructose-6-P is phosphorylated at C-1 position forming a sugar diphosphate i.e. fructose-1, 6-diphosphate under the influence of enzyme phosphofructokinase (PFK), ATP and Mg^{++} ions; *this reaction is also irreversible*. The reaction can, however, be reversed by another enzyme i.e. fructose-1, 6 - diphosphatase (Fig. 15.3). F-l, 6 diP is now cleaved under the influence of an enzyme termed aldolase as a result of which dihydroxyacetone phosphate and glyceraldehyde-3phosphate are formed. The two triose phosphates formed are convertible into each other under the influence of an enzyme called triose phosphate isomerase and these two triose phosphates can further be condensed to form fructose-1, 6-diP by the reversal of aldolase activity. Glyceraldehyde-3-P can now enter the subsequent reactions of glycolysis. The equilibrium of the reactions is such that dihydroxyacetone phosphate (DHAP) also gets changed into glyceraldehyde-3-P and enters into subsequent reactions of glycolysis. At this juncture glycerol obtained from fat degradation can also enter into the forward or backward reactions of glycolysis by first getting converted into α-glycerophosphate and then into DHAP.

Now, glyceraldehyde-3-P is oxidized to form 1,3-diphosphoglyceric acid by the action of enzyme glyceraldehyde-3-P-dehydrogenase in the presence of nicotinamide adenine dinucleotide (NAD) as hydrogen acceptor and inorganic phosphate. The phosphate group gets attached at position-l of glycerol by a high-energy bond which is formed by intramolecular rearrangement of energy during dehydrogenation. In the next reaction, high energy phosphate group at C_1 is transferred to ADP forming ATP and 3-phosphoglyceric acid (Fig 15.3) under the influence of enzyme phosphoglycerate kinase and Mg^{++} ions. Now, 3-PGA is

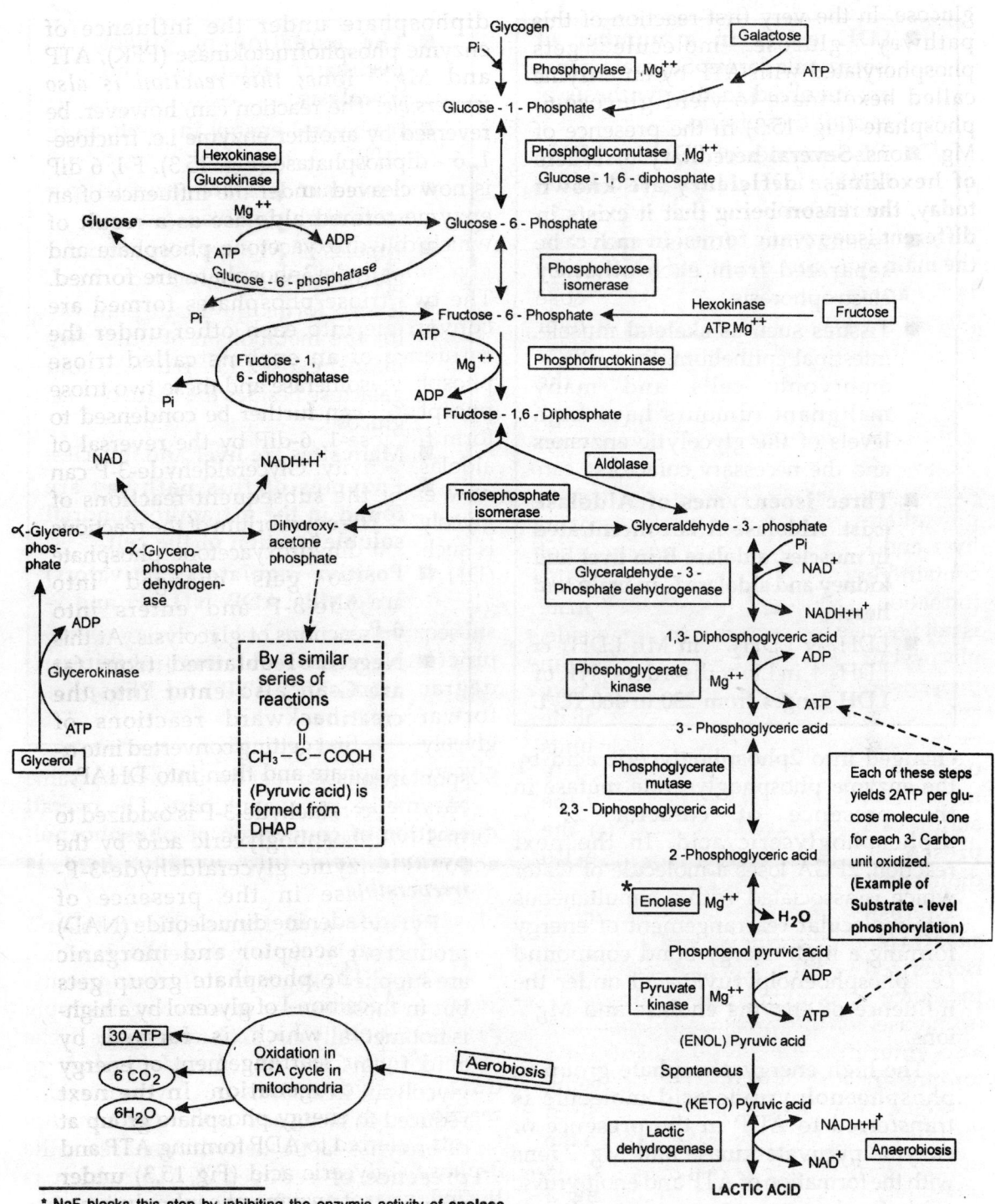

* NaF blocks this step by inhibiting the enzymic activity of **enolase**

Figure 15.3 : Glycolytic Pathway (Glycolysis)

- **LDH exists in a number of isoenzymic forms.** Separate genes are involved in the synthesis of each of these forms.
- 5 Isoenzymes of LDH i.e. LDH_1, LDH_2, LDH_3, LDH_4 and LDH_5 are known.
- Isoenzymic forms may be separated from each other by electrophoresis.
- Tissues such as skeletal muscle, intestinal epithelium, liver, RBCs, embryonic cells and many malignant tumours have high levels of the glycolytic enzymes and the necessary cofactors.
- **Three isoenzymes of Aldolase exist. Aldolase A is concentrated in muscles, aldolase B in liver and kidney and aldolase C in brain and heart.**
- LDH_1 & LDH_2 ↑ in MI; LDH_4 & LDH_5 ↑ in Liver disorders.; **NR of LDH ranges from 230 to 460 IU/1.**

- **The oxidation of glucose to pyruvate/ lactate is termed as glycolysis.**
- It liberates energy in the form of ATP.
- 8 moles of ATP are generated per mole of glucose oxidized.
- 9 moles of ATP get generated per glucosyl unit of glycogen oxidized.
- It also forms the main pathway for the metabolism of other two main hexoses i.e. fructose and galactose besides the main one i.e. glucose.
- **Main sites are liver and muscles.**
- **Enzymes of this pathway are found in the extramitochondrial soluble fraction of the cell.**
- **Positive regulators (activators) are AMP, ADP, NH_4, Pi and F-6-P.**
- **Negative regulators (inhibitors) are G-6-P, ATP and Phospho-creatine.**

changed into 2phosphoglyceric acid by the enzyme phosphoglycerate mutase in the presence of cofactor 2, 3-diphosphoglyceric acid. In the next reaction, 2PGA loses a molecule of water which is associated with a simultaneous intramolecular rearrangement of energy forming a high energy bond compound i.e., phosphoenolpyruvic acid under the influence of enzyme enolase and Mg^{++} ions.

The high energy phosphate group in phosphoenolpyruvic acid molecule is transferred to ADP in the presence of enzyme pyruvate kinase and Mg^{++} ions with the formation of ATP and enolpyruvic acid. Enol form of pyruvic acid gets changed into keto form of pyruvic acid

spontaneously under the influence of same enzyme i.e. pyruvate kinase. **The overall reaction of conversion of phosphoenol-*pyruvic acid into pyruvic acid* is *irreversible.***

Pyruvic acid forms the main end product of glycolysis in those tissues which are supplied oxygen in sufficient quantity, but in those tissues where oxygen supply is not met fully e.g. skeletal muscles, lactic acid forms the usual end-product of glycolysis. In such tissues, pyruvic acid is reduced to lactic acid under the influence of enzyme lactic dehydrogenase in the presence of reduced NAD, which is supplied by the triose-phosphate dehydro-genase reaction. Conversion of pyruvic acid into lactic acid allows glycolysis to run smoothly under anaerobic conditions.

Role of Arsenate and Fluoride in Glycolysis

Glyceraldehyde-3-P is converted to 1,3-diphos- phoglyceric acid by the enzyme **glyceraldehyde-3-P-dehydrogenase** in the presence of NAD^+ and inorganic phosphate. If *arsenate* is present, it will compete with inorganic phosphate (Pi) in the above reaction to give 1-arseno-3-phosphoglyceric acid, which hydrolyzes sponta-neously to give 3-phosphoglyceric acid along with heat, without generating ATP. This is an important example of the ability of arsenate to accomplish uncoupling of oxidation and phosphory-lation.

2-PGA is converted to phosphoenol-pyruvic acid, reaction being catalysed by enolase in the presence of Mg^{++} ions. **Enolase** is inhibited by **fluoride**, a property that can be made use of when it is required to prevent glycolysis prior to the estimation of blood glucose.

Regulation of the Glycolytic Pathway (Fig 15.4)

The irreversible reactions of glycolysis are catalysed by:

(a) **hexokinase,**

(b) **phosphofructokinase (PFK), and**

(c) **pyruvate kinase**

These are regulated by a number of allosteric modifiers as shown in Fig 15.4. Regulation of these enzymes is important in controlling the rate of glycolysis.

ENERGETICS OF GLYCOLYSIS

Glycolysis as a whole is an energy liberating process . Energy obtained from this pathway under aerobic and anaerobic conditions is different. It's also dependent

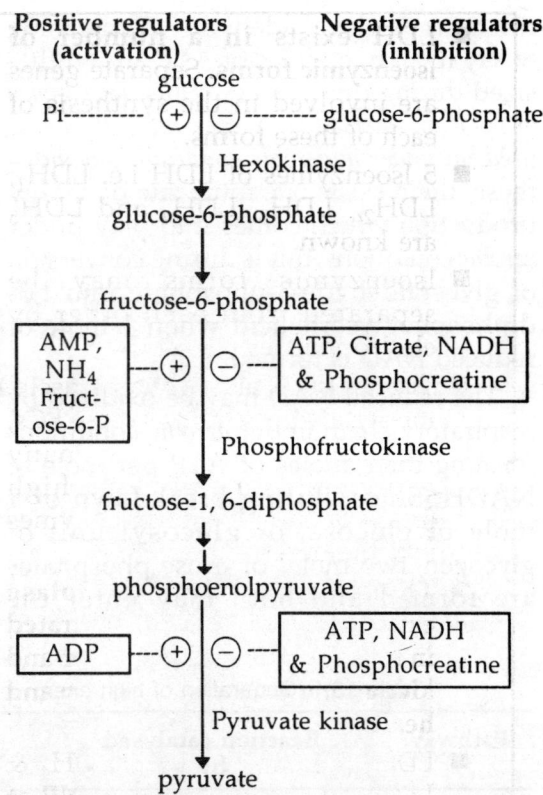

Fig. 15.4 : To show positive and negative regulators.

upon whether it is the free glucose or the glucosyl unit of glycogen which is entering into glycolysis.

In general, the sites of energy production in glycolysis are (1) during conversion of 1,3diphosphoglyceric acid (energy rich) into 3-PGA (low energy) and (2) during conversion of phosphoenol pyruvic acid (energy rich) into enolpyruvic acid (low energy). If ADP is present in these reaction systems, energy of energy-rich compounds is captured with the formation of ATP. One mole of ATP at each of the above two steps is synthesized per mole of 1, 3-diphosphoglyceric acid or phospho-enolpyruvic acid utilized for forward reaction. DHAP formed by the action of aldolase also undergoes similar series of reactions as glyceraldehyde-3-P, meaning to say in all two moles of ATP are synthesized during this process. *Thus, four moles of ATP are formed in all per mole of hexose used up under anaerobic conditions.* Besides these, there exists one more site of energy production which comes into play under *aerobic* conditions, this is during conversion of glyceraldehyde-3-phosphate into 1,3-diphosphoglyceric acid when 1 mote of reduced NAD is formed.

The reduced NAD may be oxidized by respiratory chain under *aerobic* conditions forming three moles of ATP per mole of NADH. Since, during breakdown of 1 mole of glucose, or glucosyl unit of glycogen, two moles of triose phosphates are formed and both may enter the subsequent glycolytic reactions, hence, two moles of NADH may be produced which on oxidation would give rise to 6 moles of ATP under aerobic conditions, therefore 10 i.e. (4 + 6) moles of ATP may be produced pet mole of glucose entering into glycolysis.

There are also sites in glycolysis where ATP is consumed for activation purposes. First of all, one mole of ATP is consumed in the very first reaction i.e. in the conversion of glucose to glucose-6-phosphate. However, if the starting substance is the glucosyl unit of glycogen, this step is bypassed. The second site of ATP consumption is when F-1, 6-diP is formed from F-6.P,. here too 1 mole of ATP is consumed.

Table 15.1: Generation of high-energy phosphate bonds in the catabolism of glucose

Pathway	Reaction catalysed by	Mode of -P production	Number of - P formed per mole or glucose
Glycolysis	Glyceraldehyde-3-phosphate dehydrogenase	Respiratory chain oxidation of 2NADH	6*
	Phosphoglycerate kinase	Oxidation at substrate level	2
	Pyruvate kinase	Oxidation at substrate level	2
	Allow the consumption of ATP by reactions catalyzed by Hexokinase & PFK		10
			−2
			net 8
	Pyruvate dehydrogenase	Respiratory chain oxdn of 2NADH	6
	Isocitrate dehydrogenase	Respiratory chain oxdn of 2 NADH	6
	α -Ketoglutarate dehyrogenase	Respiratory chain oxdn of 2 NADH	6
TCA cycle	Succinate thiokinase	Oxidation at substrate level	2
	Succinate dehydrogenase	Respiratory chain oxdn of 2FADH$_2$	4
	Malate dehydrogenase	Respiratory chain oxdn of 2 NADH	6
			30
Total per mole of glucose under aerobic conditions			38
Total per mole of glucose under anaerobic conditions			2

*It is assumed that NADH formed in glycolysis is transported into mitochondria via the malate shuttle. If the glycerophosphate shuttle is used, only 2 ~ P would be formed per mole of NADH, **then the total net production being 36 instead of 38.**

In order to evaluate the net gain of energy, the energy consumption has also got to be taken into consideration and must be subtracted from total energy production.

Under *anaerobic conditions;* therefore, there occurs a net gain of 3 ATP moles per glucosyl unit of glycogen and 2 ATP moles per free glucose mole broken down to lactic acid.

Under *aerobic conditions* there occurs a net gain of 9 ATP moles pet glucosyl unit and 8 ATP moles per free glucose mole broken down to pyruvic add (Table 15.1).

Energetics of Carbohydrate Oxidation

When one mole of glucose is combusted in a calorimeter to CO_2 and H_2O approximately 2,780 kJ are liberated as heat. When oxidation occurs in the tissues, some of this energy is not wasted immediately as heat but is "captured" in high-energy phosphate bonds. *On the whole* 38 *high-energy phosphate bonds are generated per molecule of glucose oxidized to CO_2 and H_2O.* Assuming each high energy bond to be equivalent to 30.5 kJ,the total energy captured in ATP per mole of glucose oxidized is 1,159 kJ, or approximately 41.7% of the energy of combustion. Most of the ATP is generated as a consequence of oxidative phosphory-lation resulting from the reoxidation of reduced coenzymes by the respiratory chain. The remainder energy is generated by phosphoryla-tion at the substrate level. Above Table indicates the reactions responsible for the generation of high energy phosphate during oxidation of glucose and the net production under aerobic as well as anaerobic conditions.

TRICARBOXYLIC ACID CYCLE (TCA CYCLE) OR KREBS CYCLE

Both the names i.e. KREBS cycle and TCA cycle are popular in use. The name 'Krebs cycle' has been given to this cycle after the discoverer's name i.e. Hans Krebs; for this brilliant discovery **Dr Hans Adolf Krebs** was given the title of **'Sir'**. He was also later on awarded **Nobel Prize in 1953 for** his brilliant research work in Physiology and Medicine. As the first product of this cycle i.e. citric acid contains three carboxyl groups, hence the name **'Tricarboxylic Acid Cycle'** has been given to this cyclic process.

This cycle may be referred to as a mechanism whereby acetyl coenzyme A may be completely oxidized to CO_2 and H_2O.

Pyruvic acid, formed from carbohydrates is an important source, but not the only source of acetyl coenzyme A Under anaerobic conditions pyruvic acid is converted to lactic acid as the chief end product of glycolysis; but under aerobic conditions, a different series of reactions occurs, which is made possible by the availability of an adequate supply of the oxidized form of NAD. In the presence of magnesium ions, NAD, FAD, thiamine pyrophosphate, lipoic acid and coenzyme A, an *oxidative decarboxylation* of pyruvic acid takes place. The products of the reaction are acetyl coenzyme A, CO_2 and reduced nicotinamide adenine dinucleotide ($NADH_2$). The series of the reactions is quite complex but the overall process may be summarized as below:

In the course of the reaction, cofactors other than coenzyme A and NAD are regenerated and reutilized. The most

The complete oxidation of 1 mol of glucose yields either 36 or 38 mol of ATP, depending upon which type of shuttle pathway is used in the transport of cytophasmic NADH to mitochondria. A list of the energy- yielding reactions of glucose oxidation is as shown below:

Energy yielding reactions in the **complete oxidation of Glucose:**

Reaction	Net moles of ATP generated per mole of glucose
Glycolysis	
(reactions catalyzed by phosphoglycerate kinase & PK yield 4 ATP, whereas 2 moles of ATP are utilized in the reactions catalysed by hexokinase & PFK, therefore, only two are left out)	2
NADH shutlle	
glycerol-phosphate shuttle (or malate-aspartate shuttle)	4 (6)
Pyruvate dehydrogenase (NADH)	6
Succinyl CoA synthetase	
(GTP is equivalent to ATP)	2
Succinate dehydrogenase	
(succinate → fumarate + FADH₂)	4
Other TCA cycle reactions	
(isocitrate → α-ketoglutarate, α-ketoglutarate → succinyl CoA, malate → oxaloacetate; total of 3NADH generated)	18
Total	36 (38)

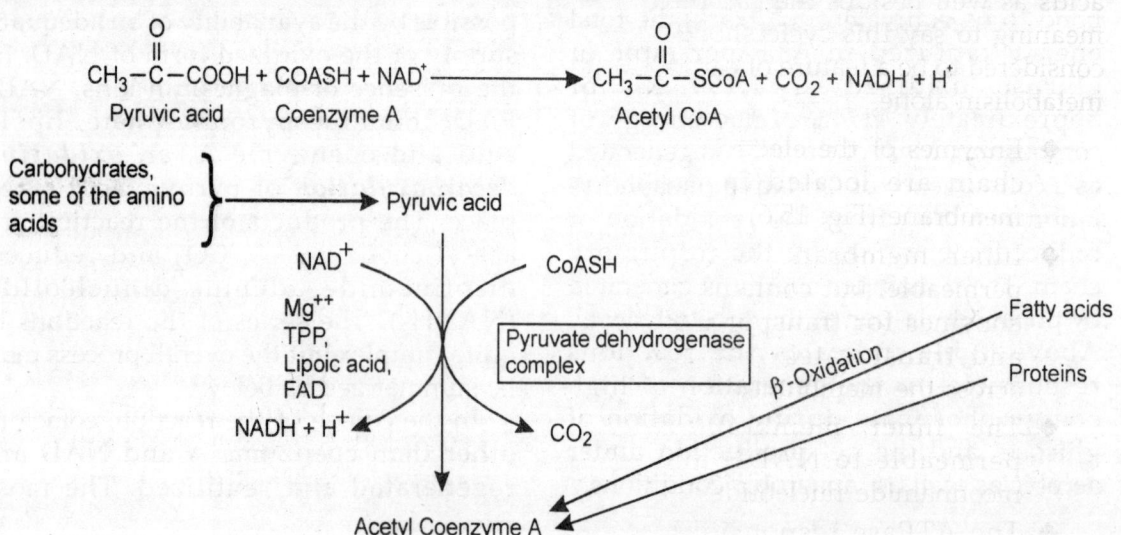

Krebs, Sir Hans Adolf (Germany/ U.K.), **a medical doctor and then Professor of Biochemistry** was awarded Nobel Prize in 1953 for his discovery of the **citric acid cycle,** also called as the tricarboxylic acid cycle or "**Krebs cycle**" which involves a series of chemical reactions. These reactions involve the conversion in the presence of oxygen, of substances formed by the breakdown of sugars, fats and protein components, to CO_2, H_2O and energy rich compounds.

Besides TCA cycle, Krebs also discovered along with the **German Biochemist Kurt Henseleit** a series of chemical reactions called the "**Urea cycle**", occurring in mammalian tissues by which ammonia is converted to urea which is far less toxic to mammalian organisms than ammonia. **The cycle also serves as the major source of amino acid arginine. Sir, Hans Krebs was a biochemist of great eminence and repute.**

important thing of the above reaction is its irreversibility.

Carbohydrates are the important sources of pyruvic acid but certain amino acids may also be converted to pyruvic acid as shown above in the reaction; besides these fatty acids, other lipid materials and proteins may eventually give rise to acetyl coenzyme A. Therefore, TCA cycle serves as the principal media for the complete oxidation of lipids and amino acids as well besides the carbohydrates, meaning to say this cycle should not be considered to be a feature of carbohydrate metabolism alone.

♦ Enzymes of the electron transport chain are located in the inner membrane (Fig: 15.6).

♦ Inner membrane is not freely permeable, but contains transport enzymes for transporting anions and translocates ATP for ADP across the membrane.

♦ The inner membrane is not permeable to NADH and other nicotinamide nucleotides.

♦ The ATPase responsible for the generation of ATP is found on

protrusions on the inside of the inner membrane.

The principal reactions of the cycle are shown in Fig 15.5. The very first reaction of the cycle which occurs in the presence of an enzyme called the condensing enzyme (citrate synthetase) is a condensation between acetyl CoA and oxaloacetic acid to form citric acid and coenzyme A. This reaction may be considered to be irreversible. The next reaction i.e. conversion of citric acid to *cis*-aconitic acid is catalysed by aconitase in the presence of Fe^{++} whereby a molecule of water is lost. Then, a molecule of water is added forming isocitric acid, reaction being catalysed by the previous enzyme i.e aconitase in the presence of Fe^{++}. Both the reactions catalysed by aconitase are reversible. Thus, we see that aconitase enzyme is a very important enzyme which

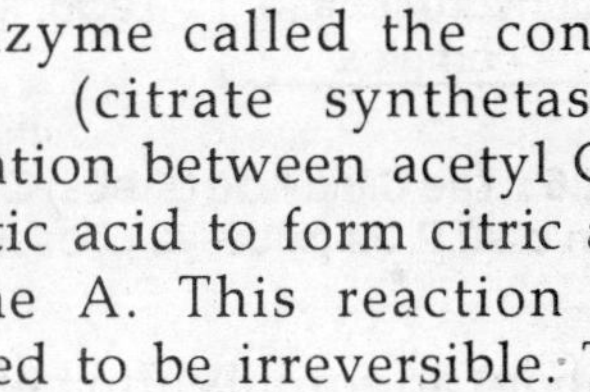

$$CH_2—COOH$$
$$|$$
$$HO—C—COOH$$
$$|$$
$$CH_2—COOH$$

Citric acid

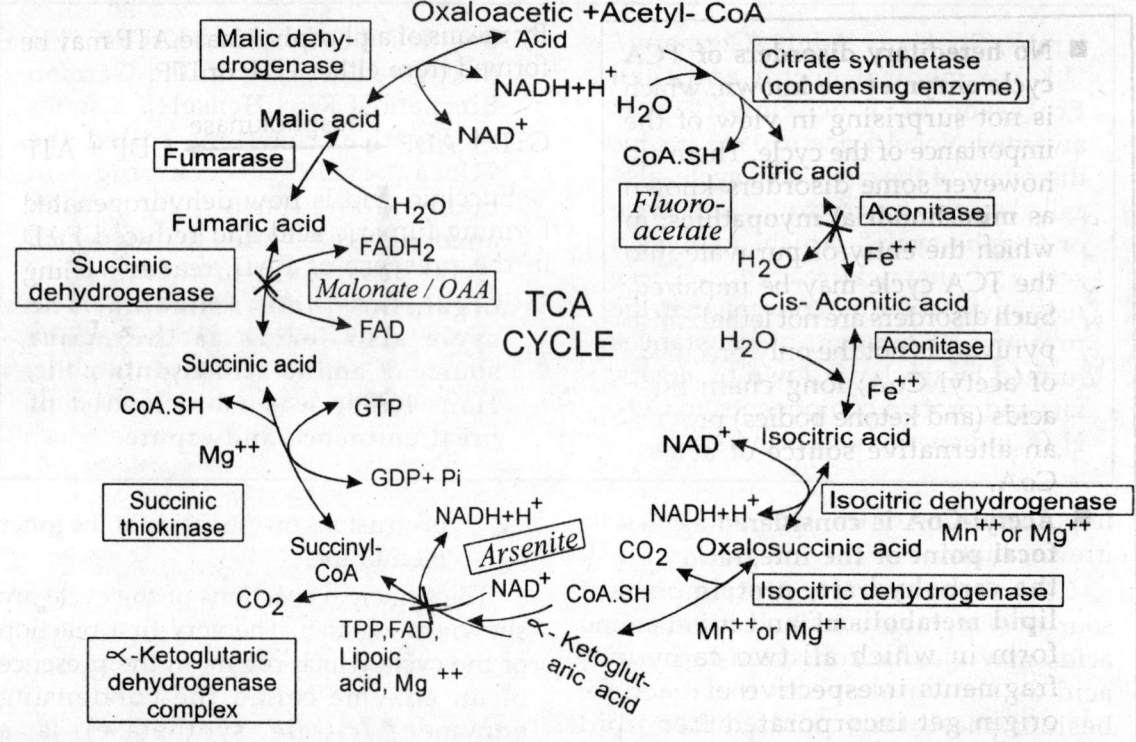

Figure 12.6 : The Citric Acid (Krebs) Cycle. Oxidation of NADH and FADH$_2$ in the respiratory chain leads to the generation of ATP via oxidative phosphorylation.

brings about an equilibrium between citric acid, *cis-* aconitic acid and isocitric acid by the removal and addition of water.

An enzyme, isocitric dehydrogenase, brings about the oxidation of isocitric acid, to oxalosuccinic acid, with, the reduction of NAD$^+$. Oxalosuccinic acid, while remaining still bound to the enzyme surface, is decarboxylated to form α-ketoglutaric acid; the reaction being catalysed by the same enzyme i.e. isocitric dehydrogenase in the presence of Mn^{++} or Mg^{++} ions. The α-keto acid' so formed now undergoes an oxidative decarboxylation forming succinyl coenzyme A in the presence of thiamine pyrophosphate, NAD$^+$, FAD, CoA, lipoic acid and Mg^{++}, in a manner exactly analogous to the

oxidative decarboxylation of pyruvic acid as shown above which is also an α-keto acid; reaction being catalysed by α-ketoglutaric dehydrogenase complex. Succinyl CoA, being a thioester, contains a high-energy bond. The equilibrium of this reaction is so much in favour of succinyl-CoA formation that the reaction must be physiologically considered as unidirectional.

Now, succinyl-CoA is converted to succinic acid by the enzyme-succinic thiokinase. The reaction requires GDP or IDP, which is converted in the presence of inorganic phosphate to either GTP or ITP. This is the only example in the whole of TCA cycle where *generation of a high-energy phosphate takes place at the substrate level.*

■ **No hereditary disorders of TCA cycle enzymes are known**, which is not surprising in view of the importance of the cycle. There are however some disorders known as **mitochondrial myopathies**, in which the entry of puruvate into the TCA cycle may be impaired. Such disorders are not lethal, since pyruvate is not the only precursor of acetyl CoA; long chain fatty acids (and ketone bodies) provide an alternative source of acetyl-CoA.

■ **Acetyl-CoA is considered as the focal point of the integration of the carbohydrate, protein and lipid metabolisms** and it is this form in which all two carbon fragments irrespective of their origin get incorporated into a common metabolic pathway.

■ **TCA cycle operates continuously in all the cells.**

■ Enzymes of TCA cycle are mainly confined in the **mitochondrial fraction of the cell. The inner membrane of the mitochondria bears the enzy-mes of the electron transport chain and oxidative phosphorylation (Fig 15.6).**

By means of a phosphokinase, ATP may be formed from either GTP or ITP.

$$GTP + ADP \xrightleftharpoons{\text{Phosphokinase}} GDP + ATP$$

Succinic acid is now dehydrogenated forming fumaric acid and reduced FAD in the presence of FAD, reaction being catalysed by succinic dehydrogenase. Enzyme succinic dehydrogenase remains bound to the inner surface of the inner mitochondrial membrane. It is the only dehydrogenation in the TCA cycle which involves the *direct transfer of hydrogen from the substrate to a flavoprotein without the participation of NAD*$^+$.

A molecule of water is added to fumaric acid to form malic acid in the presence of enzyme fumarase, and finally, malic acid is oxidized by malic dehydrogenase in the presence of NAD$^+$, resulting in the formation of reduced NAD and oxaloacetic acid. The cycle can then be repeated by the entrance of another

■ **Fluoroacetate** inhibits the conversion of citric acid to cis-aconitic acid, causing citric acid to accumulate. It is the first blockade point in the TCA cycle.

■ **Arsenite** inhibits the conversion of α-KGA to succinyl-CoA, causing α-KGA to accumulate. It is the second blockade point.

■ **Malonate or oxaloacetate (OAA)** blocks the conversion of succinic acid to fumaric acid by inhibiting the enzyme succinic dehydrogenase. It's the third and last blockade point. *Competitive inhibition* takes place here. This step results in the accumulation of succinic acid.

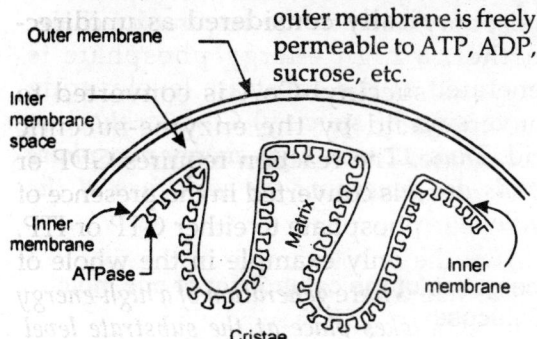

Fig. 15.6: A portion of Mitochondria

outer membrane is freely permeable to ATP, ADP, sucrose, etc.

Outer membrane

Inter membrane space

Inner membrane

ATPase

Matrix

Inner membrane

Cristae

molecule of acetyl CoA.

This process, which occurs in the mitochondria, results in the reduction of five molecules of NAD^+ or FAD (starting from pyruvate). These reduced cofactors are reoxidized by a process called the hydrogen transport system, or the electron transport system. The hydrogen, with the intermediation of a variety of cytochromes and other factors, is finally oxidized to water by combination with "activated" molecular oxygen. The reoxidized cofactors can then be reutilized in various reactions of the TCA cycle. Simultaneously, with the oxidation of hydrogen to water there occurs phosphorylation of ADP by inorganic phosphate to form ATP. The two processes, which are coupled by an unknown mechanism, are referred to as *oxidative phosphorylation*. ATP, which is the principal compound supplying energy for many reactions, such as muscle contraction, is generated in greater amount by oxidative phosphorylation than by any other means. The continued operation of this process is essential for life in aerobic organisms (cyanide, for example, is toxic because it reacts with the cytochromes, preventing their normal functioning). Since, the hydrogen transport system serves as the primary mean for the reoxidation of cofactors such as NADH, the TCA cycle is said to be an *aerobic process:* oxygen is necessary in the transport system to reoxidize NAD, FAD etc; the oxidized factors are necessary for the TCA cycle to operate.

Importance of TCA Cycle

The importance of this pathway lies in the fact that it is one of the pathways that generates the major part of the ATP and NADH in the cell.

NADPH can be formed from $NADP^+$ and NADH by a mitochondrial transhydrogenase, linked to the electron transport system and essentially irreversible.

$$NADH + NADP^+ \longrightarrow NADPH + NAD^+$$

ATP thus produced is utilized by the cell for its functions which are numerous and NADPH for the biosynthesis of fatty acids, steroids and other important substances of the human body.

Energetics of the TCA Cycle

As a result of oxidation catalyzed by dehydrogenase enzymes of the TCA cycle, 3 molecules of NADH and one molecule of $FADH_2$ are produced for each molecule of acetyl-CoA catabolized in one revolution of the cycle. These reducing equivalents are later on transferred to the respiratory chain in the inner mitochondrial membrane. During transport along the chain, each reducing equivalent from NADH generates 3 high-energy phosphate bonds by the esterification of ADP to ATP in the process of oxidative phosphorylation. However, $FADH_2$ produces only 2 high-energy phosphate bonds because it transfers its reducing power to coenzyme Q, thus, bypasses the first site for oxidative phosphorylation in the respiratory chain. Further, a high energy phosphate is generated at the substrate level during conversion of succinyl-CoA to succinic acid. *Thus, 12 new high-energy phosphate bonds are generated for each turn of the cycle.*

Energetics of the catabolism of one mole of glucose

Complete oxidation of one mole of

pyruvate through:

(a) **Acetyl-CoA,**

(b) **TCA cycle, and**

(c) **Transport system**

results in the generation of **15 moles of ATP.** The net result is the formation of CO_2 and H_2O from pyruvate, along with the ATP. Since, each mole of glucose can be converted by glycolysis to two moles of pyruvic acid, carbohydrate can be oxidized completely to CO_2 and H_2O yielding 30 moles of ATP from the reduced nucleotides and succinyl CoA formed in the Krebs cycle; 6 moles of ATP derived from the NADH formed in the triosephosphate dehydrogenase reaction of the glycolytic pathway, and a net of two moles of ATP formed from the substrates in the glycolytic pathway. Thus, **each mole of glucose oxidized** results in the production of **38 moles of ATP** (Table 12.1, given in glycolytic pathway).

Energetics of carbohydrate oxidation in terms of kilo Joules

When 1 mole of glucose is combusted in a calorimeter to CO_2 and H_2O, approximatery 2,780 kJ are liberated as heat, but when oxidation occurs in the tissues, some of this energy is not lost immediately as heat but is "captured" in high-energy phosphate bonds. On the whole, 38 high-energy phosphate bonds are generated per molecule of glucose oxidized to CO_2 and H_2O. Assuming each high-energy bond to be equivalent to 30.5 kJ, the total energy captured in ATP per mole of glucose oxidized will be 38 x 30.5 = 1159 kJ, or

approximately $\dfrac{100 \times 1159}{2780}$ = 41.69% (or 41.7%)

of the energy of combustion. Most of the ATP is formed as a consequence of oxidative phosphorylation resulting from the reoxidation of reduced coenzymes by the respiratory chain. The remainder is generated by phosphorylation at the 'substrate level'. Table 15.1 (given in glycolytic pathway) indicates the reactions responsible for the generation of high-energy phosphate during oxidation of glucose and the net production under aerobic and anaerobic conditions.

Energetics of Carbohydrate Oxidation in terms of calories

Since, each molecule of ATP can give rise to about 7,400 calories, the total energy of oxidation of glucose will be 38 x 7,400 = 2,81,200 cals but thermochemically, when a molecule of glucose is oxidized in vitro, it gives about 6,73,000 calories. Hence, the available energy from a molecule of

glucose is $\dfrac{2,81,200}{6,73,000}$ x 100 = about 42%.

The rest of the energy of oxidation is dissipated as heat.

Role of Vitamins in the TCA Cycle

There are four vitamins of the B complex group which play vital role in the functioning of TCA cycle, namely:

1. *Riboflavin* in the form of flavin adenine dinucleotide (FAD), a cofactor in the α-KGA dehydrogenase complex and in succinic dehydrogenase.

2. *Niacin* in the form of nicotinamide adenine dinucleotide (NAD), the coenzyme for 3 dehydrogenases in the cycle, i.e; isocitrate dehydrogenase, α-KGA dehy-drogenase, and malic dehydrogenase.

3. *Thiamine* (B_1) in the form of *thiamine pyrophosphate*, the coenzyme for decarboxylation in the α-KGA dehy-drogenase reaction.

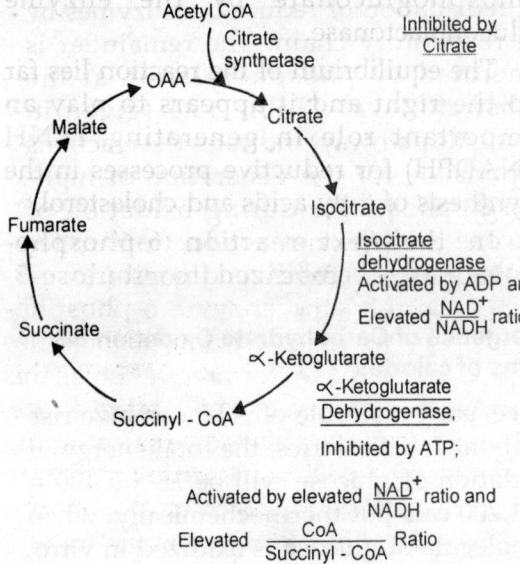

— **Alternative route for complete oxi-dation of glucose.**

— **Main sites** are adrenal cortex, testis, liver, adipose tissue, lactating mammary glands, leucocytes and erythrocytes.

— **Its enzymes** are found in the **extra-mitochondrial soluble fraction of the cell, the cytosol.**

— The enzymes of this pathway are important in providing **NADPH for the biosynthesis of fatty acids, ster-oids and other important substances.**

— This pathway also **helps in the synthesis of nucleotides** and **nucleic acids** by providing ribose sugar.

— **Two dehydrogenases** are involved in the production of NADPH:

(a) **Glucose-6-phosphate dehydrogenase.**

(b) **6-Phosphogluconate dehydrogenase.**

4. *Pantothenic acid,* as part of *coenzyme-A,* the cofactor attached to "active" acyl residues such as acetyl-CoA and succinyl-CoA.

5. **Lipoic acid,** in the reactions catalysed by pyruvate dehydrogenase complex and α-ketoglutarate dehydrogenase complex.

Regulation of the TCA Cycle

TCA cycle is regulated by the following three enzymes,
namely

(a) **Citrate synthetase,**

(b) **Isocitric dehydrogenase, and**

(c) **α-Ketoglutaric dehydrogenase**

as shown in the diagram ahead.

Both isocitrate dehydrogenase and α-ketoglutaric dehydrogenase get activated by Ca^{++}, which may be of importance in muscle in relation to contraction stimulated by Ca^{++}

The above named 3 enzymes are in non-equilibrium which means that the equilibrium of the 3 reactions catalysed by them is neither in the forward direction and nor in the backward.

HEXOSE MONOPHOSPHATE SHUNT (HMP SHUNT)
OR
PENTOSE PHOSPHATE PATHWAY (PPP)

This oxidative pathway is also known as **Warburg-Dickens-Lipmann phosphogluconate pathway** (Figures 15.7 (a) & (b)). It is quantitatively of no significance in highly glycolytic tissues such as skeletal muscles and non-lactating mammary glands, but is of considerable quantitative importance in tissues like adrenal cortex, testis, liver, adipose tissue and lactating mammary glands where fatty acids, steroids or pentoses are synthesized or L-glutamate dehydrogenase is used for L-glutamate synthesis. Besides the above tissues, it also operates in leucocytes and erythrocytes.

This pathway is an alternative route for the oxidation of glucose. The enzymes of this pathway are located in the extramitochondrial soluble portion of the cell, the cytosol.

It is a multicyclic process in which three molecules of glucose-6-phosphate give rise to three molecules of CO_2 and three-5-carbon residues namely ribulose 5 - phosphate, ribose-5-phosphate and xylulose-5-phosphate). The latter are arranged to regenerate two molecules of glucose-6-phosphate and one molecule of the glycolytic intermediate i.e. glyceraldehyde-3-phosphate. Since two molecules of glyceral-dehyde-3-phosphate can regenerate glucose-6-phosphate; glucose may be completely oxidized by this pathway. In nutshell, equation may be summarized as below: 3 glucose 6-phosphate + 6 NADP$^+$ $\longrightarrow$ 3CO$_2$ + 2 glucose - 6-phosphate +glyceraldehyde 3-phosphate + 6NADPH + 6H$^+$

By this pathway complete oxidation of glucose to CO_2 and H_2O with the formation of 36 moles of ATP per mole of sugar (glucose) oxidized takes place.

Mechanism

In the very first reaction of this pathway, oxidation of glucose-6-P to 6-phosphogluco-nolactone takes place; this reaction is catalyzed by glucose-6-phosphate dehydrogenase in the presence of NADP as a result of which NADPH is formed.

In the next reaction 6-phospho-gluconolactone is rapidly hydrolyzed to 6-phosphogluconate by the enzyme gluconolactonase.

The equilibrium of the reaction lies far to the right and it appears to play an important role in generating TPNH (NADPH) for reductive processes in the synthesis of fatty acids and cholesterol.

In the next reaction 6-phospho-gluconate is oxidized to ribulose-5-phosphate by the enzyme 6-phospho-gluconate dehydrogenase in the presence of coenzyme NADP forming NADPH; this enzyme is activated by Mg^{++} or Mn^{++} ions. NADPH so formed may serve as a reducing agent in other reactions coupled with it, such as those of fatty acid and the synthesis of cholesterol. In this reaction one mole of CO_2 is split out. This is the only step where CO_2 is formed in whole PPP.

Now, ribulose-5- phosphate is subjected to the action of two enzymes namely phospho-pentose isomerase which forms ribose-5-P and ribulose-5-phosphate epimerase which forms xylulose-5-P. Ribose-5-P so formed may be converted to ribose-1-P by the action of phospho-ribosemutase. Ribose-1-P so produced is responsible for the synthesis of nucleic acids.

In the next reaction, enzyme transketolase is involved which is responsible for the transfer of a ketol group from xylulose-5-phosphate to an aldehyde acceptor. This enzyme requires the presence of cofactor TPP and Mg^{++}.

A number of aldehydes - such as ribose-5phosphate, glyceraldehyde-3-P, glyceraldehyde, and glycolaldehyde can serve as acceptor. Thus, products formed by the action of transketolase are sedoheptulose-7-P and glyceraldehyde-3-P {Fig 12.8 (a)}, which are then subjected to the action of transaldolase forming erythrose-4-

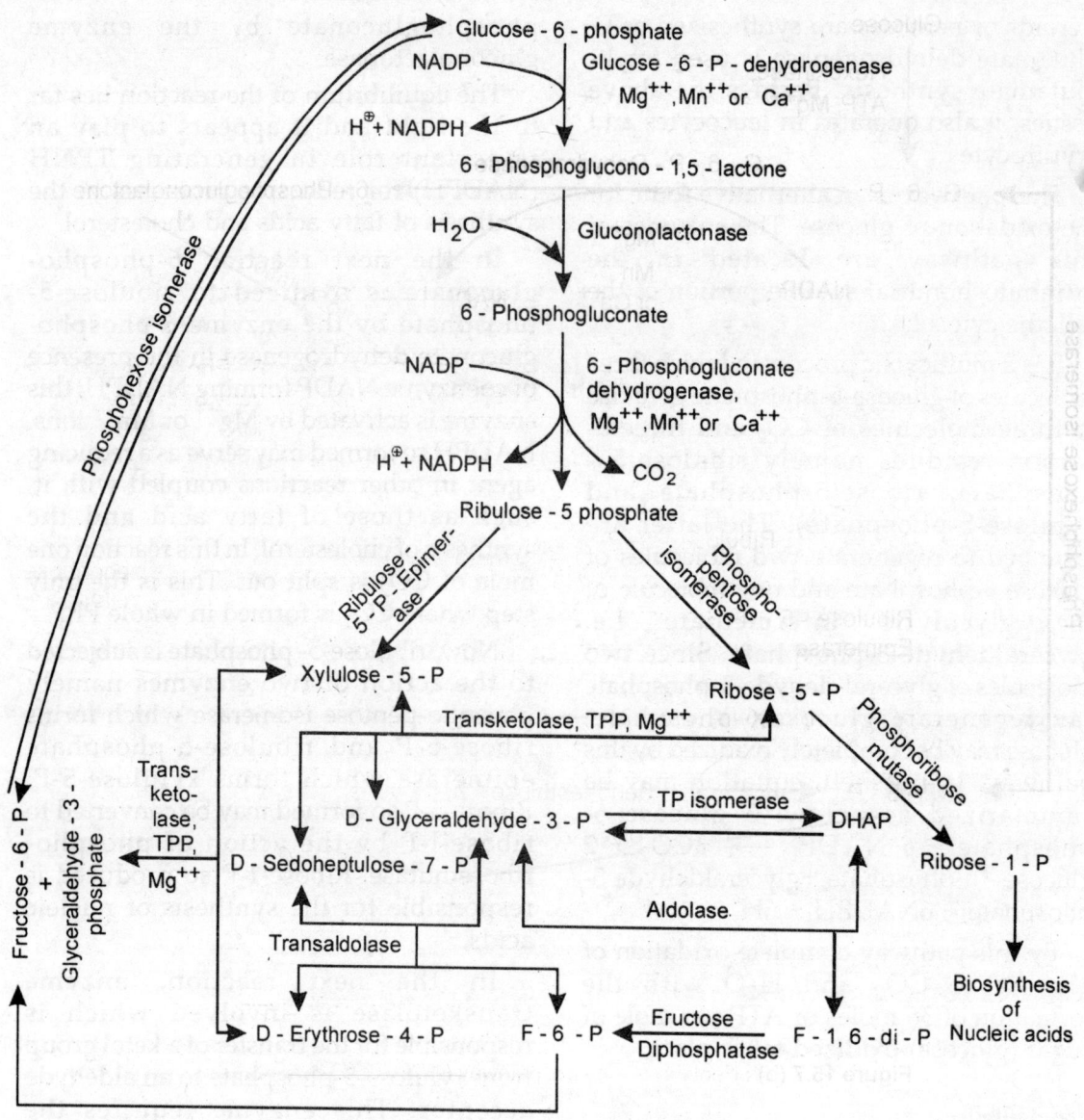

Fig. 15.7 (a) : Pentose phosphate pathway

Overall Summary of Reactions

6 hexose - PO_4 + $3O_2$ ⟶ $6CO_2$ + 6 pentose - PO_4

4 pentose - PO_4 ⟶ 2 hexose - PO_4 + 2 tetrose - PO_4

2 pentose - PO_4 + 2 tetrose - PO_4 ⟶ 2 hexose - PO_4 + 2 triose - PO_4

2 triose - PO_4 ⟶ hexose - PO_4 + inorganic phosphate

Sum : Hexose - PO_4 + $3O_2$ ⟶ $6CO_2$ + Pi 6 molecules of water would be formed in the process and 36 moles of ATP per molecule of hexose oxidized if the NADP. H formed were all converted to NAD.H (transhydrogenase) and this oxidized to NAD^+.

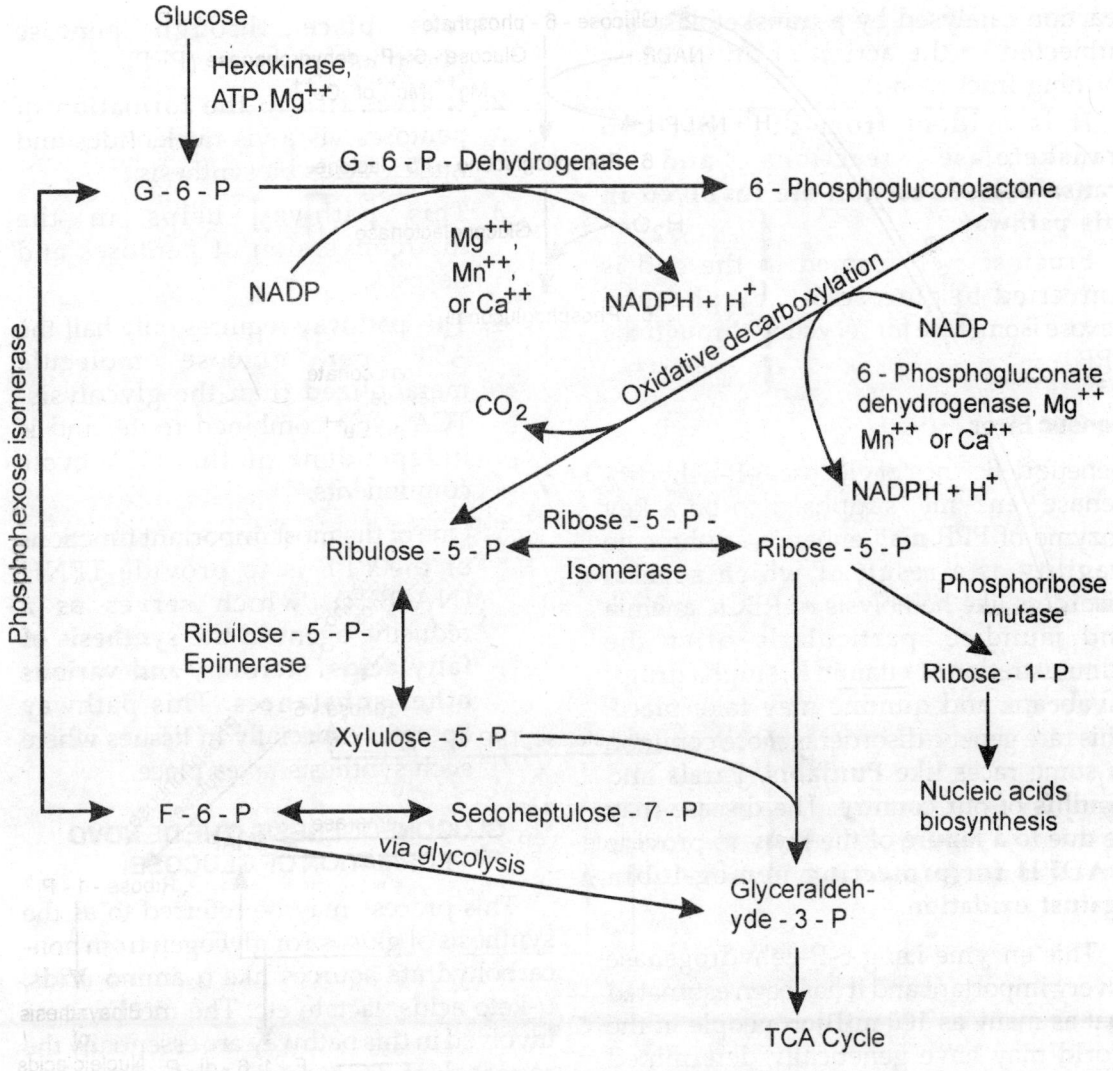

Figure 15.7 (b) : Pentose phosphate pathway (**simplified presentation**)

phosphate and fructose-6-phosphate. The function of transaldolase is to transfer a dihydroxyacetone unit from sedo-heptulose-7-phosphate (donor) to glyceraldehyde 3-P, D-erythrose-4-P, or ribose-5-P (acceptors). The enzyme appears to require no cofactors.

Now, erythrose-4-phosphate and fructose-6-P are again subjected to the

action of a transketolase forming fructose-6-P and glyceraldehyde-3-P.

Glyceraldehyde-3-P formed previously by the action of a transketolase {Fig 12.8(a)} may be converted to dihydroxyacetone phosphate by the action of a triose-P isomerase., Now, dihydroxy-acetone phosphate (DHAP) and the glyceral-dehyde-3-P formed in the last reaction catalysed by a transketolase are subjected to the action of an aldolase forming fructose-6-P.

It is evident from PPP that two transketolase reactions and a transaldolase reaction are involved in this pathway.

Fructose-6- P formed in the end is converted to glucose-6-P by phospho hexose isomerase for recycling through the PPP.

Genetic Error

Genetic deficiency of glucose-6-P-dehydro-genase enzyme, supposed to be a key enzyme of PPP may enhance erythrocyte fragility as a result of which several disorders like hemolysis of RBCs, anemia and jaundice, particularly after the administration of vitamin K, sulpha drugs, favabeans and quinine may take place. This rare genetic disorder is more common in some races like **Punjabis, Parsis** and **Sindhis** of our country. The disease may be due to a failure of the body to provide **NADPH for protecting hemog-lobin against oxidation.**

This enzyme i.e. g-6-P-dehydrogenase is very important and it has been estimated that as many as **100 million** people in the world may have genetically determined low levels of this enzyme, owing to variant forms which may be distinguished from each other by electrophoresis and various other techniques.

Significance of the Pentose Phosphate Pathway

1. A considerable proportion of glucose metabolism in various important tissues like liver, lactating mammary glands, adipose tissue, leukocytes, testis, and adrenal cortex appears to take place through pentose phosphate pathway (PPP).

2. It gives rise to the formation of pentoses vis a-vis nucleotides and nucleic acids biosynthesis.

3. This pathway helps in the interconversion of pentoses and hexoses.

4. This pathway requires only half the ATP per glucose molecule metabolized than the glycolysis-TCA cycle combined route, and is independent of the TCA cycle components.

5. One of the most important functions of the PPP is to provide TPNH (NADPH), which serves as a reducing agent **in the synthesis of fatty acids, steroids, and various other substances.** This pathway operates especially in tissues where such synthesis takes place.

GLUCONEOGENESIS (THE DE NOVO FORMATION OF GLUCOSE)

This process may be referred to as the synthesis of glucose or glycogen from non-carbohydrate sources like α-amino acids, α-keto acids, lactate etc. The mechanisms involved in this pathway are essentially the reversal of TCA cycle and glycolytic pathway (Fig 12.9). Since, some of the reactions are not reversible, such reactions do take place by alternative routes. Any substance which can form any of the intermediates of the TCA cycle or glycolysis can, therefore, easily give rise to glucose or glycogen. Such substances which are responsible for this phenomenon, are termed as gluconeogenic substances which ordinarily include several amino acids like alanine, serine, aspartic acid, valine, isoleucine, threonine, glutamic acid, histidine, arginine, proline, etc., lactate and glycerol (formed from the catabolism of fats). Main sites of this pathway are:

(a) Liver

(b) Kidneys

Out of the above two sites, liver is the main site.

Glycolytic pathway is made reversible with the help of following enzymes; such enzymes are named as **gluconeogenic enzymes:**

(a) **Glucose-6-phosphatase** (glucose-6-phosphate $\rightarrow$ glucose) is a

---

Genesis: The formation of

Neo: New

Gluco: Glucose

— **In this process glucose or glycogen is synthesized from non-carbohydrate sources like amino-acids, glycerol and lactic acid.**

— It's a useful pathway especially when an individual is consuming less carbohydrates.

— It helps in the **maintenance of blood sugar level** in its normal range.

— **It brings about proper disposal of lactic acid and glycerol.**

---

hydrolytic enzyme in the membrane of the endopl-asmic reticulum.

(b) **Fructose - 1, 6 - diphosphatase** (fructose-1, 6 - diphosphate $\rightarrow$ fructose-6-phosphate) is a hydrolytic enzyme found in the cytosol.

(c) **Pyruvate carboxylase** (pyruvate + CO_2 $\rightarrow$ oxaloacetate). This is the same enzyme as that which provides oxaloacetate for citric acid

cycle activity. It is located within the mitochondrion.

(d) **Phosphoenolpyruvate (PEP) carboxykinase** (Oxaloacetate $\rightarrow$ phosphoenolpyruvate + CO_2). It's partially located in the mitochondrion and partially in the cytosol.

Only alanine directly provides pyruvate after removal of the amino group whereas carbon skeletons of other amino acids must undergo a series of metabolic conversions to yield pyruvate (Fig. 15.8).

Lactate provides pyruvate directly after oxidation by lactate dehydrogenase. Glycerol can be converted to glucose if it is first phosphorylated (by glycerol kinase) to glycerol phosphate, which can be oxidized to dihydroxyacetone phosphate by glycerol phosphate dehydrogenase (Fig. 15.8).

Regulators of Gluconeogenesis

Regulatory system must ensure that the catabolic reactions of glycolysis are **"off"** while gluconeogenesis is taking place; otherwise the cell might engage in a futile energy-dissipating cycle:

$$glucose \rightarrow 2\ lactate + 2\ ATP$$
$$2\ lactate + 6\ ATP \rightarrow glucose$$

There are several regulators, some of

Be it known that, somehow, if there is some defect in the disposal (metabolism) of lactic acid then it goes on accumulating in blood cousing **lactic acidosis vis-a vis change in the pH of blood - a very bad sign.**

Lactic acid is a weak acid, the accumulation of which is responsible to shift the pH of blood (7.4) towards acidic side from alkaline one.

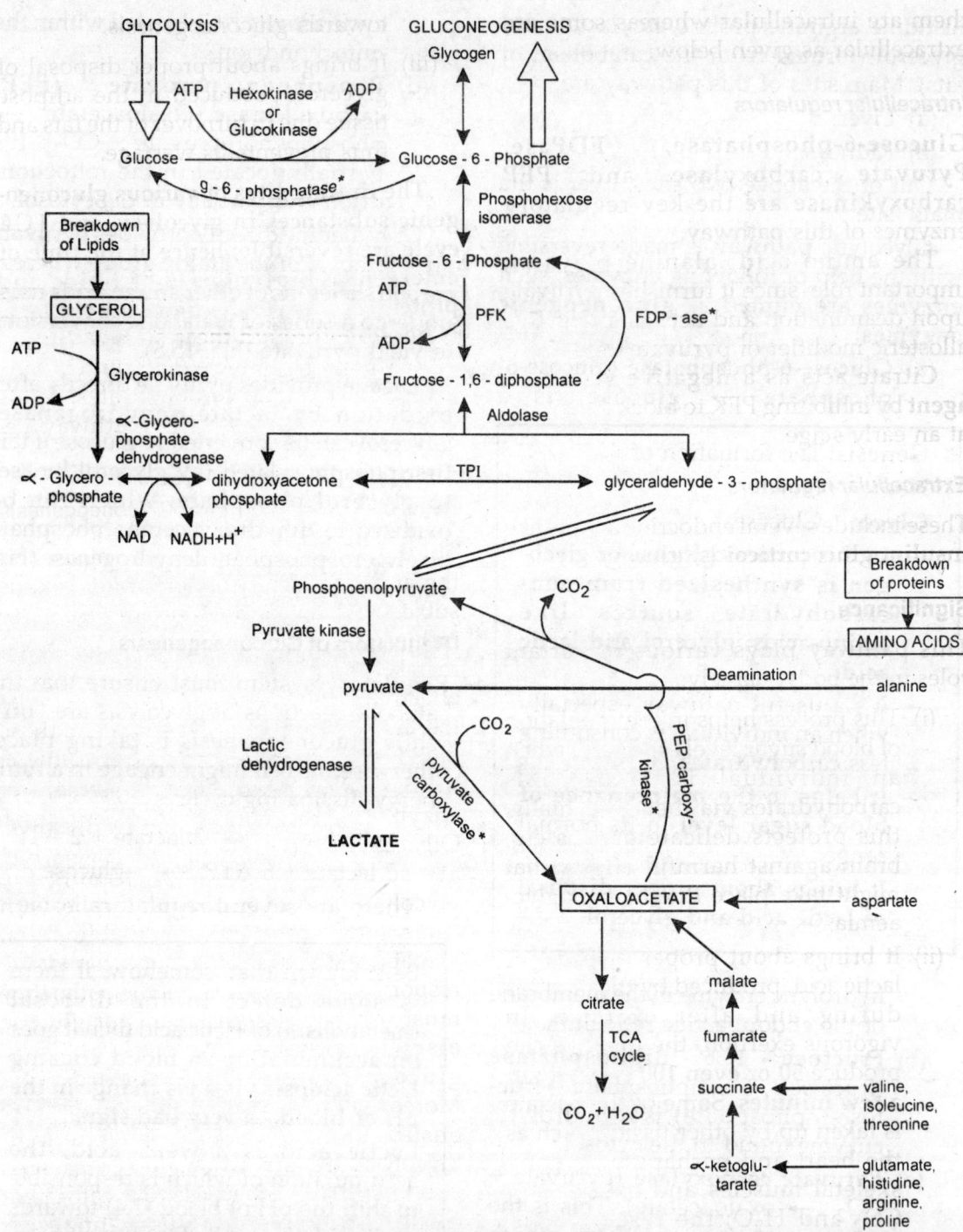

Fig. 15.8 : Pathway of gluconeogenesis showing the synthesis of glucose from (a) lactate (b) gluconeogenic amino acids and (c) glycerol. Major substrates are shown in "boxes".

* gluconeogenic enzymes.

OAA is a key intermediate

them are intracellular whereas some are extracellular as given below:

Intracellular regulators

Glucose-6-phosphatase, FDPase, Pyruvate carboxylase and PEP carboxykinase are the key regulatory enzymes of this pathway.

The amino acid, alanine plays an important role, since it furnishes pyruvate upon deamination and acts as a negative allosteric modifier of pyruvate kinase.

Citrate acts as a **negative feedback agent** by inhibiting PFK to block glycolysis at an early stage.

Extracellular regulators

These include several endocrine agents like **insulin, glucocorticoids, glucagon etc.**

Significance

This pathway plays various important roles in the body, namely:

(i) This process helps in the regulation of blood sugar level especially when an individual is taking less carbohydrates via diet. Eventually, this protects delicate organs e.g. brain against harmful effects that might take place due to hypoglycaemia.

(ii) It brings about proper disposal of lactic acid, produced by the muscles during and after exercise. In vigorous exertion, the muscles can produce **50 or even 100 g lactate in a few minutes.** Some of this lactate is taken up by other tissues such as the heart and perhaps by resting skeletal muscles and oxidized to CO_2 and H_2O; the rest diverted towards gluconeogenesis.

(iii) It brings about proper disposal of glycerol, produced in the adipose tissue due to turnover of the fats and thus prevents its wastage.

The linking sites of various gluconeogenic substances in glycolysis and TCA cycle are reversible; hence at the time of emergency, biosynthesis of lipids and proteins from carbohydrates or vice versa is possible through these sites. We mean to say that a dynamic equilibrium is thus maintained among carbohydrates, lipids and proteins through this pathway i.e. gluconeogenesis.

Regulation of Glycolysis and Gluconeogenesis

The balance between the catabolism and the anabolism of glucose in liver cells is subject to an elaborate series of regulatory influences, including the concentrations of metabolites and nucleotides as well as the effects of hormones. It should be noted that the liver cells and, to a lesser extent, those of kidney and intestinal mucosa are unique in that they contain full complement of enzymes to allow the reversal of glycolysis. Other tissues have controlling factors that are solely involved with turning the glycolytic process on or off in parallel with their own cellular energy demands. Hepatic cells, on the other hand, have large responsibilities to the rest of the body; **they must sense the requirement for glucose elsewhere and switch on the gluconeogenic reactions accordingly.** Moreover, the regulatory system must also ensure that the catabolic reactions of glycolysis are 'off' while gluconeogenesis is taking place; otherwise, the cell might engage in a futile, energy -dissipating cycle:

$$glucose \longrightarrow 2\ lactate + 2\ ATP$$
$$2\ lactate + 6\ ATP \longrightarrow glucose$$

Intracellular regulators

Substrates and intermediates play an important role in determining whether glycolysis or gluconeogenesis will predominate.

As in the case of the regulation of the citric acid cycle, the oxaloacetate concentr-ation will be rate-limiting for gluconeogen-esis. To provide an effective source of substrate for phosphoenol-pyruvate formation, the oxaloac-etate concentration must exceed that required for the cycle. The sources of oxaloacetate production, apart from the carboxylation of pyruvate are derived mainly from the catabolism of proteins and the deamination of the free amino acids to form such keto acids as oxaloacetate and α-ketoglutarate.

The amino acid, alanine, plays an important role too, since it furnishes pyruvate upon deamination and acts as a negative allosteric modifier of pyruvate kinase, thus provides a source of carbon for gluconeogenesis and prevents the operation of a futile cycle:

$$Pyruvate + ATP + GTP \longrightarrow Phosphoenolpyruvate$$

$$Phosphoenolpyruvate \longrightarrow Pyruvate + ATP$$

Citrate acts as a negative feedback agent by inhibiting phosphofructokinase to block glycolysis at an early stage. Thus, when excessive amounts of the citric-acid cycle intermediates are produced in the liver from amino-acid deamination, the brakes will be applied to the glycolytic pathway and glucose synthesis will be favoured.

Excess acetyl-CoA production will also favour gluconeogenesis, because pyruvate carboxylase requires **acetyl-CoA as a positive modifier.** Like alanine, acetyl-CoA will also inhibit pyruvate kinase activity.

Long-chain fatty acids promote gluconeo-genesis by acting as **allosteric modifiers.**

Fructose-1, 6-diphosphate exhibits a unique type of controlling influence upon the enzyme, pyruvate kinase. The latter exists under normal conditions in an inhibited state in the liver and it requires fructose diphosphate as a positive allosteric modifier. This is an example of an early intermediary in the metabolic sequence of glycolysis acting as a positive feed forward agent to ensure not only that it will not accumulate excessively, but also that its own further catabolism will be promoted.

Elevated concentrations of AMP and ADP activate phosphofructokinase, whereas elevation of ATP concentration inhibits both phosphofructokinase and pyruvate kinase.

Extracellular Regulators

Besides intracellular regulators, there are also extracellular regulators that signal the needs of the body as a whole. **Substrate availability** from the bloodstream is one such factor.

During strenuous muscular activity, for example, the production of lactate will exceed the capacity of the muscle mitochondria for pyruvate and NADH oxidation and anaerobic glycolysis will predominate over aerobic catabolism by means of the citric acid cycle and the electron-transport chain. The resulting excess of lactate will diffuse into the bloodstream and upon reaching the liver, will provide the carbon source for gluconeogenesis. The glucose produced

REGULATORS OF GLYCOLYSIS

Intracellular regulators

1. Citrate
2. Fructose-1, 6-diphosphate
3. AMP
4. ADP
5. ATP

Extracellular regulators

1. Endocrine agents like insulin, glucagon etc.

REGULATORS OF GLUCONEOGENESIS

Intracellular regulators

1. Oxaloacetate concentration
2. Amino acid alanine
3. Acetyl-CoA
4. Long chain fatty acids

Extracellular regulators

1. Lactate
2. Free amino acids
3. Endocrine agents like glucocorticoids (cortisol)
4. Glucagon, etc.

Cori, Carl Ferdinand (Czechoslo-vakia/ USA), **Professor of Biochemistry and his wife Cori, Gerty Theresa** (Czechoslo-vakia/ USA), **a biochemist** were awarded Nobel Prize in 1947 for their discoveries of the course of the catalytic conversion of glycogen.

The lack of glucose-6-phosphatase in muscle prevents the formation of free glucose in that tissue. However, muscle metabolism can contribute to blood glucose indirectly. This is known as the **Cori cycle.** Glucose-1-phosphate is known as "**Cori ester**".

---

will then pass back through the circulation to the exercising muscle, thereby constituting the so-called *Cori Cycle.*

Similar means of providing substrates for gluconeogenesis include the extrahepatic sources of free amino acids, which are produced by the catabolism of muscle and other tissue proteins.

The other group of extracellular regulators of gluconeogenesis and glycolysis in the liver consists of the endocrine agents. *Insulin,* for example, indirectly enhances the utilization of glucose by causing an increased synthesis of the ·critical enzyme, glucokinase; increased amount of the latter i.e. glucokinase will remove glucose from the circulation by converting it to nondiffusible glucose-6-phosphate within the liver cells. Hormones from the adrenal cortex with an oxygen function at position 11 of the steroid ring have profound effects upon carbohydrate metabolism and hence they are termed as the *glucocorticoids.* **Glucocorticoids, such as cortisol,** act upon the liver in the opposite direction to insulin, promoting gluconeogenesis. The mechanism of this effect is due to the induction of synthesis of several enzymes required for the gluconeogenic process, including certain transaminases, pyruvate carboxylase, phosphoenolpyruvate carboxykinase, fructose-I, 6-diphosphatase and glucose-6-phosphatase. The effects of glucocorticoids are counteracted by insulin and thus the balance between these antagonistic hormones will determine the extent of these effects.

Glucagon, which, like insulin, is a pancreatic hormone, stimulates enzyme reactions that convert pyruvate to phosphoenolpyruvate. It also indirectly increases gluconeogenesis by activating hepatic lipase, which in turn causes elevated fatty acid levels in the cells. As in the case of the effects produced by the glucocorti-coids, the action of glucagon in promoting gluconeogenesis is also antagonized by insulin.

Apparently, it is difficult to isolate the functions of individual endocrine agents upon these processes.

GLYCOGEN STORAGE DISEASES

These diseases are referred to as the diseases caused by the accumulation of polysaeharide glycogen. Tissues involved are generally liver and muscles. Such diseases are genetically transmitted from one generation to another, which means, these are hereditary.

Today, in all seven types of such diseases are known. All these are examples of *inborn errors of metabolism*. In each case, only a single enzyme appears to be missing or inactivated. These include as mentioned belew :

Type	Name	Enzyme affected
I	Von-Gierke's disease	Glucose-6-phosphatase
II	Pompe's disease	α-I$\rightarrow$4 and I$\rightarrow$ 6 glucosidase (acid maltase)
III	Cori's disease	Debranching enzyme
IV	Anderson's disease	Branching enzyme
V	Mc Ardle's disease	Muscle phosphorylase
VI	Her's disease	Liver phosphorylase
VII	Tarui's disease	Phosphofructokinase.

DIABETES MELLITUS

- Classification of Diabetes
- Prevalence
- Pathogenesis
  Type I-Insulin Dependent
  Type II-Non-Insulin Dependent

  Secondary Diabetes
  Impaired Glucose Tolerance (IGT)
- Diagnosis of Diabetes Mellitus
  Urine Sugar
  Test Paper Strips
  Hemoglobin A_{1c} (HbA$_{Ic}$)
  Clinical Signs and Symptoms
  Oral Manifestations
- Treatment of Diabetes

Diabetes mellitus is a common endocrine disease characterized by chronic hyperglycaemia and abnormalities of carbohydrate and lipid metabolism. These are caused either by an absolute or relative deficiency of insulin produced by the pancreas. Later complications of the disease involve blood vessels, eyes, kidneys and nerves. The term *diabetes mellitus* was used many centuries ago after the observation that urine of diabetics was both sweet and copious (plentiful). The relationship of the pancreas to the pathogenesis of this disorder and its overall importance in regulation of metabolism was not appreciated until the begining of the 20th century.

CLASSIFICATION OF DIABETES

Numerous conditions affect carbohydrate metabolism which include pregnancy, drug-induced changes and various diseases associated with hyperglycaemia and glucose intolerance. The following classification (Table 15.2) is based or the National Diabetes Data Group.

Prevalence

Depending upon the various diagnostic criteria employed, the prevalence of diabetes has been entimated to be between 2-4%, most of which is type II i.e., non-

Table 15.2 : National Diabetes Data Group Classification of Diabetes

I. Primary Diabetes

   A. **Type I. Insulin-dependent diabetes mellitus (IDDM)**

   B. **Type II. Non-insulin dependent diabetes mellitus (NIDDM)**

     1. **Non-obese NIDDM**

     2. **Obese NIDDM**

     3. **Maturity onset diabetes of the young (MODY)**

II. Secondary Diabetes

   A. Pancreatic disease

   B. Endocrine disease

   C. Drug induced

   D. Gestational diabetes

   E. Genetic syndromes

   F. Other

III. Impaired Glucose Tolerance (IGT)

insulin dependent diabetes mellitus (NIDDM).

It has been further seen that the prevalence within different ethnic subgroups in the general population varies markedly, for example, approximately 45% of **Pima Indians** are affected by NIDDM. Racial and environmental factors apear to play a significant role in the prevalence of *type I insulin dependent diabetes* mellitus *(IDDM)*. **Genetic studies have shown that IDDM is a disease that predominantly affects the Caucacian population.**

PATHOGENESIS

Type I. Insulin Dependent

IDDM appears by the second decade of life, although conversion from NIDDM or the state of impaired glucose tolerance may occur later in life. Onset of symptoms is usually abrupt and is characterized by a tendency for the development of **ketoacidosis and insulinopenia** (pertaining to a decrease in the level of circulating insulin). At this stage, most of the cells of the pancreas get destroyed by the autoantibodies. Pathogenic mechanisms responsible for this destruction may be viewed in a number of stages. Initially, there must be an underlying genetic susceptibility for disease to occur. Recent studies have highlighted a linkage between certain **Histocompatability leucocyte Antigen (HLA) types and IDDM.** These studies have also shown that external challange from the environment is required for the initiation of disease. The nature of this challange is not very well understood, but may be associated with the acquisition of a virus capable of infecting pancreatic β-cells. **Viruses shown to be related to the onset of IDDM are mumps, rubella virus, encephalomyocarditis virus and coxsackie B$_4$ virus.**

Epidemiological reports have shown that congenital rubella is associated with 20% of IDDM cases in **Australia**, whereas cytomegalovirus genes were found in the genome of 20% of IDDM sufferers.

The final stage in the development of IDDM is the destruction of β-cells of the pancreas by both cell mediated and humoral processes. Antibodies specific for both β-cell menbrane and cytoplasm have been identified. Presumably, the specificity of these antibodies is directed towards virally induced expression of changed or *"nonself"* β-cellular antigens.

Type II Non-Insulin Dependent

NIDDM, referred to as *"maturity onset diabetes"* affects older age group people and has a more gradual onset in comparison to IDDM. Individuals are frequently obese at the time of onset and have normal, or even high levels of circulating insulin. There is generally a decreased number of receptor sites for insulin, possibly because of destruction by autoantibodies.

Genetic studies in families with monozygote or identical twins have thrown some light on certain factors associated with the developement of NIDDM. If one twin develops NIDDM, then there is almost a 100% chance of the other twin developing the disease. This is in contrast to type I (IDDM), in which there is only a 50% chance of the second twin developing the disease. The type of the diet and the obesity may also contribute to the onset of NIDDM by overloading the insulin producing capacity of β-cells. However, it should be further noted that only a small population of obese individuals ever develop diabetes.

Secondary Diabetes

The causes of either transient or prolonged states of hyperglycaemia are many. **Pancreatic disease involving massive destruction of tissue often accompanies alcoholism.** Several endocrine disorders such as **Cushing's syndrome, Acromegaly and Pheochro-mocytoma commonly result in diabetes. Drugs involved include diuretics (e.g., furosemide), phenothiazines, catecholamines and isoniazid.**

Gestational diabetes refers to the development of hyperglycaemia during pregnancy. Blood glucose levels of such affected women generally return to normal following childbirth, but side by side such individulas are thought to have an increased risk of developing diabetes

within a 5-10 year period. This condition also increases the risk of perinatal mortality and morbidity unless the hyperglycaemic state is carefully treated. Genetic syndromes like lipodystrophies, myotonic dystrophy, and ataxia telangiectasis may occasionally be associated with impaired glucose tolerance.

IMPAIRED GLUCOSE TOLERANCE (IGT)

It occurs when plasma glucose levels are chronically higher than the normally accepted levels but are less than those required for unequivocal diagnosis of diabetes. Usually, the patient does not have fasting hyperglycaemia but has plasma glucose levels that are intermediate between normal and levels diagnostic of diabetes in an oral glucose tolerance test. IGT is usually a chance finding and is not commonly associated with clinical manifestations of diabetes.

Diagnosis of Diabetes Mellitus

Presumptive diagnosis of diabetes is often made from clinical symptoms, but laboratory confirmation of hyperglycaemia is essential for definite diagnosis. The National Diabetes Data Group has documented two specific tests relating to blood glucose levels to reach a definite diagnosis of diabetes.

1. Unequivocal (clear i.e., not doubtful) elevation of fasting plasma glucose concentration greater than 140 mg/dl on atleast two separate occasions.

2. The OGTT. This test is indicated when signs and symptoms suggest diabetes, but results of the fasting glucose tests are inconclusive. **The tolerance test is considered positive when plasma glucose**

concentration is found to be 200 *mg/dl* or higher 2 hours after a glucose load of 75 g. administered orally after dissolving it in 250-350 ml of water. Patients should be tested in the morning after 3 days of unrestricted carbohydrate diet and normal physical activity.

The main problem with the GTT is the large number of false-positive results that occur. This is thought to be associated with the sympathetic stimulation of epinephrine which blocks both the release and activity of insulin and hitherto, stimulates release of glucagon. Stimulation of the sympathetic system often occurs in patients having repeated venipuncture. Other factors that contribute to false results are the following:

(i) lack of exercise,

(ii) illness, and

(iii) inadequate diet

Urine Sugar: Testing for sugar in the urine is both insensitive and inaccurate. False-positive results are associated with the hereditary familial condition, renal glucosuria. In this condition, there is a normal plasma glucose concentration but a lower renal threshold for glucose, and therefore spillage occurs into the urine. Other inaccuracies also take place when the glucose specific glucose oxidase test is not used. Other qualitative biochemical tests may also detect other sugars such as lactose in the urine from lactating mother.

False-negative results may be reported in the early stages of diabetes when the patient has only transient episodes of glucosuria or in patients with advanced **diabetic nephropathy** when the renal threshold is markedly elevated.

Paper Strips: Strips (Dextrostix) are available for direct estimation of blood glucose levels. Blood obtained by finger-prick is applied directly to the strip which is washed 1 minute later. The subsequent colour change is compared to a standard chart to determine plasma glucose level. Results obtained by this method are generally reliable and the test has proved to be a useful screening technique for use in the office. Other strips are also available to detect glucose in the urine (e.g., clinistix) but are not as accurate.

Hemoglobin A1c (Hb A1c) i.e., Glycated Hb/ Glycosylated Hemoglobin

To monitor the degree of control of diabetes and thereby assess the efficacy of treatment regimens over a period of time, other tests have also been developed. The predominant technique currently available utilizes the fact that hemoglobin in red blood cells generally becomes glycated to form Hb A1c over a period of time. **The greater the severity of hyperglycemia, the higher the concentration of A1c in hemoglobin. Normal Hb A1c concentration averages 6% in healthy individuals whereas a range of 9-12% A1 c is found**

> Clinical manifestations of diabetes mellitus vary greatly in presentation depending upon the type of disease (i.e., type I or type II), time of onset, degree of severity at diagnosis and general condition of the patient. The usual symptoms that cause a patient to seek medical treatment are associated with mild hyperglycemia, that is,
>
> (i) **polyuria (increased frequency of urination)**
>
> (ii) **polydypsia (increased thirst)**
>
> (iii) **polyphagia (increased appetite)**

in poorly controlled chronic diabetics. Normal range of glycated Hb is from 5-7.5%.

Hb Al c levels are also useful in differentiating the hyperglycemia that often occurs after an acute myocardial infarction from that associated with diabetes. Hb A l c levels are normal after an infarction.

Clinical Sings and Symptoms

Some literal individuals become conscious and seek the advice of doctors when they come across the presence of ants after 5-10 minutes at the site (cemented floor) where they had passed the urine.

Occasionally, young patients with undiagnosed IDDM may present on the first occasion with severe **hyperglycemia** and **ketoacidosis** resulting in diabetic coma.

Onset of type I diabetes is usually abrupt and weight loss often occurs following the first bout of ketoacisdosis. Insulin levels are either very low or undetectable with a concomitant raised glucagon level. Treatment with insulin should begin immediately. Individuals with type II diabetes are usually middle-aged or older and obese, and onset of symptoms is more gradual. Insulin levels are often normal or slightly elevated.

The progress of diabetes is associated with a number of additional manifestations causing significant morbidity and almost certain premature mortality:

1. *Visual difficulties* ranging from progressive colour blindness to total blindness after the involvement of the retina is found in 90% of diabetics who have had the disease for more than 20 years.

2. *Atherosclerosis* is a common feature in long standing diabetics. This condition is fatal and contributes to the development of gangrenous infection of extremities, particularly the feet, leading ultimately to amputation.

Coronary artery disease and stroke are also frequent complications of atherosclerosis in diabetics.

3. *Diabetic nephropathy* is a major cause of death in diabetics and affects approximately 50% of type I diabetics. Fewer patients with type II diabetes have this complication, probably because the disease is of shorter duration. Unfortunately, even in controlled diabetics, there is no successful method of preventing this condition.

4. *Diabetic neuropathy:* Although neuropathy can affect the whole nervous system, peripheral neuropathy is the most common complication. Possible symptoms include numbness (deprived of feeling i.e. loss of sensation), pain, and dysesthesias (distortion of senses). When the autonomic system gets affected, gastrointestinal disturbances such as difficulty in swallowing, delayed gastric emptying and constipation may occur. This type of neuropathy also contributes to bladder infection, because the patient cannot completely empty the bladder and the chronic residual urine increases suceptibility to infection.

Much has been reported concerning causes of the complications of diabetes. Although no definite cause effect relationships have been proved, emphasis has been placed on the role of **sorbitol**, which is produced in the **polyol pathway** by the reduction of glucose. Sorbitol is toxic to tissues and has been implicated in the etiology of diabetic neuropathy, nephropathy, retinopathy and cardiovascular diseases.

Methods of prevention of diabetic complications are questionable. Close control of blood glucose concentration over long periods of time has not shown any significant effect on either preventing or slowing the development of most of the complications, except for the micro-vascular complications of the cardiovascular system. The major reason for controlling the blood sugar level is to prevent the development of ketoacidosis. This phenomenon is produced by an alternate pathway of metabolism of fatty acids in the liver, leading to an accumulation of the ketone bodies, i.e., **acetoactate, β- hydroxybutyrate, and acetone** in the blood which have a tendency to lower down the pH of blood; this is counteracted by the plasma buffer systems. If the buffer systems get exhausted, pH of blood may fall and life may be in danger. **Measurement of the severity of ketoacidosis can be done by examining the bicarborate level of blood,** since bicarborate constitutes the main plasma buffer system and becomes depleted during ketoacidosis. Additional characteristics of diabetic ketoacidosis include a lower plasma pH, hyperglycemia, and the presence of acetone and glucose in the urine. **Clinically, the ketoacidosis will, if left untreated, causes coma, commonly referred to as 'diabetic coma'.** This usually takes days to develop often in association with one or more of the following:

(i) Infection, particularly of the genitourinany tract

(ii) Dehydration

(iii) Exogenous steroids

(iv) Emotional upsets

(v) Failure to take prescribed dose of insulin

The primary treatment of diabetic coma caused by hyperglycemia is dependent upon stabilization of the pH of blood and glucose level. The term **'diabetic coma'** is also used to describe coma following *extreme hypoglycemia*. This condition usually has a rapid onset measured in hours, unlike the longer developing coma of *hyperglycemia*. The urine is commonly negative for both glucose and acetone, and blood sugar concentration is less than 40 mg/dl. Symptoms usually preceding the onset of coma are anxiousness, sweating, hunger, headache, diplopia, (the condition in which a single object is perceived as two objects i.e., double vision), convulsions and palpitations. Causes include decreased food intake, overdose of insulin, or increased exercise. Standard treatment is to administer intravenously 50 ml of 50% glucose solution or alternatively 1 to 2 mg glucagon either subcutaneously or intramuscularly and 15 minutes later.

In cases in which doubt exists whether the coma is caused by hypoglycaemia or hyperglycaemia, the first line of action should be to administer glucose or glucagon. Within minutes signs of improvement will occur if the patient was hypoglycaemic. The treatment will not appreciably worsen a hyperglycaemic coma.

Oral manifestations

In diabetics, the median rhomboid glossitis (MRG) is the main manifestation besides the one as mentioned below:

(i) **Gingivitis and periodontal disease**
(ii) **Oral candidiasis**
(iii) **Localized osteitis (dry socket) after exodontia**
(iv) **Burning tongue**

Treatment of Diabetes

In many patients with NIDDM, particularly those who are obese, dietary control towards balanced calories intake and exercise leading to weight loss is the sole treatament required. Individuals should be encouraged to initiate exercise programme, since this has been shown to have positive beneficial hypoglycaemic effects.

If dietary management proves to be ineffective in controlling hyperglycaemia, hypoglycaemic drugs may be started. These consist either of *insulin* or *oral hypoglycaemics*, namely, *the sulfonylurea group of drugs.* Sulfonylurea group of drugs act primarily by stimulating release of insulin from the pancreas and by increasing the sensitivity of cell receptor sites for insulin. First generation **(e.g. tolbutamide)** and second generation (e.g. **glyburide)** sulfonylurea drugs are now available. The dosage of the newer drugs is about one - hundreth of the first-generation drugs as far as efficacy is concerned. These oral drugs should not be used in pregnancy and have no place in the treatment of type I diabetics.

Individuals with **type I (IDDM) diabetes** require treatment with insulin. Before 1983, sources of insulin were usually from beef or pork, and serious immunologic side-effects were common place. **Since 1983,** *"human" insulin* using **recombinant DNA technology in** *Escherichia coli* **bacteria has been produced.** This type of preparation has eradicated previously recognized side-effects. **The main types of human insulin currently available include regular, protamine Hagedon (NPH), lente and the long-acting protamine zinc.** Regular insulin should be administered before meals, whereas the other preparations are usually taken once daily.

In the development stage are the insulin pumps which will enable a continuous release of insulin throughout the day. The open-loop type provides a preprogrammed insulin dose by subcutaneously implanted catheters. The closed-loop type automatically detects blood glucose level and delivers an approximate amount of insulin on a continuous basis.

DENTAL MANAGEMENT OF DIABETICS

The primary responsibility of the dentist in the management of diabetic patients is to deliver treatment in such a way so as to minimize disturbances of metabolic balance. Physical and emotional stress, infection and surgical procedures will tend to alter control of the patient's diabetes. In general, appointments should be of short duration in the morning and patients should be encouraged to maintain their standard treatment regimens. **If doubt exists on the part of the dentist as to the degree of control of blood glucose levels in diabetics, the patient's physician should be contacted before treatment is started.** Patients with type I diabetes (IDDM) are more likely to develop glucose imbalance during treatment than are those with NIDDM.

Glucose drinks should be available if patients complain of symptoms of hypoglycaemia. Following dental treatment patients should be instructed to resume their normal diet. If this proves to be impossible, medical advice should be sought immediately.

If the patient is a *brittle* (fragile) *diabetic*, experiencing sporadic (widely scattered) bouts of glucose imbalance, urine tests for the presence of glucose and acetone should be done on the day of the dental procedure and for several days after treatment depending upon the type of treatment. Again, prompt referral to a physician is recommended if the imbalance persists.

Regarding specific measures pertaining to dental treatment in diabetics, following points should be borne in mind:

- It is theoretically advisable to use local anaesthesia without epineph-

rine in dental surgical procedures.

- A physician's advice should always be sought before arranging general anaesthesia for dental treatment.

- Although some reports suggest antibiotic pro-phylaxis before dental surgery to prevent subsequent infection, there does not appear to be good evidence to support this treatment. If however, oral infection occurs after treatment/surgery, appropriate antibiotic therapy should be started at that stage.

- In general, complicated oral procedures in dental emergencies should be avoided whenever possible in uncontrolled diabetics until stabilization of blood glucose level.

CHAPTER 16

METABOLISM OF LIPIDS

> We, when metabolised, give birth to very important invaluable substances of the body, namely vitamin D, bile acids, androgenic hormones, glucocorticoid hormones, mineralocorticoid hormones and many others. We are also responsible for the generation of enormous amount of ATP which is used by the cells and body tissues for various biochemical reactions/processes.

Blood lipids

The normal level of total serum cholesterol is from 150-200 mg/dl; normal level of HDL-cholesterol in serum is from 30-63 mg/dl (men) and 35-75 mg/dl (women); normal level of VLDL is upto 28 mg/dl, normal level of LDL-cholesterol in serum is upto 150 mg/dl; normal level of serum triglycerides is from 30-140 mg/dl; normal level of total lipids in serum is from 400 -

700 mg/dl; even then the intake of lipids via diet is very essential for various reasons. However, periodical checkup of various lipid fractions (Lipid profile) in blood is also very essential and demand of the day especially in the society 40+in age because of the alarming rising trend in the incidence of cardiovascular disorders/diseases.

In contrast to the blood glucose level,

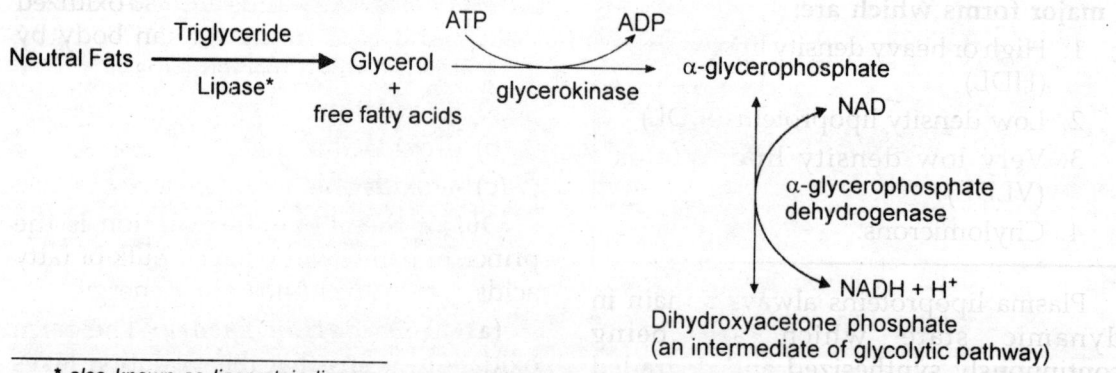

* also known as lipoprotein lipase

the normal fasting level of total blood lipids of about 500 mg/100 ml may be subject to much wide fluctuations ($\pm$ 200 mg/100 ml) and will return much more slowly to baseline levels after a meal.

Since probably no absolute tissue demand for blood lipids exists, the consequences of lowered lipid levels are insignificant in comparison to the effects of hypoglycaemia. The pathology of the disorders in blood lipid metabolism tends to be related, rather, to excessive concentrations of lipids i.e., **hyperlipidemia.**

Plasma Lipoproteins

Virtually, all the phospholipids in liver or other tissues exist in the membranes, with very few of them occurring in the form of solutions or micelles.

Lipids are water insoluble and are transported in the body in an aqueous medium in combination with various specific proteins. This results in lipid: protein complex called as lipoproteins, synthesis of which takes place in the liver.

Lipoproteins (phospholipid-carrier protein complex) are the important vehicles for the transfer of phospholipids.

Plasma lipoproteins occur in four major forms which are:

1. High or heavy density lipoproteins (HDL)
2. Low density lipoproteins (LDL)
3. Very low density lipoproteins (VLDL)
4. Chylomicrons.

Plasma lipoproteins always remain in dynamic state which are being continuously synthesized and degraded with rapid exchange of both lipid and protein among themselves. **Two enzymes namely, lecithin cholesterol acyl transferare (LCAT) and lipoprotein lipase (also called triglyceride lipase)** play a significant role in the catabolism of lipid fraction of lipoproteins.

Tangier Disease: An inability to carry normal amount of phospholipids and cholesterol in the blood is encountered in Tangier disease, which results from a congenital defect in the formation of a transport protein by the liver. A deficiency in the liver's capacity for the synthesis of albumin; which causes **analbuminemia**, leads to a decrease in the plasma's capacity to carry the fatty acids released from the fat depots.

OXIDATION OF FATTY ACIDS

The action of hormonally controlled lipase results in the hydrolysis of neutral fats to glycerol and free fatty acids. Glycerol enters the glycolytic pathway as shown below via the formation of glycerophosphate:

Fatty acids tightly bound with albumin are carried to various tissues for oxidation via blood.

Fatty acids oxidation takes place in *mitochondria*. Fatty acids are also oxidized to CO_2 and H_2O in the human body by the following three mechanisms:

(a) β-**oxidation**

(b) α-**oxidation, and**

(c) ω-**oxidation**

Out of the above, β-oxidation is the principal pathway, by which bulk of fatty acids gets oxidized liberating energy.

(a) β-*Oxidation Theory:* The term oxidation means that the oxidation takes

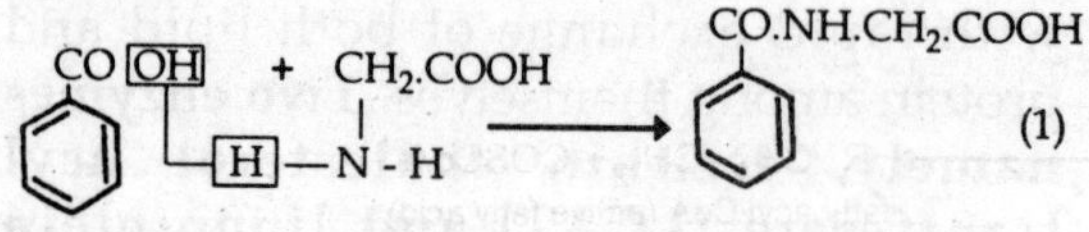

Benzoic acid   glycine   Hippuric acid   (1)

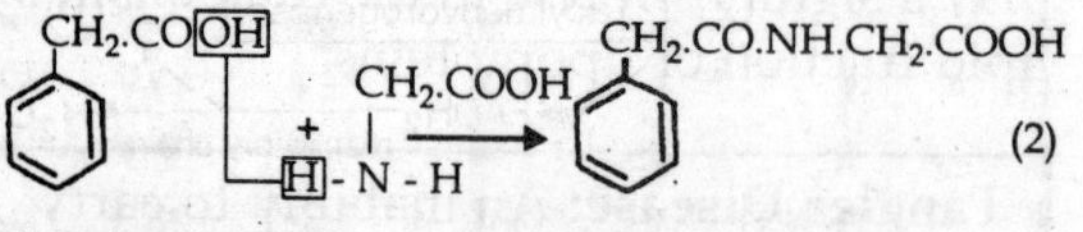

Phenylacetic acid   glycine   Phenylaceturic acid   (2)

place in the β-carbon of the fatty acid with the removal of two carbon atoms at a time from the carboxyl end of the molecule.

Fatty acids containing both the even number and the odd number of carbon atoms and as well as unsaturated fatty acids are oxidized by this theory. **Knoop** was the first who in 1904 invented this theory. In order to study the fate of fatty acids, he prepared a homologous series of phenyl fatty acid derivatives, which he fed to the animal; then he was able to isolate the phenyl labelled compounds in the urine. The simplest is benzoic acid, which is eliminated in the form of hippuric acid after combination with glycine. However, the next higher derivative i.e. phenylacetic acid is eliminated as the corresponding glycine derivative i.e., phenylaceturic acid.

With higher fatty acids, the products isolated were either hippuric acid (1) or phenylaceturic acid (2) for example,

$C_6H_5.CH_2 CH_2 COOH$ yields   (1)
$C_6H_5.CH_2. CH_2. CH_2. COOH$ yields   (2)
$C_6H_5.CH_2. CH_2. CH_2. CH_2.COOH$ yields   (1)
$C_6H_5.CH_2.CH_2.CH_2.CH_2.CH_2.COOH$ yields   (2)
etc.

From the results, he was able to draw the conclusion that oxidation of fatty acids occurred in such a way that at each stage in the degradation process there was a loss of two carbon atoms because of the oxidation at the β carbon atom, for example (Figure 16.1).

Mechanism of β-Oxidation of fatty acids

Five reactions are involved in the β-oxidation process as described below. All these reactions take place in the mitochondria of the cell.

1. Activation: The very first reaction consists in the formation of an acyl coenzyme A derivative from the free fatty acid; this reaction is catalysed by a *thiokinase* which required the presence of ATP and CoA. (Fig. 16.2).

2. Desaturation : Once the fatty acid has been activated, it can now be dehydrogenated in the α, β position by *acyl dehydrogenase* in the presence of FAD.

3. Hydration: In next reaction, a molecule of water is added across the double bond; this reaction is catalyzed by *enoyl hydrase* as a result of which a β-hydroxyacyl CoA derivative is formed.

4. Oxidation: Now, the hydroxyl group of the β–hydroxyacyl CoA derivative is oxidized to a keto group in the presence of an enzyme known as β-*hydroxyacyl dehydrogenase* and NAD.

5. Thiolytic cleavage: The final step in

$$\overset{\beta}{C_6H_5.CH_2}\overset{\alpha}{.CH_2.COOH} \longrightarrow C_2H_5 COOH$$
$$\overset{\beta}{C_6H_5.CH_2}\overset{\alpha}{.CH_2.CH_2.COOH} \rightarrow C_2H_5 CH_2.COOH$$
$$\overset{\beta}{C_6H_5.CH_2}\overset{\alpha}{.CH_2.CH_2.CH_2.COOH}$$

$$\overset{\beta}{C_6H_5.CH_2}\overset{\alpha}{.CH_2.COOH}$$

$$C_6H_5.COOH$$

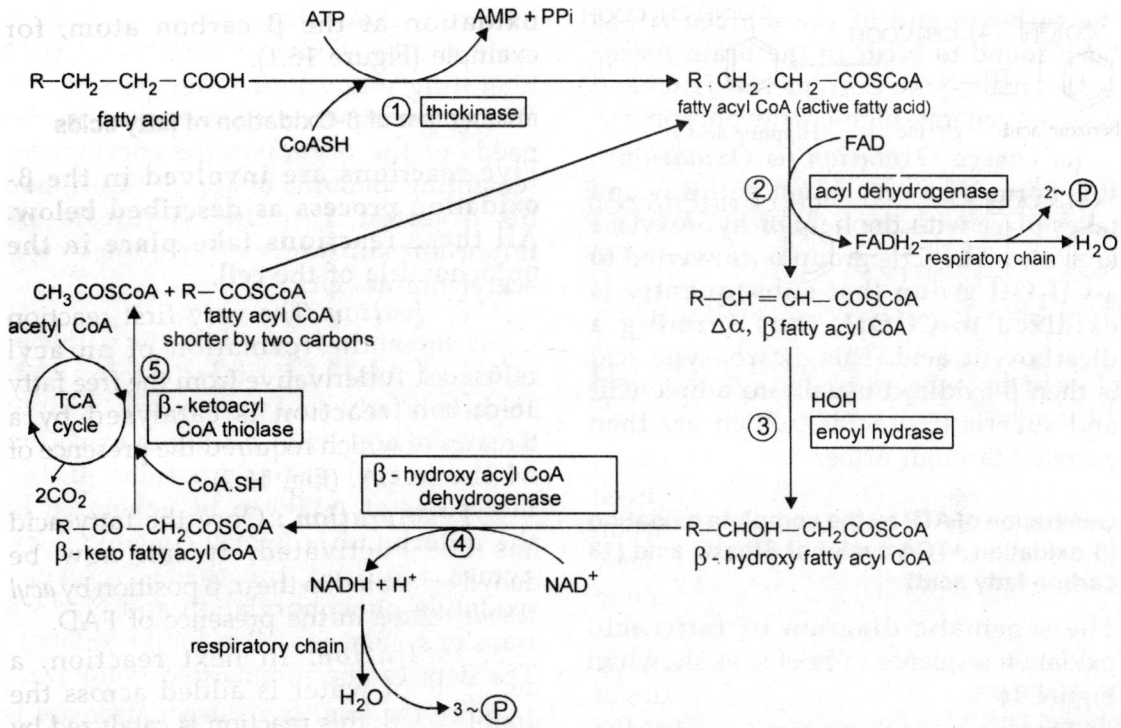

Fig 16.1 : Schematic diagram of β–oxidation of fatty acids (removal of one acetyl CoA unit from a fatty acid may be seen). Also known as **Fatty Acid Cycle.** [FADH$_2$ and NADH$_2$, when oxidized by the mitochondrial electron transport chain, **generate two and three moles of ATP per mole of FADH$_2$ and NADH$_2$ respectively].**

the process of β-oxidation is the cleavage of the β-keto derivative by a molecule of coenzyme in the presence of enzyme β-*ketoacyl CoA thiolase.*

The products of the reactions are a molecule of acetyl CoA and a molecule of an activated fatty acid which is two carbon shorter than the fatty acid at the start. Now, the activated fatty acid can be further degraded by repititions of the process, starting at the second reaction; reaction no. 1 i.e. activation step is not necessary at all. By the successive repititions of the process, entire fatty acid chain can be converted to acetyl CoA. The acetyl CoA so formed now mixes with the acetyl CoA pool derived from the metabolisms of carbohydrates and amino acids and

participates in a variety of biological processes of the body.

The fatty acid residue, of the first turn of the cycle, is released as the CoA derivative and may be acted upon by the acyl dehydrogenase system (reaction no. 2) without further activation.

It appears that once a fatty acid e.g. palmitic acid, is activated and enters the β-oxidative system, the products are 8 acetyl CoA units and the appropriate amounts of reduced cofactors.

(b) α-*Oxidation:* Quantitatively, β-oxidation has been found to be the most important pathway for the oxidation of fatty acids. However, α-oxidation, i.e. the removal of one carbon at a time from

the carboxyl end of the molecule, has been found to occur in the brain tissue. It does not require CoA intermediates and does not generate high-energy phosphates.

(c) *Omega Oxidation (ω-Oxidation)* : It is normally a very minor pathway and takes place with the help of hydroxylase enzymes. The CH_3 group is converted to a-CH_2OH group that subsequently is oxidized to-COOH, thus forming a dicarboxylic acid. This dicarboxylic acid is then β-oxidized usually to adipic (C_6) and suberic (C_8) acids, which are then excreted through urine.

Generation of ATP by the complete oxidation (β-oxidation +TCA cycle) of Stearic acid (18 carbon fatty acid)

The schematic diagram of fatty acid oxidation sequence in brief is as shown in Figure 16.3.

The net overall reaction involved in degrading a fatty acid by two carbons can be represented as follows:

By repeatition of these reactions, the entire fatty acid molecule gets converted

Steps	Moles of ATP
1. Stearate + ATP + CoASH	
↓	
Stearyl~SCoA ----------------------------	- 1
2. Stearyl~SCoA → 9 Acetyl-SCoA	
(a) 8 $FADH_2$ → 8 FAD (8 x 2=16)	
(b) 8 NADH → 8 NAD^+ (8 x 3=24)---	+ 40
3. 9 Acetyl~SCoA + 18 O_2	
(9 x 12=108)	
↓	
18 CO_2 + 9 H_2O + 9 CoASH ----------------	+ 108
	+ 147

Overall reaction

$C_{17}H_{35}$ COOH + 18O_2 +147 ADP +147 Pi

Stearic acid   ↓

18CO_2 + 18H_2O + 147 ATP

into acetyl CoA, which may enter the TCA cycle and be oxidized to CO_2 and H_2O liberating many molecules of ATP for energy purposes. Depending upon the needs of the organism for energy, the remaining amounts of acetyl~SCoA may be diverted for the synthesis of important substances like cholesterol, acetylcholine, etc.

As shown in figure 16.3, the pathway is used a total of 8 times to convert an 18-carbon fatty acid (e.g., stearic acid) to 9 moles of acetyl S~CoA. Upon oxidation of the acetyl groups, a total of 147 molecules of ATP can be generated in the mitochondria, which contain all enzymes required for the TCA cycle, oxidative phosphorylation and electron transfer system as well as for β–oxidation. The steps can be summarised as follows:

Since the total free energy decrease is nearly 2600 kcal per mole, the "efficiency" of conversion of energy to ATP is :

$$\frac{147 \times 8}{2600} \times 100 = 45\%$$

GENERATION OF ATP BY THE COMPLETE OXIDATION (β-OXIDATION + TCA CYCLE) OF PALMITIC ACID (16-CARBON FATTY ACID) :

If an even numbered fatty acid is taken into consideration e.g. palmitic acid (C_{16}), it gets split completely into 8 acetyl units in 7 rounds. On completion of each round, one mole of $FADH_2$ and mole of NADH are produced which are equivalent to 2+3=5 moles of ATP. In seven cycles (7 rounds), therefore, 35 moles of ATP are synthesized.

Each acetyl unit is oxidized by Krebs cycle to CO_2 and H_2O generating 12 moles of ATP. Thus, the total number of ATP generated during oxidation of 8 moles of acetyl conenzyme A would be 12x8=96.

$$CH_3(CH_2CH_2)_n - COOH + ATP + (n + 1) CoASH + nNAD^+ + nFAD + nH_2O$$

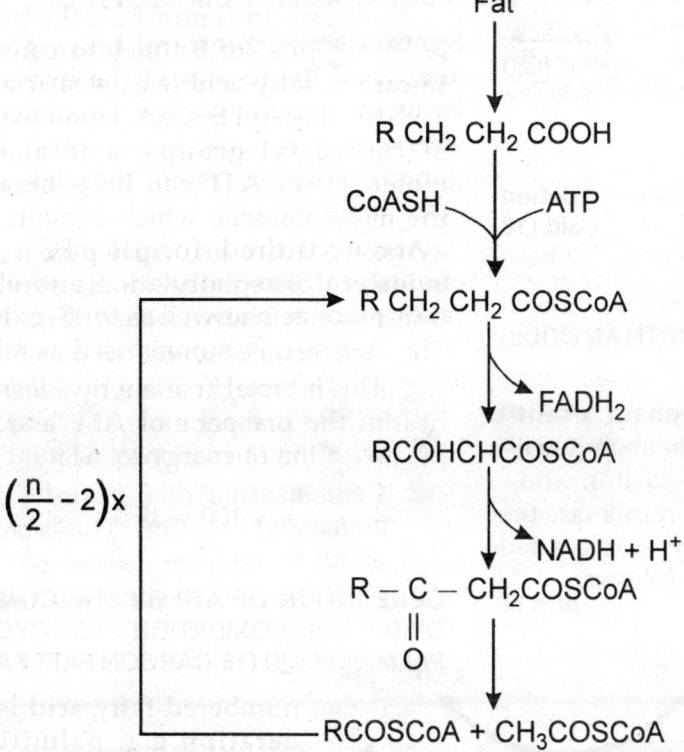

$$(n + 1) \; \overset{\overset{\displaystyle O}{\|}}{CH_3 C} \sim SCoA + \left.\begin{array}{l} (ADP + Pi) \\ (AMP + PPi) \end{array}\right\} + n \; NADH + nH^+ + nFADH_2$$

Fat

R CH$_2$ CH$_2$ COOH

CoASH   ATP

R CH$_2$ CH$_2$ COSCoA

FADH$_2$

RCOHCHCOSCoA

NADH + H$^+$

$$R - \overset{\overset{\displaystyle }{}}{\underset{\underset{\displaystyle O}{\|}}{C}} - CH_2COSCoA$$

$\left(\dfrac{n}{2} - 2\right)x$

RCOSCoA + CH$_3$COSCoA

Fig. 16.2 : Fatty acid oxidation sequence. The pathway is used (n/2-1) times for each fatty acid. For instance, an 18 carbon chain would go through the cycle 8 times, i.e., once through and 7 repeats-to yield the nine two - carbon fragments as acetyl CoA.

In total, 35+96=131 moles of ATP are generated per mole of palmitic acid oxidized. Since, the initial activation reaction requires the consumption of 1 mole of ATP, therefore, the net gain of ATP per mole of palmitic acid oxidized would be 131-1=130. The steps of palmitic acid (C$_{15}$H$_{31}$ COOH) oxidation can be summarised as flollows:

When palmitic acid is oxidized, the free energy change is 2,340 k cal. Using the value of 7.0 kcal for the free energy of hydrolysis of ATP to ADP and Pi, the formation of 130 ATP by the biological oxidation of palmitic acid yields, 130x7.0 or 910 kcal, therefore, the "efficiency" of

Steps   **Moles of ATP**

1. Palmitate+ATP+CoASH

         ↓

    Palmityl CoA ----------------------   -1

2. Palmityl CoA →   8 acetyl CoA
   (a) 7 FADH$_2$ →   7 FAD (7x2=14)
   (b) 7 NADH → 7 NAD$^+$ (7x3=21)-------   **+35**

3. 8 Acetyl CoA+16 O$_2$
         (8 x 12 = 96)

         ↓

 16CO$_2$ + 8H$_2$O + 8CoASH -----------------   **+96**

Overall Reaction   **+130**

C$_{15}$H$_{31}$COOH+130ADP+130Pi→16CO$_2$+130ATP+ 148 H$_2$O

conversion of energy to ATP is :

$$\frac{130 \times 7}{2340} \times 100 = 39\%$$

OXIDATION OF FATTY ACIDS WITH AN ODD NUMBER OF CARBON ATOMS

In natural fats, the straight-chain, even-carbon fatty acids are found in abundance but they also contain odd carbon and branched chain fatty acids in minor quantity. The odd-carbon fatty acids e.g. propionic acid is oxidized as follows:

Succinyl CoA, so formed can now be oxidized via succinic acid and the TCA cycle to CO$_2$ and H$_2$O.

Heart mitochordria cannot oxidize propionyl CoA. The involvement of biotin in the CO$_2$ fixation reaction is a clear example of the function of this vitamin as a coenzyme.

BIOSYNTHESIS OF CHOLESTEROL

Synthesis of cholesterol takes place in almost all the tissues of the body, liver being the most active site. Less important sites serially include skin, adrenal glands, gonads, adipose tissue, muscles, aorta, adult brain etc.

Acetate is the principal precursor of cholesterol biosynthesis. Its synthesis takes place as shown below (Fig. 16.3) :

1. *Activation of acetate to acetyl CoA :* This is brought about by a *thiokinase* in the presence of ATP and CoA with the formation of acetyl CoA.

2. *Condensation of 2 acetyl CoA to acetoacetyl CoA :* This is brought about by enzyme *thiolase*.

3. *Formation of β-hydroxy-β-methylg-*

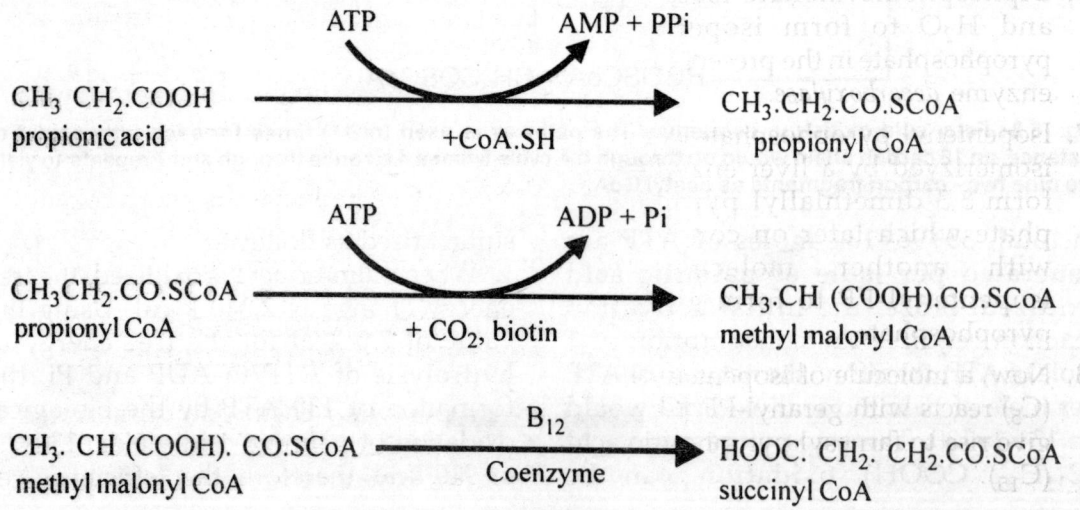

CH$_3$ CH$_2$.COOH $\xrightarrow{\text{ATP} \quad\quad \text{AMP + PPi}}$ CH$_3$.CH$_2$.CO.SCoA
propionic acid   +CoA.SH   propionyl CoA

CH$_3$CH$_2$.CO.SCoA $\xrightarrow{\text{ATP} \quad\quad \text{ADP + Pi}}$ CH$_3$.CH (COOH).CO.SCoA
propionyl CoA   + CO$_2$, biotin   methyl malonyl CoA

CH$_3$. CH (COOH). CO.SCoA $\xrightarrow[\text{Coenzyme}]{\text{B}_{12}}$ HOOC. CH$_2$. CH$_2$.CO.SCoA
methyl malonyl CoA   succinyl CoA

lutaryl CoA : Acetoacetyl CoA further condenses with another molecule of acetyl CoA in the presence of HMG CoA synthetase forming β-hydroxy-β-methyl glutaryl CoA.

4. *Formation of mevalonic acid:* Now, β-hydroxy β-methyl glutaryl CoA is reduced to mevalonic acid; the reaction is catalysed by the enzyme *HMG-CoA reductase* in the presence of reduced NADP.

Side-by-side, β-OH- β-methyl glutaryl CoA (HMG−CoA) may also give rise to ketone bodies.

5. *Phosphorylation of mevalonic acid:* Mevalonic acid is phosphorylated to 5-phosphomevalonic acid in the presence of ATP and Mg^{++} ions. Reaction is catalysed by *mevalonate kinase*.

   5-phosphomevalonic acid is further phosphorylated to form 5-diphosphomevalonic acid in the presence of ATP and Mg^{2+}; the reaction is catalysed by the enzyme *phosphomevalonate kinase*.

6. Diphosphomevalonate loses CO_2 and H_2O to form isopentenyl pyrophosphate in the presence of an enzyme *decarboxylase*.

7. Isopentenyl pyrophosphate is now isomerizyed by a liver enzyme to form 3,3-dimethlallyl pyrophosphate which later on condenses with another molecule of isopentenyl-PP to form geranyl pyrophosphate.

8. Now, a molecule of isopentenyl-PP (C_5) reacts with geranyl-PP (C_{10}) to give rise to farnesyl pyrophosphate (C_{15}).

9. Now, in the presence of *squalene synthetase* reduced pyridine nucleotide and Mg^{++}, Mn^{++}, or Co^{++}, two moles of farnesyl-PP condense to form squalene.

10. Squalene in the presence of *oxydocyclase I* and a pyridine nucleotide undergoes cyclization process forming a steroid like structure called *lanosterol* (Fig. 16.3).

11. Now, lanosterol is finally converted to *cholesterol* through a number of intermediates.

In this way, molecule of cholesterol is synthesized. Of the 27 carbon of cholesterol molecule, 15 arise from the methyl and 12 from the carboxyl of acetate. The first phases of synthesis involve activation of intermediates through union with CoASH, whereas the later stages of synthesis involve participation of phosphates.

Mevalonic acid and squalene are prime intermediates in this pathway.

Synthesis of cholesterol is the only example of a basic biosynthetic process in nature that involves condensation of isoprenoid (C_5) units and the formation of the active intermediate namely isopentenyl pyrophosphate.

High blood cholesterol level may be associated with increased risk of atherosclerosis.

HMG-CoA reductase is a key enzyme that regulates the activity of the pathway of cholesterol biosynthesis.

REGULATION OF CHOLESTEROL BIOSYNTHESIS AND ITS BLOOD LEVEL

1. Fats/oils rich in polyunsaturated fatty acids (PUFA) have been found to lower the level Of blood

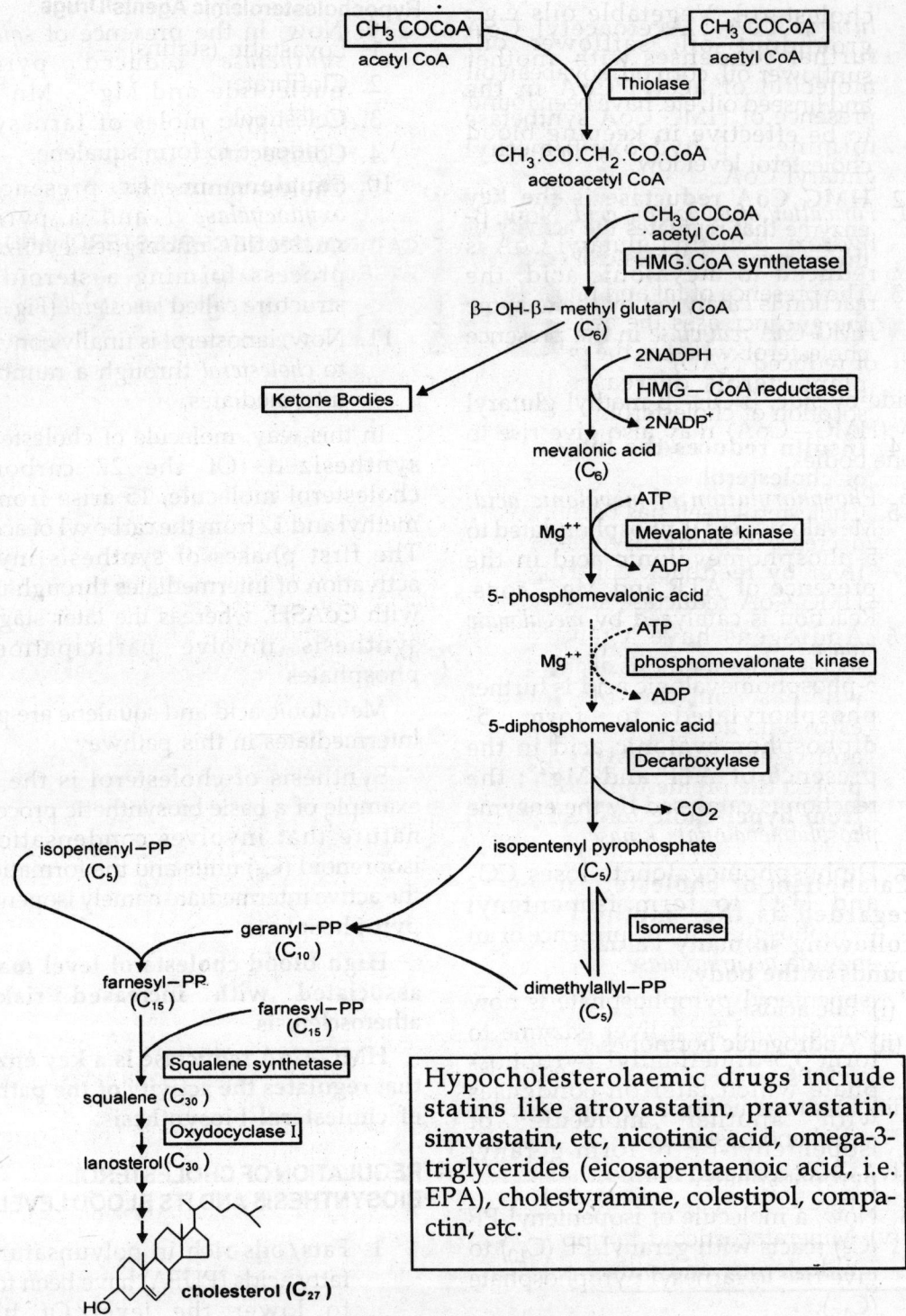

Hypocholesterolaemic drugs include statins like atrovastatin, pravastatin, simvastatin, etc, nicotinic acid, omega-3-triglycerides (eicosapentaenoic acid, i.e. EPA), cholestyramine, colestipol, compactin, etc.

Fig. 16.3 : Biosynthesis of Cholesterol

cholesterol. Vegetable oils e.g., groundnut oil, safflower oil, sunflower oil, corn oil, soyabean oil and linseed oil, etc. have been found to be effective in keeping blood cholesterol level low.

2. **HMG CoA reductase is the key enzyme that regulates the activity of the pathway for cholesterol synthesis.**

3. The presence of fat and bile acids in the gut increases the absorption of cholesterol, whereas the presence of plant sterols decreases the absorption of cholesterol.

4. **Insulin reduces the biosynthesis of cholesterol.**

5. Cholesterol itself has been found to decrease its own biosynthesis in the liver by feedback control at the HMG-CoA reductase stage.

6. Androgens have a tendency to increase the synthesis of cholesterol, whereas, on the other hand, estrogens have opposite effect to androgens, thus **estrogens also protect the premenopausal women from hyper-cholesterolemia.**

Catabolism of cholesterol may be regarded as the "mother" of the following so many valuable compounds of the body.

(i) Bile acids

(ii) Androgenic hormones, e.g. testosterone

(iii) Oestrogenic hormones, e.g. oestradiol and oestrone

(iv) Glucocorticoid hormones, e.g. cortisol

(v) Mineralocorticoid hormones, e.g. aldosterone and others.

Hypocholesterolemic Agents/Drugs

1. Lovastatin (statins)
2. Clofibrate
3. Colestipol
4. Compactin
5. Cholestyramine, etc.

CATABOLISM OF CHOLESTEROL AND ITS EXCRETION

Cholesterol is formed by many tissues of the body, but is catabolized by only a few tissues. The main catabolic fate of cholesterol is its oxidation to cholanic acids (cholic acids) and side by side, the main route of excretion is into the GI (gastrointestinal) tract via bile or through mucosal cells. Besides, gonads and the adrenals also utilize cholesterol for the biosynthesis of hormones (Figure 16.4 a & b).

The formation of bile acids from cholesterol in the liver represents the most important fate of cholesterol. Nearly, 80-90% of body's cholesterol is ultimately

---

Level of cholesterol gets increased in the following conditions:

(i) Diabetes mellitus

(ii) Hypothyroidism

(iii) Obstructive jaundice

(iv) Cirrhosis of liver

(v) Nephrotic syndrome

(vi) Atherosclerosis, etc.

And gets decreased in :

(i) Acute hepatitis

(ii) Malnutrition

(iii) Anaemia

(iv) Occasionally in hyperthyroidism

(v) Gaucher's disease, etc.

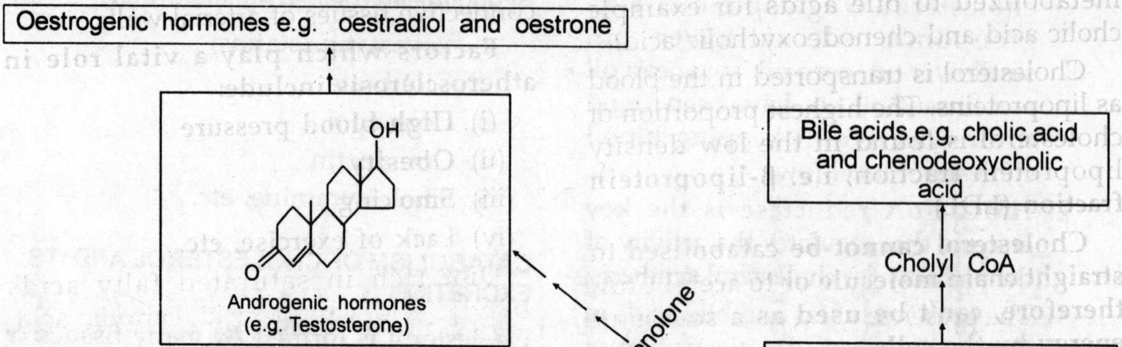

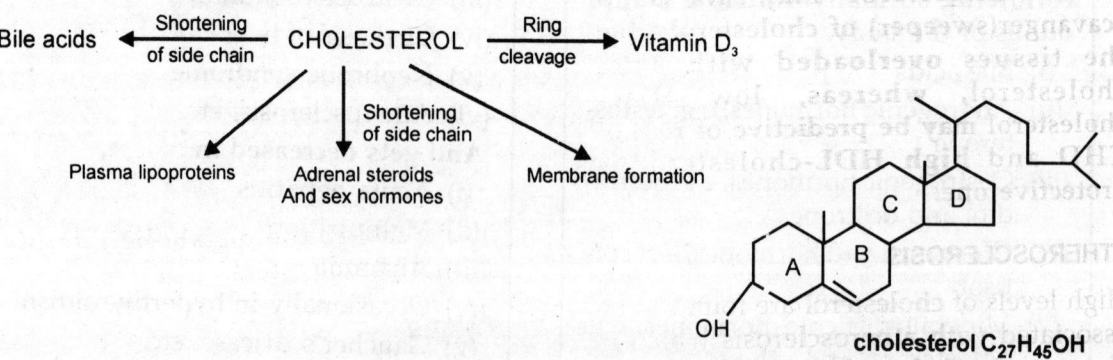

Oestrogenic hormones e.g. oestradiol and oestrone

Androgenic hormones (e.g. Testosterone)

Bile acids, e.g. cholic acid and chenodeoxycholic acid

Cholyl CoA

cholesterol

Sunlight

Vitamin D (cholecalciferol)

Pregnenolone

Progesterone

Glucocorticoid hormones (e.g. Cortisol)

Mineralocorticoid hormones (e.g. Aldosterone)

Fig. 16.4 (a) : Catabolism of cholesterol, end products of which are several very important substances like **vitamin D, bile acids, androgenic hormones, glucocorticoid hormones and mineralcorticoid hormones** (main substances are in boxes)

Bile acids $\xleftarrow[\text{of side chain}]{\text{Shortening}}$ CHOLESTEROL $\xrightarrow[\text{cleavage}]{\text{Ring}}$ Vitamin D_3

Shortening of side chain

Plasma lipoproteins

Adrenal steroids And sex hormones

Membrane formation

cholesterol $C_{27}H_{45}OH$

Fig. 16.4 (b): Catabolism of cholesterol

metabolized to bile acids for example cholic acid and chenodeoxycholic acid.

Cholesterol is transported in the blood as lipoproteins. The highest proportion of cholesterol is found in the low density lipoprotein fraction, i.e. β-lipoprotein fraction (LDL).

Cholesterol cannot be catabolised to straight chain molecule or to acetyl CoA, therefore, can't be used as a source of energy by the cells.

The combined risk factors of coronary heart disease (CHD) can be determined following the estimations of serum cholesterol and HDL-cholesterol. The ratio of cholesterol to HDL-cholesterol has predictive value in determining the risk of CHD more accurately. For normal males, the ratio of 5 : 1 and for normal females the ratio of 4.5 : 1 are considered as average risk. Lower ratios significantly reduce the risk, whereas ratios 9.5 : 1 and 7:1 for males and females respectively, are believed to double the risk of CHD. An inverse relationship has been observed between the risk of CHD and the concentration of HDL-cholesterol.

HDL-cholesterol represents approximately 20-25% of the total cholesterol in serum.

HDL-cholesterol may act as a scavanger(sweeper) of cholesterol from the tissues overloaded with extra cholesterol, whereas, low HDL-cholesterol may be predictive of risk of CHD and high HDL-cholesterol is protective one.

ATHEROSCLEROSIS

High levels of cholesterol are found to be associated with atherosclerosis which is characterized by the deposition of cholesterol ester and other lipids in the connective tissues of arterial walls.

Factors which play a vital role in atherosclerosis include:

  (i) **High blood pressure**

  (ii) **Obesity**

 (iii) **Smoking**

 (iv) **Lack of exercise, etc.**

Diet rich in saturated fatty acids (butyric acid, caproic acid, caprylic acid, palmitic acid, stearic acid, etc.) increases the plasma cholesterol concentration, whereas diet rich in polyunsaturated fatty acids (PUFA) such as linoleic acid, linolenic acid and arachidonic acid decreases the plasma cholesterol concentration.

Corn oil, linseed oil, soyabean oil, peanut oil, cottonseed oil, sunflower oil etc. have a tendency to lower blood cholesterol level whereas butter fat and coconut oil, etc. raise it.

PUFA exert their effect by :

  (i) **stimulating the excretion of cholesterol into the intestines.**

  (ii) **stimulating the oxidation of cholesterol to bile acids.**

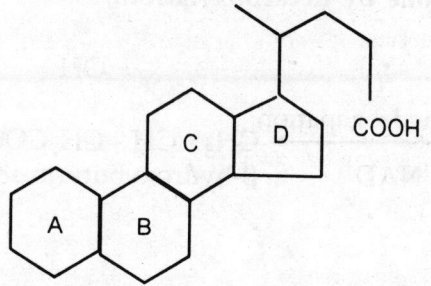

 (iii) **increasing the metabolic rate of cholesterol esters.**

BILE ACIDS

Bile acids are the following three, namely:

(i) Cholic acid

(ii) Deoxycholic acid, and

(iii) Lithocholic acid.

They remain present in the bile in conjugation with glycine and taurine as glycocholic and taurocholic acids. Bile acids are the derivatives of cholanic acid.

Cholic acid is 3,7,12 trihydroxy cholanic acid; deoxycholic acid is 3,12 dihydroxy cholanic acid; and lithocholic acid is 3-hydroxy cholanic acid.

Salts of bile acids have a tendecny to lower the surface tension and are good emulsifying agents and hence play an important role in the absorption of fats from the intestines.

KETONE BODIES (ACETONE BODIES)

Ketone bodies are the three, namely:

(i) acetoacetic acid

(ii) β-hydroxybutyric acid, and

(iii) acetone

The principal ketone body is acetoacetic acid which gives rise to β-hydroxybutyric acid by reduction and acetone by decarboxylation.

$$CH_3COCH_2COOH$$
acetoacetic acid

dehydrogenation / NAD^+ →
$$CH_3 - CH - CH_2COOH$$
$$\overset{|}{OH}$$
β-hydroxybutyric acid

decarboxylation / $-CO_2$ →
$$CH_3COCH_3$$
acetone

Ketone bodies are acidic in nature and when produced in excess over long period, as happens in diabetes mellitus, causes *ketoacidosis* which is ultimately fatal.

Ketone bodies are the intermediate breakdown products of fatty acid metabolism. Under normal conditions, fatty acids are oxidized to CO_2; these intermediates do not appear to any great extent either in the blood or urine.

KETOSIS

Significant accumulation of ketone bodies in the blood (ketonemia) and their excretion in urine (ketonuria) give rise to a condition known as **ketosis.**

Normal level of ketone bodies in blood is upto 3 mg per 100 ml and upto 50 mg in urine per day.

Under certain metabolic conditions such as starvation, high fat diet, severe diabetes mellilus, more fat is metabolized for energy purposes giving rise to increased formation of ketone bodies.

Increased fatty acid oxidation is a characteristic of starvation and diabetes mellitus, leading to the production of ketone bodies by the liver.

Under normal metabolic conditions, most of the acetyl CoA formed from the oxidation of fatty acids, puruvate and other sources get condensed with oxaloacetic acid and oxidized through the TCA cycle. However, in circumstances when the metabolism of carbohydrate gets impaired or operating at a low level, such as in the diabetes mellitus, starvation, or prolonged living on a low carbohydrate diet, the fate of acetyl CoA gets altered for two reasons.

1. the oxaloacetate available to condense with acetyl CoA is in

limited supply, and

2. a much greater proportion of the body's energy needs is being supplied by the oxidation of fatty acids, leading to the production of acetyl CoA in greater than normal amounts.

Because of this combination cicumstances (large amount of acetyl CoA and small amounts of oxaloacetate), the metabolism of acetyl CoA (Fig 16.5) instead of a normal route takes place via a different route which consists of the condensation of the two molecules of acetyl CoA to form acetoacetyl CoA. Now, by the action of deacylase present in the liver, acetoacetyl CoA is hydrolyzed to coenzyme A and acetoacetic acid. Acetoacetic acid may be reduced to β -hydroxybutyric acid or decarboxylated to produce acetone (Fig. 16.5).

Ketone bodies are normal end products of fatty acid oxidation in the liver, but the

> The three compounds, namely acetone, acetoacetic acid and β-hydroxybutyric acid are called as **'ketone bodies'** or **'acetone bodies'** and the process of their formation is known as 'ketogenesis'.

amount formed is relatively small.

If adequate carbohydrate is available, the liver apparently prefers carbodydrate

> **Normal level of ketone bodies in blood is upto 3 mg per 100 ml. In diabetes mellitus as much as 300 to 400 mg per 100 ml and over has been reported.**
>
> **In normal urine upto 50 mg of acetone bodies** (as acetone) **may be excreted daily**, whereas in diabetics **10 to 50 g per litre** may be found, the greater proportion being that of β-OH butyric acid.

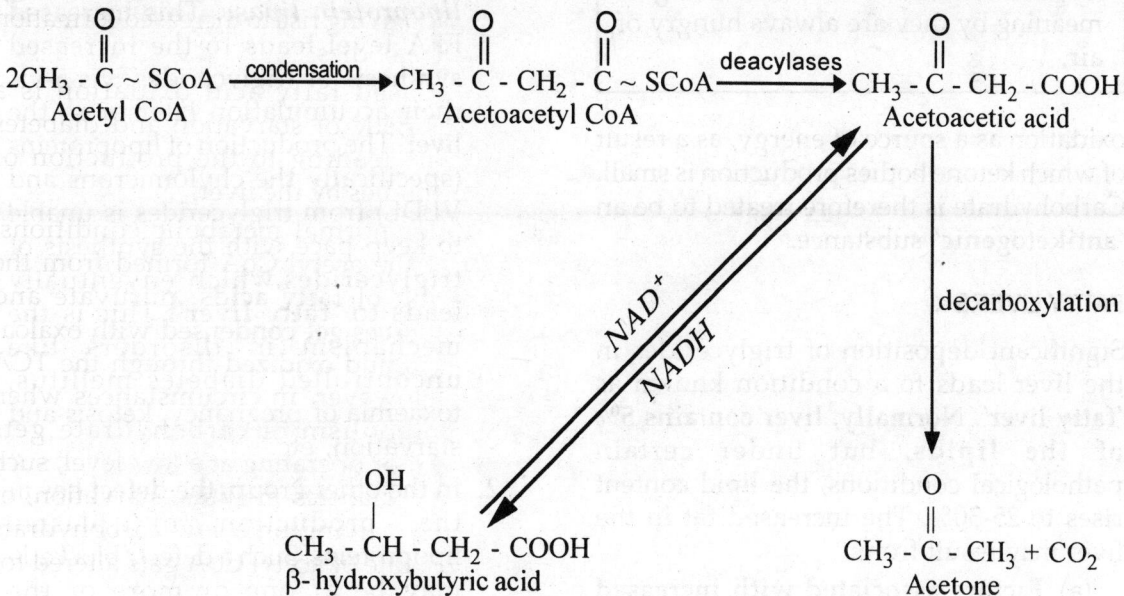

$$2CH_3 - \overset{\overset{\textstyle O}{\|}}{C} \sim SCoA \xrightarrow{\text{condensation}} CH_3 - \overset{\overset{\textstyle O}{\|}}{C} - CH_2 - \overset{\overset{\textstyle O}{\|}}{C} \sim SCoA \xrightarrow{\text{deacylases}} CH_3 - \overset{\overset{\textstyle O}{\|}}{C} - CH_2 - COOH$$

Acetyl CoA   Acetoacetyl CoA   Acetoacetic acid

NAD^+ $NADH$

decarboxylation

$$CH_3 - \overset{\overset{\textstyle OH}{|}}{CH} - CH_2 - COOH$$

β- hydroxybutyric acid

$$CH_3 - \overset{\overset{\textstyle O}{\|}}{C} - CH_3 + CO_2$$

Acetone

Fig. 16.5 : Formation (synthesis) of Ketone bodies

Danger of Ketone bodies

An increase in ketone bodies is the result of both i.e. (i) increased fatty acid metabolism in liver producing excessive amount of ketone bodies and (ii) a markedly decreased capacity to oxidize the ketone bodies by the muscles of the diabetics. The ketone bodies lead to severe acido is, a condition called as' ketoacidosis' in which the ketone bodies (which are acidic in nature) neutralize the alkalinity of the blood and tilt the pH Qf the blood towards acidic side which is a verydapgerous state. This dangerous state leads to coma and 'finally'death ensues within 4-14 days.

The typical breathing (sl11ell of acetone) found in the cases of diabetic coma i.e. cases of *uncontrolled diabetes mellitus* is known as *Kussmaul breathing* which is due to the effect of enol form of the acetoacetic acid on the respiratory centre. Such patients exhibit hyperventilation i.e. air-hunger, meaning by they are always hungry of air.

oxidation as a source of energy, as a result of which ketone bodies production is small. Carbohydrate is therefore treated to be an **'antiketogenic'** substance.

FATTY LIVERS

Significant deposition of triglycerides in the liver leads to a condition known as **'fatty liver'. Normally, liver contains 5% of the lipids**, but under certain pathological conditions, the lipid content rises to 25-30%. The increased fat in the liver may result from:

(a) **Factors associated with increased free fatty acids (FFA) level are:**

(i) **Diabetes mellitus (severe uncontrolled)**
(ii) **Starvation**
(iii) **Ketosis**
(iv) **Toxaemia of pregnancy,** etc.

Here, the increased mobilization of FFA leads to the increased synthesis of triglycerides and then their accumulation.

(b) Due to the deficiency of lipotropic factors such as choline, lecithin, methionine, vitamin E, vitamin B_6 i.e. pyridoxine, etc.

(e) Other intoxicating agents like $CHCl_3$, CCl_4, phosphorus, arsenic, lead, alcohol, etc.

BIOCHEMICAL BASIS OF FATTY LIVER

1. In one group, there is some primary factor which causes an increase in the FFA either due to increased mobilisation from adipose tissue or increased hydrolysis of lipoproteins or chylomicrons by the enzyme *lipoprotein lipase.* This increased FFA level leads to the increased synthesis of triglycerides, vis-a-vis their accumulation later or in the liver. The production of lipoproteins (specifically the chylomicrons and VLDL) from triglycerides is unable to keep pace with the synthesis of triglycerides,which enventually leads to **'fatty liver'.** This is the mechanism in disorders like uncontrolled diabetes mellitus, toxaemia of pregnancy, ketosis and starvation, etc.

2. In the other group, the defect lies in the production of plasma lipoproteins. Such a defect/blockade may be at one or more of the following sites:

(i) **Synthesis of apoproteins.**

(ii) **Synthesis of lipoproteins from lipid and apoproteins.**

(iii) **Synthesis of lipids-specifically the phospholipids.**

(iv) **Secretory mechanism of the lipoproteins.**

Substances which have got the capability to prevent or relieve such abnormal deposition of lipids in the liver are termed as **lipotropic factors** which are as mentioned just above.

Role of liver in the Metabolism of lipids:

Liver is the main site for the metabolism of lipids because it contains complete enzyme systems to carry out the following major activities as follows:

(i) **Synthesis of triglycerides**

(ii) **Synthesis of phospholipids**

(iii) **Synthesis of plasma lipoproteins such as VLDL, HDL, etc.**

(iv) **Synthesis of cholesterol and its derivatives such as bile acids, etc.**

(v) **Synthesis and degradation of fatty acids (β- oxidation)**

(vi) **Formation of ketone bodies**

CHAPTER 17

METABOLISM OF PROTEINS

Metabolism of ours includes the metabolism of 20 amino acids atleast. When we (amino acids) are metabolised, we participate in the synthesis of very important and invaluable substances of the body- to name a few are purines, haems, bile acids, creatine, glucose, acetyl CoA, melanin pigment, epinephrine, norepinephrine, T_3, T_4 and many more. We also include in ourselves the major pathway of nitrogen excretion i.e., 'Urea Cycle'.

The total protein turnover of an adult male is estimated to be around 400 g/day, of which 50 g. is accounted for the synthesis of digestive enzymes and another 15 g for the synthesis of haemoglobin.

On an overall, 20 amino acids are present in dietary proteins. These amino acids remain present in L-configuration. L-form of the amino acids is the physiological active form of the amino acids. The transport of such amino acids is energy dependent and requires ATP, Na^+, K^+, Mn^{++} and vitamin B_6.

Whereas D- form of amino acids is physiologically inactive and is transported by the phenomenon of diffusion.

DIGESTION AND ABSORPTION

Two important features of digestion are:

(1) It breaks down the non-diffusible larger molecules into smaller diffusible molecules which are commonly known as amino acids.

(2) During digestion, the biological specificity of the proteins gets destroyed as a result of which they are no longer antigenic in nature, thus avert allergic reactions to food.

Digestion of Proteins by various enzymes

Proteins are hydrolysed to their constituent amino acids by the action of a battery of enzymes found in the body, namely:

1. *Pepsin:* Responsible for the conversion of proteins to proteoses and peptones. It is secreted in the gastric juice as an inactive precursor i.e., pepsinogen. Pepsin is a very acidic protein and acts at pH between 1.5-2.5.

2. *Trypsin:* Responsible for cleaving peptide bonds involving carboxyl groups of arginine and lysine.

3. *Chymotrypsin:* Responsible for cleaving peptide bonds iinvolving carboxyl groups of phenylalanine, tyrosine and tryptophan.

4. *Carboxypeptidases:* The two carboxyp-eptidases are secreted as precursor *procarboxypeptidases*. They cleave proteins and peptides from the carboxyl end.

5. *Aminopeptidases:* Responsible for cleaving proteins and peptides from the amino end.

6. *Dipeptidases:* Responsible for the cleavage of dipeptides.

Absorption

It is known that absorption is very rapid in man. The extent of hydrolysis of the food protein is low in the stomach which is nearly 10-15% but quickly reaches upto 50-60% in the duodenum. In the duodenal contents, the enzymes trypsin and chymotrypsin remain present at the concentrations of 200-800 µg per ml of fluid within a short time of stimulation. These high concentrations of enzymes are capable of rapidly hydrolyzing food proteins to small peptides. Absorption of protein fragments takes place in the duodenum and the jejunum, most of it is absorbed as di-and oligopeptides.

L- form of the amino acids is absorbed at much faster rate than the D-form. All amino acids are absorbed by active process which requires ATP, Na^+, K^+, Mn^{++} and pyridoxal phosphate.

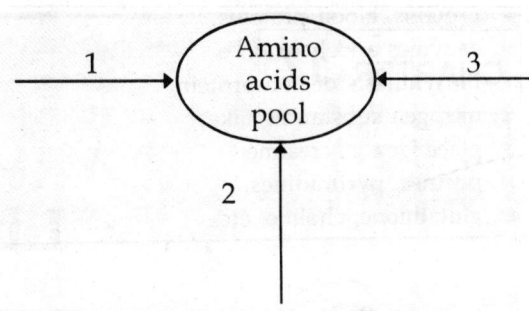

Sources of amino acids in the body pool include:

1. Dietary proteins
2. Intracellular synthesis
3. Tissue protein breakdown

}Metabolism (Table 17.1)

Transport of Amino Acids into Cells

The absorption of L-amino acids and some L– peptides is an active process and requires the metabolism of the mucosa to be intact. This absorption is interfered with by the presence of the D-isomers. Two mechanisms are known to exist:

1. The major mechanism is by carriers that are Na^+ dependent, so, the amino acids are not taken up unless Na^+ is also present in the lumen. The Na^+ then has to be pumped out of the mucosal cell by a Na^+/K^+ pump.

2. The glutamyl-transfer mechanism. This is a widespread mechanism and not confined to mucosal cells, but it is not easy to estimate what proportion of amino acids absorbed from gut, or in general transferred across cell membranes. Indirectly, it is highly energy dependent, since

Table 17.1 : Metabolism of Amino acids within the cell

Anabolic phase	Catabolic phase
It is a synthetic process	**It is a breakdown process**
1. Biosynthesis of proteins which includes tissue proteins, blood proteins, enzymes and hormones	1. Transamination
	2. Decarboxylation
	3. Oxidative deamination
	4. Utilization of nitrogen residue i.e.,
2. Biosynthesis of non-protein nitrogen substances takes place for e.g., creatine, purines, pyrimidines, glutathione, choline, etc.	(i) Synthesis of glutamine
	(ii) Urea cycle

glutathione—the glutamyl donor has to be completely resynthesized after each transfer.

Transamination

It is a combined process of deamination and amination according to which the amino group of one amino acid may be reversibly transferred to the keto acid of an other amino acid, thus effecting amino acid-keto acid interconversion. This phenomenon was for the first time discovered by two scientists namely *Braunstein* and *Kritzmann*.

The process represents intermolecular transfer of amino groups without the splitting of ammonia. The reaction is reversible and is catalyzed by *transaminase enzymes,* which remain confined to almost every tissue or the animal but the major sites are heart, brain, kidney, testicle and liver.

The general process of transamination may be represented as follows:

It was earlier found that glutamic acid and its keto acid i.e., α - ketoglutaric acid participate in a large proportion of transamination reactions but now it has

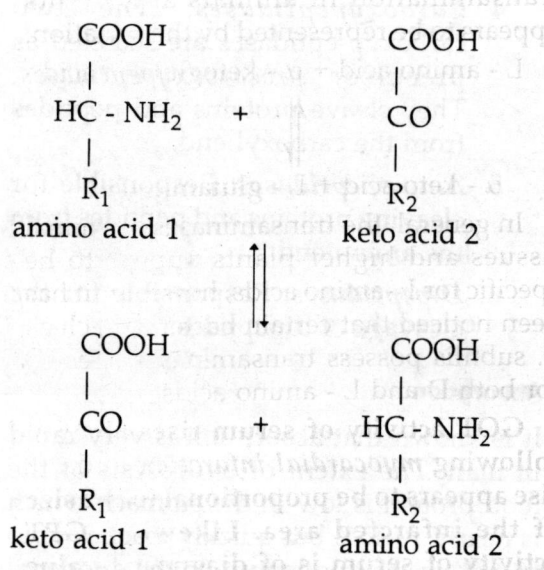

been concluded that all naturally occurring amino acids participate in transamination reactions.

There are two very important transaminases viz., glutamic-oxaloacetic transaminase i.e., GOT (AST) and glutamic-pyruvic transaminase i.e., GPT (ALT) which catalyze the following reactions:

The transaminases require pyridoxal phosphate as cofactor. GOT is the most

L - glutamic acid + pyruvic acid

$\updownarrow$ transaminase

α - ketoglutaric acid + L - alanine

L - glutamic acid + oxaloacetic acid

$\updownarrow$ transaminase

α - ketoglutaric acid + L - aspartic acid

active and widely distributed of the transaminases. The most general type of transamination in animals and plants appears to be represented by the equation:

L - amino acid + α - ketoglutaric acid

$\Updownarrow$

α - keto acid + L - glutamic acid

In general, the transaminases of animal tissues and higher plants appear to be specific for L -amino acids, however, it has been noticed that certain bacteria, such as B. subtilis possess transaminases specific for both D and L - amino acids.

GOT activity of serum rises sharply following *myocardial infarction* and the rise appears to be proportional to the size of the infarcted area. Likewise, GPT activity of serum is of diagnostic value in liver disorders.

All available evidence indicates great importance of the transamination reaction in amino acid and protein metabolism. It represents a mechanism for the deamination of amino acids and also for the synthesis of amino acids from keto acids and glutamic acid. The key role of glutamic acid and α - ketoglutaric acid in amino acid and protein metabolism is obvious.

DECARBOXYLATION

Amino acids are decarboxylated to produce amines. Such reactions are catalysed by enzymes known as decarboxylases which are found in liver, kidney and brian. These enzymes also require pyridoxal phosphate as a cofactor. Pyridoxamine phosphate is not required. The process is very important in the human body as it gives rise to important substances i.e., *biologically active amines as follows:*

Tyrosine $\xrightarrow{\text{decarboxylation}}$ tyramine

Tryptophan $\xrightarrow{\text{decarboxylation}}$ tryptamine

Histidine $\xrightarrow{\text{decarboxylation}}$ histamine

Glutamic acid

$\downarrow$ decarboxylation

γ–aminobutyric acid (GABA)

5-Hydroxytryptophan

$\downarrow$ decarboxylation

hydroxytryptamine (serotonin)

OXIDATIVE DEAMINATION

This process may be referred to as the liberation of ammonia oxidatively from amino acids, approximately two mols of NH_3 are formed for each molecule of O_2 taken up:

$$R - CH(NH_2) - COOH + 1/2O_2 \rightarrow R.CO\text{-}COOH + NH_3$$

Enzymes which bring about oxidative deamination are known as D- & L - amino acid oxidases; these act upon D - and L - amino acids respectively.

The D - amino acid oxidases are flavoproteins containing FAD, whereas L - amino acid oxidases are also flavoproteins but contain FMN (flavin mononucleotide).

The D - amino acids are not found in the tissues whereas L - amino acids are found which means that animal tissues are devoid of corresponding enzyme i.e., D - amino acid oxidases but contain L - amino acid oxidases. Both D - and L - amino oxidases are found in microorganisms. The functioin of D - oxidases is not yet known. .

The mechanism of oxidative deamination may be represented by the following equations:

$$R - \underset{\underset{\text{amino acid}}{\underset{\text{NH}_2}{|}}}{CH} - COOH + \underset{\underset{\text{enzyme}}{\text{flavoprotein}}}{FP} \rightarrow R - \underset{\underset{\underset{\text{acid}}{\text{imino}}}{\underset{\text{NH}}{||}}}{C} - COOH + \underset{\underset{\text{enzyme}}{\text{reduced}}}{FP. H_2}$$

$$R - \underset{\underset{\text{imino acid}}{\underset{\text{NH}}{|}}}{C} - COOH + H_2O \rightleftharpoons R - \underset{\underset{\text{keto acid}}{\underset{\text{O}}{||}}}{C} - COOH + NH_3$$

Protein Biosynthesis

All the different RNA's, t RNA, mRNA, and rRNA (as part of the ribosome), are involved in the synthesis of proteins. The process of protein biosynthesis is called **translation** because information must be transferred from the four-letter language of the nucleic acids to the twenty-four language of the amino acid constituents of the proteins.

There are twenty genetically important amino acids. These are listed

with the genetic code in Table, 17.1. All other amino acids in proteins are derived from the set of twenty; **for example, the hydroxyproline found in collagen is formed from prolyl residues after they become part of the protein chain.**

The ribosome: site of protein synthesis

Aminoacyl-tRNA's are condensed into protein on ribosomal particles, not in solution. The functional ribosome consists of two rather large particles. In animal

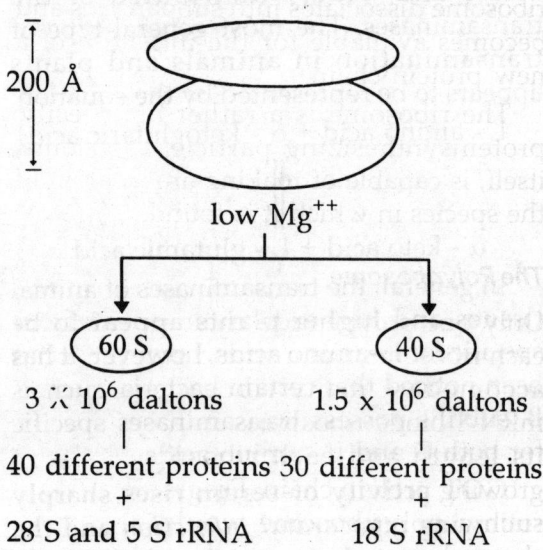

Fig. 17.1 : Composition of mammalian ribosomes

cells, these subparticles have sedimentation coefficients of 40 S and 60 S. In bacteria and mitochondria, the subparticles sediment at 30 S and 50 S. The subunits are derived from the functional particle, which is 80 S in all parts of the mammalian cell except the mitochondria, where it is 70 S. Even though these particles are quite large (about 200 Å in diameter), high-speed ultracentrifuges are required to sediment them. Figure 14.1

shows the composition of a mammalian ribosome. The particle as a whole is about half protein and half rRNA. The 40S subparticle contains a single RNA that sediments at 18S and about thirty different proteins. The larger 60 S subparticle contains two RNA's that sediment at 28 S and 5 S. The entire sequence of the 5 S RNA is known, but there are few clues as to how it functions. In addition, the larger subunit contains about 40 different proteins.

A single peptide chain grows from 80 S ribosome. On completion of the chain, the ribosome dissociates into subparticles and becomes available for the initiation of a new protein chain.

The ribosome is a rather nonspecific proteinsynthesizing particle. Ribosome, itself, is capable of making any protein of the species in which it is found.

The Polyribosome

Only one polypeptide chain grows from each ribosome, but a strand of mRNA can accomodate many ribosomes. Such a mRNA binds ribosomes in proportion to its length and each ribosome holds a growing protein chain. Diagrammatically, such a polyribosome would appear as shown below:

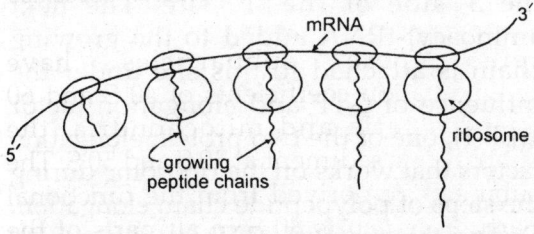

Protein synthesis starts by attaching a ribosome at or near the 5' end of mRNA. Recall that this is the end of the mRNA that is first synthesized from the DNA template.

As a ribosome directs the addition or aminoacyl groups to a growing peptidyl-tRNA, it moves along the message, decoding it from the 5' to the 3' end until it has moved far enough for another ribosome to be bound onto the initiating site just vacated. Soon the messenger is completely loaded with ribosomes. These polyribosomes can be seen with the electron microscope and the number of ribosomes on them can be counted. The number of ribosomes on a polyribosome is proportional to the size of the protein being synthesized. Thus, a globin chain for hemoglobin consists of about 150 amino acid residues and its polyribosome holds five ribosome monomers. A major chain of myosin contains about 1,800 amino acid residues and its polyribosome holds 60 to 100 monomeric ribosomes.

Initiation of Protein Synthesis (Fig. 17.2)

Protein synthesis starts at the amino end of the peptide and progresses by the addition of amino acids at the carboxyl end.

All protein chains start with the same amino acid, methionine, at the N-terminal position. Very often the methionine residue is cleaved off after the growing polypeptide chain has been somewhat extended; consequently, proteins isolated from cells contain amino acids other than methionine at their N-terminals. Methionine has two acceptor tRNA's, tRNA^M and tRNA^F. Only Met-tRNA^F is involved in the initiation.

A diagram of the initiation reactions is shown in Fig. 17.2. Despite much experimentation, little is known of the early steps in protein synthesis initiation. One view proposes that messenger RNA first binds to the smaller ribosomal subunit.

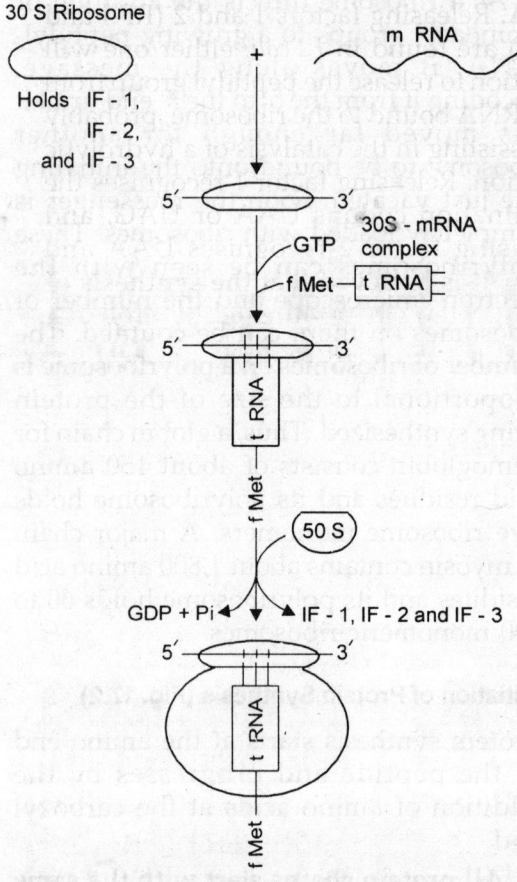

Fig. 17. 2: Initiation of Protein Synthesis. IF-1, IF-2 and IF-3 refer to initiation factors 1, 2 and 3 from *E. coli.*

In this scheme the 30 S subunit carries initiation factor 3 (IF-3). On subsequent addition of IF-2 and GTP, fMet-tRNA binds to an AUG sequence on the mRNA forming a stable complex. More recent experiments suggest that the 30 S ribosome first interacts with fMet-tRNA, not mRNA. In a later step, the messenger RNA binds. The message is bound in a functional way in a reaction that also requires the other two initiation factors.

The larger subunit is added in a reaction in which GTP is split to give GDP and inorganic phosphate; initiation factor 2

acts as the guanosine triphosphatase in this reaction. The hydrolysis of GTP in this process produces a conformational change in the 50 S particle so that the final initiation complex is accommodated to accept the attachment of the succeeding aminoacyl-tRNA programmed by the messenger.

Messenger RNA binding to ribosomes

A messenger RNA is attached to the ribosome so that the initiating sequence is presented in the proper reading frame. **The first amino acid inserted into peptide linkage is a methionyl residue coded by an AUG or GUG codon.** Not every AUG sequence in a mRNA programs the start of a new protein chain, since AUG sequences also code for methionyl residues that occur at internal positions of the polypeptide chain.

Protein chain elongation

There are two sites for tRNA attachment on the ribosome: One usually contains the peptidyl-tRNA; it is closest to the 5' end of the mRNA and is called the 'P' site. After the initiation reactions shown below in Fig. 14.3, tMet-tRNA is in the 'P' site. The other site, the aminoacyl-tRNA or 'A' site, is on the 3' side of the 'P' site. The next aminoacyl-tRNA added to the growing chain is attached to this site under the influence of GTP and elongation factor 1(EF-1), one of the two protein elongation factors that works on the ribosome during the steps of polypeptide chain elongation. During this reaction, GTP is split to GDP + Pi.

The formyl-methionyl group, or in subsequent steps the peptidyl moiety, is transferred to the nucleophilic amino group of the aminoacyl-tRNA in the 'A' site. This reaction is catalyzed by the ribosome itself, specifically by protein (s) of the larger subunit. The result is peptidyl-tRNA, now one amino acid longer, resting in the 'A' site while the 'P' site contains the deacylated tRNA that formerly held the peptidyl chain. This deacylated tRNA is removed in a reaction that requires elongation factor 2(EF-2) and GTP and that is concomitant with the translocation to the 'P' site of the new peptidyl-tRNA still hydrogen bonded to its codon on the mRNA. The cycle is now completed and a new codon is brought into apposition with the 'A', site. These reactions are shown diagrammatically in Fig. 17.3.

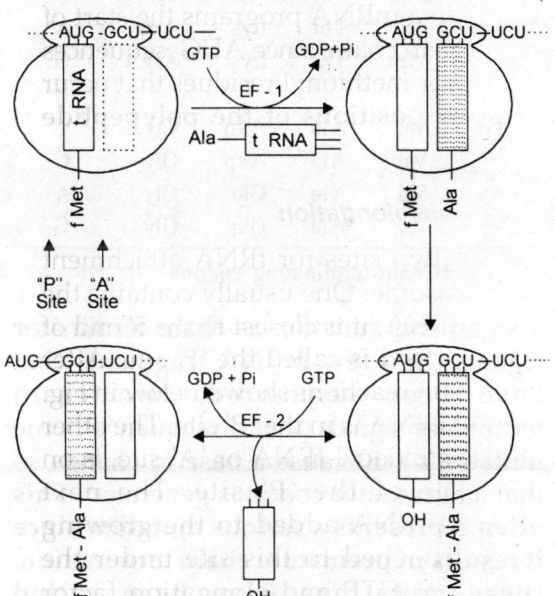

Fig. 17. 3: Peptide chain elongation

Termination of Protein Synthesis

Termination of protein synthesis in both animal and bacterial system requires GTP and one or more protein releasing factors. The releasing factors recognize the termination codons UAA, UAG, and UGA. Releasing factors 1 and 2 (RF-l and RF-2) are found in *E. coli;* either one will function to release the peptidyl group from the tRNA bound to the ribosome, probably by assisting in the catalysis of a hydrolytic reaction. Releasing factor 1 recognises the termination codons UAA or UAG, and releasing factor 2 recognises UAA and UGA. **It is believed that the synthesis of most proteins is terminated by the UAA signal, so that either factor might serve to stop the synthesis of most proteins.** Only a single releasing factor has been isolated from mammalian cells. No special tRNA's are required for termination. The peptidyl transferase of the ribosome may be involved, since in the presence of the antibiotic puromycin, it can carry out chain elongation in the absence of the releasing factor.

Strategies for the Biosynthesis of Proteins

The protein synthesizing activity of the body is subdivided among various tissues, e.g.

* **Mammary gland makes *milk proteins.***
* **Muscle makes *contractile proteins.***
* **Liver makes *serum proteins.***
* **Lymphocytes make *antibodies.***

Antibiotics and Protein Synthesis

Several antibiotics recognize differences between animal and bacterial protein synthesis by specifically inhibiting one or the other. The health scientist is most interested in those antibiotics that act specifically against bacteria. Table 17.2 lists a **few important commonly used antibiotics and the step in protein synthesis they inhibit.**

Diphtheria toxin, although it is not an

Table 17.2: Antibiotics that inhibit Protein Synthesis

Sl. No.	Antibiotic	Step inhibited
1.	Chloramphenicol	Ribosomal peptidyl transferase
2.	Streptomycin	Initiation; causes misreading of code
3.	Tetracycline	Prevents aminoacyl tRNA attachment to ribosome
4.	Puromycin (also inhibits animal cells)	Accepts growing peptidyl chain in place of aminoacyl-tRNA; chain terminates prematurely also
5.	Cycloheximide (inhibits animal cells only)	Ribosomal peptidyl transferase

Table 17.3: Genetic Code

First Position (5' end)	Second Position				Third Position (3' end)
	U	C	A	G	
U	Phe	Ser	Tyr	Cys	U
	Phe	Ser	Tyr	Cys	C
	Leu	Ser	Term*	Term*	A
	Leu	Ser	Term*	Trp	G
C	Leu	Pro	His	Arg	U
	Leu	Pro	His	Arg	C
	Leu	Pro	Gln	Arg	A
	Leu	Pro	Gln	Arg	G
A	Ile	Thr	Asn	Ser	U
	Ile	Thr	Asn	Ser	C
	Ile	Thr	Lys	Arg	A
	Met	Thr	Lys	Arg	G
G	Val	Ala	Asp	Gly	U
	Val	Ala	Asp	Gly	C
	Val	Ala	Glu	Gly	A
	Val	Ala	Glu	Gly	G

*Chain-terminating codons

antibiotic is another substance that inhibits protein synthesis. The toxin is an enzyme that is exceedingly deadly even in small amounts.

Genetic Code

Three nucleotide bases are required to specify the insertion of an amino acid into a polypeptide chain. Each series of three bases is read in a linear sequential manner without using a particular base more than once. Because there are four different bases in RNA, the maximum number of three letter code words are 4^3, or 64. Sixty-one of these words are used to specify the 20 amino acids, and essentially the same code word dictionary is used in all species tested. **Consequently, the genetic code is said to be triplet, nonoverlapping, degenerate, and universal. Table 17.3 lists the codon assignments for the 20 amino acids. Notice, that the first two letters of a code word are very specific but that often the same amino acid is coded regardless of the third nucleotide.**

The three codons without amino acid assignments function as chain terminator signals. In a few mRNA fragments that have been sequenced, two chain terminator signals occur in sequence. Some mutations will cause a base to change so that a terminator codon is generated. **This often represents a serious mutation since it results in premature chain termination; these mutations have been called "nonsense" mutations because a code word has been made for which there is no amino acid. A mutation that changes a base so that a new amino acid is now specified by the code is called a "missense" mutation. Missense mutations often result in altered or reduced enzymatic activity, and not necessarily in a complete absence of**

activity. Considering the degeneracy of the code, one can predict that almost one third of all base replacements will probably cause no change at all in the protein made since they will occur in the third nucleotide of the codon.

The genetic code assumes that each codon base pair is in antiparallel fashion with the anticodon of the tRNA's that are specific for the amino acid corresponding to the code word. It was found, however, that when purified tRNA's became available, a single tRNA could recognize several code words. For example, tRNA for alanine recognises GCU, GCC and GCA. The anticodon for this tRNA is IGC and the base-paired structures would be:

5'――――――――――――――――――――― 3'

```
  G C U       G C C       G C A
  ‖ ‖ ‖       ‖ ‖ ‖       ‖ ‖ ‖
  C G I       C G I       C G I
```

3'――――――――――――――――――――― 5'

Notice, that the nonstandard base pairing is the third position of the codon, the position that has the least effect on specifying a particular amino acid. **Crick** has proposed a hypothesis to account for these data. It is called the **"Wobble hypothesis** because it predicts that a "Wobble" in the base pairing in the third position of the code word might account for the lessened specificity. Based on the analysis of several other tRNA's, Crick proposed the rules shown below.

Third Position of anticodon in tRNA	Third Position of codon in mRNA
U or ψ	A or G
C	G
A	U
G	C or U
I	C, U or A

Assuming that the Wobble hypothesis is valid, one can see that while all sixty-one possible code words might be read when they occur in mRNA, it is not necessary to have as many as 61 different types of tRNA to read them.

The genetic code for the most part seems to be universal. The codon assignments established for *E. coli* are consistent with the known amino acid replacements in a large number of abnormal human hemoglobins and mutant coat proteins of the tobacco mosaic virus.

Salient Features (Characteristics) of Genetic Code

Base sequences. of DNA constitute coded messages which determine hereditary characters; such coded messages are later on transcribed into complementary base sequences of mRNA, obeying the **base-pairing rule**. The sequence of such bases in a part of the m-RNA molecule thus constitutes a **'genetic code'** which is translated into a particular sequence of amino acids in the peptide chain synthesized on that part of the mRNA strand. The genetic code is made up of many units which are called as codons, each directs the incorporation of a specific amino acid in the peptide. **Each codon is a triplet of bases (Table 17.4) present in three ribonucleotides set consecutively in the m-RNA strand. The genetic code has the following four characteristics:**

1. *Universality:* Each particular amino acid is coded by the same codon or codons in all species of organisms.

2. *Degeneracy:* Except methionine and tryptophan, each amino acid is coded by more than one codon and any of the latter may incorporate that amino acid in the peptide; **L-valine, for instance, is coded by**

Table 17.4 Genetic code

Sl. No.	Amino acids	
1.	Ala	GCU, GCC, GCA, GCG
2.	Arg	CGU, CGC, CGA, CGG, AGA, AGG
3.	Asn	AAV, AAC
4.	Asp	GAU, GAC
5.	Cys	UGU, UGC
6.	Gln	CAA, CAG
7..	Glu	GAA, GAG
8.	Gly	GGU, GGC, GGA, GGG
9.	His	CAU, CAC
10.	Ile	AUU, AUC, AUA
11.	Leu	UUA, UUG, CUU, CUC, CUA, CUG
12.	Phe	UUU, UUC
13.	Ser	UCU, UCC, UCA, UCG, AGU, AGC
14.	Lys	AAA, AAG
15.	Thr	ACU, ACC, ACA, ACG
16.	Met	AUG*
17.	Pro	CCV, CCC, CCA, CCG
18.	Trp	UGG
19.	Tyr	UAU, UAC
20.	Val	GUU, GUC, GUA, GUG
	Terminator codons	UAA, UAG, UGA

* AUG is an initiator codon also

four codons, i.e., GUU, GUC, GUA and GUG (Table 14.3); isoleucine by three codons, namely AUU, AUC and AUA; tyrosine by two codons, namely, UAU and UAC; whereas, methionine by only one codon i.e., AUG. and tryptophan also by only one codon i.e., UGG (Table 14.3).

3. *Non-overlap:* Consecutive codons of an mRNA strand are separate from each other and also independent of each other and thus do not overlap—the same base cannot thus function as a common member of two codons.

4. *Commalessness:* There is no intervening nucleotide between two consecutive codons.

Genetic code ensures the dependence of the primary structure of a protein on the base sequence of a particular segment of the DNA strand.

It has been established so far that procaryotic m-RNA is *polycistronic,* i.e., it carries more than one genetic code; whereas eukaryotic m-RNA is *monocistronic,* i.e., it carries only one genetic code.

Codons are always read in the 5'-3' direction (usually shown as left-right) along the m-RNA strand. Out of the total of 64 codons, three do not incorporate any amino acid in the peptide but act as terminator codons for ending the translation, whereas the remaining one code for 20 different amino acids (Table 14.3). One of the terminator codons, viz; UAA, UAG or UGA, is the last codon at the 3' end of the row of codons in a genetic code and is preceded on its 5' side by the codon coding for the c-terminal amino acid of the peptide.

Translation always begins with a chain initiator codon, i.e., AUG, which forms the first codon at the 5' end of the genetic code. AUG codes for methionine with which the translation starts from the N-terminal end of the peptide. Besides this, AUG may occur at intermediate sites of the code for incorporating methionine in the middle of the peptide.

UREA CYCLE
(KREBS-HENSELEIT CYCLE/ORNITHINE CYCLE)

Urea is the main end product of protein metabolism in the body. The deamination of amino acids produces ammonia which is toxic. By this cycle, it is converted to urea, a non-toxic compound, which is transported via blood to the kidneys and then excreted in the urine. Urea formation takes place in the liver. Two molecules of ammonia and one molecule of CO_2 are converted to urea for each turn of the cycle.

Various stages of urea cycle include:

1. Formation of carbamoyl phosphate
2. Formation of citrulline from ornithine
3. Fomation of urea from arginine

1st stage: i.e. Formation of carbamoyl phosphate.

The first stage in the synthesis of urea in animals may be considered to be the formation of carbamoyl phosphate, the reaction is catalysed by the enzyme known as carbamoyl phosphate synthase (Fig. 17.4).

Carbamoyl phosphate is a reactive high energy compound. The enzyme requires an acyl glutamate such as N-acetylglutamate as a cofactor.

IInd stage i.e. Formation of citrulline from ornithine

Ornithine is converted to citrulline by the action of carbamoyl phosphate; this reaction is catalysed by the action of enzyme ornithine transcarbamoylase. **This**

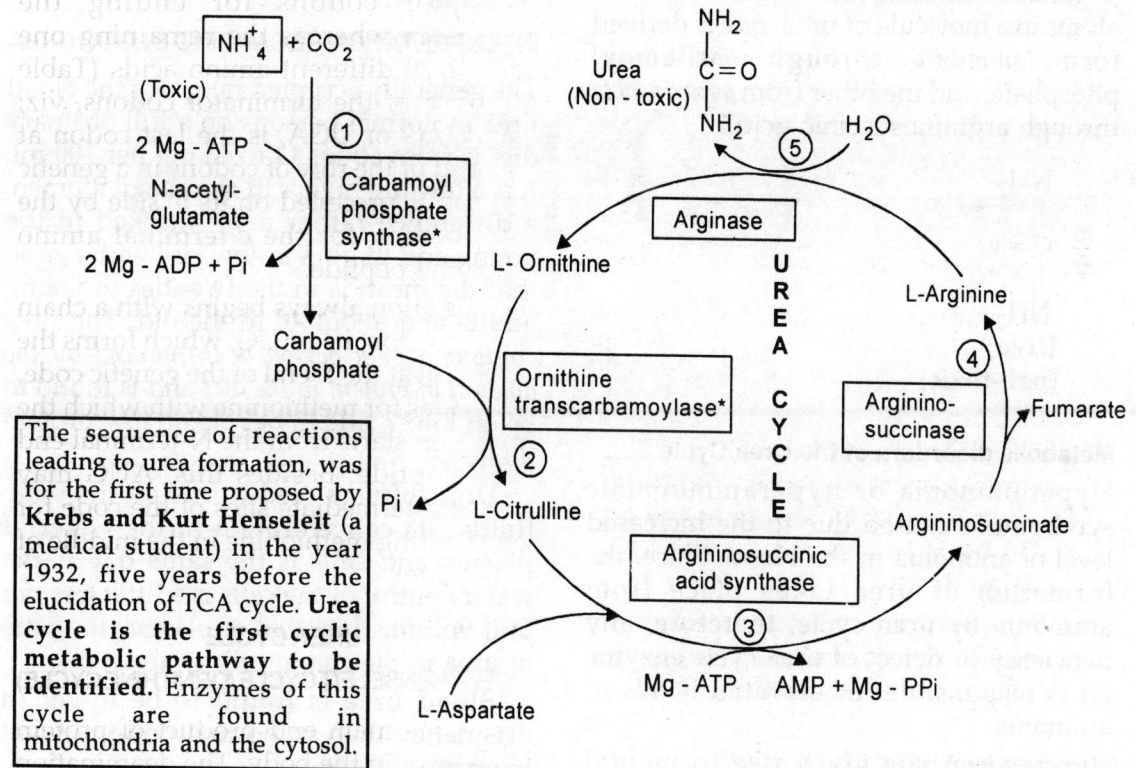

> The sequence of reactions leading to urea formation, was for the first time proposed by **Krebs and Kurt Henseleit** (a medical student) in the year 1932, five years before the elucidation of TCA cycle. **Urea cycle is the first cyclic metabolic pathway to be identified.** Enzymes of this cycle are found in mitochondria and the cytosol.

* *Mitochondrial enzymes*

Fig. 17.4 : Reactions and intermediates of Urea Cycle (biosynthesis)

reaction is not reversible.

IIIrd stage i.e. Formation of arginine from citrulline

The syntheis of arginine from citrulline takes place in two stages. The first stage is the condensation of citrulline with aspartic acid to form argininosuccinic acid by the enzyme argininosuccinate synthetase. The argininosuccinate gets then split into arginine and fumarate by the cleavage enzyme known as argininosuccinase. (Fig. 17.4).

IVth and last stage i.e. Formation of urea from arginine

Arginine is hydrolyzed to ornithine and urea by the enzyme arginase.

It has been observed that of the two N atoms in a molecule of urea, one is derived form *ammonia* through carbamoyl phosphate, and the other from *aspartic acid* through argininosuccinic acid.

$$
\begin{array}{c}
NH_2 \\
| \\
C = O \\
| \\
NH_2 \\
\textbf{Urea} \\
\textbf{(non-toxic)}
\end{array}
$$

Metabolic disorders of the Urea Cycle

Hyperammonia or hyperammonemic syndrome is caused due to the increased level of ammonia in the blood. Since, the formation of urea takes place from ammonia by urea cycle, therefore, any deficiency or defect of urea cycle enzyme (s) is responsible for elevated levels of ammonia.

Hyperammonemia gives rise to mental retardation.

There are five disorders:

1. *Hyperammonemia type I:* In this type there is found **absence of enzyme carbamoyl phosphate synthetase.**

2. *Hyperammonemia type II:* In this type there is found **absence of enzyme ornithine trans carbamoylase.**

3. *Citrullinemia:* There is found **absence of enzyme argininosuccinate synthetase (synthase) in this type.**

4. *Argininosuccinic aciduria:* There is found **absence of enzyme argininosuccinase in this type.**

5. *Hyperarginemia:* In this type, there is found **absence or deficiency of enzyme arginase.**

INTERPRETATION REGARDING BLOOD UREA

The generally accepted range for the blood urea in normal persons on a full ordinary diet is from about 14 to 43 mg per 100 ml. It is a few mg higher in men than women, a difference rather more marked in the young and there is a slow rise with age so that the mean is in the twenties in young adults and about 40 in the old. The urea *content over a period is influenced by the amount of protein in the diet* and is found to be on lower side in people on low protein diets.

Urea diffuses readily into all the body fluids Its concentration in the water of plasma and cells is the same but as the water control of the cells is a little less per unit volume than that of plasma, the ratio of urea in plasma to cells is about 5:4.

Blood urea is found to be lower in pregnancy than in normal non-pregnant women.

Increases in the level of blood urea may

1. Ammonia is produced in deamination, deamidation, desulphuration, trans-amination involving amino acid amides and transdeamination.
2. The principal source of NH_3 is the oxidation of glutamate by glutamate dehydrogenase, present in liver mitochondria and other tissues.
3. These reactions take place chiefly in the liver.
4. Ammonia is highly toxic to the human body, hence, it's earliest removal/excretion is very essential.
5. Toxic ammonia is converted into harmless water-soluble urea in the liver by the operation of the Krebs- Henseleit cycle.
6. While the TCA cycle is 'revenue' to the body, the urea cycle is 'expenditure', ATP molecules are produced in the former while they are spent in the latter.
7. Urea produced from ammonia during the metabolism of amino acids is excreted in the urine.
8. Daily excretion of urea is **20-30 g.**
9. Blood urea level is an index of kidney functioning and its normal level is about 14-43 mg %.
10. When the kidney functioning is impaired as in acute nephritis, the blood urea level rises due to retention.
11. **Brain and mammary glands are the other two very minor sites for the synthesis of urea from ammonia.**

occur in a number of diseases in addition to those in which the kidneys are primarily involved. For increases, three states may be responsible, namely:

(a) **Pre-renal**
(b) **Renal and**
(c) **Post- renal**

(a) *Pre-renal* : In this state, kidneys are not involved. In this state, blood urea level gets increased in cases of dehydration due to severe and protracted vomiting **as in pyloric and intestinal obstruction;** in chronic intestinal obstruction without vomiting; in diarrhoea; etc. *Very high values* of blood urea are encountered in these conditions if they are allowed to go untreated. Thus, in *pyloric stenosis* **with severe vomiting, the blood urea may exceed 200 mg/dl,** and even occasionally be over **300** and can be quite rapidly brought down to normal with satisfactory treatment.

It may also exceed 300 mg/dl in ulcerative collitis with severe chloride loss.

In diabetic coma, it may be found in the range of 50 to 150 *mg*/dl, returning to normal as soon as the coma has been treated.

It may also be found elevated **i.e., in the range of 50 to 100 mg/dl or even higher in the cases of** *Addison's disease* **(hypoadrenalism).**

Other conditions in which blood urea may be found to be elevated include:

(a) Haematemesis,
(b) Shock due to severe burns,
(c) Post-operative state,
(d) Cardiac failure, etc.

(b) *Renal:* In this state, kidneys are involved as a result of which level of blood urea gets increased **in all types of kidney diseases** which include:

(i) Acute glomerulonephritis

(ii) Ellis's Type II nephritis

(iii) Malignant hypertension

(iv) Chronic pyelonephritis

(v) Murcury poisoning

(vi) Hydronephrosis

(vii) Congenital cystic kidneys

(viii) Renal tuberculosis

(ix) Hyperparathyroidism

(x) Hpervitaminosis D

(c) *Post - renal:* Post renal diseases lead to increased blood urea level, are those in which there is obstruction to the flow of urine. **This causes retention of urine.** If prolonged, irreversible kidney damage results. **Most important among these is** *enlargement of the prostate,* in which estimation of blood urea is an essential part of the assessment of the condition. **Besides prostate, other conditions include:**

(i) **stones in the urinary tract**

(ii) **stricture of the urethra**

(iii) **tumour of the bladder affecting the ureters, etc.**

METABOLISM OF THE INDIVIDUAL AMINO ACIDS

According to the metabolic fate of their skeletons, amino acids have been classified in the following categories:

(a) Glycogenic or glucogenic amino acids

(b) Ketogenic amino acids

(a) Glycogenic (Glucogenic) amino acids:

These are those amino acids which may be responsible for the synthesis of glucose (see gluconeogenesis pathway). These include glycine, alanine, serine, threonine, valine, aspartic acid, glutamic acid, cysteine, cystine, methionine, proline, hydroxyproline, arginine and histidine.

Table 17.5 : Classification of glycogenic and ketogenic amino acids

Glycogenic or glucogenic	Ketogenic only	Glycogenic and ketogenic i.e., both
glycine, alanine, serine, threonine, valine, aspartic acid, glutamic acid, cysteine, cystine, methionine, proline, hydroxyproline, arginine and histidine	leucine	isoleucine, lysine, phenylalanine, tyrosine and tryptophan

(b) Ketogenic amino acids

Amino acids which have the capability to synthesize *acetate* or *acetoacetate* (the intermediates formed during fatty acid metabolism) are known as ketogenic amino acids. These include leucine, isoleucine, lysine, phenylalanine, tyrosine and tryptophan (see Table 17.5).

Glycine

It is one of the glycogenic (glucogenic) amino acids. It is a non-essential amino acid and is synthesized by the living cells. It contains no asymmetric carbon atom, hence does not exist in D or L form.

$$\begin{array}{c} NH_2 \\ | \\ H - C - COOH \\ | \\ H \end{array}$$

glycine

Glycine, (Fig 17.5 (a) & (b), the simplest of the amino acids, to date has been found to be utilized in more different ways in the animal body than pratically any other amino acid. It is a very important and useful amino acid as its metabolism gives rise to several important substances as follows:

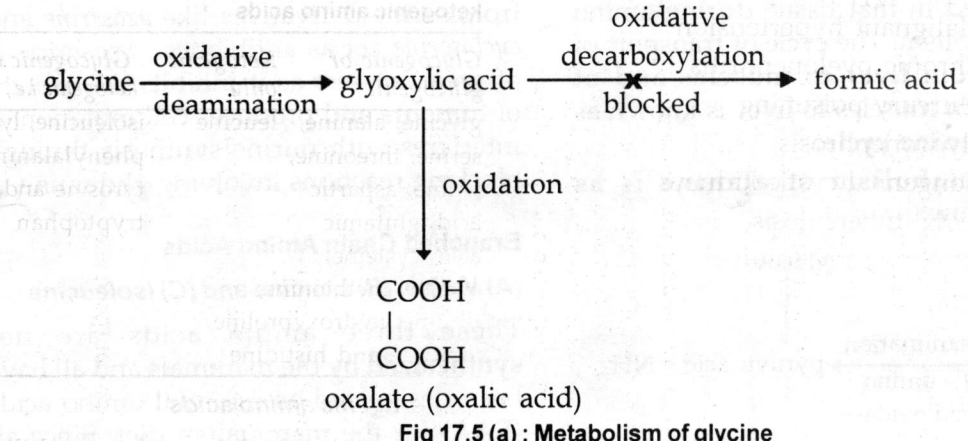

Fig 17.5 (a) : Metabolism of glycine

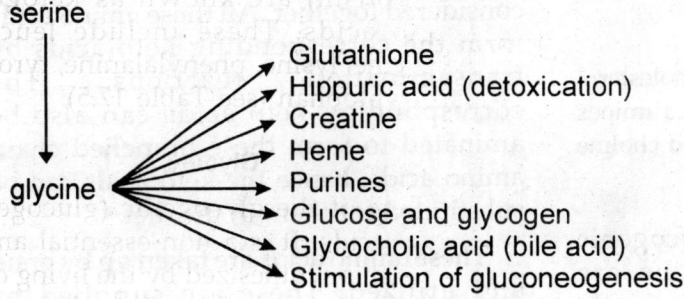

Fig. 17.5 (b): Metabolism of glycine

Abnormalities of glycine metabolism

1. Primary Hyperoxaluria

The metabolism defect in this disease in due to the disorder of glyoxylate metabolism where in glyoxylic acid is not oxidised to formic acid but is converted to oxalate, thus, giving rise to increased excretion of **Oxalates** in urine.

2. Glycinuria

There is decreased tubular reabsorption of glycine in the kidneys as a result of which appreciable amount of glycine is found in the urine of such individuals.

ALANINE

This is also a non-essential glycogenic amino acid. Deamination or transamination produces pyruvic acid which can be readily converted to glucose or oxidized in citric acid cycle. β - alanine is a constituent of pantothenic acid.

Formation of alanine from pyruvate in

muscles also helps in removing some of the NH_3 formed in that tissue during amino acid metabolism. The cycle of transport of glucose from liver to muscles and of alanine from muscles to liver is known as **glucose alanine cycle.**

The metabolism of alanine is as shown below:

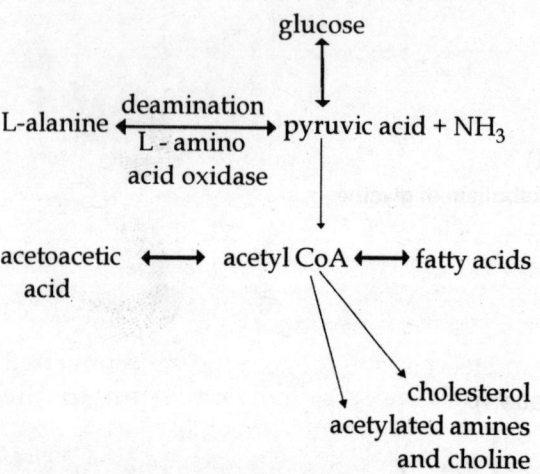

Serine

This is also a non-essential glycogenic amino acid. Serine and glycine are interconvertible in the body, as previously indicated. The metabolism of serine is as follows:

It is of interest to note that certain molds from serine derivatives like *azaserine* and *cycloserine* act as antibiotics. Azaserine is of great interest as it inhibits the growth of tumours and produces cell mutation. It interferes with purine synthesis through blocking reactions involving glutamine.

Branched Chain Amino Acids

(A) Valine, (B) Leucine and (C) Isoleucine

These three amino acids are not **synthesized** by the mammals and all have been designated as essential amino acids **(EAA)** for the mammalian diet. Since all of them contain branched chain aliphatic groups and have metobolic features in common, therefore, their metabolisms are considered together. All these amino acids form the corresponding keto acids by transamination reactions. The corresponding keto acids can also be aminated to form these branched chain amino acids, hence the keto acids can be substituted for them in the diet.

These amino acids are taken up by brain and utilized. These are supplied by absorption from the gastrointestinal tract following a meal and are preferentially

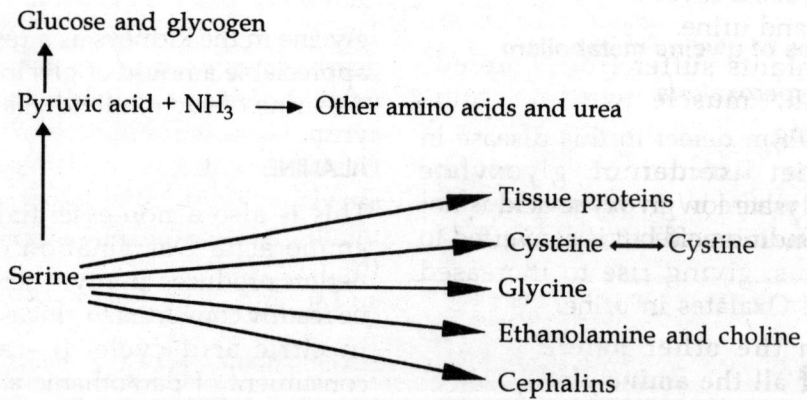

taken up by the brian and the muscles. In the post absorptive state, they are supplied by protein breakdown in the muscles.

(A) Valine

It's glycogenic, on deamination, it forms α-keto isovaleric acid and later on succinyl Co-A. It's metabolism in brief is as follows:

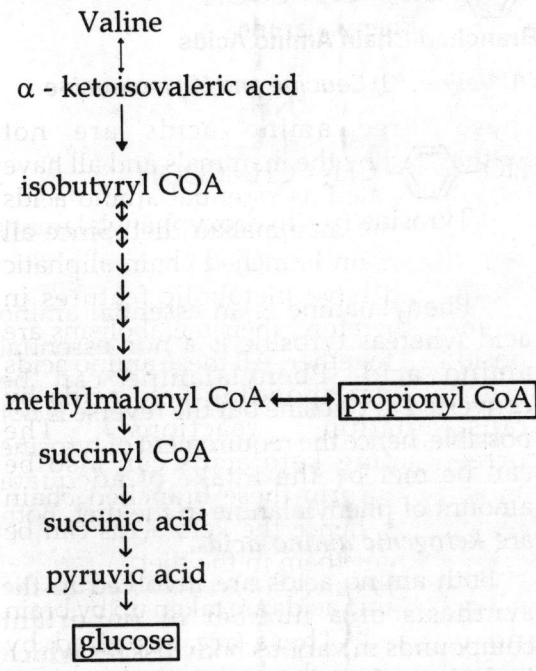

Valine
↓
α - ketoisovaleric acid
↓
isobutyryl COA
↓
↓
↓
↓
↓
↓
methylmalonyl CoA ⟷ propionyl CoA
↓
succinyl CoA
↓
succinic acid
↓
pyruvic acid
↓
glucose

Hypervalinemia

1. In this abnormal conditioin one finds raised level of valine in the blood and urine.
2. The infants suffer from stunted growth, muscle wasting and vomiting
3. A diet containing protein hydrolysate low in valine prevents this condition effectively.

(B) Leucine

Leucine, on the other hand is most ketogenic of all the amino acids, i.e., it forms the ketone bodies. Its metabolism

in short may be represented as follows: Acetyl Co-A once formed may give rise to ketone bodies.

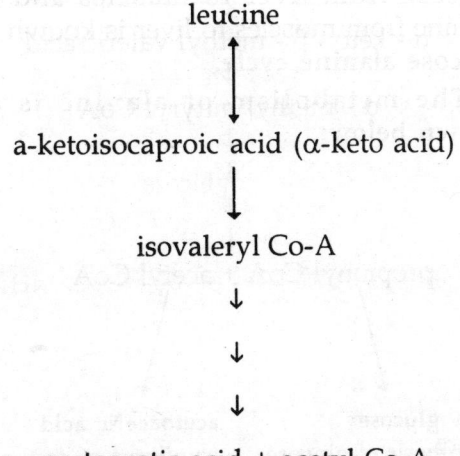

leucine
↓
a-ketoisocaproic acid (α-keto acid)
↓
isovaleryl Co-A
↓
↓
↓
acetoacetic acid + acetyl Co-A

In step (2), the α - keto acid is converted by oxidative decarboxylation to the corresponding Co-A derivative (with one carbon less) i.e. isovaleryl Co-A. This reaction is catalysed by branched chain 2-keto acid dehydrogenase complex in the presence of TPP, lipoic acid, FAD, NAD and coenzyme - A as cofactors. The deficiency of this enzyme causes **maple syrup urine disease.** In this disease, there is metabolic defect involving the branched chain amino acids which results in the excretion of their keto acids in the urine. The defect is in step (2), the oxidative dearboxylation of the α- keto acids. **The urine is said to have the odour of maple syrup. There is rapid deterioration in the first two months of life. If the child survives, he or she manifests serious mental retardation. It's a serious disease, the treatment of which is not available so far.**

(C) Isoleucine

The metabolism of **isoleucine** may be

represented in brief as follows:

isoleucine

↓

α - keto - β - methyl valeric acid

↓

α - methyl butyryl CoA

↓
↓
↓
↓
↓

propionyl CoA + acetyl CoA

glucose
(synthesis of glucose takes place, which means isoleucine is glycogenic)

acetoacetic acid
(synthesis of acetoace tic acid takes place which means isoleucine is ketogenic)

From the pathway of isoleucine metabolism, it is conclusive that two carbon atoms may lead to the formation of acetyl CoA and three carbon atoms to the formation of glucose.

Metabolism of Phenylalanine and Tyrosine

Both phenylalanine and tyrosine are aromatic amino acids. Tyrosine is hydroxylated phenylalanine. The structure of these are:

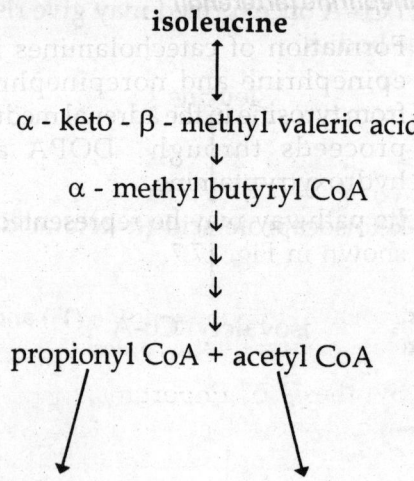

Phenylalanine

Tyrosine (p - hydroxyphenylalanine)

Phenylalanine is an essential amino acid whereas tyrosine is a non-essential amino acid. Phenylalanine can be converted to tyrosine but the reverse is not possible, hence the requirement of tyrosine can be met by the intake of adequate amount of phenylalanine in the diet. Both are *ketogenic amino acids*.

Both amino acids are involved in the synthesis of a number of important compounds in various body tissues **which include melanin pigment, epinephrine, norepinephrine, T₃ and T₄ (thyroxine) etc. as shown below:**

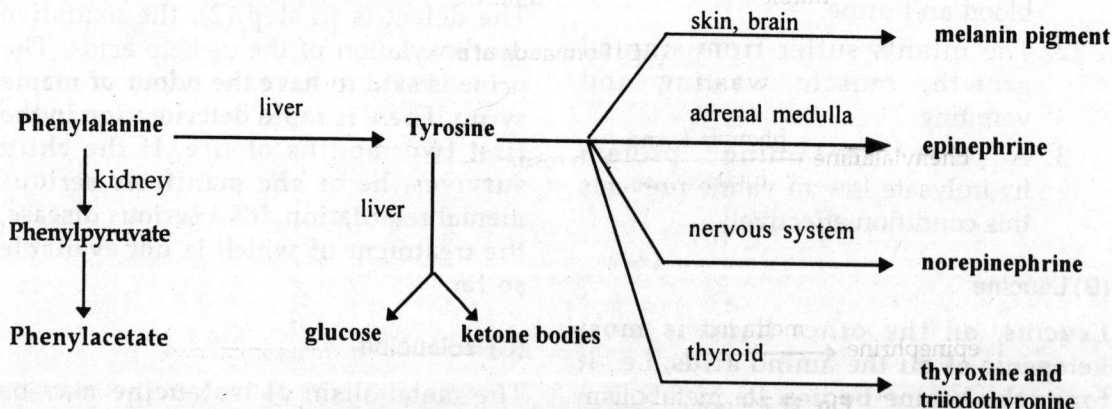

(a) Formation of melanin

(a) Melanins represent the dark pigments of the skin, hair and retina of the eye and are formed from 3, 4 - dihydroxyphenylalanine (DOPA) through a complex series of reactions.

(b) Melanin forms a reversible oxidation reduction system in which the reduced form is tan and the oxidized form is black.

(c) Melanins are produced in pigment - forming cells, the *melanocytes*.

(d) Melanins are very complex substances of high molecular weight and are insoluble in most solvents.

(e) The pathway of melanin formation is given below in Fig. 17.6.

(b) Formation of epinephrine (adrenaline) and norepinephrine (arterenol)

(a) Formation of catecholamines i.e., epinephrine and norepinephrine from tyrosine in the adrenal medulla proceeds through DOPA and hydroxytryptamine.

(b) Its pathway may be represented as shown in Fig. 17.7.

(c) Formation of triiodothyronine (T_3) and thyroxine i. e. tetraiodothyronine (T_4)

(a) Synthesis of important hormones like T_3 and T_4 takes place in the thyroid gland from phenylalanine and tyrosine (Fig. 17.7).

(b) Phenylalanine is converted to tyrosine which on iodination forms monoiodotyrosine; this on further iodination gives rise to diiodotyrosine.

(c) Coupling of two molecules of

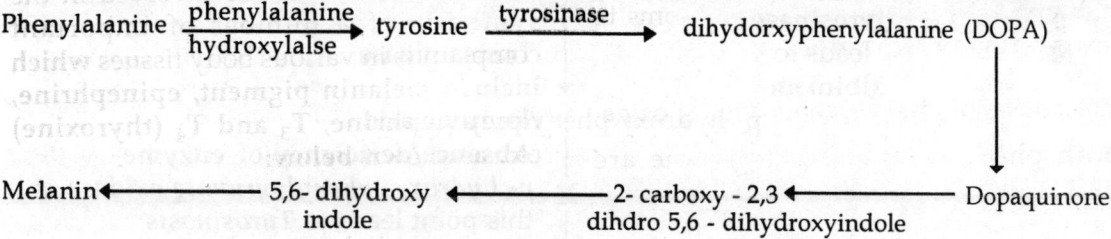

Fig. 17.6 : Formation of melanin

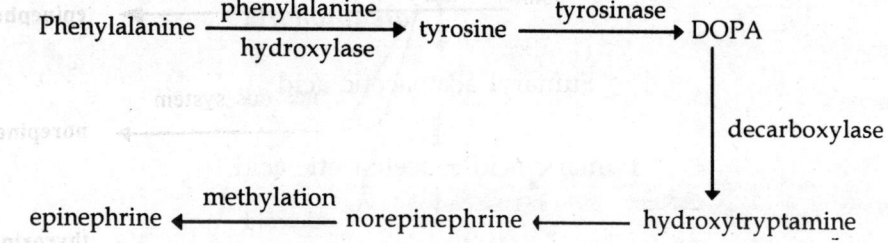

Fig. 17.7: Formation of epinephrine and norepinephrine

The steps are as shown below :

Phenylalanine

   | phenylalanine
   | hydroxylase

Tyrosine

   | iodination

Monoiodotyrosine

   | iodination

Diiodotyrosine

   | 2 mols coupling

Thyroxine + Alanine

Monoiodotyrosine
   +
Diiodotyrosine

Triiodothyronine(T₃)

Fig 17.8 : Formation of T₄ and T₃

diiodotyrosine yields thyroxine (Fig. 17.8).

(d) Coupling of 1 mol. of monoiodotyrosine and 1 mol. of diiodotyrosine yields triiodothyronine (Fig. 17.8).

Inborn errors of the metabolism of Phenylalanine and Tyrosine (Hereditary defects in phenylalanine and tyrosine metabolism).

There are number of metabolic abnormalities which are congenital and remain present throughout life. These disorders are hereditary (Fig. 17.9). Four well established hereditary defects in the metabolism of phenylalanine and tyrosine include **phenylketonuria (phenylpyruvic oligophrenia), tyrosinosis, alkaptonuria and albinism;** In each case the defect is

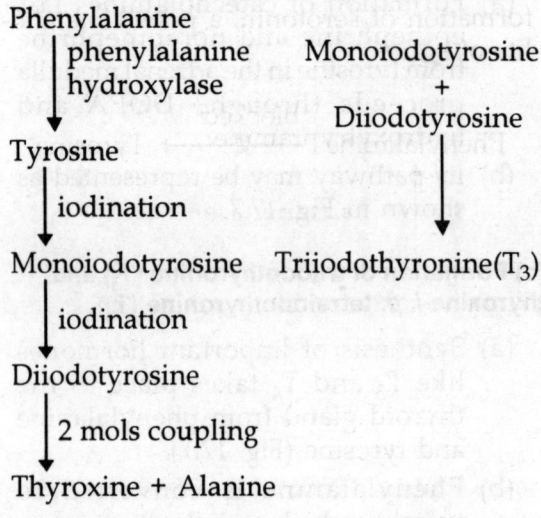

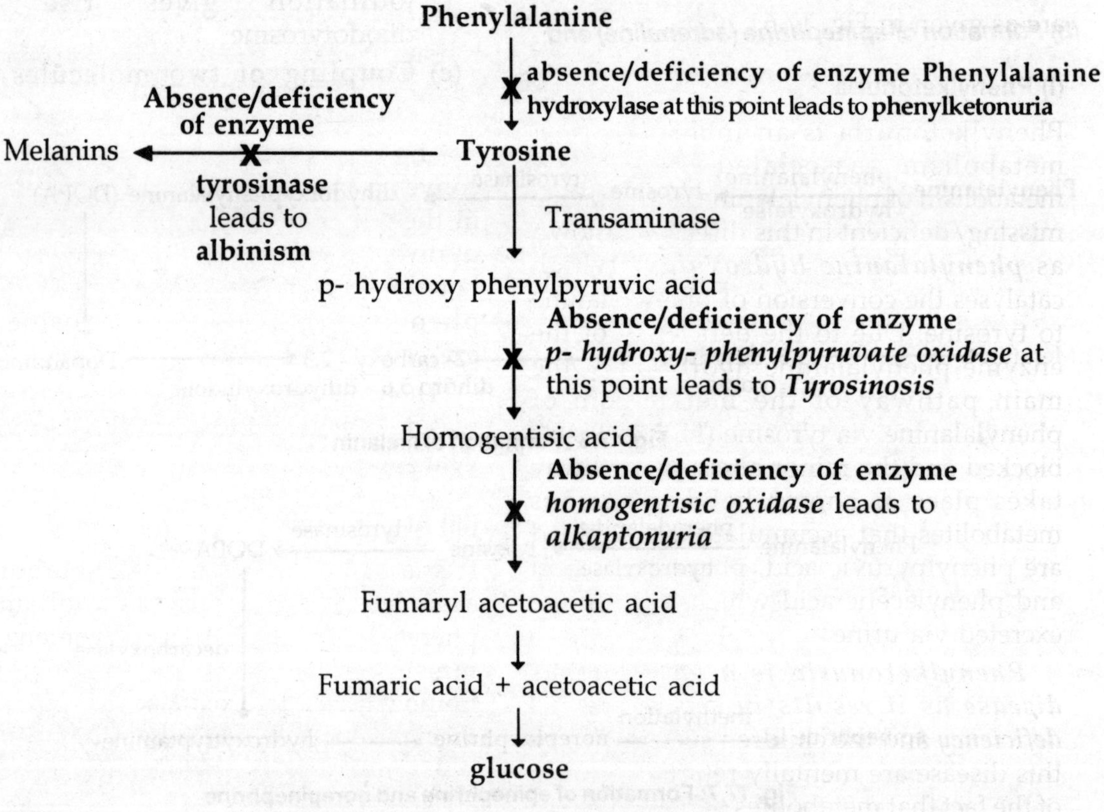

Phenylalanine

absence/deficiency of enzyme Phenylalanine hydroxylase at this point leads to phenylketonuria

Melanins ← **Absence/deficiency of enzyme** **X** ← Tyrosine

tyrosinase leads to **albinism**

Transaminase

p- hydroxy phenylpyruvic acid

Absence/deficiency of enzyme *p- hydroxy- phenylpyruvate oxidase* at this point leads to *Tyrosinosis*

Homogentisic acid

Absence/deficiency of enzyme *homogentisic oxidase* leads to *alkaptonuria*

Fumaryl acetoacetic acid

Fumaric acid + acetoacetic acid

glucose

Fig. 17.9: Catabolism of Phenylalanine and Tyrosine

Inborn error	Enzyme defect
(i) Phenylketonuria	Phenylalanine hydroxylase
(ii) Tyrosinosis	p-hydroxyphenylpyuvate oxidase
(iii) Alkaptonuria	Homogentisic acid oxidase
(iv) Albinism	Tyrosinase

due to hereditary absence or deficit of a specific enzyme involved in a specific reaction. These conditions belong to what **Scientist Garrod called 'inborn errors of metabolism.**

Various blocks (checks) in the metabolism of phenylalanine and tyrosine give rise to different inborn errors of metabolism taking place either due to absence or deficiency of an enzyme which are as given in Fig. 17.6.

(i) Phenylketonuria

Phenylketonuria is an inborn error of metabolism associated with the metabolism of phenylalanine. The enzyme missing/deficient in this disease is known as *phenylalanine hydroxylase* which catalyses the conversion of phenylalanine to tyrosine. Due to the deficiency of the enzyme phenylalanine hydroxylase, the main pathway of the metabolism of phenylalanine via tyrosine (Fig. 17.9) gets blocked and the minor alternate pathway takes place as shown below . Various metabolites that accumulate in the blood are phenylpyruvic acid, phenyllactic acid and phenylacetic acid which later on are excreted via urine.

Phenylketonuria is a very serious disease as it results in severe mental deficiency and the children suffering from this disease are mentally retarted because of the fact that metabolites of phenylketon-

uria i.e. phenylpyruvic acid, phenyllactic acid and phenylacetic acid inhibit the formation of serotonin, a potent metabolite of brain.

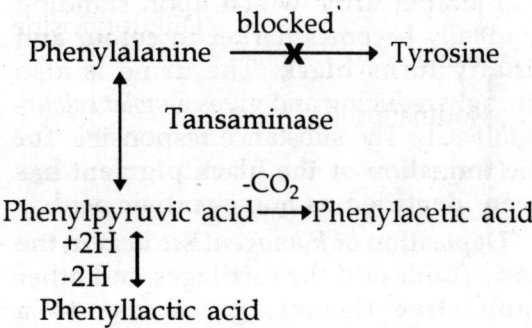

(ii) Tyrosinosis

This is an inborn error of metabolism associated with the metabolism of phenylalanine and tyrosine. The enzyme missing/deficient in this disorder is known as p - hydroxyphenyl pyruvate oxidase; due to the deficiency of this enzyme p - hydroxyphenylpyruvic acid is not converted to homogentisic acid resulting in the deposition of p - hydroxyphenyl-pyruvic acid in the blood. It's a very rare hereditary disorder in which p - hydroxy-phenylpyruvic acid and tyrosine are excreted in the urine.

The first authentic case of *tyrosinosis* was described by the scientist *Medes* in the year 1932.

(iii) Alkaptonuria

It's an inborn error of metabolism associated with the metabolism of phenylalanine and tyrosine. The enzyme missing/deficient is known as **homogentisic acid oxidase**; as a result of the deficiency of this enzyme homogentisic acid is not catalysed to form fumarylaceto-acetic acid. The net result is the accumulation of homogentisic acid in the blood and other body fluids which is later on excreted via urine.

Alkaptonuria is characterized by the excretion of urine which upon standing gradually **becomes darker in colour and finally turns black**. The urine is also strongly reducing and gives a *violet colour-with* FeCl$_3$. The substance responsible **for the formation of the black pigment has been identified as homogentisic acid.**

Deposition of *homogentisic acid* **in the body fluids and the cartilages and other connective tissues, gives rise to a condition known as** *ochronosis.*

(iv) Albinism

This is also an inborn error of the metabolism of phenylalanine and tyrosine. The enzyme missing/deficient is known as *tyrosinase,* the deficiency of which does not catalyse the formation of melanins from tyrosine. **In this disorder, the natural melanin pigments of hair, skin and eyes are not formed.**

Total albinism is a hereditary condition in which there is complete absence of pigment in the skin, eyes and hair. It is due to absence of enzyme *tyrosinase* in the melanocytes and is transmitted as a simple recessive. **There are known various types of hereditary albinism in which pigment is only found to be lacking from certain parts of the body, such as the eye, areas of the skin and areas of the hair.**

Metabolism of Tryptophan

It's an aromatic amino acid and it is the only amino acid which contains indole ring in its structure. It is an essential amino acid. Omission of tryptophan from the diet of human beings is promptly followed by tissue wasting and negative nitrogen balance. Tryptophan has the metabolic distinction of giving rise to nicotinic acid, serotonin and indoles on the one hand and glucose and ketone bodies on the other hand as shown below:

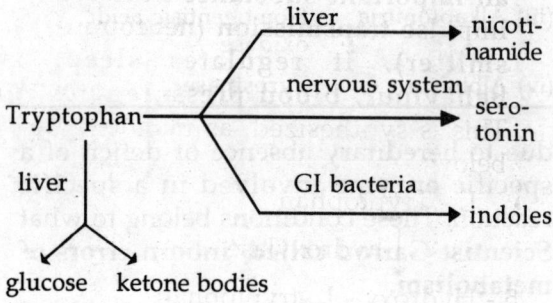

Tryptophan is metabolised in the following way:

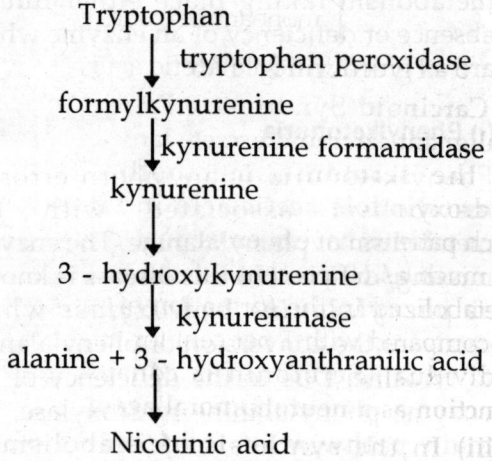

Salient features of this pathway are:

(i) **This pathway gives rise to the synthesis of niacin. 60 mgs of tryptophan gives rise to 1 mg of nicotinic acid in the human body.** In human diet, tryptophan is not in so much amount to meet the requirement of this vitamin.

(ii) **In the synthesis of serotonin: The vasoconstrictor substance 5 -**

hydroxy tryptamine or serotonin is synthesized which remains present in the blood, particularly in the gastric mucosa, intestine, brain, mast cells and blood platelets. **It is an important substance in nerve impulse transmission (neurotransmitter). It regulates sleep, behaviour, blood pressure, etc.** This is synthesized, as mentioned below:

L - Tryptophan

$\downarrow$ hydroxylase

5 - Hydroxy - L -tryptophan

$\downarrow$ decarboxylase

5 - Hydroxytryptamine (serotonin)

$\downarrow$ monoamine oxidase (MAO)

5 - Hydroxyindole acetic acid

Carcinoid Syndrome : Patients with malignant carcinoid excrete large amounts of the serotonin metabolite i.e. 5-hydroxyindole acetic acid in the urine. Such patients have been estimated to utilize as much as 60 percent of the tryptophan metabolized in the formation of serotonin as compared with 1 per cent for the normal individual. **Serotonin is considered to function as a neurohumoral agent.**

(iii) In the synthesis of indole and skatole : This is the minor pathway by which tryptophan is metabolized as a result of which indole, indole acetic acid and skatole are formed in the large intestine due to action of certain bacteria. The foul smell of the feces is due to these substances. These are excreted via urine or faeces.

Hartnup disease: This is an inbron error of metabolism associated with *tryptophan metabolism.* It has been named after the first detected family. **The enzyme deficient is *tryptophanperoxidase.*** This disease is characterized by the following three main symptoms:

(i) **Pellagra like dermatitis, the affected victims display skin lesions.**

(ii) **Sensitivity to sunlight**

(iii) **Motor ataxia characteristic of cerebellar dysfunction.**

Treatment: The treatment of patients with Hartnup disease consists in supplementing the diet with additional amount of niacin to alleviate the dermatological and neurological lesions together with protection from sunlight and the periodic sterilization of the gastrointestinal tract with antibiotics to reduce the formation of the bacterial breakdown products of tryptopban that may exert toxic effects.

got the capability to further hydrolyze
nucleosides to form D-ribose, D-
deoxyribose, purine and pyrimidine bases
are known as nucleosidases which are

Bios
Puri
con
nucl
Diph
syn
B)
con
syn

CHAPTER 18

DIGESTION AND ABSORPTION OF NUCLEOPROTEINS AND METABOLISM OF NUCLEIC ACIDS

> We play special role in body. Ours importance is tremendous. When the enzymes of our metabolism are either missing or deficient, then we cause havoc in the body, for eg; excessive production of uric acid and abnormalities of central nervous system which include mental retardation, spasticity, choreoathetosis (irregular, jerky, explosive, involuntary movements), xanthine stones, fatigue, exercise- induced muscle- aches, loss of immune system and even death at an early age.

Digestion and Absorption of Nucleoproteins

The protein part of the nucleoproteins is easily hydrolyzed by the following two types of enzymes viz:

(i) **gastric enzymes,**

(ii) **intestinal enzymes**

As a result of hydrolysis, the protein portion of nucleoproteins is broken down to its constituent amino acids; whereas the remaining part of nucleoproteins i.e., nucleic acids is not broken down in the stomach but is acted upon by pancreatic nucleases in the intestine. Ribonuclease found in pancreatic juice hydrolyzes ribonucleic acid (RNA) splitting off particularly pyrimidine mononucleotides.

Another enzyme which hydrolyzes deoxyribonucleic acid (DNA) to oligonucleotides (composed of a few mononucleotides) is a pancreatic deoxyribonuclease. **Besides these two important enzymes, other enzymes, found in intestinal mucosa are known as nucleases such as phosphodiesterase which hydrolyzes the nucleic acids completely to mononucleotides** which are further hydrolyzed by intestinal phosphatases (nuclotidases) to inorganic phosphate and nucleosides. It appears that nucleosides are not further hydrolyzed in the intestine but are absorbed as such.

Corresponding enzymes which have

got the capability to further hydrolyze nucleosides to form D-ribose, D-deoxyribose, purine and pyrimidine bases are known as nucleosidases which are found in the extracts of various tissues of the body like liver, kidney, bone marrow etc. Some examples are given below:

uracil riboside + H_2O $\xrightarrow{\text{nucleosidase}}$ uracil + ribose
(uridine)

guanine riboside + Pi $\xrightarrow[\text{phosphorylase}]{\text{nucleoside}}$ guanine + (guanosine) α-D-ribose-1-P

. Nucleoside phosphorylase found in liver and other tissues acts upon various nucleosides.

Biosynthesis of Purines

Purines like adenine. guanine and their corresponding ribo and deoxyribo nucleosides are not synthesized as such in higher organisms, instead they are synthesized as nucleotides.

> Body does not require purines and pyrimidines in the diet but has got the capability to synthesize them *de novo(from* the begining) from the products of carbohydrate and protein metabolism.
> Site of synthesis of purine nucleotides is liver.

Biosynthesis of Purine Nucleotides

Various components of the purine ring are derived from the following i.e.,:
 (i) formate,   (ii) CO_2,
(iii) glutamine   (iv) aspartic acid, and
 (v) glycine
    as shown in Figure 18.1

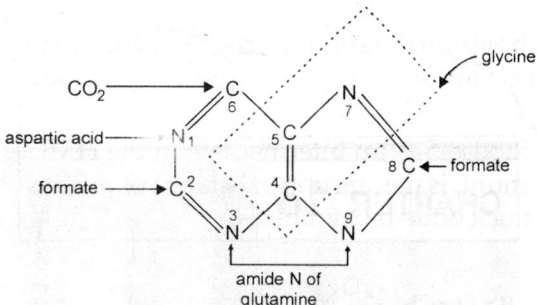

Fig. 18.1 : To show various sources of the purine ring

> ## WHY IS THE BIOSYNTHESIS OF NUCLEOTIDES IMPORTANT?
>
> - Adenine nucleotides like AMP, ADP and ATP are centrally involved in cellular metabolism.
> - ATP is the biological "quantum" of energy.
> - Nucleotide coenzymes like NAD, NADP and coenzyme A contain nucleotide moieties as part of their structures.

The purines are synthesized *de novo* not as free purines but first of all as the nucleotide inosinic acid (hypoxanthine-ribose-5'-phosphate), which is later on converted to adenine and guanine nucleotides. Purine ring gets built on to ribose-5'phosphate through many intermediates to form inosinic acid as shown below:

Biosynthesis of purine nucleotides involves 10 steps in all as shown below:

Step 1

Synthesis of inosinic acid begins with D-ribose 5-phosphate which is formed during pentose phosphate pathway (HMP shunt). D-ribose-5-P in the presence of ATP and Mg^{++} ions is converted into 5-

phosphoribosyl-1-pyrophosphate; the reaction is catalyzed by PRPP synthetase.

> Ribose-5-P, an intermediate in the HMP shunt, is the starting substance of purine nucleotide biosynthesis.

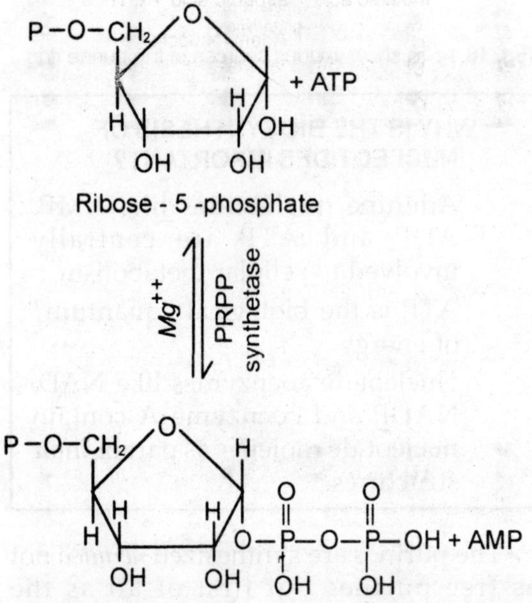

Ribose - 5 -phosphate

5 -Phosphoribosyl - 1 - pyrophosphate (PRPP)

Step 2

5- phosphoribosyl-1-pyrophosphate then reacts with glutamine to replace the pyrophosphate group (PP) by an -NH$_2$ group as a result of which 5-phosphoribosyl-1-amine is formed; this reaction is catalysed by the enzyme 5-phosphoribosyl pyrophosphate amidotrans-ferase.

Step 3

Now, 5-phosphoribosyl-1-amine in the presence of glycine and ATP is converted to glycinamide ribotide; the reaction being

catalyzed by the enzyme 2-amino-N-ribosylacetamide -
5'- phosphate kinosynthase (glycinamide ribotide kinosynthase).

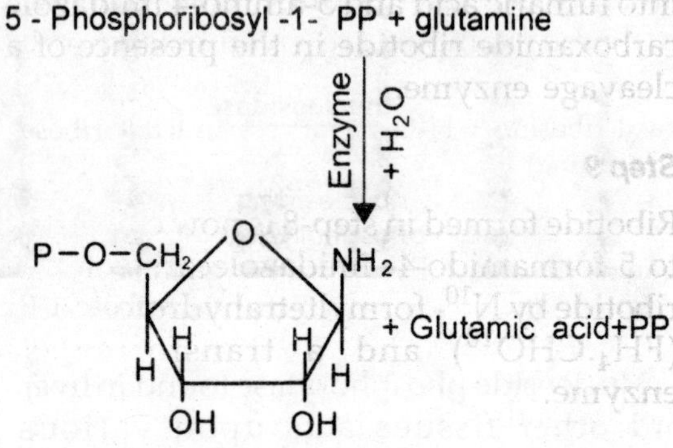

5 - Phosphoribosyl -1- PP + glutamine

5 -Phosphoribosyl - 1 - amine

Step 4

Glycinamide ribotide is now converted to formylglycinamide ribotide in the presence of N^5, N^{10} - anhydroformyltetrahydrofolic acid; the reaction is catalyzed by glycinamide ribotide transformylase.

Step 5

Now formylglycinamide ribotide reacts with glutamine and ATP forming a new product known as formylglycinamidine ribotide, which then undergoes ring closure to form 5 -amino-imidazole ribotide.

Step 6

5- aminoimidazole ribotide is then carboxylated to form 5-amino-4-imidazole carboxylic acid ribotide by the enzyme aminoimidazole ribotide carboxylase.

Step 7

In this step, 5 - amino- 4 imidazolecarboxylic acid ribotide reacts with aspartic acid and ATP to form the product 5-amino-4-imidazole- N-succinocarboxamide ribotide.

Step 8

Ribotide formed in step 7 is then cleaved into fumaric acid and 5-amino-4 imidazole carboxamide ribotide in the presence of a cleavage enzyme.

Step 9

Ribotide formed in step-8 is now converted to 5-formamido-4- imidazolecarboxamide ribotide by N^{10}- formyltetrahydrofolic acid ($FH_4.CHO^{10}$) and a transformylase enzyme.

$$5 - Amino - 4 - imidazolecarboxamide$$
$$ribotide + FH_4.CHO^{10}$$

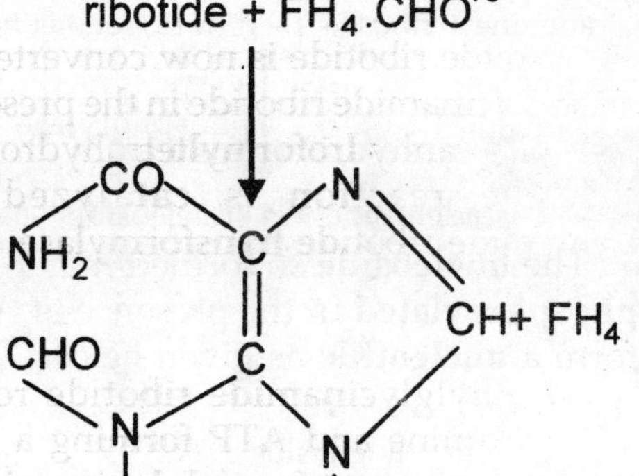

5 - Formamido - 4 - imidazole - carboxamide ribotide

Step 10

Now,. the ribotide formed in step 9 is converted to inosinic acid by the action of enzyme inosinicase. In this reaction, the product formed contains complete closed ring which is known as a hypoxanthine ring. This is a very important step in which complete hypoxanthine ring is formed.

Step 11

Formation of Adenylic Acid (adenosine -5'-phosphate)

It involves two steps i.e., steps 11 & 12. In this step, inosinic acid in the presence of aspartic acid and GTP is converted to adenylosuccinic acid as shown below:

Inosinic acid + aspartic acid + GTP

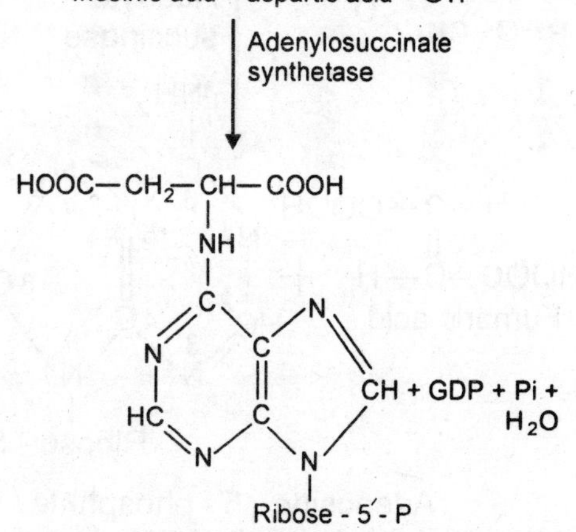

Adenylosuccinic acid

Step 11a

Formation of Guanylic Acid (guanosine-5'-phosphate):

The mononucleotide guanylic acid is synthesized from inosinic acid (Step-10) through xanthylic acid:

Inosinic acid

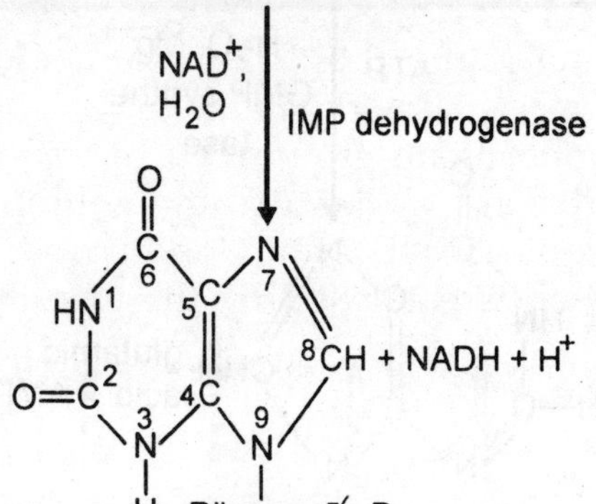

Xanthosine - 5' - monophosphate ie, XMP (xanthylic acid)

Step 12

Now, adenylosuccinic acid gets split into fumaric acid and adenylic acid by the action of enzyme adenylosuccinase.

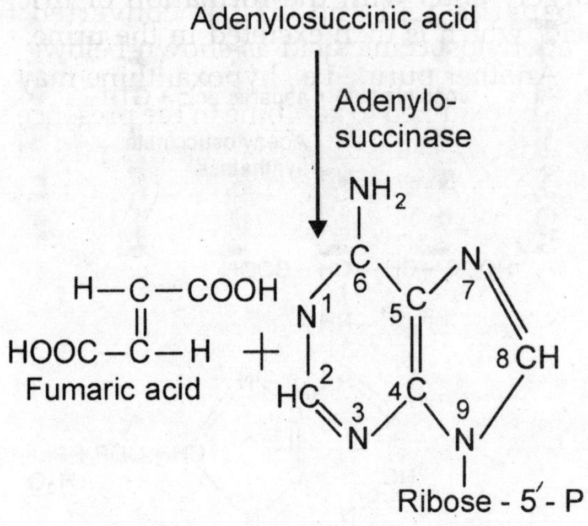

Adenylosuccinic acid

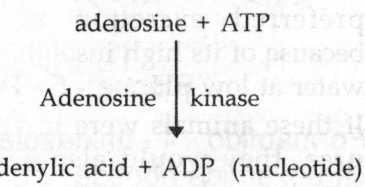

Adenylo-
succinase

NH_2

H–C–COOH

HOOC–C–H
Fumaric acid

Ribose - 5′- P

Adenosine - 5′- phosphate
(adenylic acid)

Step 12a

Xanthylic acid may now be aminated in the 2nd position in the presence of glutamine and ATP to form guanylic acid.

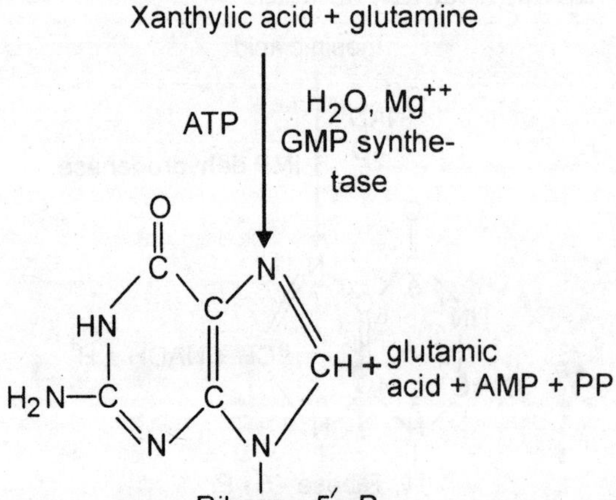

Xanthylic acid + glutamine

ATP H_2O, Mg^{++}
GMP synthe-
tase

CH + glutamic
acid + AMP + PP

Ribose - 5′- P

Guanosine - 5′- phosphate
(guanylic acid)

Salvage Pathways of Nucleotide Synthesis

Nucleosides and nucleotides may be synthesized from purine bases by the reactions as shown below:

adenine + phosphoribosyl - pyrophosphate
(nitrogenous base) (phosphorylated sugar i.e., ribose)

↓ enzyme

adenylic acid + PP
(a nucleotide; combination of
a nitrogenous base, sugar & phosphate)

Similar reactions are given by guanine and hypoxanthine.

Nucleosides may be formed by the reaction with ribose-1-phosphate as shown below:

adenine + ribose - 1 - P (nitrogenous base)

↓ phosphorylase

adenosine + Pi (nucleoside)

The **nucleoside** so formed may then be **phosphorylated in** the presence of ATP to form **a nucleotide** as given below:

adenosine + ATP

Adenosine | kinase

adenylic acid + ADP (nucleotide)

In this way, adenylic acid may be formed in animals by a so-called salvage pathway from adenine and then incorporated into nucleic acids but on the other hand this is not the case with guanine.

PURINE CATABOLISM

The end products of purine catabolism vary widely with different animal species;

for instance man and other primates, birds and certain reptiles convert purines to **uric acid whereas mammals other than primates and gastropods have a tendency to carry the breakdown still farther and thus allantoin is the end product of purnies catabolism in them. Allantoin is formed by the action of uricase upon uric acid.**

Enzyme adenase appears to be absent from the tissues of man, hence the conversion of adenine to hypoxanthine is not possible in man. However, this enzyme is found to be present in some animals like cow, etc., hence, the conversion of adenine to hypoxanthine is possible in them.

- Uric acid is quite insoluble in water, but contrarily, urea is highly soluble in water.
- Birds and fishes (**uricotelic animals**) excrete uric acid rather than urea as the end product of nitrogen catabolism. The urine of these animals is acidic and contains a high proportion of crystalline uric acid.
- Uric acid is apparently the preferred excretion product because of its high insolubility in water at low pH.
- If these animals were to excrete urea, they would also have to excrete very large amount of water which had been fatal to them.
- **Thus, conservation of water is the main advantage of uric acid excretion.**

Enzyme guanase is found to be present in various tissues of the human body like liver, kidneys, spleen, pancreas etc, which deaminizes guanine to xanthine (Fig. 18.2).

Now, in the next reaction, enzyme xanthine oxidase (found in the liver of man and several other organs) oxidizes xanthine to uric acid (enol form). In man and other primates, purine catabolism largely ends with the formation of uric acid, which is then excreted in the urine.

Another purine i.e., hypoxanthine may also be oxidized to xanthine in the presence of enzyme xanthine oxidase (Fig 18.2) which then enters the main pool.

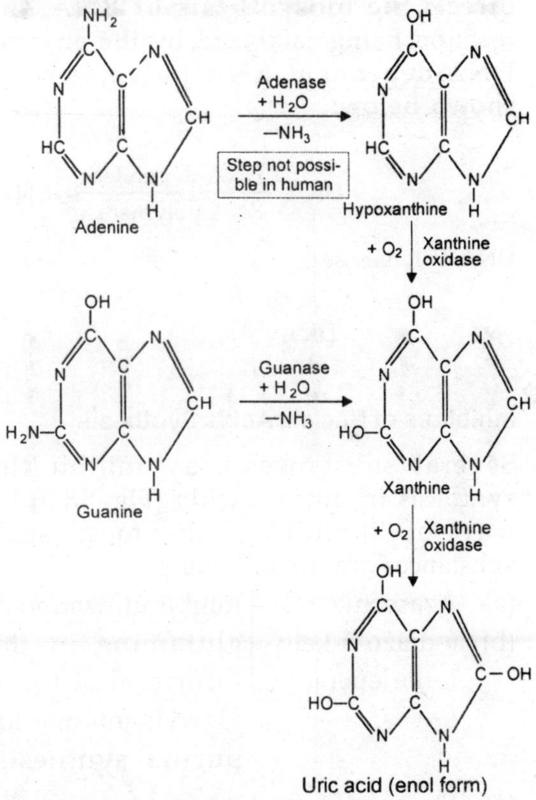

Note: Adenine, guanine, hypoxanthine and xanthine are purines.

Fig. 18.2 : Purine Catabolism

BIOSYNTHESIS OF NUCLEIC ACIDS

According to general view, the relationship between DNA and RNA during cell division and cell growth is as follows:

$$DNA \xrightarrow{\text{transcription}} RNA \longrightarrow Protein$$

$$\text{replication} \downarrow$$

$$DNA$$

The relationship shown in the diagram above suggests that DNA directs its own synthesis which is carried out by the enzyme DNA polymerase. The diagram also suggests that DNA also directs the biosynthesis of RNA; the reaction being catalyzed by the enzyme DNA-dependent RNA polymerase as shown below:

$$DNA \xrightarrow[\text{RNA polymerase}]{\text{DNA-dependent}} RNA$$

$$\text{DNA-Polymerase} \downarrow$$

$$DNA$$

Inhibitors of Nucleic Acids Synthesis

Several substances may inhibit the synthesis of nucleic acids (Fig. 18.3) by way of inhibiting enzymes; such substances are the following:

(a) Azaserine ⎤ inhibit utilization of
(b) 6-diazo-5-keto- ⎟ glutamine in the
    L-norleucine ⎦ formation of form-
                   ylglycinamidine for
                   purine synthesis.

(c) Pteroylglutamic interferes with the
    acid (structural formylation reacti-
    analogue of ons involved in
    folic acid) purine and pyrimi-
                   dine synthesis.

(d) 8-azaguanine
    (purine derivative)

(e) 6-mercaptopurine
    (purine derivative)

(f) 4-azathymine
    (pyrimidine struc-
    tural analogue)

(g) Antibiotic-Anthra- ⎤ inhibit replication
    mycin ⎟ by respectively
                   covalent and
(h) Antibiotic-Actino- ⎟ noncovalent
    mycin-D ⎦ binding with the
                   DNA template
                   strand.

(i) Antibiotic- prevents replication
    Mitomycin by 'intrastrand cross-
                   links' in DNA
                   strands.

(j) Antibiotic-Nov- **blocks superhelical**
    obiocin **tertiary structures**
                   of bacterial DNA
                   by inhibiting DNA
                   gyrases.

Because, the growth of tumor cells is closely related to the rapid synthesis of the nucleic acids i.e., DNA and RNA, therefore, aim should always be to check the synthesis of these nucleic acids vis-a-vis the growth of the tumor cells should then be automatically checked. Various inhibitors of nucleic acids synthesis which possess low toxicity to the normal cells should be employed with full watch. Unfortunately, most of the substances exhibit toxicity, some less and whereas some more. Chemical structures of some of the inhibitors are as given over here:

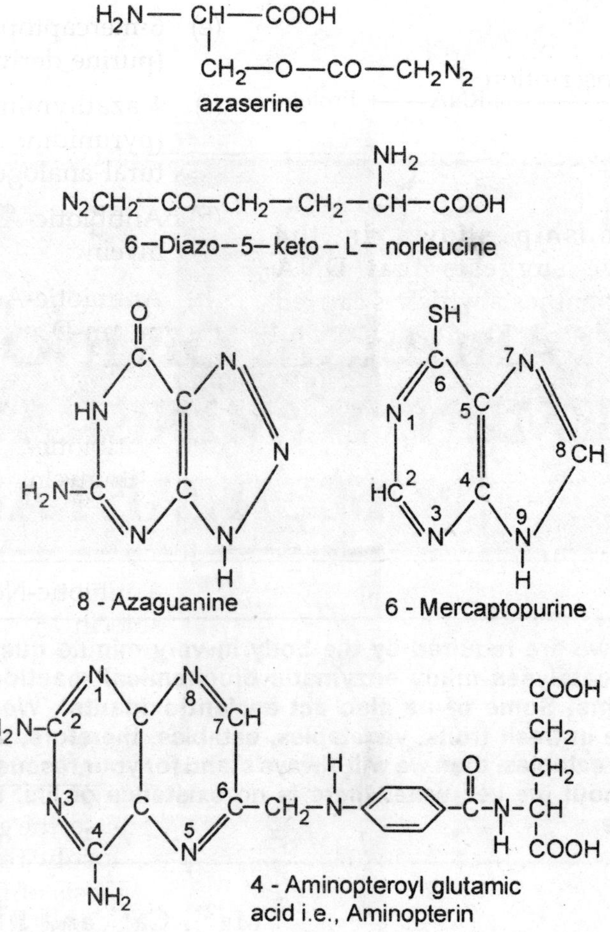

Fig 18.3 : Chemical structures of some inhibitors of nucleic acids synthesis

---

Adenosine Deaminase (ADA) Deficiency and Purine Nucleoside Phosphorylase (PNP) Deficiency

ADA deficiency and PNP deficiency are two autosomal recessive traits that cause immune system dysfunction. Both enzymes function in conversion of adenosine and deoxyadenosine to hypoxanthine. PNP is also involved in conversion of guanosine and deoxyguanosine to guanine. In ADA or PNP deficiency, the appropriate substrates accumulate along with other alternative products to cause toxic effects on the cells of the immune system.

Patients with ADA deficiency lack both T- and B-lymphocyte-mediated functions, namely, cellular and humoral immunity, respectively, and exhibit a severe combine immunodeficiency (SCID) disorder. Other genetic defects can cause SCID, but ADA deficiency is responsible for about one-third of patients who have SCID. PNP deficiency is associated only with T-lymphocyte dysfunction.

In general,
only i
Se is
perox
In body
prov
norm
be ad
Water as

present in the main nudear fluid
concentration it
whethe of

METABOLISM OF INORGANIC ELEMENTS (MINERALS) AND WATER METABOLISM

Although, we are required by the body in very minute quantity but ours presence catalyses many enzymatic biochemical reactions of various metabolisms. Some of us also act as 'antioxidants'. We are found in abundance in fresh fruits, vegetables, eatables, therefore, if you will love the natural eatables, then we will always stand for your rescue against many odds. Without me i.e., water there is no existence of life. Life is in peril without me.

MINERALS

The main minerals that are required by the human body are listed below in the Table 19.1 along with the daily requirement and the deficiency symptoms. Main minerals are sodium, potassium, magnesium, calcium, iron, copper, chloride, phosphate, iodine and fluoride. Requirement for Na^+ and Cl^- reflects the fact that these are the main ions excreted in urine and sweat; whereas requirement for iron is determined largely by the rate of its excretion in the faeces. The ions are digested in a number of ways. The bulk of Na^+ and Cl^- is eaten in the form of salt. The other ions are present either as free salts in food and water, examples K^+,

Mg^{2+}, Ca^{2+} and F^- or bound to other molecules, for examples Fe^{2+}, Zn^{2+}, PO_4^- and I^-.

Each ion performs a number of functions in the body.

A requirement for chromium has been reported, **and in animals selenium is required for satisfactory reproduction but is toxic if taken in excess.**

The most important inorganic requirements for the human beings are Na, K, Ca, Mg, Fe, Cu, Zn, Mo, Cl, I, and P. (Table 19.1). Sulphur as sulphate is essential for the formation of certain body constituents, but it is always organic sulphur, in the form of sulphur-containing amino acids, which is oxdized to sulphate

Table19.1: Mineral requirements and deficiency symptoms

Sl. No.	Ion	Approximate Daily requirement	Deficiency symptoms
1.	Na^+ (Sodium)	5g; 200 m mol	Dehydration, acidosis
2.	K^+ (Potassium)	3g; 75 m mol	Acidosis, renal damage, cardiac arrest
3.	Mg^{2+} (Magnesium)	0.3g; 15 m mol	Muscular tremor, mental depression
4.	Ca^{2+} (Calcium)	0.8g; 20 m mol	Rickets in children and osteomalacia in adults
5.	Fe^{2+} (Iron)	10 mg; 200 μmol	Anaemia
6.	Zn^{2+} (Zinc)	15mg; 200 μmol	Anaemia, stunted growth
7.	Cu^{2+} (Copper)	3mg; 50 μmol	Anaemia (hypochromic), various nervous lesions
8.	Cl^- (Chloride)	7g; 200 mmol	Alkalosis
9.	Phosphate	0.8g; 30mmol	Renal rickets
10.	Iodine	0.1 mg; 1 μmol	Endemic goitre (hypothyroidism)
11.	F (Fluoride)	2mg; 100 μmol	Dental caries

in vivo. Co, as far as known at present, is only necessary in the form of vitamin B_{12}. Se is a constituent of glutathione peroxidase. The involvement of Cr and V in normal human physiology is not yet proven. Fluoride does not form part of the normal body requirements, but it should be added regularly in traces to drinking water as a preventive factor of dental caries.

Potassium is the main inorganic cation present in the intracellular fluid, as distinct from plasma and extracellular water. Its concentration is about 3.2 g (80 meq) per kg (muscle). It also occurs to the extent of about 4 meq per litre in plasma. Since it is universally abundant in foodstuffs, whether of plant or animal origin, there is usually no difficulty in supplying the daily requirements, probably in the order of 1 g per day (20-30 meq). Disturbances of potassium metabolism may occur, particularly in derangements of the adrenal cortical gland.

Besides the main minerals as mentioned above, our body also requires large number of elements called as 'trace elements' in minor quantity for proper functioning. These include sulphur, zinc, manganese, cobalt, molybdenum, selenium, chromium etc.

SODIUM

It is the main ion of the plasma and other extracellular fluids. Under normal dietary conditions, human beings are not subject to the deficiency of sodium. However, excessive diarrhoea, pernicious vomiting or extreme sweating over a long period may bring about the deficiency of sodium and chloride. Now a days, it is a common practice to supply extra amount of sodium chloride either in the form of salt water or salt tablets to those, who are subjected/exposed to excessive heat like labourers, workers, rikshaw pullers etc. Normal sodium chloride consumption of an individual is nearly 10g per day (about 4g of sodium) which is supplied easily by the dietary ingredients. This is many times the actual requirement. In health, excess salt consumed is excreted by the kidneys.

Main functions of sodium are:

(a) It maintains the osmotic pressure i.e. osmolarity throughout the body. Osmolarity is maintained at approximately 0.3 mol/l (it is approximately made up of 0.15 mol/l of Na^+ and 0.15 mol/l of Cl^-).

(b) It maintains the normal state of acid-base balance.

(c) It maintains the normal state of water balance.

(d) It plays a role in gaseous transport.

An average adult requires about 4 g Na^+ per day (150-200 meq), of which about 1g (50 meq) is in foodstuffs before flavouring is added. Intakes lower than 50 meq may be tolerated with difficulty, but the requirement may be greatly increased in many circumstances, particularly when a hot climate or prolonged exercise have caused a considerable loss of Na^+ in perspiration. Insufficient Na^+ intake can give rise to heat exhaustion or heat stroke, characterized by muscular weakness, nausea and fever. The excretion of sodium is carefully regulated by renal mechanisms under the control chiefly of aldosterone, and may be abnormal in the diseases of the adrenal gland.

(e) It maintains the muscle and nerve irritability at the proper level.

(f) In blood plasma sodium chloride has got an outstanding function of keeping the globulins in physical solution. It also regulates the degree of hydration of the plasma proteins, vis-a-vis the viscosity of blood.

(g) Gastric HCl is derived from the sodium chloride of the blood.

Saline depletion causes cramps, weakness and faintness and clinical features of 'dehydration', diminished tissue turgor, hypotension and peripheral circulatory failure.

Saline overloading is most often the result of a primary disturbance of the function of the heart, kidneys, or liver which leads to complex causes like oedema and raised central venous pressure. Occasionally, it is caused by the excess intravenous infusion of saline.

POTASSIUM

It is a very important mineral for various functions of the human body. Under normal dietary conditions, human beings do not suffer from potassium deficiency. The human potassium intake is around 2 to 4 g per day which is supplied easily by the dietary items that we eat daily. Again this is far more than our requirement, and the excess is excreted in the urine. It is the principal cation of intracellular fluid. Its metabolism is regulated by the hormone named as *aldosterone.*

Important functions of potassium in human body are as given below:

(a) It maintains the osmotic pressure (osmolarity) in its normal range throughout the body.

(b) It helps in maintaining the normal state of acid base balance.

(c) It maintains water balance.

(d) It plays an important role in gaseous transport.

(e) It helps in maintaining muscle and nerve irritability at the proper level.

(f) Like sodium chloride, potassium chloride has also an outstanding function of keeping the globulins in physical solution and also helps in the regulation of the degree of hydration of the plasma proteins which is eventually very important for proper viscosity of the blood:

(g) Potassium is required by several enzymes of glycolysis and other pathways. It may be required for nuclear activity and also for protein synthesis.

Hypokalaemia causes tiredness, **muscle weakness, paralysis, mental confusion and polyuria. It is commonly noticed after the prolonged administration of powerful diuretic drugs.** Such drugs provoke an increased flow of urine by inhibiting the activity of enzymes in the renal tubules that are responsible for the absorption of Na^+ and Cl^-. When, however, there is low dietary intake of Na^+ and high level of circulating aldosterone, these diuretics promote the exchange of Na^+ for K^+ in the distal tubule and thus lead to an increased excretion of K^+. Chronic diarrhoea and repeated vomiting also are responsible for **hypokalaemia.**

Potassium is toxic in high amounts (hyperkalaemia) by virtue of the fact that it stops the heart beat and thus leads to death. Besides, hyperkalaemia also causes small bowel ulcers.

MAGNESIUM

Adult human body contains nearly 20-25 g magnesium. It is an indispensable constituent of all living cells. About 60 percent of the magnesium of the body remains present in the bones. In muscles magnesium exceeds calcium as regards amount, whereas in blood, the reverse is true. In blood it remains very constant.

Biological Functions: Magnesium ions act as activator for number of enzymes such as hexokinases, phosphorylases enolase, alkaline phosphatase, DNA polymerase, phosphoglu-comutase, etc.

Absorption and excretion: About one-third or less of the magnesium in the diet is absorbed. In a state of balance, the amount of magnesium in the urine equals that absorbed, which in normal men has been found to average 162 ± 45 mg per day. Faecal magnesium represents that which remains unabsorbed. High dietary intake of fat, calcium and phosphorus reduces its absorption and so is the condition with alkaline food.

It is excreted both in urine and faeces. Nearly 70% of it is excreted via faeces. Intake of alkaline food reduces its excretion via urine.

Urine is the principal route of its excretion; most magnesium filtered by the glomeruli is reabsorbed by the renal tubules.

Requirement:

Its daily requirement is 250 - 300 mg.

Sources:

It is found in such amount in plant foods and meat that there is little possibility of the diet being inadequate in it. However, the main sources include meat, eggs, green leafy vegetables potato, cereals, fruits, etc.

Deficiency symptoms: These may be observed in chronic alcoholics, uraemics, tetany, children suffering from kwashiorkor, pregnancy (particularly toxaemia of pregnancy), rickets, diabetic acidosis, diarrhoea and vomiting. Its deficiency causes depression, hyperirritability (muscle spasm or convulsions), cardiac arrhythmias, muscular weakness and convulsions. Its normal level in blood is from 1-3 mg/dl.

Hypermagnesemia: Excess magnesium in the body can occur when absorption from the gut exceeds excretion by the kidneys, as happens in renal insufficiency. Its pharmacological effects are characterized by:

(i) Depression of the central nervous system

(ii) Depression of the cardiovascular system

(iii) Depression of the blood pressure.

IRON

Introduction and Storage:

Our body contains nearly 4 g iron; nearly 70% of which remains present in blood in the form of **haemoglobin** or similar structures such as **myoglobin. Small amount of iron acts as cofactors in many enzyme reactions, notably those of oxidation. The remaining, about 25% is stored in the following:**

(i) Liver

(ii) Reticuloendothelial system

(iii) Spleen, and

(iv) Bone marrow, bound to protein.

Nearly 3 mg of iron is found in transit in blood plasma which remains bound largely to a β-globulin called as **transferrin.** Iron is found in the body in two forms, i.e., the essential iron and the storage iron.

Absorption: Its absorption occurs mainly in the stomach and the duodenum. Normally nearly 6.5% of the dietary iron is absorbed. The absorption may be increased by 20 percent in mensurating and pregnant women. Its absorption from the food depends upon several factors such as the form of iron and other constituents present in the diet. **Alcohol, hydrochloric acid, Vitamin C, etc promote its absorption while tea decreases it.** The amount absorbed depends upon the individual's need for iron.

The well known mechanism for absorption of iron in the mucosal cells is known as **mucosal block theory.** After digestion, iron present in the diet gets converted into the ferrous form (Fe^{2+}) by the H^+ and the reducing substances, such as vitamin C present in the intestinal lumen. It is the only form in which iron is absorbed. Transfer of iron from the intestinal lumen into mucosa is an energy dependent process. After absorption Fe^{2+} is oxidised to Fe^{3+} and combines with apoferritin which is converted to ferritin. Apoferritin has got a very rapid turnover which is degraded and reformed when the absorption of iron takes place. The high concentration of ferritin in the mucosal cell further blocks the absorption of iron.

Iron from ferritin (Fe^{3+}) is reduced to Fe^{2+} and passes into the blood capillaries which is again oxidised to Fe^{3+} and combines with apotransferrin for its conversion to transferrin, the form in which iron is transported in plasma. The excess of iron which cannot be stored as ferritin is then stored in liver as **haemosiderin.** When excessive hemoglobin iron is given repeatedly to an indvidual by transfusion then it results into excess storage **(haemosiderosis).** In iron-deficiency anaemia, utilization of iron is increased considerably; under this condition average absorption of dietary iron increases to 20% as compared to nearly 6.5% under normal conditions.

The oxidation of Fe^{2+} to Fe^{3+} is catalysed by ferroxidase I (ceruloplasmin) and ferroxidase II. Ferro-reductases reduce Fe^{3+} iron to Fe^{2+} form. This oxidation and reduction of iron is essential as it remains present in the Fe^{2+} form in hemoglobin whereas in the Fe^{3+} form in ferritin and transferrin.

Iron is used with great economy in the body. Daily destruction of the red blood cells (RBCs) contributes nealy 25 mg of iron to the iron pool which is stored as ferritin and reused whenever required for the synthesis of hemoglobin.

Excretion of iron gets increased particularly in the hot moist climate which causes **iron deficiency anaemia.** Normally, its excretion takes place through the following routes:

a) Faecal: (The unabsorbed iron is excreted via faeces which is nearly 90% of the food iron).

b) Renal: (Nearly 0.05 mg/day through urine).

c) Dermal : (0.5 - 1.8 mg/day through sweat)

d) Menstrual : (35-70 ml per period, average daily loss would amount to 0.5 to 1.0 mg/day)

e) Gestational, and (iron is lost by mother during pregnancy. About 300 mg of iron is transferred to the foetus).

f) Lactational: (0.5 - 0.7 mg if 400 - 600 ml milk is lactated.)

Besides the above, iron loss also occurs through hair clippings, combing and nail clippings which amounts to nearly 1.2 mg per year (1 to 5 µg/day).

Plasma Iron level and its variations

a) Males: 80 to 175 µg per 100 ml
b) Females: 60 to 160 µg per 100 ml

An increase in the concentration is often found in **haemochromatosis,** acute infective hepatitis, etc. whereas its low values are found in iron-deficiency anaemias.

Biological functions:

It plays indispensable role in human body. Its main functions are:

(i) It is involved in the transport of oxygen by hemoglobin and hemoerythrin.

(ii) It is involved in the electron transfer reactions including oxidative phosphorylation.

(iii) It is involved in the synthesis of DNA (as an essential component of ribonucleotide reductase).

(iv) It is involved in the catalysis of oxidation by oxygen and hydrogen peroxide.

(v) It is involved in the decomposition of harmful derivatives of oxygen notably peroxide and superoxide.

(vi) Besides, it also plays a very important role in the fixation of nitrogen and hydrogen.

(vii) It is a component of several proteins such as hemoglobin, myoglobin, peroxidases, catalases, cytochromes and iron requiring enzymes, e.g. xanthine oxidase, acyl CoA **dehydrogenase** and NADH reductase.

(viii) It is also required as a cofactor for various enzymes like aconitase, succinic dehydrogenase, ribonucleotide reductase, etc.

Body Iron: It remains present in the body as a part of several compounds which play role in respiration. Its total amount varies from 2-6 g in healthy adults.

Transport: It is transported in the body by a specific iron binding β_1-globulin called as transferrin (siderophilin). It performs the functions of selective removal of iron from reticuloendothelial cells and intestinal mucosa and selective delivery of iron to the erythron and placenta. It is a glycoprotein having a molecular weight of 80,000 and binds two atoms of ferric iron. The average transferrin content of plasma is about 250-350 mg per 100 ml. Since each gram of transferrin can bind about 1.25 mg of iron, therefore, the total iron binding capacity is approximately 250-450 µg/ 100 ml of plasma.

Storage: It is stored intracellularly as **ferritin** and **hemosiderin,** mainly in the liver, spleen and bone marrow. Approximately 25% of iron (600 to 1500 mg) in the body is in the form which does not participate in active metabolic process but represents a reserve which can be mobilised whenever there is acute need.

Hook warm infestation leading to chromic blood loss is an important cause of iron deficiency especially in the rural population engaged in agricultural work. Each worm causes a loss of nearly **0.3 ml blood per day. This may be one of the important causative factors in the tribal areas of India.**

It is stored in the ferric form but the release of iron appears to be in the ferrous form.

Iron toxicity: The presence of the excess of iron in the body results in its deposition as **ferritin** and **hemosiderin** in various tissues such as liver, spleen, bone marrow, skin etc which is called as **hemosiderosis.**

Deficiency disorders (iron deficiency):

It is the result of an imbalance between iron assimilation and its loss. Deficiency of iron leads to anemia which is a common feature in children, adolescent girls and females of the child bearing age, particularly in the developing countries like India.

Bantu siderosis

In the African tribe Bantus, iron deficiency anemia even in women is unknown, absorption of food iron is very high and considerable hemosiderin is present in liver (siderosis). This has been explained on the basis of the facts that their staple diet is corn (high iron, low phosphate) **which is cooked in iron pots (high in iron) and they consume lot of alcohol which enhances iron absorption.**

Following are the signs and symptoms of anemia:

(a) Dullness

(b) **Inactiveness**

(c) Loss of appetite

(d) Poor growth

(e) Fatigueness

(f) Decreased excrecise tolerance

(g) Weakness

(h) Palpitations

(i) Irritability, and

(j) Headache

Children become dull, inactive, lose appetite and exhibit poor growth. Deficiency in females reduces their work capacity and feel fatigueness and breathlessness upon doing work.

Hemochromatosis

It is a genetic disease transmitted by autosomal recessive gene in which the afflicted person has inherited ability to absorb much greater percentage of food iron which is then deposited in the **skin, pancreas,** and **liver,** giving rise to **bronze colouration, diabetes mellitus** and **cirrhosis** respectively.

Although breast milk is a poor source of iron. Prolonged lactation results in a serious drain on the **iron reserves**. The output of the breast milk during the first two years of lactation is nearly 400-600 g per day and average iron content is 0.12 mg/100 g which gives a daily excretion of 0.5 - 0.7 mg iron through the milk for several months. Thus menstrual irregularities, repeated pregnancies and prolonged lactations apart from dietary inadequacy are the chief causes of iron deficiency anemia in Indian women.

Significant anemia is usually notable **for its pallor pale** face which has long been recognised as a sign of severe iron deficiency anemia which was initially known as **chlorosis.**

Sources: Meat, fish, chicken, liver, green leafy vegetables, etc, are good sources of iron in which its concentration is from 15-20 mg/100g.

Cereals, legumes, potatoes, carrots are also fair sources in which its concentration ranges from 10-15 mg/100g.

Fruits (guava, banana, papaya, etc) generally are poor sources and so are eggs, rice, milk, etc. in which its concentration ranges <5.0 mg per 100 g.

Requirement:

(a) Adult males   : 10 mg per day
(b) Adult females   : 15 mg per day
(c) Pregnant females : 20 mg per day
(d) Children   : 8-15 mg per day depending upon age

Infants are born with additional iron reserves to carry them through the nursing period, for milk contains less than 0.1 mg iron per 100 g. Therefore, iron containing foods are required by the time they are one year old.

Iron deficiency anemia is ranked second only to protein calorie malnutrition including Kwashiorkor. There are two main functions of iron in the body because it is the active centre of the haem group. It is required for:

(i) The functions of hemoglobin, and
(ii) The functions of cytochromes

COPPER

Copper is essential for both plants and animals. It is widely distributed in all human tissues with highest concentrations in liver, brain, heart and kidney.

It is transported by serum albumin hemocuprein and ceruloplasmin to various tissue stores; excess is excreted via bile and to a small extent via the intestinal wall. **Copper does not ordinarily accumulate in the human body with age.**

Physiological functions

(i) It is required in small amounts for the synthesis of normal haemoglobin.

(ii) It is required for the synthesis of;
   (a) Phospholipids,
   (b) Melanin, and
   (c) Collagen.

(iii) It plays role in the formation of bone.

(iv) It maintains the integrity of myelin sheath in the nerve fibres

(v) It is a cofactor of several oxidative enzymes:
   (a) Tyrosinase,

(b) Cytochrome oxidase,

(c) Ascorbic acid oxidase,

(d) Uricase,

(e) Monoamine Oxidase,

(f) Ceruloplasmin (ferroxidase-I)- a blue copper-protein complex,

(g) Non-ceruloplasmin ferroxidase- a yellow copper-protein complex, etc.

(vi) It is also found in some proteins, namely erythrocuprin, cerebrocuprin; and hepatocuprin, which remain present in red blood cells, brain and liver respectively.

Disorders of copper metabolism

Wilson's disease, (hepatolenticular degeneration) is a rare hereditary disorder of copper metabolism which is caused due to an autosomal recessive genetic defect. Following disorders are observed in this disease:

(a) Absorption of copper from the intestine gets increased (nearly 50 per cent); whereas 2-5 per cent copper is absorbed in normal ones.

(b) Ceruloplasmin formation is very less.

(c) The disease is characterized by low plasma copper, low biliary copper, poor serum ferroxidase activity, high urinary copper, excessive deposition of copper in liver, pancreas, kidney, cornea and brain, and consequent symptoms like abnormal muscular movements **(like Parkinson's disease)**, diabetes mellitus, renal tubular damage, a **visible brown ring** *(Kayser-Fleischer ring)* **at the margin of the cornea, hepatic cirrhosis; dementia, jaundice etc. The patient may ultimately die of hepatic** failure.

Menke's disease (Kinky hair syndrome) is characterized by skeletal malformations, immunological deficiency, mental retardation, and defective thermoregulation.

Hypochromic microcytic anaemia takes place in milk-fed infants due to the deficiency of copper.

Copper deficiency may cause atrophy of myocardium. The elastic tissue of aorta, coronary and pulmonary artery gets deranged; these vessels may rupture as a result of which end comes into death.

Copper Toxicity: Its excess casuses Wilson's disease in which there is a positive copper balance due to the deficient synthesis of ceruloplasmin in liver. There is also a defect in the incorporation of Cu into newly synthesized apoceruloplasmin to form ceruloplasmin. Thus excess of copper gets deposited in tissues mainly in liver and basal nuclei of the brain. Besides, it also causes increased excretion of copper which causes renal tubular damage and generalised aminoaciduria.

Sources

Liver, lentils, nuts, dry legumes, fish, oysters, etc. Milk is a poor sources of copper.

Daily Requirement

Adults: 2.5 mg; children: 0.5-2.5 mg.

Normal range

Normal range for plasma/serum copper is within the limits of 75 to 160 μg/100 ml.

Treatment

Treatment consists in the administration of some copper chelating agent such as penicillamine which has got the

capability of removing excess copper from the tissues.

Calcium and its Metabolism

Distribution : This element is the most abundant of all the elements found in the human body. Adult human body contains nearly 1.5. kg of calcium, which is the largest amount for any cation; 99% of this remains present in bones and teeth and the remaining in the body fluids..

In older subjects, especially in the women, bone resorption exceeds bone loss and there is progressive loss of calcium from the skeleton which leads to 'Osteoporosis' in them. This phenomenon is universal in Eastern and as well as Western communities.

Functions:

1. It is required for the formation of bones and teeth

2. Ionic calcium is of great importance in blood coagulation

3. It is required for neuromuscular activity

4. It is required for muscle contractility

5. It is required for myocardial activity

6. It is required for the function of the permeability of membranes

7. It is required for the activity of certain enzymes.

Sources and Dietary Calcium

(i) Milk and cheese are the most important dietary sources of calcium, because the calcium and phosphorus ratio in them is optimal for the absorption of this element.

(ii) Other good sources are egg yolk, beans, lentil, nuts and green leafy vegetables like cabbage, cauliflower, etc.

In Eastern countries, good source of it is through eating of betel leaves in which calcium hydroxide is used invariably along with catechu (kattha). A good satsifactory proportion of the society consumes betel leaves in some of the eastern countries.

Drinking water is not a good source of calcium but very hard water may provide up to 200 mg per day.

At one time it was thought that dietary lack of calcium was a factor countributing to poor development of bone and teeth. This may be true in some very underprivileged communities of the World but the body has a remarkable facility for adapting to a low calcium intake and it is unlikely that calcium intake of as little as 200 mg/day may have any harmful effects in otherwise normal subjects. More calcium than usual is required during period of rapid growth (during

Table 19.2 : Approximate concentrations of Ca, P and Mg in various routine edibles (per 100 g)

Edibles	Ca (g)	P (g)	Mg (g)
Almonds	0.239	0.465	0.251
Beef (lean)	0.007	0.218	0.024
Beans(dried)	0.160	0.470	0.156
Cheese	0.931	0.680	0.037
Corn meal	0.018	0.190	0.084
Cottonseed meal	0.265	1.193	0.462
Eggs	0.067	0.180	0.011
Egg yolk	0.137	0.524	0.016
Linseed meal	0.413	0.741	0.432
Milk	0.210	0.093	0.012
Oranges	0.045	0.021	0.012
Potatoes	0.014	0.058	0.028
Spinach	0.067	0.068	0.037
Wheat	0.045	0.423	0.133

adolescence), pregnancy and lactation.

Since calcium, phosphorus and magnesium are very important minerals for the humans, hence it's in the interest of all of us to be aware of their concentrations in different routine edibles per 100 g (Table 19.2).

From the above Table no. 19.2, it's evident that amongst the routine edibles which we generally take daily, the best sources of calcium are cheese, milk and egg yolk.

Calcium remains distributed in blood as shown below in Table 19.3.

Table 19.3 : Distribution of calcium in blood of humans in milligrams per 100 ml.

Substance	Normal (Mean value)
Total serum calcium	10.3
Diffusible calcium	5.4
Non diffusible calcium	4.9

Level of calcium in blood remains as shown below in certain pathological conditions which may be of diagnostic value (Table 19.4).

Table 19.4 : Blood calcium level in certain pathological conditions

Disease	mg per 100 ml.
Rickets	9.0
Parathyroid tetany	7.9
Hyperparathyroidism	15.9

Regulation of blood Calcium and Phosphorus :

Calcium is reabsorbed in the tubules, therefore, only small amount is excreted via urine (200 mg). Unabsorbed calcium is passed is faeces. Parathyroid hormone (PTH) increases serum calcium whereas calcitonin (CT) hormone of the thyroid decreases it. The main features of the regulation of blood calcium are as shown below in figure 19.1.

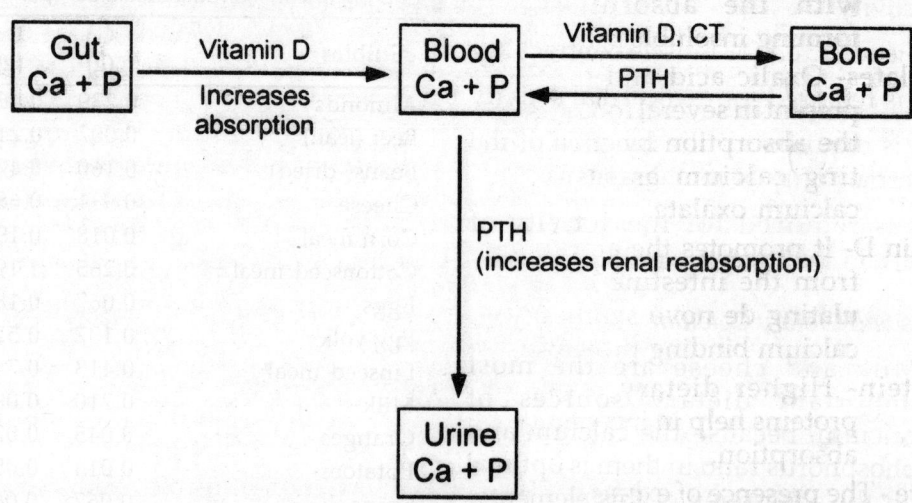

Fig. 19.1 : Regulation of blood calcium and phosphorus

Calcium absorption

It is absorbed in the intestine under the influence of vitamin D. The active form of vitamin D i.e., 1, 25- dihydroxychole-calciferol (1, 25 - DHCC) is taken up by the intestinal mucosal cells, where it stimulates the production of specific m - RNA, which remains concerned with the production of calcium binding proteins; besides this, there are several other factors which affect calcium absorption as mentioned below. Many of these are common to the absorption of another divalent cation, i.e., ferrous iron.

Factors:

1. **pH -** Calcium absorption is very good at the normal pH of the intestinal contents; if the pH becomes more alkaline, then the absorption gets suppressed.

2. **Phosphate-** Excess of phosphate lowers calcium absorption by forming insoluble calcium phosphate.

3. **Phytic acid-** Phytic acid found in good amount in cereals interferes with the absorption by forming insoluble salt.

4. **Oxalates-** Oxalic acid and oxalates present in several foods lower the absorption by precipitating calcium as insoluble calcium oxalate.

5. **Vitamin D-** It promotes the absorption from the intestine by stimulating de novo synthesis of calcium binding proteins.

6. **Protein-** Higher dietary levels of proteins help in increaing the absorption.

7. **Fibre -** The presence of excess of fibres in the diet decreases its absorption and has been found to be associated with negative balance of calcium, magnesium and zinc.

8. **Fatty acids -** Free fatty acids (formed as a result of impaired fat absorption) lower its absorption by forming insoluble calcium soaps.

Metabolism

There remains virtually no calcium present in red blood cells; all remains present in plasma. Normal level of total calcium ranges from 9 - 11.5 mg%. Calcium exists in plasma in two fractions, viz.

a) Diffusible (50-60% of total) which includes ionized calcium and

---

Calcium as the chief consituent of bone remains present as a salt resembling minerals of the hydroxyapatite group: $3Ca_3(PO_4)_2.Ca(OH)_2$. Around 99 percent of the total calcium of the body is found in the bones. Smaller amounts are found in teeth (dentine and tooth enamel). Bone formation (ossification) involves impregnantion with calcium salts of organic material, similar to collagen, and held together by **mucopoly-saccharides and mucoproteins.**

Calcium is found exclusively in the plasma portion of blood, where it occurs to the extent of 9 to 11.5 mg% ; its 3 forms are found in the plasma, namely;

   i) ionized calcium,

   ii) diffusible, but not ionic- e.g. as calcium citrate.

   iii) nondiffusible, combined mostly with the albumin of serum calcium complexed with citrate and phosphate, and

b) Non- diffusible (40-50%) or protein bound.

Plasma calcium is chiefly used for the formation of bone salts. Bone is not the static deposit of calcium and phosphorus. These ions from plasma exchange with those on the surface of bones, and complete exchange of plasma calcium occurs in a very short time i.e., within 2-3 minutes.

Urinary Excretion of Calcium

About 15 g calcium daily passes into the glomerular filtrate from the diffusible fractions of the plasma calcium. 50 to 200 mg is reabsorbed in the tubules but the exact amount is not yet known. Calcium reabsorption gets diminished in the deficiency of vitamin D and in the presence of sodium diuresis.

The calcium lost in the sweat is very variable which ranges from 20-350 mg/day

Factors affecting the plasma Calcium level

Calcium is found exclusively in the plasma portion of blood: its normal range in plasma is from 9 to 11.5 mg%. Three forms of calcium are recognized in the plasma, i.e.,

(i) ionized calcium

(ii) diffusible, but not ionic, e.g., as calcium citrate,

(iii) non-diffusible, combined mostly with serum albumin.

It's the ionizable fraction of the total plasma calcium which is most important physiologically; this fraction remains in equilibrium with calcium level of other tissues. It is this fraction which participates in the following very important activities of human body, namely:

i) Coagulation of blood,

ii) Neuromuscular activity,

iii) Muscle contractility and

iv) Myocardial activity

The non- diffusible calcium in plasma

For the proper calcification and eruption of teeth, the diet must contain adequate amount of calcium and phosphorus and certain vitamins.

In the developing tooth, dietary deficiency of vitamin C leads to the impairment of the **odontoblasts** and retarded dentine deposition. The pulp becomes hemorrhagic and is filled with calcified tissue.

Vitamin D regulates absorption of calcium.

Normal dental growth requires an adequate supply of thyroxine. Hypothyroidism in children causes retardation in dental development. In hyperthyroidism, in children which is relatively rare in them, there is early shedding of the deciduous teeth and accelerated dentition.

Deficient parathyroid function may interfere with calcium and phosphorus metabolism to such an extent that growing teeth fail to calcify properly.

The pituitary plays an important role in the eruption of the teeth which gets accelerated in hyperpituitarism, whereas in hypopituitarism the teeth are normal but eruption gets retarded and the teeth get crowded in the arch due to retardation of bone development.

In hypergonadism, the eruption of the teeth is accelerated. Estrogen in the human has no effect on the teeth; **whereas large doses of adrenal steroids favour osteoporosis.**

remains bound to protein.

Low ionized calcium level may lead to **tetanic spasms** which may be fatal. Side by side, if the plasma calcium level is high, then it disturbs cardiac functions and may be deposited in kidney or other tissues.

Physicochemical factors: If EDTA (Ethylene diamine tetra acetic acid, a calcium complexing agent) is injected intravenously into man or dog then the plasma calcium falls rapidly but returns to normal level within a few hours. If EDTA is given after removal of the parathyroid glands, the plasma calcium again returns to the preinfusion value (7 to 8 mg%) but not so rapidly. Thus chemical equilibrium between the **labile** part of the bone mineral and the interstitial fluid, quite independent of the parthyroid glands, keeps the plasma calcium upto 7 to 8 mg%. In intact animals, parathyroid hormone is responsible for maintaining the normal serum calcium level around 10 mg%.

Parathyroid hormone: The parathyroid glands develop from the third and fourth pharangeal pouches of the embryo. They lie in the neck immediately adjacent to the posterior surface of the thyroid gland with which, however, they have no physiological relationship. As a rule, they consit of four oval bodies about 6 mm long each weighting 20 to 50 mg, but they are variable in number, size and position. Accessory parathyroid tissue is not uncommon lower in the neck or even in the thorax. The secretory cells are arranged in cords, separated into imperfect lobules by the thin septa of connective tissue. There are two types of **chief cells** with large nuclei nearly filling the cells and **oxyntic cells** with small nuclei with small nuclei and acidophil granules in the cytoplasm.

The vascular supply is rich but the nervous connections are scanty.

PTH is a 84 amino acid single chain peptide (MW 9,500) that contains no carbohydrate (Fig 19.2). PTH_{1-34} has full biologic activity. The region 25-34 is primarily responsible for receptor binding.

PTH secretion apparently ceases when the plasma calcium exceeds 12 mg%. Plasma calcium appears to be the sole stimulus of PTH secretion. Since the half-life of the hormone in the blood is about 20 minutes, changes in hormone secretion may play an important role in minute to

1
H_2N–Ala–Val–Ser–Glu–Ile–Gln–Phe–Met–His–Asn–Leu–Gly–Lys–

15
His–Leu–Ser–Ser–Met–Glu–Arg–Val–Glu–Trp–Arg–Lys–Lys–Leu–

30   34
Gln–Asp–Val–His–Asn–Phe–Val–Ala–Leu–Gly–Ala–Ser–Ile–Ala–

45
Tyr–Arg–Asp–Gly–Ser–Ser–Gln–Arg–Pro–Arg–Lys–Lys–Glu–Asp–
Asn–

60
Val–Leu–Val–Glu–Ser–His–Gin–Lys–Ser–Leu–Gly–Glu–Ala–Asp–Lys–

75   84
Ala–Asp–Val–Asp–Val–Leu–Ile–Lys–Ala–Lys–Pro–Gln–COOH

Fig. 19.2 : Amino acid sequence of bovine PTH. The fragment 1 to 34 is biologically active, in vivo and in vitro, on both bone and kidney receptors.

minute regulation of the plasma calcium.

Quite independent of its action on blood calcium, PTH has effects on bone and kidney, and probably also on the gastrointestinal tract and on the mammary glands during lactation. The effects on the bone and intestine, but not on the kidney, require the presence of vitamin D. PTH exerts its action on bone by stimulating osteoblasts to mobilize bone. PTH decreases the reabsorption of phosphate by the kidney tubules, and therefore increases the excretion of phosphate. It also increases the urinary excretion of sodium, potassium and bicarbonate and decreases the excretion of hydrogen ions. In the intestine, PTH enhances calcium absorption. The exact mechanism of action of PTH is not very well understood so far but recent evidences suggest the involvement of 3', 5'- AMP.

Clinical disorders of both excess and deficiency of parathyroid activity are known. Actively secreting tumors of the parathyroid glands produce excessive amount of PTH_1 and the resulting disturbance of phosphorus and calcium metabolism leads to withdrawl of large amount of these elements from the bones which therefore become weak and deformed and liable to be fractured (Fig 19.3).

The absorption of calcium from the gut is increased. **The serum calcium may reach upto 16 mg% or even more and the urinary excretion may be greatly raised so that stones may form in the kidneys.**

Parathyroid deficiency sometimes occurs after accidental removal of parathyroid glands during thyroidectomy. Neuromuscular excitability and muscular spasm (tetany) are the main symptoms. **The condition improves after the**

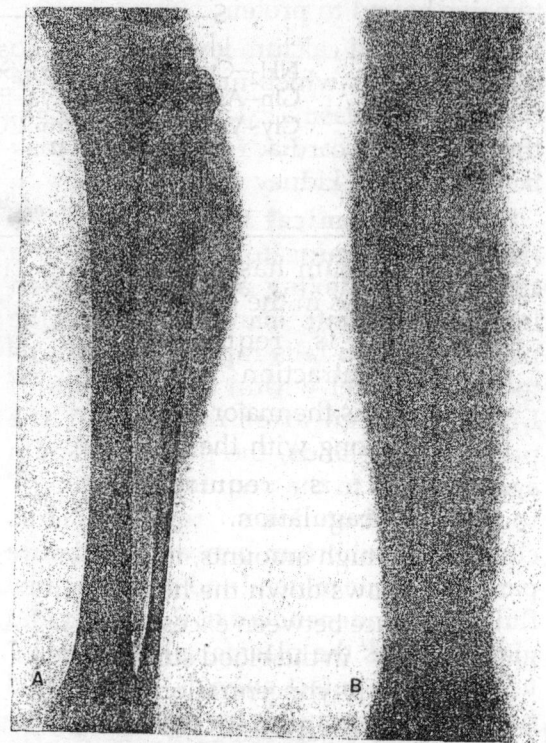

Fig.19.3: X-ray photograph of the right lower legs of the two women, age 25. A is from a normal subject, B from a patient with a parathyroid tumour. In B the fibula is deformed and both bones cast a poor shadow because of extensive resorption of calcium salts.

administration of PTH but large doses of vitamin D are given for longer period.

Calcitonin: In 1962 Copp and his colleagues produced evidence for the existence of a hormone which lowered the plasma calcium level. He named it as calcitonin. **The hormone is a lipophilic single chain polypeptide of 32 amino acids (Fig 19.4).**

In man calcitonin is secreted by the cells of the thyroid, parathyroids and the thymus. The parafollicular (C cells) of the thyroid have been known since 1932. They contain geranules which increase in number during a period of prolonged

$$S \text{-----------------------------------} S$$

$$
\begin{array}{c}
| \qquad\qquad\qquad\qquad 5 \qquad | \qquad\qquad\qquad\qquad\qquad 13\\
NH_2-Cys-Gly-Asn-leu-Ser-Thr-Cys-Met-Leu-Gly-Thr-Tyr-Thr-\\
Gln-Asp-Phe-Asn-Lys-Phe-His-Thr-Phe-Pro-Gln-Thr-Ala-Leu-\\
Gly-Val-Gly-Ala-Pro-CONH_2\\
32
\end{array}
$$

Fig 19.4: Human Calcitonin.

Calcium has got very important functions in the body, namely :

(i) It is required for muscle contraction

(ii) It is the major constituent of bone along with the phosphate.

(iii) It is required for blood coagulation.

In high amounts, it is toxic and like K^+ slows down the heart beating. The balance between excess and deficiency of Ca^{2+} in the blood stream is a delicate issue. Its concentration is regulated by the antagonistic action of two hormones, viz; **parathormone** and **calcitonin**.

hypocalcaemia. Calcitonin has been identified within these cells by the immunofluorescent antibody technique.

Calcitonin secretion is stimulated by hypercalcaemia. Calcitonin reduces bone resorption even in the absence of parathormone and promotes phosphate and sodium excretion through the kidneys. Its secretion is also stimulated by gastrin, pancreozymin and glucagon. Therefore, as calcium is absorbed from a meal, there is little or no rise is the level of blood calcium.

As elevation of calcitonin level is found in the patients with medullary- cell carcinomas of the thyroid. So far, no convincing evidence of a syndrome due to calcitonin deficiency is known.

1, 25 - Dihydroxycholecalciferol

This hormone, a metabolite of vitamin D is produced by the kidneys. It promotes the absorption of calcium in the intestine.

Other hormones affecting Calcium Metabolism

An adequate supply of growth hormone from the anterior pituitary is necessary for the proliferation of the cells of the epiphyseal cartilage and therefore, for the growth in length of a long bone. In hypophysectomized amimals, epiphyseal activity is much reduced or even absent; which can be restored by the administration of grwoth hormone (GH)

Increased loss of bone is a feature of Cushing's syndrome due to excessive activity of the adrenal cortex.

Variation in blood Calcium level in Health and Diseases

Normal level of calcium in plasma/ serum is from 9 to 11.5 mg% (4.5 to 5.8 meq/litre).

Hypercalcemia (rasied level of serum calcium) is of diagnostic value in several disorders, like;

a) Hyperparathyroidism (level between 12 to 22 mg%)

b) Multiple myeloma (level normal to 20 mg% due to destruction of bone with liberation of its mineral)

c) Cancer (level remains usually normal but values as high as 22 mg% may be obtained in cases of tumors which cause rapid bone destruction.

d) Bronchogenic carcinoma (hypercalcemia due to secretion of parathyroid hormone precursors or its homologues).

e) Vitamin D poisoning

f) Excessive ingestion of milk

g) Excessive intake of alkali by patients with peptic ulcer.

Signs of hypercalcemia include:

a) Thirst,

b) Tiredness,

c) Weakness, and

d) Mental disturbances, and if severe, then coma and death.

Untreated hypercalcemia causes renal damage.

Hypocalcemia (low level of serum calcium) is of diagnostic value in several disorders, like:

a) Hypoparathyroidism

b) Tetany (In this disorder it's usually between 7-8 mg% in latent tetany patients and 4-6 mg% in manifested tetany patients).

c) Nephrotic syndrome
   (low due to loss of non- diffusible protein bound calcium in urine)

d) Rickets and osteomalacia (in early cases serum calcium level is normal, afterwards it falls. If the intake of calcium is low, hypocalcemia occurs which gives rise to tetany)

e) Pregnancy (It may be low during late pregnancy or lactation owing to increased demand of calcium, phosphorus and vitamin D)

f) Chronic renal failure : Fall in the level of serum calcium (4-6 mg%) is due to retention of phosphate (12-20 mg%) by kidneys. Tetany may

also occur.

g) Steatorrhoea (Defective absorption of fat, fatty acids and vitamin D is the cause of hypocalcemia of steatorrhoea).

Daily Requirement

WHO/FAO (1962) and ICMR (1981) have recommended similar requirement of calcium as follows:

Age Group	Mg / day
Infants (0-12 months)	500-600
Children (1 to 9 years)	400-500
Children (10-15 years)	600-700
Children (16 to 19 years)	500-600
Adults	400-500
Pregnancy and lactation	1000

CHLORIDE

It is the main ion of plasma and other extracellular fluids and is responsible for maintaining osmolarity at approximately 0.3 mol/l.

Sources

Sources for chloride include table salt, cheese, butter, pickles, salted fish or meat, salted nuts, etc.

Daily Requirement

Daily requirement of chloride for various categories is as follows:

Adults: 1.5 to 5 g; **infants:** 0.25 to 1 g; **children:** 0.5 to 4 g. **Adult human body contains about 70-80 g chloride** and the excretion of chloride per day is 7-8 g via urine. It is reabsorbed by diffusion from the proximal and distal tubules and the thin segment of the ascending limb along

Chloride

It's the chief anion present in the body, particularly in the extracellular fluid. The excretion in urine is slightly higher than that of Na^+, which would put the average daily intake at about 7g Cl^- (200 meq). However, the kidney is capable of secreting a urine almost free of Na^+ and Cl^-, although this is often an indication of incipient heat exhaustion.

the electrical gradient developed by the reabsorption of Na^+. Apart from this, some Cl^- also gets actively reabsorbed from the thick segment of the ascending limb. Cl^- reabsorption is indirectly helped by aldosterone as Cl^- is alwyas reabsorbed along with Na^+.

Some Cl^- is secreted in saliva, gastric juice, tear, sweat, pancreatic juice, etc. During profuse sweating, Na^+ and Cl^- are lost in greater quantity. Secretion of aldosterone hormone reduces the Na^+ and Cl^- concentrations in sweat.

Functions

1. *Acid-base balance:* Chloride helps in maintaining acid-base balance. Cl^- has a role in buffering CO_2; some of the HCO_3^- formed from CO_2 in *RBCs* passes out into the plasma in exchange of Cl^- which enters the erythrocytes (chloride-shift phenomenon).

2. *Cl^- in HCl secretion:* Plasma Cl^- is the source of Cl^- for the formation of gastric HCl.

3. *Osmotic pressure regulation:* It is also responsible for maintaining osmotic pressure i. e. osmolarity throughout the body which is maintained at about 0.3 mol/l by the joint effect of Na^+, K^+ and Cl^-.

Clinical Condition

Intense vomiting may cause Cl^- depletion due to the loss of Cl^- with the gastric contents as a result of which plasma Cl^- level gets decreased. Some of the lost Cl^- is replaced by HCO_3^- in the ECF and **metabolic alkalosis may result. In several diseases like Addison's disease, primary aldosteronism, Cushing's syndrome, serum Cl^- changes are similar to those of serum Na^+.**

Phosphorus

The mean phosphorus content of an adult man is 800 g; four- fifths of this is found in the bones, the remaining being in the cells as phosphates or nucleic acids. The concentration of inorganic phosphorus in the plasma in fasting adults is between 2.5 and 4.5 mg/dl. Higher values are found in infants. Almost all the inorganic phosphate is dialysable, only nearly 12 percent being protein bound. At normal pH i.e., 7.4, 85% of the ionized inorganic phosphate remains present as HPO_4^{2-} and 15% as $H_2PO_4^-$. Small amounts of the phosphate may be bound to calcium and magnesium. It has been estimated that the amount of non-ionized phosphate may be 50% of the dialysable phosphate.

Since the greater part of the phosphorus of the body is associated with calcium in bone, the metabolism of these two elements is to a considerable extent parallel to each other.

Phosphorus, however, is abundant also in many of the softer tissues of the body and plays various important roles in life-processes.

Functions:-

It has the following main functions in the human body, namely:

(i) **Constituent of bones and teeth:** It is a very important mineral for the development of bones and teeth. It is required in greater amount during infancy and childhood when there is growth of every tissue. It is the major constituent of the bone as **calcium phosphate or hydroxyapatite.**

(ii) **Enzyme action:** Phosphate remains present in nucleotides, a majority of which functions as coenzymes, for instance pyridoxal phosphate, nicotinamide coenzymes, flavin coenzymes, thiamine pyrophosphate, etc.

(iii) **Intermediary metabolism:**

(a) Through the intermediary formation of lecithins, it is concerned with fat metabolism

(b) Through the formation of hexosephosphates, of adenylic acid, and of creatine phosphate, it plays a primary role in the carbohydrate metabolism of animals as well as in fermentation processes.

(c) It participates in intermediary metabolism in the form of organic phosphates; the most important of these is ATP. Phosphorylation is essential for many reactions like those of glycogenesis, glycolysis, etc.

(iv) Phosphates play a role in the neutrality regulation of the organism.

(v) Phosphates are concerned with the absorption of sugars from the intestine and the reabsorption of glucose in the kidney tubules.

(vi) Phosphorus is a constituent of the phospoholipids present in all tissues. Phospholipids are found in abundance in nervous tissues.

(vii) It remains present in nucleoproteins of the chromatin material of cells and in phosphoproteins such as casein.

(viii) It has been suggested that most of the phosphorus, as well as the fat of milk, arises from the lecithin of the blood of the lactating animal.

(ix) **Acid- Base regulation:** A very important property. Mixtures of monobasic and disbasic phosphates ($H_2PO_4^-$ and HPO_4^{2-}) constitute the phosphate buffer which plays role in the maintenance of pH of the body fluids.

(x) **Energy transfer:** Free energy produced by various metabolic reactions is stored as high energy phosphates like adenosine triphosphate and is liberated by their hydrolysis for other energy-requiring pathways/ reactions.

Absorption and Depletion:

Inorganic phosphates are absorbed from the middle third of jejunum. Vitamin D increases the absorption of phosphate. Ninty percent of the phosphorus filtered at the glomerulus is reabsorbed in the tubules.

Depletion of phosphate may occur with tubular defect and a high plasma phosphate may be a consequence of renal i.e., glomerular failure. **Besides, phosphate depletion may also occur in** patients who consume excessive amout of aluminium hydroxide (an antacid) which binds phosphorus present in gut.

Requirement

Indian Council of Medical Research states that the daily allowance of phosphorus should be equal to that of calcium for the children and women during pregnancy and lactation.

Daily requirement of phosphorus for:

(i) adult man/women: 500 mg

(ii) pregnant or lactating women: 1 g

(iii) infants and children : 400- 600 mg

Sources:

(i) Milk is an excellent source of phosphorus, nearly 750 ml of intake a day for children which contains 0.88 g of phosphorus is O.K. in all respects for them. Milk contains 93 mg of phosphorus per 100ml.

(ii) Meat (average 175 mg per 100 g)

(iii) Eggs (200 mg per 100 g)

(iv) Cheese (480 mg per 100 g)

(v) Nuts (400 mg per 100 g)

(vi) Whole cereals (as whole wheat, 375 mg per 100 g)

(vii) White flour (about 90 mg per 100 g)

(viii) Polished rice (about 90 mg per 100 g)

Too high a ratio of calcium to phosphorus in the diet, however, is unfavourable to phosphorus absorption. **Diets high in beryllium or strontium also inhibit the absorption of phosphorus and give rise to rickets.**

Since phosphorus remains present in all animal and vegetable cells, therefore, dietary deficiency of it never occurs in man.

Regulation

Various substances like vitamin D, plasma proteins, hormones like calcitonin and parathormone regulate phosphorus metabolism.

Calcitonin lowers serum calcium and phosphate by reducing their mobilization from bones and thus maintains the bone minerals; whereas parathormone (PTH) has a tendency to increase serum Ca^{2+} and lower serum phosphates.

Clinical Conditions

Phosphate deficiency is not very common as most of the naturally occurring foods contain phosphate in one or the other form. However, **there are some diseases like rickets and osteomalacia which may be caused due to the deficiency of calcium, phosphorus or vitamin D.** These diseases are characterized by reduced calcium and phosphate absorption, low serum Pi, rise in urinary phosphates, demineralization of bones and negative calcium balance.

Serum calcium is, however, almost normal in rickets although it falls sometimes in osteomalacia. Serum calcium level may be elevated by *hypervitaminosis D*; whereas *hyperparathyroidism* **causes demineralization of bones, rise in serum calcium, fall in serum Pi, high urinary calcium and phosphate** and metastatic calcifications of soft tissues.

Hypoparathyroidism **is responsible for lowering serum calcium, urinary calcium and urinary Pi; raises serum Pi moderately and produces hypocalcaemic tetany.**

Besides the above, X-linked genetic disorders of phosphate metabolism is responsible for the onset of *vitamin D-resistant rickets* and *idiopathic osteomalacia* which eventually lead to reduced intestinal and renal absorptions of phosphates, low serum phosphate, high serum alkaline phosphatase activity, high urinary Pi and poor mineralization of bones.

IODINE

Introduction

The thyroid gland produces two hormones i.e., 3, 5, 3'- triiodothyronine (T_3) and 3, 5, 3', 5'- tetraiodothyronine (T_4, thyroxine) which have long been recognized for their importance in regulating general metabolism, development and tissue differentiation. These hormones, whose structures are as given below (Fig 19.5) regulate gene expression using mechanisms similar to those employed by steroid hormones.

About 20 mg of iodine remains present in adult human body and nearly two- third of it remains present in the thyroid gland. Small doses of it are important in the prevention of **'goitre'** in areas where it is endemic.

Iodine remains present in thyroxine. Under normal conditions almost all the blood iodine is in the plasma, less than a third of this remains present as inorganic iodine compounds, the remainder being organic which remains bound to the protein known as protein bound iodine i.e., PBI.

This element for the first time was discovered by **Courtois** in seaweed and as early as in 1820, it was postulated that iodine was a curative factor of **'goitre'**. Since at that time iodine deficiency goitres were common in many parts of the world, the news spread like a wild fire as a result of which the use of iodine and iodine-containing substances like burnt sponge,

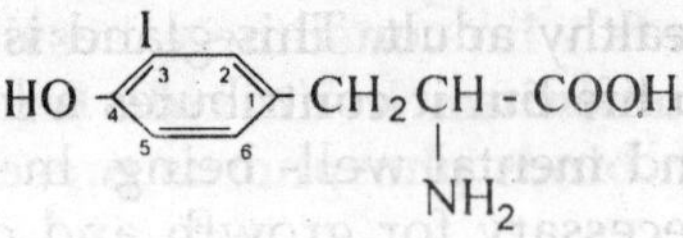

3 - Monoiodotyrosine (MIT)

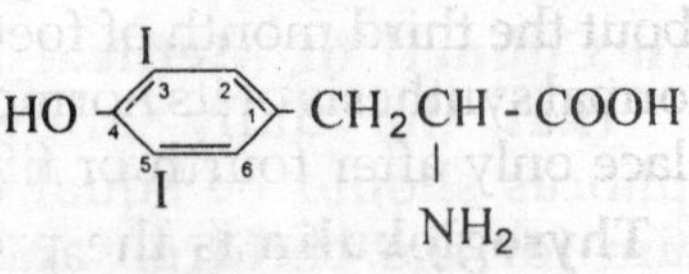

3, 5 - Diiodotyrosine (DIT)

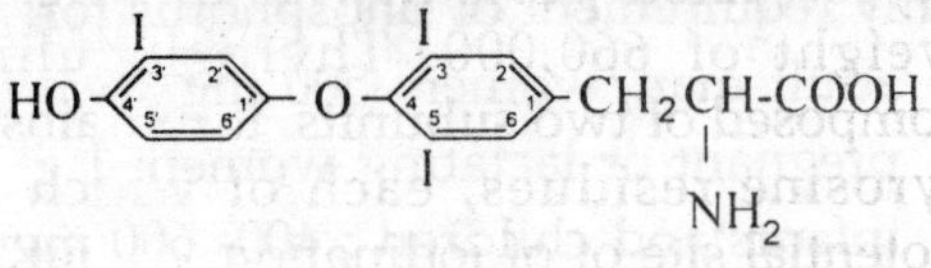

3,5,3' - Triiodotyrosine (T_3)

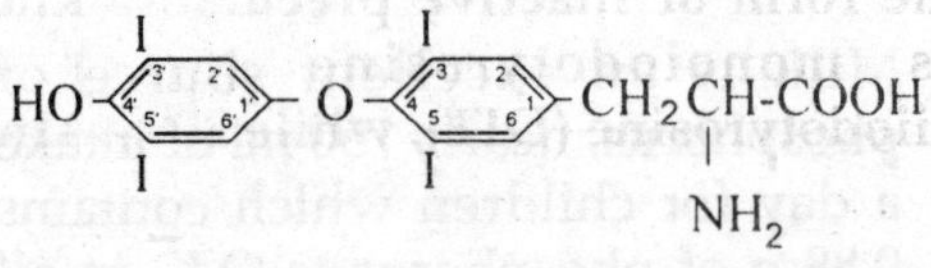

3,5,3',5' - Tetraiiodotyrosine (thyroxine, T_4)

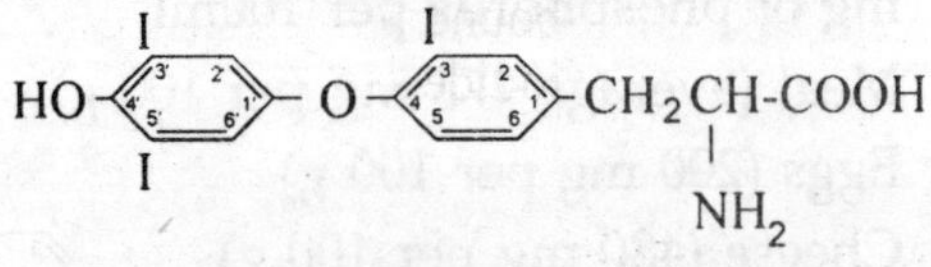

3,3',5' - Triiodothyronine [reverse T_3 (rT_3)]

Fig.19.5: Structures of thyroid hormones and related compounds.

etc. became very popular for the treatment of goitres. With the time as the knowledge advanced, discrimination in the use of this **'wonder drug'** came forward as a consequence of which, the beneficial effect of salts rich in iodine advanced the prophylactic and therapeutic treatment of goitre.

The thyroid gland in the adults lies at the neck infront of the upper rings of the trachea which sometimes is prolonged in to the thorax behind the sternum. Weight of the thyroid gland is nearly 25 g in a healthy adult. This gland is not essential to life but it contributes a lot to physical and mental well- being. In humans, it is necessary for growth and development. The thyroid begins to trap iodine from about the third month of foetal life but the normal synthesis of its hormones does take place only after fourth or fifth month.

Thyroglobulin is the precursor of T_3 and T_4. It is a large, iodinated and glycosylated protein with a molecular weight of 660,000. Thyroglobulin is composed of two subunits. It contains 115 tyrosine residues, each of which is a potential site of of iodination. **About 70% of the iodide in thyroglobulin exists in the form of inactive precursors known as monoiodotyrosine (MIT) and diiodotyrosine (DIT), while 30% is in the** iodotyronyl residues i.e., T_3 and T_4.

The thyroid gland contains a large amount of iodine (0.06 percent), almost all of which remains firmly bound to a protein called as **thyroglobulin**. On hydrolysis thyroglobulin yields:.

(i) Several iodine containing derivatives of tyrosine

(ii) Monoiodotyrosine

(iii) Diiodotyrosine

(iv) T_3, &

(v) T_4

Biosynthesis

The biosynthesis of thyroid hormones proceeds as shown below in figure 19.6. The first step in their synthesis is the concentration of inorganic iodide within

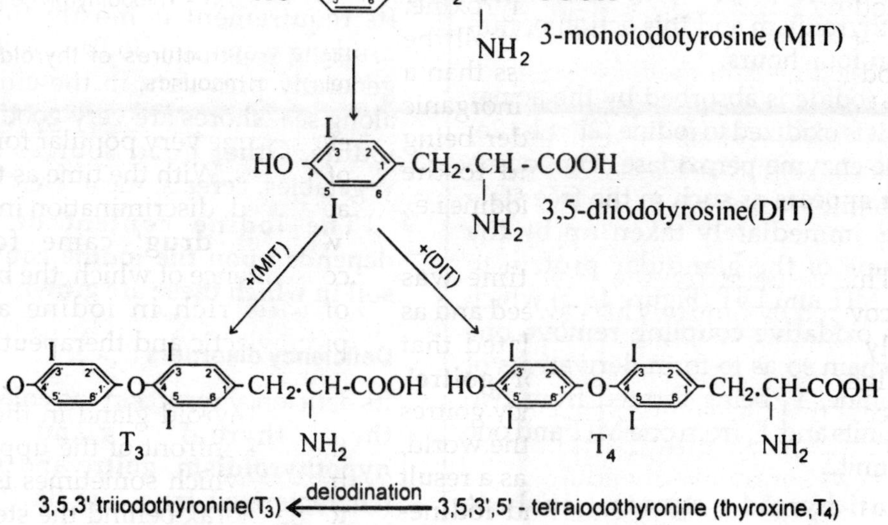

Fig. 19.6 : Biosynthesis of thyroid hormones

the thyroid gland (iodide trapping). The next major steps involve **oxidation** and **organic iodination.** The thyroid iodide is oxidized to iodine via a peroxidase enzyme. In the next reaction tyrosine in the presence of iodine (iodination occurs) forms monoiodotyrosine(MIT) and then diiodotyrosine (DIT).

Now, two molecules of diiodotyrosine are coupled to form one molecule of thyroxine (T_4) with the loss of one alanine side chain. Triiodothyronine (T_3) is synthesized either by the coupling of diiodotyrosine with one molecule of monoiodotyrosine (Fig 19.6) or from the deiodination of thyroxine.

All The compounds taking part in the synthesis of thyroid hormones are found in thyroglobulin, a specialized storage glycoprotein with a molecular weight of about 6,80,000. The **action of proteases causes the release of MIT, DIT, T_3 and**

T_4; the latter two being available for discharge into the blood stream. Deiodination of the iodotyrosines (MIT, DIT) conserves thyroidal iodine for reuse.

Absorption and Excretion

Iodine is quickly absorbed from food and water as inorganic iodide by the alimentary canal. Depending upon the activity of the thyroid gland, a portion of the absorbed iodide in taken up by the gland. For more information regarding 'absorption', see box.

Most of the iodine in blood is found in plasma, nearly 90% of which is found in the organic form bound to protein and is called as protein bound iodine (PBI).

Inorganic iodine is mostly excreted via urine whereas nearly 10% of the circulating organic iodine is excreted via faeces.

Requirement

100-150 µg/day is sufficient to prevent goitre.

Sources

Its requirement is mostly fullfilled by drinking water and iodized salt. Seafoods generally prevalent in the cities located along sea- shores are very good sources of iodine. Other good sources are fruits, vegetables, cereals, meat, etc.

The iodine content of the food depends upon the iodine content of the soil in which these are grown/cultivated.

Deficiency disorders :

Its deficiency results in the enlargement of the thyroid gland causing **hypothyroidism, goitre** and **myxedema** (characterized by a low BMR, thickness and puffing of the skin, coarse and brittle hair and fingernails and a general mental

---

T_3 possesses all the biological properties of T_4 and is 3-5 times more potent than T_4 in raising the oxygen consumption of patients with hypothyroidism and this action occurs within four hours.

As iodide is absorbed by the acinar cells, it is oxidized to iodine ($2I^- \rightarrow I_2 + 2e$) by the enzyme peroxidase. The iodine never appears as such in the free state but is immediately taken up by the tyrosine of the glandular protein to form MIT and DIT (Figure 19.5) which upon oxidative coupling remove one side chain so as to form derivatives of thyronine, T_4 being formed from two DIT units and T_4 from one MIT and one DIT unit.

Antithyroid agents include thiouracil, thiourea etc.

and physical lethargy).

In hypothyroidism, the child becomes a **dwarf** or **cretin** who grows slowly (stunted growth) and has a low mental status (low IQ), his/ her hair are scanty and coarse and his skin is thick and dry and low BMR.

Toxicity of iodine may result in **thyrotoxicosis (hyperthyroidism),** one of the most servere condition of which is **Grave's disease (exophthalmic goitre).** It results in weight loss, typical protrusion of the eye-balls and elevated BMR.

Goitrogenic foods:

Vegetables/ Foods which if cosumed in abundance may cause **goitre,** these are the following:

(i) Cauliflower,

(ii) Brocooli,

(iii) Cabbage,

(iv) Rutabagas,

(v) Turnip, etc.

Chemical Name of the goitrogenic substance (goitrin) isolated from rutabagas is 1-5- vinyl - 2 thiooxazolidone.

FLUORINE (Fluoride)

Traces of fluoride (F) are present in human tissues mainly in bones, teeth, thyroid gland, skin, etc.

Physiological functions

1. This element is essential for the growth of teeth and bones and is required in minute quantities.
2. Fluoroacetate is a powerful inhibitor (it virtually blocks) of TCA cycle.
3. In combination with vitamin D, it is required for the treatment of bone disease i.e. osteoporosis which is characterized by softening of bone as a result of excessive absorption of bone elements.
4. Sodium fluoride acts as a powerful inhibitor of the glycolytic enzyme enolase, therefore, it's used as a blocker of glycolytic pathway while collecting blood samples for the determination of sugar.
5. It forms a protective layer of acid-resistant fluoroapatite with hydroxyapatite crystals of the enamel.
6. Fluoride ions inhibit the metabolism of oral bacterial enzymes and also restrict the local production of acids which are responsible for dental caries.

Sources

1. Drinking water is the chief source for the human beings.
2. Tea and sea fishes are the only other significant sources of fluorine in the diet.

Distribution and daily requirement

Fluorine remains present in animal soft tissues in amounts ranging from 0.2 to 1.5 mg per 100 g of the dry material. Bones and teeth contain larger amounts (20 to 30 mg per 100 g ash); whereas dentine may contain more than the enamel of teeth. Drinking water containing 1 to 2 parts per million of fluorine is sufficient to meet all the requirements of the body and thus prevents dental caries without producing any ill effect.

Absorption

Soluble fluorides are rapidly absorbed by

the small intestine.

Excretion

It's excreted via: (a) sweat, (b) urine, and (c) intestinal mucosa.

Abnormalities

1. Excessive intake of fluoride (3 to 5 parts per million) in childhood is responsible for "**dental fluorosis** (mottled enamel Fig. 19.7 & 19.8),

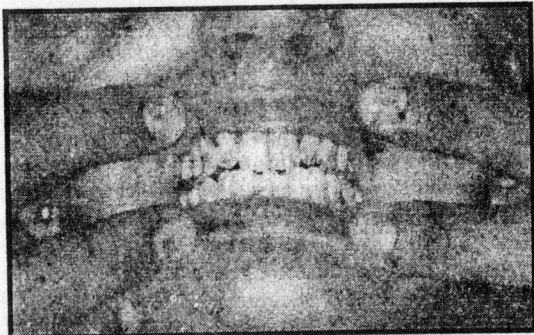

Fig. 19.7 : Dental fluorosis

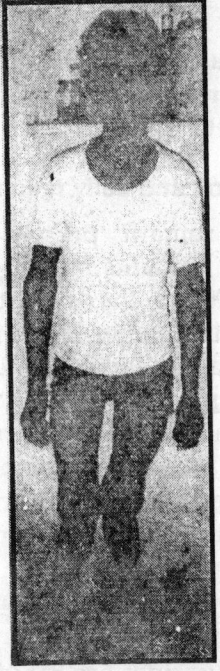

Fig. 19.8 : Skeletal fluorosis

in which enamel of the teeth loses its lustre and becomes rough Chalky white patches with yellow or brown staining do appear over the surface of the teeth which may be easily distinguished by naked eyes. In this disease, enamel becomes weak and in severe cases there is found great loss of enamel with 'pitting' and other depressions **give the surface a corroded appearance.**

2. Highly excessive intake of fluorine (over 10 ppm) may be responsible for increased density and hypercalcification of the bone of spine, pelvis and limbs. The attack most of the times is so serious that even the ligaments of the spine and the collagen in the bone become calcified. Its severity is fatal and may cause neurological disturbances as a result of which such individuals become crippled and can not do normal daily routine work, such as, bending, squatting etc; as the joints become stiff; this is all due to fluoride toxicity which is not very common but its patients may be seen once in a while.

3. Drinking water containing less than 0.5 ppm fluorine causes dental caries amongst children. **Therefore, fluorine is considered to be a caries preventive agent, that is why these days the manufacturers of tooth-paste indiscriminately add it.**

4. Excessive amount of fluoride (> 10 ppm) in drinking water causes skeletal fluorosis (Fig 19.7 & 19.8). There is pain in the back, ligaments and collagen are calcified, bending of the back/spine, "**knock knee**", and bow legs occur which cripple the person. **The treatment of water**

with lime and alum is recommended to remove excess fluoride from it.

Prevention of fluorosis

It can be prevented by removing excessive fluorides from the water by treating it with activated carbon or by some other appropriate absorbents. Local district water department/health department may be informed and consulted without any delay in cases of suspicion.

Mechanism

The mechanism by which fluorine inhibits caries production is not very well understood.

Fluoridation

It is a very important aspect if by chance it comes to knowledge that the drinking water contains less fluorine than the recommended standards; the fact must be brought to the notice of local water/health/competent authorities so that such water gets fluoridated. **Deliberate fluoridation of water supply in such cases is very useful.**

Fluoride Toxicity:

Fluoride toxicity results in **fluorosis** which is common in many parts of the world where its concentration in water is found over 5 PPM. **In India, fluorosis is common in north where water contains over 10 PPM of fluoride.**

In fluorosis, there is mottling of teeth. The dental enamel loses its lustre and becomes rough. Bands of brown pigmentation are seen. Mottling is best seen on the incisors of the upper jaw. There is also loss of appetite and osteoporosis of the bones particularly of the spine, pelvis and limbs. In addition ligaments of the spine become calcified.

SULPHUR

In the diet, greater part of sulphur remains present in proteins in the form of two well known amino acids namely cystine and methionine. Besides, it's also found in some non-protein organic sulphur compounds. It may also be found in inorganic sulphur compounds as sulphates. Most of the sulphur present in proteins is finally converted to **inorganic sulphate;** some of which gets excreted in that form and some as **ethereal sulphates** and the remainder in the form of **phenolic compounds such as indoxyl and skatoxyl sulphates** which are formed from indole and skatole produced in the intestine by the action of microorganisms on proteins. Important compounds of the body which contain sulphur are:

(a) Insulin,

(b) Glutathione, and

(c) Thiamine

In blood, sulphur remains distributed in the following forms:

(a) inorganic sulphur: About 1mg per 100ml;

(b) ethereal sulphate sulphur: 0.5mg per 100ml; and

(c) neutral sulphur: 1.9 mg per 100 ml

In this way total sulphur in blood averages nearly 3.4 mg per 100 ml.

Determination of these sulphur compounds in blood has not so far found any diagnostic application in the diseased state. Some types of sulphur compounds are found in urine where also they are not of any diagnostic significance.

ZINC

An average human body contains nearly 2 gm of zinc.

The importance of zinc as a micronutrient has received increasing attention. Normal animals absorb only 3-10 percent of dietary zinc.

Sources

Liver, legumes, milk, unmilled cereals, maize, meat, spinach, lettuce, yeast, oysters and egg etc. High concentrations are found in the prostate, eye , liver, bone and skin.

Daily requirement

(i) Adult men/women: 15 mg;

(ii) Pregnant/lactating women: 20-25 mg;

(iii) Infants and children; 3-10 mg.

Deficiency

(i) Its deficiency in man causes poor growth and hypogonadism (retarded genital development).

(ii) It is also responsible for low carbonic anhydrase activity in red blood cells.

(iii) It also causes **alopoecia.**

(iv) Its deficiency **lowers spermato-genesis in males and menstrual cycle gets also disturbed in the females.**

(v) Its deficienty is characterized by lesions in the (a) skin (b) mucocutaneous junctions and (c) epithelial structures.

(vi) Wound healing: Its deficiency was found to be associated with poor healing of surgical wounds and burns.

Absorption and Excretion

Nearly 20% of the dietary zinc is absorbed. Its absorption takes place in duodenum and ileum. Phytates and other components of the dietary fibre affect its absorption by increasing the faecal excretion.

Zinc toxicity : When consumed in excess, it causes toxicity which depresses growth and interferes with the utilisation and functions of copper and causes anaemia.

Physiological Functions

(i) Role in enzyme action: It is a cofactor for many metalloenzymes like carboxypeptidase A, cytoplasmic superoxide dismutase, carbonic anhydrase, alcohol dehydrogenase phosphatases, etc.

(ii) Role in vitamin A metabolism: Zn^{2+} may stimulate the release of vitamin A from the liver into the blood, thus plays a role in vitamin A metabolism.

(iii) Zinc therapy has been found to be useful in some cases of atherosclerosis.

(iv) It has been found to play a vital role in the healing of wounds.

(v) It is essential for normal growth and reproduction in animals.

(vi) It is required in the commercial preparation of **'insulin'** hormone. It increases the duration of insulin action in diabetics when given to them by injection, that is why, preparations of zinc-insulins (also known as crystalline insulins) or **zinc-protamine insulin is more common and popular.**

(vii) Perhaps, its most vital function may be concerned with the synthesis of **ribonucleic acids.**

(viii) It is also required for the maturation of spermatozoa.

(ix) Zinc is a component of many metalloenzymes which include carbonic anhydrase, carboxypeptidase, alcohol dehydrogenase, alkaline phosphatase, DNA polymerase, RNA polymerase, etc.

(x) As a constituent of DNA polymerase and RNA polymerase, zinc indirectly plays very important role in the metabolism in general and in nucleic acid metabolism in particular. Apart from this, zinc is essential for the preservation of tertiary structure of ribosomes.

Manganese

The kidney and the liver are the chief storage places for manganese in the body. In blood it varies from 0.004 to 0.020 mg per 100 ml. It is largely excreted via faeces.

Sources

It is also an essential element required by the body. Average diet contains nearly 4 mg manganese. Its important sources include cereals, vegetables, nuts, tea, fruits, whole grains, etc.

Daily requirement

Adult men/women: 2.5-5 mg; infants and children: 0.5-3 mg.

Functions

1. **Enzyme action.:** Manganese acts as a cofactor in a number of enzymic reactions. It's also a constituent of number of enzymes, e.g. arginase, isocitrate dehydrogenase, cholinesterase, pyruvate carboxylase, acetyl-CoA carboxylase, glycosyl transferases, etc.

2. **Proteoglycan synthesis:** It plays some role in the synthesis and deposition of proteoglycans in many tissues including bones.

3. **Porphyrin synthesis:** It may help aminolevulinic acid (Am Lev) synthetase **in porphyrin synthesis.**

4. It is also required for the **biosynthesis of long chain fatty acids.**

5. It has been reported to exhibit **lipotropic effect.**

6. It also stimulates the biosynthesis of cholesterol and fatty acids. For example, the biosynthesis of cholesterol from accetate depends upon the presence of a manganese containing enzyme i.e., mevalonic kinase.

Normal Range

4-20 µg per 100 ml blood.

Deficiency symptoms:

Its deficiency leads to bone deformities, poor growth and ataxia in several aminal species. Its deficiency has also been shown to affect the synthesis of oligosaccharides, glycoproteins and proteoglycans.

Manganese Toxicity: Manganese toxicity may occur in the mine workers of manganese who then develop **madness with severe psychotic symptoms and parkinsonism.**

COBALT

Not much is known about the metabolism of cobalt. Adult human body contains only about 1-2 mg cobalt.

Functions

1. It may act as a cofactor for several

enzymes, e.g. glycylglycine dipeptidase which is found in intestinal juice.

2. It forms a component of vitamin B_{12}.

3. It also occurs in cobamide coenzymes.

4. It helps in erythropoiesis. Cattles grazing in cobalt-deficient fields are found to develop macrocytic anemia which is easily curable either by vitamin B_{12} or cobalt sulfate administration. It may also increase the production *of* erythropoietin **and may be a cofactor- for aminolevulinic acid synthetase in the synthesis** *of* **heme.**

Cobalt toxicity

Cobalt, if administered to man/animals in large quantity, becomes toxic as a result of which polycythemia (increased number of red blood cells in blood) takes place.

Sources

It is found in daily edible routine items.

Daily requirement

It is required by the human beings in very less quantity. It is required in the form of vitamin B_{12}. As little as 1-2 µg of B_{12}, containing 0.045-0.09 µg cobalt is sufficient to maintain normal bone marrow functioning in pernicious anaemia.

MOLYBDENUM

The element is readily absorbed as molybdate, excreted mainly in the urine, like other anions, concentrated in liver, kidney and adrenal. Human serum contains about 3 mcg per 100 ml and urine about 56 mcg per day.

Sources

Cereals and dry legumes supply more than 50 µg per day. Liver and kidney are also good sources.

Daily requirement

(i) Adults : Nearly 0.5 mg

(ii) Children: 0.05 - 0.3 mg.

Functions

1. Role in enzyme action: Some of the flavoproteins, such as xanthine oxidase and aldehyde oxidase contain traces of molybdenum in their prosthetic group where it is believed to play an important role in the electron transport.

2. A trace of molybdenum may help in the utilization of copper.

Toxicity

Excess intake of it is responsible for toxicity known as **"molybdinosis",** in which there occurs anaemia, growth retardation, loss of weight, diarrhoea, skeletal deformities, etc.

SELENIUM

Sources

It is found in different daily edible routine foodstuffs. The variation depends upon the differences of selenium content of the soil of that particular place. Fish, meat and cereals are the rich sources of selenium.

Daily requirement

(i) Adults : 0.2 mg

(ii) Children: 0.02 - 0.1 mg.

Absorption and Excretion

It is mainly absorbed in the duodenum and is taken up by β-lipoproteins, myoglobin, cytochrome C and nucleoproteins. It is excreted mainly in the faeces and expired air.

Functions:

1. It is constituent of **glutathione peroxidase** which catalyzes the breakdown of hydrogen peroxide in RBCs. Deficiency of selenium in human beings is not yet well established.

2. **Tocopherol sparing action**: Se has got close metabolic relationship with vitamin E. It reduces the requirement of vitamin E in more than one way (i) Se-containing glutathione peroxidase destroys acyl hydroperoxides, thus, lowers the need for antioxidant action of vitamin E in preventing peroxidative damages. (ii) Se may probably help in retaining vitamin E in lipoproteins.

3. It is involved in the mitochondrial ATP synthesis, ubiquinone synthesis and immune mechanisms.

4. It has been reported to be a **cancer protecting agent**.

Deficiency symptoms: Selenium deficiency may lead to liver necrosis muscular atrophy, necrosis of the cardiac muscle and dilatation of the heart.

Toxicity

(i) Its toxicity is fatal which generally occurs in the workers of paint, electronics, ceramic industries and glass factories etc.

(ii) Areas of high selenium have higher prevalence of dental caries.

Chromium

Very small amounts of chromium i.e. 0.01 mcg with insulin promote the conversion of acetate into glucose and fat. It is poorly absorbed from foods. Human serum contains about 6-20 mcg% and daily urinary excretion varies from <0.05 to 1 mcg.

Sources

Cereals, meat, yeast, milk, liver and other dietary foods.

Daily requirement

0.02 - 0.15 mg

Functions:

(i) Chromium plays an important role in carbohydrate, lipid and protein metabolism.

(ii) It is responsible for increasing sugar tolerance, probably by increasing the sensitivity of the peripheral tissues to insulin. **It is known as a *glucose tolerance factor*.**

(iii) It maintains the normal cholesterol level in blood in rats.

(iv) It regulates the incorporation of certain amino acids, mainly α-amino, isobutyric acid, glycine, serine and methionine in heart muscle in rats.

So far, no specific chromium deficiency disease in human beings is known today.

Absorption & Excretion:

Chromium is absorbed in the small intestine and combines with β- globulin in plasma. It's mainly excreted via urine.

Chromium Toxicity: Toxicity of chromium may be observed in occupational exposure to chromium dust **which is responsible for the cancer of lungs.**

WATER AND MINERALS

Everybody, whether plants or animals or human beings, is very familiar with the water from the day life starts in them. **Human body contains about 60- 70% water and nearly 8.5% minerals.** Minerals include relatively larger quantities of sodium, potassium, calcium, magnesium, phosphorus, chlorine and sulphur; whereas those required comparatively in small amounts are iron, copper, cobalt, manganese, zinc, selenium, iodine, fluorine, chromium, cadmium, molybdenum etc.

Water Metabolism

Importance of water than the food is evident from the fact that the deprivation of water brings about death much more rapidly than the deprivation of food. When water is completely withheld, death takes place in a few days after the body has lost only 10 to 20 per cent of its water content. If, however, water is given but no food, life may continue for several weeks inspite of the loss of most of the body fat and about 50 per cent of the tissue proteins.

Water is so important that its importance can not be ignored as most tissues contain more than 70 per cent water; even bone possesses nearly one third water and adipose tissue (fat) contains large quantity of water in the connective tissue and in the spaces between the fat cells. About half of the body water is to be found in muscle which accounts for about one-third of the body mass.

Sources

Body water comes through main three channels:

1. *Food water:* Nearly 700 - 1000 ml of water comes from food daily.
2. *Water in drinks:* Human beings receive at least 600 ml of water daily through various kinds of drinks like water itself, tea, coffee, milk, beverages etc. On an average, the amount comes around 1200 ml per day.
3. *Metabolic water:* Nearly 300-400 ml of water is formed daily within the body itself by way of oxidation. Each gram of carbohydrate, lipid and protein yields 0.55, 1.06, and 0.45 g of water respectively on complete oxidation.

Losses

Water is lost daily by several ways:

1. **Insensible losses;** About 1000-1200 ml of water may be unconsciously lost daily .from the human body. These *obligatory losses* occur irrespective of the availability of water.
   (a) **Insensible cutaneous evaporation:** Man loses nearly 600 ml of water daily by way of cutaneous diffusion and evaporation, excluding that by sweating.
   (b) **Pulmonary evaporation:** Normally about 400 ml of water gets evaporated from pulmonary alveoli and respiratory passages and eliminated with expired air every day.
2. *Loss via sweat:* In extreme hot circumstances, a man may lose upto 10 litres per day of sweat containing as much as 30 g of salt. If water and salt are not taken at frequent intervals under such hot circumstances, then the blood

Table 19.5 : Balance sheet of water (per day)

Water intake			Water loss		
(a)	By food water	: 850 ml	(a)	By lungs	: 400 ml
(b)	By drinks	: 1,200 ml	(b)	By skin	: 700 ml
(c)	By oxidation of foods	: 400 ml	(c)	By urine	: 1,250 ml
			(d)	By faeces	: 100 ml
	Total	2,450 ml		Total	2,450 ml

becomes concentrated which eventually affects the circulation, which may even fail. On an average, the loss is nearly 700 ml per day.

Sweat is a slightly acidic, watery fluid of variable composition but always hypotonic with respect to blood plasma. It contains 0.5 per cent solids only, mainly sodium chloride. The sodium content of sweat is also affected by aldosterone.

3. *Faecal loss:* Normally, about 100-200 ml may be *obligatorily* lost via faeces due to osmotic effects of faecal constitutents. Diarrhoea increases the faecal loss.

4. *Renal loss;* About 14 litres of fluid is filtered by the renal tubules in 24-hours, but nearly 99% of the water is reabsorbed leaving behind 1000-1500 ml of urine only.

Water balance

An equilibrium is maintained by different factors between the intake and output of water in the body (Table 19.5). In addition to other factors, certain hormones like anti-diuretic hormone (ADH), vasopressin, oxytocin and aldosterone also influence the regulatory mechanism of the body water.

An animal is said to be in *water equilibrium* when the total loss of water is in toto replaced by the amount obtained from various sources. When more water

is eliminated from the body than what is taken in, the body is said to be in negative water balance, e.g., in less consumption of water, diarrhoea, excessive and frequent vomiting and excessive sweating. If the loss of water is less than the amount received from various sources, the body is said to be in *positive water balance,* **e.g., during growth and pregnancy.** The balance sheet of water is as given in Table 19.5.

Physiological functions of water

1. *Solvent action:* The most important role of water is that it acts as a solvent both around and inside the cells. That is why, both, the extracellular and intracellular fluids are aqueous solutions. Water acts as a solvent for many biomolecules and also forms the medium where they may intermix and interact easily. Water donates H^+ and OH^- for many biochemical reactions, a beautiful property of water. It is also a reactant in hydrolysis and hydration.

2. *Ionization:* This property is very important from the point of view that water itself ionizes into H^+ and OH^- to provide a specific H^+ concentration in the biological fluids: Besides this, ionization of mineral salts in aqueous body fluids provides mineral ions like Na^+, K^+ and Cl^-,

which are required for electrical conductivity of body fluids and membrane polarization and depolarization.

3. *Homeostasis:* Homeostasis or constancy of internal environment is largely maintained with the help of body water.

4. *Fluid exchange:* Small molecules and polar nature of water enable its molecules to pass through the hydrophilic pores of membranes.

5. *Lubricating action:* Water also acts as a lubricant in the body so as to prevent friction in joints, pleura, peritoneum and conjuctiva.

6. *Latent heat of evaporation:* Water has the highest latent heat of evaporation than any other liquid. A certain amount of water can, therefore, cause maximum cooling by evaporation; so that the temperature of body does not rise so easily.

Regulation of Water Metabolism

There are several factors which regulate the water metabolism in the body; they are as follows:

1. *Antidiuretic hormone or Vasopressin:* Posterior pituitary releases ADH which has got the property to enhance water reabsorption in the distal tubules and collecting ducts. Water permeability gets increased.

2. *Hypothalamus:* There is a centre in hypothalamus known as a *thirst centre;* whenever there is dehydration in the body, osmoconcentration of plasma takes place which eventually stimulates the thirst centre producing thirst as a result of which animal gets provoked to drink the required amount of water. Besides this, osmoconcentration of plasma also stimulates supraoptic and paraventricular nuclei of hypothalamus; nerve impulses from them are responsible to increase the release of vasopressin from neurohyp-ophysis into the blood. Lesions in the supraopticoparaventricular region or in the neurohypophysis produce *diabetes insipidus* in which large volume of dilute (hypotonic) urine is passed, may be 10 litres or so a day. *Diabetes insipidus* **is due to the abnormalities in the ADH secretion. In primary diabetes insipidus, there is less secretion of the ADH hormone** which is usually due to the destruction of the hypothalamic-hypophyseal tract either from a basal skull fracture, or tumor, or infection. **Besides, diabetes insipidus may be hereditary also.**

3. *Adrenal Cortex and Water loss:* Loss of electrolytes and the loss of water from the body are closely interlinked. Adrenal cortex plays a very important role in governing the reabsorption of water by the renal tubules. **The excretion of sodium and potassium by the kidneys is controlled by a steroid hormone called *aldosterone* which is secreted by the zona glomerulosa of the adrenal cortex.** In man, aldosterone first increases the elimination of potassium and hydrogen ions and then decreases the excretion of sodium without any change in GFR. Aldosterone acts mainly at the distal tubule but its

effect on sodium reabsorption may be partly at the proximal tubule. Apart from its action on the renal tubule, aldosterone increases the reabsorption of sodium from the secretions of the intestinal mucosa and of the salivary and sweat glands. Thus, the body content of Na^+ rises and that of K^+ decreases.

Aldosterone is not the only cortical hormone affecting water balance. The diuretic response to a water load gets impaired in patients whose adrenal glands are destroyed by diseases like Addison's disease or are removed after operation. The ability to deal normally with water is, however, restored by the administration of cortisone or hydrocortisone.

4. *Rennin-Angiotensin system:* **This system is also involved in the regulation of blood pressure and electrolyte metabolism. The primary hormone involved - is** *angiotensin II,* **an octapeptide formed from angiot-ensiongen.** A decrease in circulating blood volume stimulates rennin secretion from kidneys which in turn promotes angiotensin formation in plasma. Angiotensin II stimulates the synthesis and secretion of aldosterone and the release of vasopressin, and thereby increases renal absorption of Na^+ and H_2O.

5. *Prostaglandins:* They are also believed to help maintain glomerular filtration inspite of hypotension, by causing renal vasodilation. They may also increase urinary loss of water by inhibiting the antidiuretic effect of vasopressin and by increasing the urinary sodium.

6. *Solutes:* Osmotic effect of Na^+ helps to retain water in extracellular fluids. Elevation in plasma Na^+ raises the ECF volume in primary aldosteronism while an increase in urinary Na^+ raises the urinary water output in Addison's disease. K^+ helps to retain water in the cells, whereas, plasma proteins do help to retain water in the body by their osmotic effects. Increase in urinary urea or excretion of glucose in urine increases osmotically the urinary loss of water **(osmotic diuresis).**

Dehydration

Dehydration may be defined as a state in which loss of water exceeds that of intake, as a result of which body's water content gets reduced. In this state, the body is in negative water balance.

Causes

1. *Primary- dehydration:* There is purely water depletion and no salt depletion. It occurs in following states:

   (a) Due to deprivation of water as generally happens during desert travelling.

   (b) In mental patients who refuse to drink water/fluids.

   (c) In those who keep such a 'fast' in which water/fluid is completely restricted.

   (d) It occurs more quickly during fever or in the high temperature of the environment.

   (e) Excessive water loss due to vomiting, prolonged diarrhoea, gastroenteritis.

   (f) Due to excretion of large quantities of urine or sweat.

This type of dehydration raises the concentration and osmotic pressure of extracellular fluid as a result of which there is consequent outflow of the intracellular water to the ECF; thus, ECF volume gets largely restored but there becomes deficiency of water inside the cells as a result of which they suffer from osmoconcentration; symptoms of which include dry tongue, poor salivation, dry shrunken skin, nausea, reduced sweating and intense thirst.

When the blood becomes hypertonic, it lowers the urinary output and also makes the urine concentrated as a result of which there is less elimination of NPN and other acids which leads to acidosis and eventually coma. Death occurs in man due to renal failure, acidosis, intracellular hyperosmolarity, circulatory collapse or neural depression, when body water falls by 20%.

Drinking of concentrated saline like sea-water or failure of Na^+ excretion (e.g., in Cushing's syndrome and Primary aldosteronism) may cause hypertonicity of ECF which in turn is responsible for withdrawal of water from tissue cells, dehydration of tissues, but a rise in ECF volume. Mg^{2+} of sea-water may be responsible for an increased intestinal loss of water due to its osmotic effect in the intestinal lumen.

2. *Secondary dehydration:* The concentration of the electrolytes of the body fluids is maintained constant either through The elimination or retention of water. The reduction or elevation in the total electrolytes, which affects the basic radicals chiefly i.e. Na (extracellular) and K (intracellular) and the acid radicals HCO_3 and Cl are accompanied by a corresponding increase or decrease in the volume of body water which is eventually the cause of intracellular edema; as a result of which there is slowing of circulation and impairment of urinary functions. All this causes an individual to become weak bodily.

3. *Dehydration due to injection of hypertonic solution:* When a highly concentrated solution of sugar or salt is injected into the body of an individual, the osmotic pressure of blood will increase which results in the flow of fluid from the tissues into the blood unless an equilibrium is reached. Consequently, the blood volume increases. This increased blood volume soon returns to normal by the loss of excess material through excretion which finally causes a net loss of body water producing dehydration.

Effects of dehydration

There are various side effects of dehydration as follows, which may be overcome as soon as the body gets hydrated; otherwise the consequences are serious and may even lead to death.

1. Disturbance in acid-base balance.

2. Loss of body weight due to the reduction in tissue water.

3. Rise in nonprotein nitrogen (NPN) of blood.

4. Dryness, wrinkling and looseness of the skin.

5. Elevation in the plasma protein concentration and chloride.
6. Rise in the temperature of body due to reduction of circulating fluid.
7. Increased pulse rate and reduced cardiac output.
8. Exhaustion and collapse i.e. death.

Correction of dehydration

1. Ordinarily, sodium chloride solution may be given parenterally to compensate the loss.
2. In several disorders like diarrhoea, gastroenteritis, pancreatic or biliary fistulas, etc., a mixture of two-thirds isotonic saline solution and one-third sodium lactate solution (M/6) should be administered intravenously.
3. **Dehydration is a burning problem in several disorders like diabetes mellitus, Addison's disease, uremia, shock and extensive burns** which is difficult to correct by the above two ways.

Water Intoxication

This condition is generally caused due to the retention of excess water in the body and can occur due to renal failure, excessive administration of fluids parenterally and hypersecretion of ADH. Symptoms of water intoxication include nausea, headache, muscular weakness, etc.

Poisoning by Trace Elements

Poisoning by trace elements can either be acute or chronic. Meal poisoning can take place due to over exposure to metals like lead or mercury.

Lead poisoning can take place due to industrial exposure or due to paints which have a high lead content. Main symptoms of lead poisoning are neurological signs, anemia, renal failure etc.

Mercury poisoning is also relatively common which can take place due to the ingestion of inorganic and organic compounds containing mercury. In Japan, an outbreak of mercury poisoning known as **Minemata disease** resulted from the ingestion of fish which had incorporated mercury compounds from the food chain. The original source was industrial waste.

Likewise, lithium is used therapeutically as an antidepressant, the overdose of which can produce toxicity.

CHAPTER 20

ENZYMES AND ISOENZYMES

> Voluminous books have been written on us; without ours participation in chemical reactions 'biochemistry of any living organism' is never possible. End of ours shall never come. We are still being discovered by the scientists. We are organic compounds and complex molecules. Ours classification is very systematic. We play very important role in making the diagnosis foolproof for physicians/ surgeons, thus make the treatment part to the point and we are also of tremendous use therapeutically.

ENZYMES

Enzymes are biological catalysts (biocatalysts) which bring about chemical reactions in living cells. They accelerate the rate of the reaction and are usually present in very small amount in various cells. They can also exhibit their activity when they have been extracted from the source. They are organic compounds and a number of them have been obtained in crystalline form. **Today, more than 840 enzymes are known.**

General properties of the enzymes:

1. They are proteinous in nature.
2. They accelerate the rate of the reaction by:
   (a) not altering the reaction equilibrium.
   (b) being required in minute quantity.
   (c) being not consumed in the overall reaction.
3. They act as catalysts, deficiency of which may diminish the rate of a particular reaction; whereas complete absence of it may completely block a particular reaction.
4. They are very specific for their substrates.
5. They possess active sites at which interaction with substrate occurs.

> Pyridoxal phosphate, a slightly modified form of vitamin B_6 (pyridoxine), is an essential cofactor or coenzyme, for an important group of enzymes known collectively as *transaminases*. As the name implies, these enzymes transfer α-amino group from an amino acid to a α-keto acid.

6. They are responsible for lowering the activation energy.
7. **Some enzymes are regulatory in function.**

Enzyme Cofactors, Coenzymes, Prosthetic Groups

In addition to the protein component, many enzymes require nonprotein constituents for their proper functioning. In some cases these components, broadly described as cofactors, may be metal ions and, in other cases, organic molecules of relatively low molecular weight. When the small organic molecules are tightly bound either by covalent or coordinate bonds, they are called as **prosthetic groups. The heme group of the cytochromes is an example of a prosthetic group.**

Coenzymes

Coenzymes are organic molecules, often derived from the B vitamins, that participate directly in enzymatic reactions. Some coenzymes are attached to their companion enzymes as tightly bound prosthetic groups, whereas others can be easily removed by dialysis. The complete functional complex of enzyme and cofactors is called a *holoenzyme;* the protein part, free of the cofactors, is called an *apoenzyme.*

Characteristics of coenzymes:

1. They are stable towards heat.
2. Generally derived from vitamins.
3. Function as co-substrates.
4. They participate in:
   (a) Electron transfer reactions, e.g. NAD$^+$, NADH, FMN, FAD, etc.
   (b) Group transfer reactions e.g., CoA, TPP, pyridoxal phosphate, tetrahydrofolic acid, etc.

Coenzymes	Functions performed
1. NAD$^+$	Hydrogen transfer
2. NADP$^+$	Hydrogen transfer
3. FAD	Hydrogen transfer
4. FMN	Hydrogen transfer
5. TPP(Thiamine pyrophosphate)	Acetyl group transfer
6. PP (Pyridoxal phosphate)	Amino group transfer
7. Biotin	Carboxyl group transfer
8. Coenzyme A	Acyl group transfer

Nicotinamide nucleotides

NAD$^+$, NADP$^+$ and their reduced forms are involved in a great variety of

*NADP$^+$ has PO$_4$ here

Nicotinamide adenine dinucleotide (NAD); NADP is nicotinamide adenine dinucleotide phosphate.
* NADP$^+$ has got PO$_4$ in place of OH

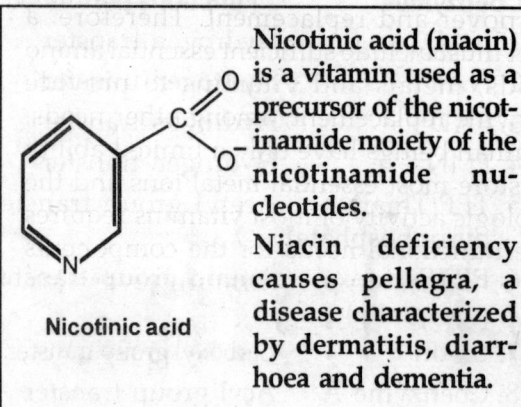

Nicotinic acid (niacin) is a vitamin used as a precursor of the nicotinamide moiety of the nicotinamide nucleotides.

Niacin deficiency causes pellagra, a disease characterized by dermatitis, diarrhoea and dementia.

Nicotinic acid

dehydrogenase reactions in the mitochondria, cytosol and endoplasmic reticulum of the cell. They are water soluble, and are usually free to diffuse away from the enzyme after conversion to the oxidized or reduced form, to take part in another dehydrogenase reaction catalysed by another enzyme.

Flavin nucleotide coenzymes:

FAD is the coenzyme of a class of dehydrogenases known as flavoproteins. The flavin moiety of the molecule is derived from riboflavin (vitamin B_2).

Flavin mononucleotide (FMN) is an important coenzyme in some flavoproteins, including NADH coenzyme Q reductase, etc.

FMN consists of riboflavin phosphate (i.e., FAD without the adenosine monophosphate moiety).

Flavin coenzymes remain tightly bound to the enzyme protein throughout the reaction, in contrast to the nicotinamide coenzymes that bind reversibly to the enzyme.

A number of mitochondrial dehydrogenases are flavoproteins; for example, NADH dehydrogenase, succinate dehydrogenase and fatty acyl CoA dehydrogenase.

Thiamine pyrophosphate

Thiamine (Vitamin B_1) is the precursor of thiamine pyrophosphate, the coenzyme for some important oxidative decarboxylation reactions (pyruvate dehydrogenase, oxoglutarate dehydrogenase).

In oxidative decarboxylation, loss of CO_2 is accompanied by oxidation of an aldehyde to an acid.

Deficiency of thiamine causes the disease beriberi, a disease associated with neuropathy and cardiopathy. Experimental deficiency causes **neurological symptoms** (pigeons fail to hold their head erect) that can readily be reversed by administering the vitamin.

Pyruvate dehydrogenase enzyme has a complex mechanism involving binding sites for pyruvate, NAD^+, thiamine pyrophosphate and lipoic acid.

Pyridoxal phosphate

Pyridoxal phosphate (derivative of vitamin B_6) acts as a coenzyme in transamination and decarboxylation reactions. In a transamination reaction the aldehyde group of pyridoxal phosphate first forms a Schiff's base with the amino group of the amino acid, which is then converted to keto acid. Pyridoxal phosphate is thereby converted to pyridoxamine phosphate which transfers the amino group to another keto acid to form an amino acid.

Pyridoxal phosphate also acts as a coenzyme in decarboxylation reactions of amino acids such as :

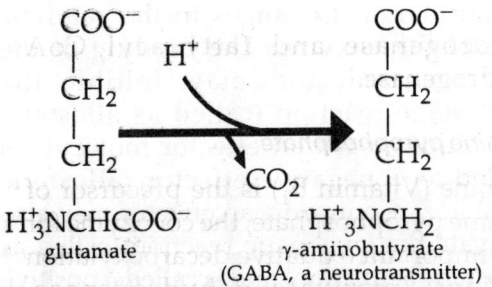

glutamate → γ-aminobutyrate
(GABA, a neurotransmitter)

> Vitamin B_6 deficiency is rare in man, because the vitamin is widely distributed in common foodstuffs and in addition is synthesized in appreciable quantities by intestinal flora. The main abnormality seen in B_6 deficiency is dermatitis which is readily cured by the administration of the vitamin.

Biotin

It is an essential food factor and is a coenzyme for carboxylation reactions (e.g. pyruvate carboxylase). These reactions involve ATP, which is necessary in the first step of the reaction; this is the conversion of biotin to carboxybiotin by the addition of CO_2 to C-1 of biotin.

> Pantothenic acid is an essential food factor which forms part of coenzyme A.

Coenzyme A

It is a complex molecule which contains a free sulfhydryl (-SH) group. This group can react with a carboxyl group to form a thioester. Such thiolesters are involved in many reactions involving acyl groups, including acetyl and fatty acyl groups.

Enzyme and cofactor turnover

Like all biologic materials, enzymes have a finite half-life; that is, they are subject to turnover and replacement. Therefore, a diet must include sufficient essential amino acids, metals and vitamins to provide enzyme replacement, among other needs. Human beings have only a limited ability to store most essential metal ions and the biologic activity of most vitamins requires the nutritional needs for the components of enzymes on a continuing everyday basis.

Zymogens or proenzymes

Most of the intracellular enzymes are secreted in their active forms known as **Zymase** form of the enzyme but side by side few enzymes are secreted in their inactive forms known as **proenzymes** or **zymogens**.These enzymes (proenzymes/zymogens) have a tendency to undergo prior change in structure after coming into contact with certain activating agents.Activating agent may be H^+, another enzyme on the active form of the zymogen itself. For instance gastric juice contains pepsin which is secreted by pepsinogen (a zymogen). **Pepsinogen (Fig 20.1) is changed into its active form pepsin** by H^+ of the gastric juice. Once formed pepsin itself acts on pepsinogen and catalyses its own conversion into pepsin;such a process is called as **autocatalysis** (Fig 20.1).

Thus, **zymogens** are inactive precursors of enzymes that are primarily concerned with proteolytic activity. The important

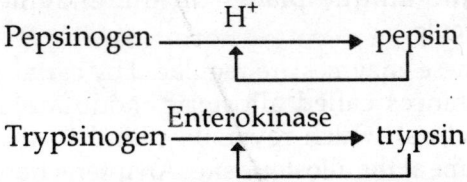

Fig. 20.1 : Activation of a zymogen

examples of this category are the enzymes found in the gastrointestinal tract that act on dietary proteins. This unique process is probably involved with the protection of tissues from digestion by their own proteolytic enzymes.

Important examples of the enzymes that occur as zymogens are as follows:

Zymogem	activator	active enzyme
Pepsinogen	H⁺, pepsin	pepsin
Trypsinogen	trypsin, enterokinase	trypsin
Chymotrypsinogen chymotrypsin		trypsin
Procarboxy-peptidase	trypsin	carboxy-peptidase
Proelastase	trypsin	elastase
Prorennin	H⁺, rennin	rennin

> **Pepsin is the major proteolytic enzyme found in the stomach. Pepsinogen has a M.W. of 42,500 and is converted by acid or pepsin itself to active pepsin with a M.W. of 34,500.** The conversion is accompanied by the removal of one-fifth of the peptide chain(in the form of six peptides).

Allosteric Enzymes

Some of the enzymes possess additional sites known as allosteric sites (Greek:allo-other) besides the active site. Such enzymes are known as allosteric or regulatory enzymes. The allosteric sites are the unique places on the enzyme molecule.

These enzymes are regulated by certain substances called allosteric modulators (effectors) which reversibly bind to the enzyme at the allosteric site. An interaction with the effector molecule brings about conformational changes in the catalytic site of the enzyme. The binding of the effector molecule may inhibit the enzymatic reaction (called as allosteric inhibition); such an effector molecule is called as a negative effector (allosteric inhibitor). Contrarily, an effector may also activate the enzymatic reaction (called as allosteric activation) and is called a positive effector (allosteric activator).

Examples of this category are (i) HMG CoA reductase is a regulatory enzyme of cholesterol biosynthesis, where as aspartate transcarbamoylase is the regulatory enzyme for pyrimidine synthesis.

If the effector substance is the substrate itself then it is called as **homotropic effect;** contrarily, if the effector molecule is a substance other than the substrate then it is called as the **hetrotropic effect.** Removal of inhibition can be brought about by increasing the amount of the inhibitor. Mechanism of action of allosteric enzymes can be very well understood by the following Figure 20.2.

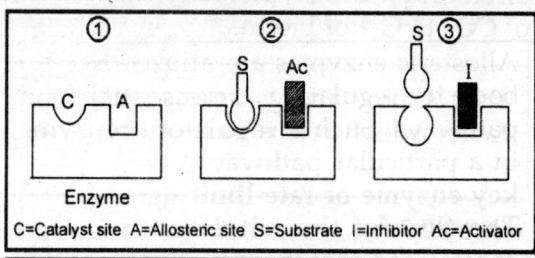

C=Catalyst site A=Allosteric site S=Substrate I=Inhibitor Ac=Activator

Fig. 20.2 : Action of allosteric enzymes: (1) The enzyme has separate catalytic (C) and allosteric (A) sites (2) When activator (Ac) is fixed, the catalytic site assumes correct three dimensional structure, so that substrate(S) can combine, (3) When inhibitor (I) is attached, catalytic site is altered, so that substrate is not engaged.

A few examples of allosteric enzymes are as follows:

(a) succinylCoA+glycine $\xrightarrow{\text{ALA synthase}}$ δ-amino-levulinic acid (ALA)

This is the first step in the synthesis of heme. Here the end product i.e., heme will allosterically inhibit the enzyme ALA synthase which is the key enzyme of heme synthesis.

(b) Carbamoyl phosphate + asparate

$$\downarrow \text{Asparate transcarbamoylase}$$

carbamoyl asparate

This is the first step in the biosynthesis of cytidine triphosphate (CTP). Here ,the end product i.e.,CTP will allosterically inhibit the enzyme asparate transcarbamoylase.

(c) Inhibition of enzyme HMG CoA reductase by cholesterol (the end product of cholesterol biosynthesis) is another example of allosteric inhibition.

(d) **Phosphofructokinase (PFK) which catalyzes the phosphorylation of** fructose-6-phosphate to fructose-1, 6 -diphosphate is the rate limiting enzyme of glycolysis. This enzyme is allosterically inhibited by ATP and citrate but allosterically activated by AMP and fructose-6-phosphate.

Feedback inhibition

Feed back inhibition (Fig 20.3) refers to the inhibition of the enzyme by the end product of the reactions, for e.g., when a substrate (A) is converted to a product (P) through various intermediates (B, C,D, E, etc), the end product of the reaction inhibits the first enzyme of the pathway (Fig 20.3). In this type of inhibition, the accumulation of the end product slows down the whole reaction sequence and since the end product continues to be consumed, its synthesis continues. Since it is partially competitive, both V_{max} and K_m are altered.

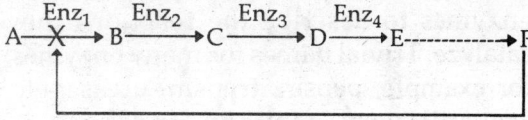

Fig. 20.3 : Feedback Inhibition

As it is a mixed type of inhibition, the inhibitor binds to the enzyme at a site other than the active site called as **allosteric site** which is encountered in **allosteric enzymes.**

Feedback inhibition is a type of regulatory mechanism which has been identified in many instances and is especially interesting since it is a self-regulatory device allowing a cell to adjust the rate of synthesis of a metabolic intermediate to its everchanging needs. One important classical example of it involves the synthesis of CTP in

---

Allosteric enzymes are utilized by the body for regulating various metabolic pathways. Such a regulatory enzyme in a particular pathway is called as a **key enzyme or rate limiting enzyme.** The flow of the whole pathway is constrained as if there is a bottle- neck at the level of the key enzyme. The allosteric inhibitor is most effective when substrate concentration is low. This is metabolically very significant. When more substrate molecules are available, automatically there is less necessity for stringent regulation. In this way, the whole pathway can be easily regulated.

Escherichia coli. Early in this reaction sequence, carbamoyl phosphate is converted to carbamoyl aspartate by the enzyme **aspartate transcarbamoylase.** This reaction is crucial, since its inhibition affects the subsequent reactions leading to CTP. This enzyme is sensitive to inhibition by CTP. As the reaction sequence produces CTP, and when the CTP is not used rapidly enough in subsequent reactions (e.g., incorporation into nucleic acids), a critical concentration of CTP is reached, which inhibits aspartate transcarbamoylase. The result is a decrease in the synthesis of CTP until its concentration is lowered below the level at which the enzyme is inhibited.

Classification of Enzymes

As per international classification, **the enzymes have been classified into six major classes,** each with several subclasses; within each subclass, formal names have been assigned to the known enzymes to describe the reactions they catalyze. Trivial names for many enzymes, for example, pepsin, trypsin, urease, etc. are still very common and easy to remember as well. Many enzymes are still easier to recognize them by their trivial names. The newer nomenclature has been less widely adopted due to its own complications.

Six major classes are:

1. *Oxidoreductases:* They catalyze a wide variety of oxidation-reduction reactions and frequently employ coenzymes such as NAD^+, $NADP^+$, FAD, or lipoate as the hydrogen acceptor. Other acceptors include coenzyme Q or molecular oxygen. **Common trivial names include dehydrogenase, oxidase, peroxides, and reductase.**

2. *Transferases:* They catalyze various kinds of group transfers. Many important steps in metabolism require transfer from one molecule to another of amino, carboxyl, carbonyl, methyl, acyl, glycosyl, or phosphoryl groups. **Common trivial names include amino transferase (transaminase), acyl carnitine transferase and transcarboxylase.**

3. *Hydrolases:* They catalyze cleavage of bonds between a carbon and some other atom by addition of water. **Some common trivial names include esterase, peptidase, amylase, urease, phosphatase, pepsin, trypsin and chymotrypsin.**

4. *Lyases:* They catalyze breakage of carbon-carbon, carbon-sulphur and certain carbon-nitrogen (excluding peptide bonds. **Common trivial names include decarboxylase, aldolase, citrate lyase and dehydratase.**

5. *Isomerases:* They catalyze racemization of optical or geometric isomers and certain intramolecular oxidation-reduction reactions. **Trivial names include epimerase, racemase, and mutase.**

No.	Major classes	Examples
1.	Oxidoreductases	Alcohol dehydrogenase, xanthine oxidase.
2.	Transferases	Hexokinase, etc.
3.	Hydrolases	Glucose-6-phosphatase, pepsin, carboxypeptidase
4.	Lyases	Aldolase, pyruvate decarboxylase
5.	Isomerases	Phosphotriose isomerase, phosphoglucomutase
6.	Ligases	Glutamine synthetase, glutathione synthetase

6. *Ligases:* These catalyze the formation of bonds between carbon and oxygen, sulphur, nitrogen and other atoms. The energy required for bond formation is frequently derived from the hydrolysis of ATP. **Some trivial names include synthetase and carboxylase.**

Isomeric enzymes or isoenzymes or isozymes (Multiple molecular forms of enzymes)

A particular enzyme obtained from different times often has certain physicochemical properties which are characteristic of the tissue of origin, although the same chemical reaction is catalyzed in each case. Electrophoresis and chromatography in particular are the two techniques which are most frequently used to separate and 'finger print' these multiple molecular forms. Different physicochemical properties of the enzymes frequently affect their catalytic activity, so that they often differ in such properties as their Km, sensitivity to heat, effect of inhibitors and reactions with coenzyme or substrate analogues.

The term **"isoenzyme"** is used to describe the multiple form of an enzyme which are distinct proteins, such as those

Examples of Isoenzymes are:
1. Lactate dehydrogenase (LDH)
2. Creatine phosphokinase (CPK or CK)
3. Alkaline phosphatase (ALP)
4. Malate dehydrogenase
5. Carbonic anhydrase
6. Hexokinase
7. Phosphorylase
8. Glucose-6-phosphate dehydrogenase, etc.

of lactate dehydrogenase, creatine phosphokinase, alkaline phosphatase etc. A single tissue may contain more than one form of an enzyme, for instance, kidney contains isoenzymes of alkaline phosphatase which may be separated from each other with the help of column chromatography on diethylaminoethyl-cellulose (DEAE-Cellulose).

Lactate dehydrogenase which has thoroughly been studied is composed of four subunits. There are two different subunits that can be combined into tetramers in five ways. The possible combinations can be separated by electrophoresis as shown in Figures 20.4 and 20.5. If one subunit type is identified as "M" (the major form found in muscle or liver) and the second as "H" (the major form found in heart), then the tetramers could have the compositions M_4, M_3H, M_2H_2, MH_3, or H_4. These can be separated from each other by electrophoresis.

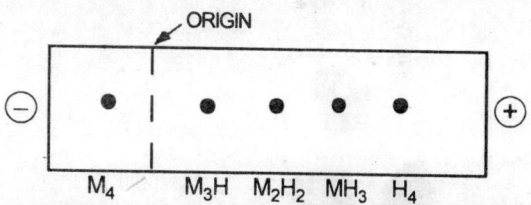

Fig. 20.4: Electrophoresis of lactate dehydrogenase isoenzymes at pH 8.6

In man, the content of several isoenzymes differs in heart and liver. Although the reason for this is not known, use is made of the fact in diagnostic differentiation of diseases of the liver and myocardium. In both types of disease states, lactate dehydrogenase leaks out of the damaged cells and increases the concentration of the enzyme in blood serum. Differentiation can be based in part on the pattern that appears on electrophoresis and in part on the fact that some of the isoenzymes from the myocardium are more resistant to heat denaturation than the corresponding hepatic isozymes. In the simpler differential test situation, a serum sample may be analyzed twice, once before and once after heat denaturation under carefully controlled conditions.

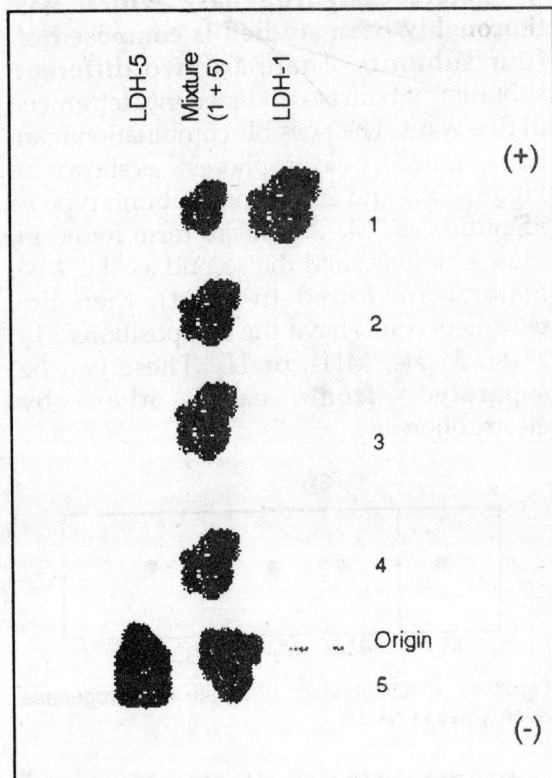

Fig. 20.5: This photograph shows the LDH isozymes in each of three preparations after electrophoretic resolution in starch gel. On the right is LDH-1, on the left LDH-5, and in the middle are the isozymes resulting from a mixture of equal quantities of these two preparations. All five isozymes were generated in the mixture in the approximate ratio of 1 : 4 : 6 : 4 : 1, the expected distribution after random reassociation of subunits. The total enzyme activity in the mixture was the sum of the activities of the single isozyme preparations. All three preparations were placed in 1 M NaCl and frozen overnight before electrohoretic resolution.

Clinically Important Enzyme Inhibitors

Enzymes may also be inactivated or denatured by a variety of chemical means, several of which have clinical importance. Many enzymes depend on essential sulfhydryl groups, which form tight covalent bonds with various heavy metals. For this reason mercury, lead, silver, etc are extremely toxic. **Even iron and copper, although they are classed as essential minerals, can produce intoxication when ingested in excess.**

Another class of inhibitors affects enzymes by introducing foreign alkyl groups into the structure. Most of these substances were initially developed as chemical warfare agents and are highly toxic in nature. Two best known are:

(a) diisopropylfluorophosphate (DFP), and

(b) the so called nitrogen mustards, for example, methachloramine and 2, 2'-dichloro-N-methyldiethylamine.

These, so called, nitrogen mustards are now employed clinically as enzyme inhibitors in the treatment of certain types of neoplastic diseases.

Enzyme inhibitors are:
1. Mercury
2. Lead
3. Silver
4. DFP
5. Various insecticides used in agriculture
6. Nitrogen mustards

The organic phosphates, of which DFP is only one example, are particularly good inhibitors of acetylcholinesterase, which breaks down the neurotransmitter substance known as acetylcholine. **Inactivation of acetylcholinesterase produces violent spasms of the pulmonary system and interferes with normal neuromuscular and cardiac functions.** Similar agents employed as insecticides in agriculture may be severely or fatally toxic.

Enzyme Inhibition

The rate of an enzyme-catalyzed reaction can be decreased by specific inhibitors, i.e., compounds that combine with the enzyme and prevent normal enzyme substrate interactions in the active site, thus diminishing the rate of the reaction. Certain enzymic inhibitors are poisonous for living organisms, including cyanide, hydrogen sulfide and carbon monoxide. Many drugs are also inhibitors of metabolic reactions and molecular pharmacology is largely dependent on the knowledge of inhibition of enzymes.

Application of enzyme inhibition

1. Studies on enzyme inhibition have led to the development of hundreds of new drugs for use in medicine and veterinary science.

2. Enzyme inhibition studies have been directed specifically toward increasing our understanding of specific reactions or metabolic pathways in animals and plants.

3. Enzyme inhibition studies have also led to the development of nerve gases, insecticides and herbicides (weed killers).

Types of Inhibition

Many substances inhibit enzymes and reduce the initial velocity (increase $1/v$). The Lineweaver-Burk plots reveal the mechanism of the inhibition. **Following four types of inhibitions are known:**

1. **Competitive inhibition,**
2. **Non-competitive inhibition,**
3. **Partially competitive inhibition, and**
4. **Uncompetitive inhibition.**

1. Competitive Inhibition

In this type of inhibition (Fig. 20.6), competitive inhibitors can combine reversibly with the active site of the enzyme and compete with the substrate at the active site. While the site is thus occupied, it is unavailable for the binding of the substrate. The combination of a competitive inhibitor I with enzyme E can be written in the same manner as

$$E + I \rightleftharpoons EI$$

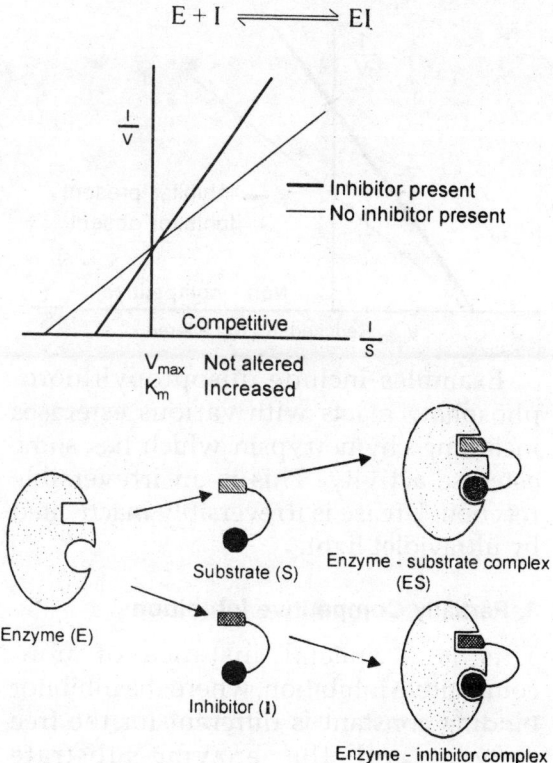

Fig. 20.6 : Showing Competitive Inhibition of an enzyme

combination with substrate, although the inhibitor is not chemically transformed to products.

One classical example of this type of inhibition involves malonic acid as an inhibitor of succinic dehydrogenase. This enzyme forms complexes and with the proper concentrations of reactants, succinate is not dehydrogenated (oxidized) to fumaric acid. On the other hand, with sufficient succinate present, the inhibition by malonate can be completely overcome.

2. Noncompetitive Inhibition

In this type, inhibition occurs when the inhibitor binds to a site on the enzyme other than the active site or binds irreversibly to the active site.

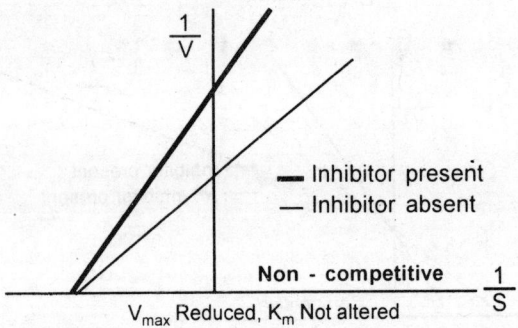

Examples include diisopropylfluorophosphate reacts with various esterases including chymotrypsin which has some esterase activity. This is an irreversible reaction. Urease is irreversibly inactivated by ultraviolet light.

3. Partially Competitive Inhibition

This is a special instance of noncompetitive inhibition, where the inhibitor binding constant is different for the free enzyme and the enzyme-substrate complex. Two alternatives are indicated by

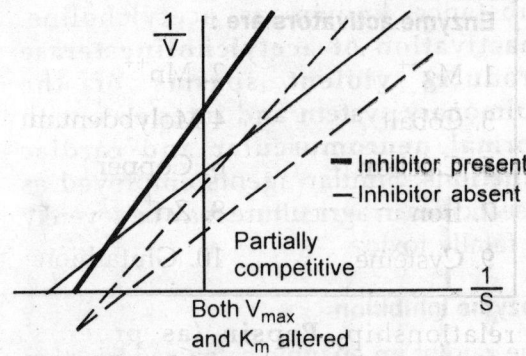

the solid and broken lines.

4. Uncompetitive Inhibition

It occurs when the inhibitor binds after the substrate has bound to the enzyme, and then stops the reaction from occurring; eventually no product is formed. This type of inhibition is not reversed by increasing substrate concentration. This type of inhibition is most frequently found in enzymic reactions with two or more substrates.

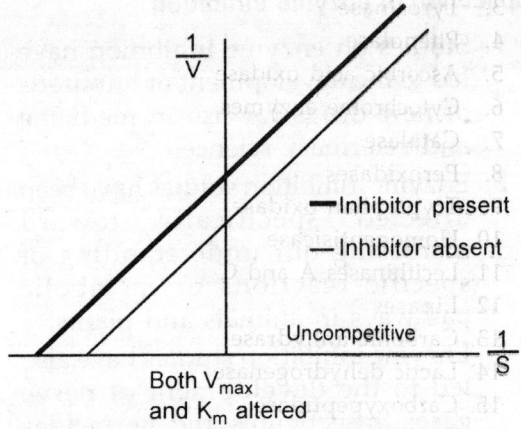

Enzyme Activators

Many ions and molecules have the capacity to activate some enzymes. Metal ions are activators of a number of enzymes. Following Table 20.1 shows this

Enzyme activators are :

1. Mg^{++}	2. Mn^{++}
3. Cobalt	4 Molybdenum
5. Calcium	6. Copper
7. Iron	8. Zn^{++}
9. Cysteine	10. Glutathione

relationship. **Pepsin (as proenzyme pepsinogen) is activated by H^+ to form the active enzyme.** Many reducing agents (cysteine, glutathione) act as enzyme activators of-SH enzymes. Enzymes themselves activate other enzymes or proenzymes; i.e., enterokinase activates trypsinogen to form active trypsin.

Many enzymes require a metal ion (Table 20.1) for activity. In some cases, the requirement is specific for a particular metal. Carbonic anhydrase shows no activity upon removal of zinc, and no other metal is known to replace zinc in this enzyme. In other cases, more than one metal is able to bring about activation; for example, Mg^{++}, Mn^{++}, or Zn^{++} activate enolase (2-phosphoglycerate→phosphoenolpyruvate + H_2O). In a few cases it appears that two metal ions may be required by the enzyme; for example, pyruvate phosphokinase requires both Mg^{++} and K^+ (pyruvate + ATP→phosphopyruvate + ADP).

Enzyme inhibitors are those which have a tendency to inhibit/ retard or stop the activity of an enzyme.

Some important examples of enzyme inhibitors are as given in Table 20.2:

Table 20.1: Metalloenzymes

(Enzymes either contain metal or are activated by it)

Sl. No.	Enzyme	Metal
1.	Xanthine oxidase	Mo
2.	Nitrate reductase	Mo
3.	Tyrosinase	Cu
4.	Phenolase	Cu
5.	Ascorbic acid oxidase	Cu
6.	Cytochrome enzymes	Fe
7.	Catalase	Fe
8.	Peroxidases	Fe
9.	Tryptophan oxidase	Fe
10.	Homogentisicase	Fe
11.	Lecithinases A and C	Ca
12.	Lipases	Ca
13.	Carbonic anhydrase	Zn
14.	Lactic dehydrogenase	Zn
15.	Carboxypeptidase	Zn
16.	Peptidases	Mg
17.	Phosphatases	Mg
18.	ATP-enzymes, such as hexokinases	Mg
19.	Arginase	Mn
20.	Phosphoglucomutase	Mn
21.	Dipeptidases	Mn
22.	Peptidases	Co

Table 20.2 : Enzymes and their inhibitors

Enzyme	Inhibitors
Arginase	Ornithine, lysine, L- amino acids
Alkaline phosphatase	Chelating compounds, arsenate, F^-
Carboxylase	HCHO, CH_3CHO, C_6H_5CHO
Cholinesterase	Physostigmine, neostigmine
Carbonic anhydrase	CO, sulfanilamide
Cytochrome oxidase	CN^-, H_2S, CO, azide
Carboxy-peptidase	Iodoacetate, S^{--}, CN^-
α-Ketoglutaric oxidase	Parapyruvate
Lipase	Benzaldehyde, some metal ions
Succinic dehydrogenase	Malonate, hematin, Se
Urease	Heavy metals, o-quinone

Factors Affecting Enzyme Activity

Major factors responsible to affect the enzymic activity are the following:

1. Concentration of substrate
2. Concentration of enzyme
3. Concentration of reaction products
4. Effect of pH
5. Effect of temperature and
6. Effect of time

Substrate concentration

It is sometimes found that as the substrate concentration is increased, the reaction velocity increases, but then falls at high substrate concentrations. This is known as substrate inhibition (Fig. 20.7).

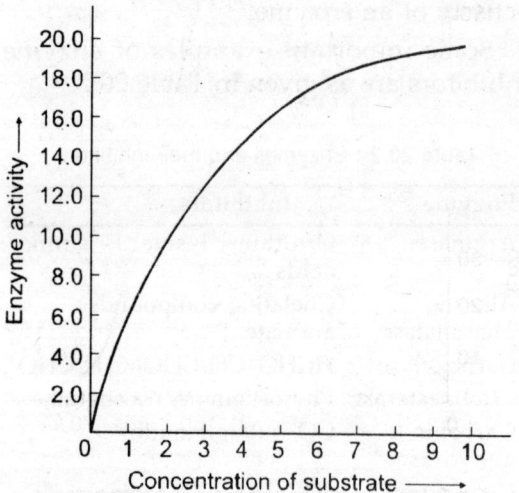

Fig. 20.7 : Effect of substrate concentration on enzyme activity

Liver alcohol dehydrogenase, which has a mechanism in which NAD^+ binds first, is inhibited by high concentrations of the second substrate, alcohol.

Concentration of enzyme

Within fairly wide limits the speed of an enzymatic reaction is proportional to the enzyme concentration. This can be shown to hold for many enzyme systems, provided interfering conditions do not develop and the substrate concentration is maintained constant (Fig. 20.8).

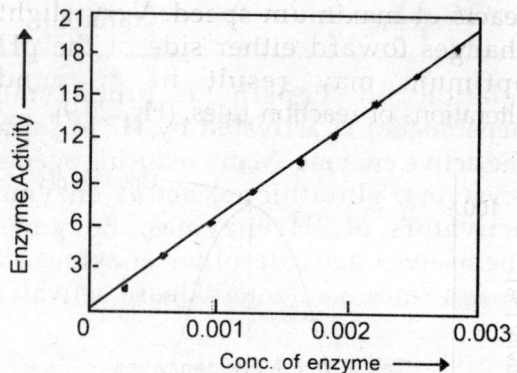

Fig 20.8 : Effect of enzyme concentration on enzyme activity

Concentration of reaction products

An enzyme-product complex is part of the reaction sequence of enzyme-catalysed reactions. In the presence of large concentrations of product, this complex is dominant and product inhibition is observed. This is one of the reasons why the velocity of the reaction falls as the equilibrium is approached and it is of physiological importance in controlling pathways by negative feedback. In single-product enzymes as shown below in equation, addition of the product causes reversal of the reaction, but if there are two or more products, both are needed for reversal to occur, so inhibition of the forward reaction by each can be studied separately.

$$E + S \underset{k_2}{\overset{k_1}{\rightleftharpoons}} ES \xrightarrow{k_3} E + P$$

Usually each product is competitive with the substrate from which it is derived, e.g. see 'box'

Effect of pH

Each enzyme has a pH optimum- i.e., a H^+ concentration at which the enzyme reacts at maximum speed. Very slight changes toward either side of the pH optimum may result in profound alterations of reaction rates, (Fig. 20.9).

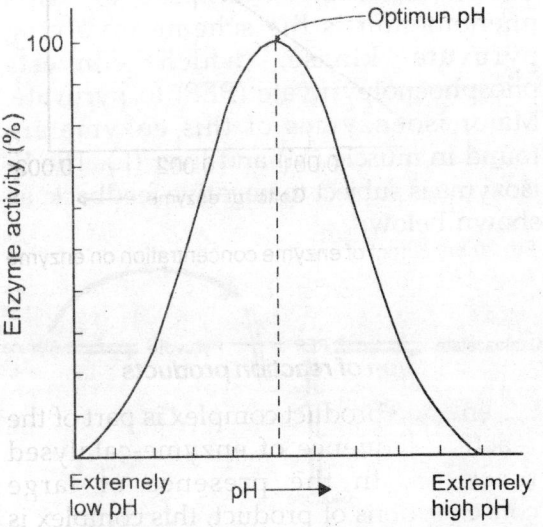

Fig. 20.9 : Effect of pH on enzyme activity

Hexokinase reaction is an example of product inhibition. In this reaction, ADP is competitive with ATP, and glucose -6- phosphate is competitive with glucose.

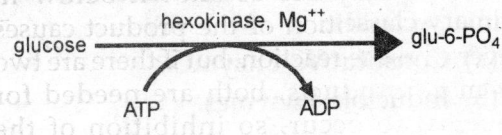

G-6-P may also act as a product inhibitor if it is not removed rapidly.

Effect of temperature

Chemical reactions, both catalyzed and noncatalyzed proceed at a faster rate as the reaction temperature is increased. This is true of enzymatically catalysed reactions in general only up to about 50°C. Above this temperature, heat inactivation of enzymes becomes a more important factor than the increased reaction rate and in all but a few exceptional cases, the speed of reaction slows and ceases around 70^0 to 80°C.

The optimum temperature of an enzyme is that temperature at which the greatest amount of substrate is changed in unit time. (Fig. 20.10).

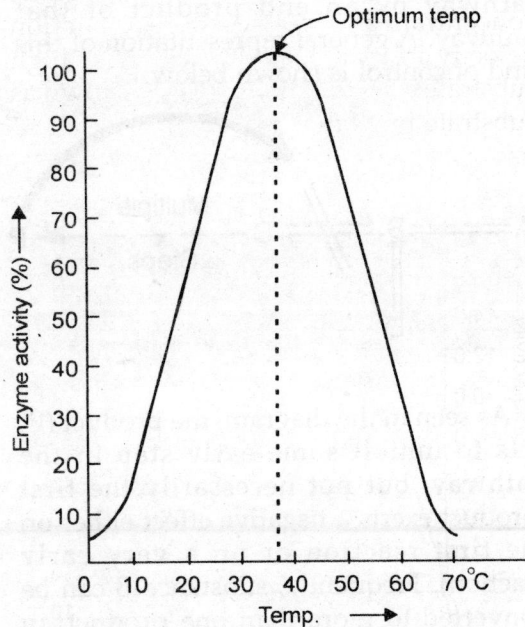

Fig 20.10: Effect of temp. on enzyme activity

Effect of time

Scientist Gortner points out that the element of time is generally not given sufficient consideration in discussing factors that affect the rate of enzyme action. He states, there cannot be an optimum hydrogen ion concentration or an optimum temperature independent of time. He indicates further that the optimum temperature of many enzymes from warm blooded animals is approximately 37°C only if time is measured in hours. It has been established that the time element is important in defining other conditions which regulate the rate of enzyme action.

Feedback Inhibition or Feedback Control

A significant control mechanism operating in living cells is known as feedback inhibition or control of enzymes. Specifically, this refers to the inhibition of the activity of an enzyme in a biosynthetic pathway by an end product of that pathway. A general representation of this kind of control is shown below:

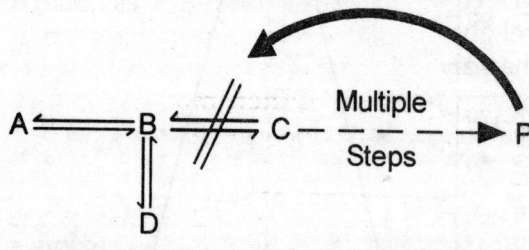

As seen in the diagram, the product (P) acts to inhibit some early step in the pathway, but not necessarily the first (product exerts a negative effect either on the first reaction or on a very early reaction). Frequently, substance B can be converted to more than one product; in this case the intermediate products are C and D. By feedback control it is possible not only to inhibit the production of P, but also to divert the flow of B from one pathway to another.

Several examples of this type have been studied in some detail. One of these systems involves the synthesis of pyrimidines. In this case, cytidine triphosphate (CTP) is an end product in a

series of reactions and CTP markedly inhibits the enzyme concerned with the first specific step in this biosynthesis, namely, aspartate transcarbamoylase, which catalyzes the reaction between aspartate and carbamoyl phosphate to form ureidosuccinate. A series of further reactions leads to the synthesis of cytidine triphosphate.

Cholesterol synthesis is also regulated by feedback inhibition.

Yet another example of this phenomenon is the scheme involving pyruvate kinase, which converts phosphoenolpyruvate (PEP) to pyruvate. Major isoenzymes of this enzyme are found in muscle (M) and liver (L). The L-isozyme is subject to negative feedback, as shown below:

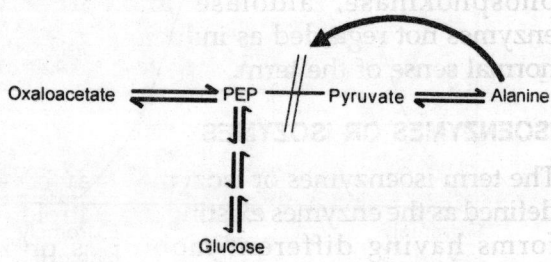

Alanine is a feedback inhibitor of pyruvate kinase and diverts the flow of pyruvate from alanine to glucose.

Enzyme Induction

Cellular enzymes can be divided into two primary classes:

(a) Constitutive Enzymes,
(b) Inducible Enzymes.

Constitutive enzymes

Enzymes of this class are present at virtually a constant concentration during the life of the cell. Presumably this is caused by a more or less constant relationship between the processes of enzyme synthesis and those of enzyme degradation.

Inducible enzymes:

Enzymes of this class are variable in the cell and as the need for the particular enzyme increases, the rate of synthesis gets increased or induced with respect to the rate of enzyme degradation. Thus, some of the enzymes responsible for glucose metabolism may be induced by increasing the load of glucose that an animal is required to metabolize. **Similarly, some of the enzymes involved in amino acid metabolism are inducible either by loading doses of the amino acid itself or by certain hormones.** During the wasting process, it is possible to measure increased serum concentrations of creatine phosphokinase, aldolase and other enzymes not regarded as inductive in the normal sense of the term.

ISOENZYMES OR ISOZYMES

The term isoenzymes or isozymes may be defined as the enzymes existing in multiple forms having different mobilities on electrophoresis, different relative activities

> **Examples of isoenzymes are:**
> 1. lactic dehydrogenase (LDH),
> 2. Alkaline phosphatase **(ALP)**
> 3. Creatine phosphokinase (creatine kinase), **CPK or CK**
> 4. Acid phosphatase, **(ACP)**
> 5. Amylase
> 6. Malate dehydrogenase,
> 7. Cholinesterase,
> 8. Hexokinase,
> 9. Phosphoglucomutase,
> 10. Pyruvate kinase, etc.

towards different substrates, and being differently depressed by inhibitors.

It has been shown that the relative amounts of the isoenzymes of a particular enzyme differ in different organs so that in diseases different enzyme patterns are found according to the organ from which they have come. Examples of isoenzymes are cited in 'box'.

In clinical biochemistry till date most of the work has been done on the following isoenzymes:

(a)   Lactic dehydrogenase (LDH),

(b)   Alkaline phosphatase (ALP) and

(c)   Creatine kinase i.e. creatine phosphokinase (CK or CPK)

Today, nearly 100 enzymes have been detected to exist as 'isoenzymes'. Starch gel gives a clear electrophoretic separation than any other media. The vertical form is recommended. Other media include cellulose acetate, agar gel, etc.

Clinical significance of enzymes

The relative abundance of certain enzymes or their isoenzymes in serum has found application in the diagnosis of several diseases as mentioned below:

Alkaline Phosphatase

Measurement of the activity of alkaline phosphatase in serum in the investigation of bone diseases constituted one of the earliest applications of enzyme tests in diagnosis and has remained one of the most useful. The value of serum alkaline phosphatase assays in various disorders of bone has been confirmed by more than 50 years' experience, while isoenzyme studies have demonstrated that bone is indeed the source of the raised serum enzyme activity in these conditions. In contrast, no other enzyme test has emerged of comparable value in bone diseases, inspite of the systematic attention which has been devoted to the development of diagnostic enzymology in recent years.

Raised serum alkaline phosphatase was shown to accompany rickets of various aetiologies, **Paget's disease**, and **hyperparathyroidism with skeletal involvement.**

> **γ-glutamyl transferase is probably the most sensitive enzymic test of liver function yet described.**
> The normal range of serum alkaline phosphatase activity in adults is usually taken as **3-13 King-Armstrong units/ 100 ml.**

The serum alkaline phosphatase activity of the new-born infant is rather above the normal adult level, and it rises rapidly to as much as two and a half to three times the adult upper limit of normal during the first year of life. The activity falls somewhat by the end of the second year to values which are of the order of one and a half to two and a half times of 20-30 King-Armstrong units/100ml. These elevated values are maintained approximately constant throughout childhood and early adolescence with perhaps some upturn at the onset of puberty, typically declining to adult levels during the later teenage years.

When hepatobiliary disease is suspected, it is advisable to resort to an alternative enzyme test. The activities of several enzymes in serum reflect impaired biliary function in ways similar to (but not completely identical with) the behaviour of alkaline phosphatase in this situation. These enzymes typically show normal activities in osteoblastic bone disease. **Two such enzymes, i.e., 5'-nucleotidase and**

γ-**glutamyltransferase**, have been shown to exhibit serum activities within the adult normal range in children and their use has therefore been recommended as a liver function test in young patients.

The highest serum alkaline phosphatase levels are generally encountered in Paget's disease of bone (Osteitis deformans) and the raised enzyme activity is often the only abnormality in the composition of the serum seen in this condition. The activity in serum may reach levels of 100-200 King-Armstrong units/100 ml or more, **the higher values being associated with cases in which a greater proportion of the skeleton is involved.**

While, determination of serum **alkaline phosphatase activity is of great value in the detection of osteomalacia and rickets,** the same is not true of hyperparathyroidism, in which an increased serum alkaline phosphatase is only seen in those cases in which bone changes are present.

Successful treatment of hyperparathyroidism (e.g. by the removal

---

ISOENZYMES OF ALKALINE PHOSPHATASE (ALP)

On careful electrophoresis of plasma, four isoenzyme bands of ALP can be distinguished (liver, placenta, intestine, bone), but unfortunately there is a major difficulty in distinguishing the bone enzyme from the liver enzyme, as they migrate very close together in the support systems used. With these difficulties ALP isoenzyme detection has so far had to remain as a semi research procedure.

of a parathyroid adenoma) is followed by a fall in serum alkaline phosphatase activity which may, however be preceded by an initial rise due to healing of the bony lesions: this contrasts with the immediate fall in serum calcium.

Infiltration of the bones by malignant disease is accompanied by a rise in serum alkaline phosphatase activity whenever the process stimulates osteoblastic activity.

Acid Phosphatase

Acid phosphatase is an important enzyme and is found to be in abundance in adult prostate and seminal fluid, while significant amounts are found in several other tissues such as red cells, liver, kidney, bone, spleen and pancreas.

Normal Range

1 to 3.5 K.AU./100 ml or

1.8 to 6.5 I.U./litre

Most of the activity in normal serum is nonprostatic in origin and is found in both sexes at all stages. Less than 0.8 K.A. units is tartarate labile and so represents prostatic fraction.

Elevation

Clinical significance of acid phosphatase is chiefly in metastatic cancer of prostate, both in detection and following the progress of disease. **Raised values mostly between 5 to 50 K.A.U. are seen in over 75% cases of metastasizing prostatic carcinoma. Some times, values over 100 and very rarely even over 1,000 may be found.** Most of the increased enzyme activity is tartarate labile. Very high levels may be found in some cases of malignant prostate with secondaries (most often in bones).

A small increase has also been found in acute retention and following prostate massage, but values soon return to normal. Similar increases are noticed in Paget's disease and carcinoma of breast but in such cases the determination is not of much clinical significance.

If the increase in tartarate labile fraction is not significant and the total level is found raised, the increase may be due to red cells or other sources of acid phosphatase.

Isoenzymes of Acid Phosphatase

By polyacrylamide gel electrophoresis, various isoenzymes designated arbitrarily as 0, 1, 2, 3, 3b, 4 and 5 have been identified from different sources in normal and disease conditions. Zero represents the slowest moving and 5 the fastest moving fraction. Most of these isoenzymes are labile even at the room temperature and become inactivated. Therefore, in the serum only stable isoenzyme is found. The isoenzyme pattern in the leukocytes found is as follows:

Isoenzymes	Sources
1,2,4	in neutrophils
1,4	in monocytes
3	in lymphocytes and platelets
3b	in primitive blasts
5	in reticulum cells of leukaemic reticuloendothelosis

> **ISOENZYMES OF ACID PHOSPHATASE (ACP)**
>
> **At the most, there do exist 14 isoenzymes on electrophoresis. One finds clear cut 14 bands on electrophoretogram. The only isoenzyme of clinical importance is prostatic acid phosphatase.**

Normal plasma contains a tartarate resistant isoenzyme 5.

In variety of diseases, other isoenzymes

may appear in plasma.

In metastatic prostatic cancer, changes in plasma enzyme activity are due to the presence of isoenzyme 2, which is tartarate labile.

Many acid phosphatase isoenzymes are cell specific i.e. derived from a specific type of cell.

Aminotransferases (Transaminases)

The enzymes which are involved in the transfer of an amino group (CH_2-NH_2) from an alpha amino acid to a alpha keto acid are called as transaminases and the process is called as transamination. Transamination reaction is an important step in the metabolism of amino acids.

Two enzymes occur in human tissues which catalyze reaction of this type:

(a) Aspartate aminotransferase, popularly known as **GOT** (glutamicoxaloacetic transaminase) and

(b) Alanine aminotransferase, popularly known as **GPT** (glutamicpyruvic transaminase).

Both transaminases are widely distributed in human tissues, GOT activity almost always being greater than GPT activity.

Serum GOT and GPT catalyse the following reactions of transaminations respectively:

$$\alpha \text{ KG + Aspartic acid}$$
$$\updownarrow \text{GOT}$$
$$\text{Glutamic acid + Oxaloacetic acid}$$

$$\alpha \text{ KG + Alanine}$$
$$\updownarrow \text{GPT}$$
$$\text{Glutamic acid + Pyruvic acid}$$

Interpretation

The normal range for serum GOT is 4-17 IU/l or 8-40 units/ml and for GPT 3-15 IU/l or 5-35 units/ml.

According to Wroblewski, in the newborn, values upto 120 units for GOT and 90 units for GPT must be considered normal.

Determination of GOT is particularly useful in myocardial infarction (M.I.) when ECG findings are not very clear. GOT rises rapidly after myocardial infarction; peak values which may be 2-20 times of normal, are reached within 24-48 hours and return to normal levels typically within 3-5 days.

Elevated level of GOT has been observed in almost 97% clinically proved cases of M.I.

Normal values have been reported in heart conditions without infarction, such as angina and pericarditis, in patients with pulmonary embolism and also in patients with acute abdominal attacks.

Foulk and Fleisher found an increase in over 50% patients with acute pancreatitis.

SGPT is not usually elevated in M.I. unless the lesion is a large one or there is associated liver damage.

Both the enzymes exhibit raised levels in hepatocellular damage e.g. due to hepatotoxic drugs, infective hepatitis and primary or secondary liver cancer. Raised levels are also seen in **Lannec's cirrhosis**, biliary cirrhosis and obstructive jaundice. In infective hepatitis, the increase is particularly marked and highest values are obtained. In early stage GOT is more increased than GPT, but SGPT exceeds SGOT in advanced stage. In infective hepatitis, estimation of serum transaminases is the most sensitive diagnostic index.

Very high values are obtained in toxic hepatitis due to carbontetrachloride poisoning.

Serum transaminases particularly SGOT gets elevated in certain muscular disorders, e.g. progressive muscular dystrophy, dermatomyositis and also following extensive muscle trauma, but is usually normal in progressive muscular atrophy, myasthenia gravis and rheumatoid arthritis.

Recommendations on the Use of Serum Enzyme Assays in the Diagnosis of Acute Myocardial Infarction

1. A single set of cardiac enzyme values in the emergency room is not sufficiently sensitive to exclude myocardial infarction. **Although a single, markedly positive CK-MB value will greatly increase the probability of acute infarction,** data are insufficient to support or reject a policy whereby low-risk patients, who otherwise would be sent home, would be observed until one or more CK-MB values are obtained.

2. If a myocardial infarction is inspected, then samples of total CK andCK-MB levels should be measured on admission and about 12 and 24 hours later, although condensed versions of this strategy may ultimately prove to be equally efficacious and more cost effective. If MI may have occurred more than 24 hours before admission, and if CK and CK-MB levels are not diagnostic, a total LDH level should be ordered. If the total LDH level is elevated, an assay of LDH isoenzymes should be obtained. If the first LDH_1/LDH_2 ratio is only

slightly less than 1.0, a second assay is probably indicated.

3. If chest pain occurs after admission, CK and CK-MB assays should be done at 0, 12 and 24 hours.

4. **Routine use of enzyme assays other than those for CK, CK-MB, and LDH isoenzymes is not recommended.**

5. If more than 2 hours may pass before CK isoenzymes will be assayed, the serum sample should be preserved on ice.

Other Laboratory Measurements

Blood sugar

Hyperglycemia occurs frequently following AMI (acute myocardial infarction), not only in diabetic patients, in whom ketoacidosis may be precipitated, but also (with a lower frequency) in nondiabetics, in whom several weeks may elapse before carbohydrate tolerance returns to normal.

Serum lipids

These are often determined in patients with AMI. However, the results may be misleading, since numerous factors that can alter the values are operating at the time of the patient's admission to the hospital; for example, **stress increases serum cholesterol, whereas recumbency (the state of taking rest by lying down) decreases it.** Serum triglycerides are affected by calorie intake, intravenous and recumbency.

During the first 24-48 hours after admission, total cholesterol and HDL cholesterol remain at or near baseline values but generally fall precipitously after that. The fall in HDL cholesterol after AMI is greater than the fall in total cholesterol, thus the ratio of total cholesterol to HDL cholesterol is no longer useful for risk assessment early after MI. Therefore, unless values are obtained very early in patients admitted for AMI, it is the best to defer determinations of serum lipid levels until at least 8 weeks after the infarction has occurred.

Serum Amylase

Amylase is a starch splitting enzyme which hydrolyses starch and other high molecular dextrins to maltose at an optimum pH of 7.1. It is present in the pancreas and parotid gland. The major activity of this enzyme, called amylopsin, is in pancreatic juice, some is also found in saliva.

Interpretation

Normal range of serum amylase is given as 80-180 Somogyi units/100 ml. **The clinical significance of this enzyme chiefly lies in the diagnosis of acute pancreatitis in which values frequently exceed 2000 units.** Usually activities over

---

ISOENZYMES OF AMYLASE

Although techniques are becoming available for the separate estimation of amylase isoenzymes (pancreatic, salivary), the measurement of isoenzymes is unlikely to resolve the major diagnostic problem of differentiating acute pancreatitis from nonpancreatic abdominal emergencies (perforated peptic ulcer, gut obstruction, etc.). This is because in the later situation, the pancreatic amylase that is normally present in the gut lumen leaks through the intestinal wall into the peritoneal cavity and from there it is absorbed into the blood stream.

---

550 units strongly suggest a diagnosis of acute pancreatitis. The rise is rapid and transient, reaching a peak within the first 12-24 hours after the onset and returning to normal usually in 2 to 3 days.

In chronic disease of the pancreas, whether due to neoplasm or due to chronic pancreatitis, such high values are not seen (rarely exceeds 200 units/ 100 ml). In these conditions either duct obstruction is more gradual or progressive destruction of secreting tissues largely counteracts its effect.

High activities may also occasionally occur in variety of conditions in which pancreatic damage is secondary to other abdominal disturbance such as perforated gastric ulcers, peritonitis, intestinal obstruction. In these conditions values over 500 units may be found. These usually develop 5 to 10 days after the onset of symptoms and appear to be due to increased pressure on pancreatic duct.

Drugs such as morphine which cause contraction of sphincter of oddi increase serum amylase.

Creatine Kinase (CK or CPK)

CPK is a dimer consisting of one subunit which is found in the brain (designated as B) and another in muscle (designated as M). It exists in the following three isozymic forms namely:

1. **MM (found in skeletal and heart muscle)**
2. **MB (found in cardiac muscle, also found in striated muscle)**
3. **BB (found in brain and a variety of other tissues)**

About 15% of the heart CK is in the form of MB isoenzyme, the remaining 85% being MM. It should be noted that skeletal muscle also contains some MB isoenzyme

(<0.4%). The amount of MB isoenzyme increases in the plasma after a myocardial infarct, and therefore in theory provides a fairly specific test.

> **MB isoenzyme of CK increases in plasma after a myocardial infarction.**

The most useful application of estimating plasma MB activity is in the investigation of those patients suspected of having an infarct.

Heart and skeletal muscles are the richest sources of serum creatine phosphokinase, an enzyme which reversibly catalyzes the phosphorylation of creatine with ATP to form adenosine diphosphate and creatine phosphate.

$$\text{Creatine Phosphate + ADP} \underset{}{\overset{\text{CPK}}{\rightleftharpoons}} \text{Creatine + ATP}$$

This enzyme is also found in cerebral tissue. Consequently, damage or disease (e.g. myocardial infarction, acute cerebrovascular disease, muscular dystrophy or injury) of these tissues will result in elevated serum CK levels.

High levels of CPK are also found after

> **In the wake of myocardial infarction, CK activity begins to rise within 4 to 6 hours; reaches to peak between 18 to 30 hours and returns to normal by the third day.** Marginally increased levels may be found due to severe exercise and by large multiple intramuscular injections. **Besides the diagnostic importance in M.I, it's also of diagnostic importance in progressive muscular dystrophy of Duchenne type, polymyositis and in other muscular dystrophies.**

severe exercise, in hypothyroidism, acute cerebrovascular accidents and strokes and motor neuron disorders.

Normal levels in men and women differ with the methods employed. Normal values in men and women according to the method of Hughes (modified) are as given below:

Men	:	20 - 50 IU/litre
Women	:	10 - 37 IU/litre

The magnitude of elevation of CK in M.I. is found to be greater than those of SGOT and LDH elevations. CPK may be a more sensitive indicator of myocardial ischaemia than the other enzymes and may be potentially more useful in subendocardial infarctions. No increase in activity is noted in heart failure cases.

CPK activity is not elevated in liver disease, blood dyscrasia, chronic pulmonary diseases and chronic renal diseases. Minimal elevation has been infrequently noted in isolated cases, of pulmonary infarction. Rarely, positive reactions have been reported associated with gangrene of the gallbladder, carcinoma of the pancreas, and diabetic acidosis. CPK activity levels may be altered by the presence of thyroid disease. Extremely high enzyme values are found more frequently in severe myxoedema than in the milder forms. When the disease is controlled with thyroid hormone, the enzymic activity returns to the normal range.

In contrast to SGOT and LDH, CPK is not elevated in patients with primary hepatic disease or with hepatic congestion from heart failure. In rare instances of pulmonary embolism or pulmonary infarction, one may find abnormal serum CPK activity, but the elevation in CPK is slight and may be due to local irritation of skeletal muscle by phlebitis.

Lactic Dehydrogenase (LDH or LD)

Lactic dehydrogenase is an enzyme which catalyzes the reversible conversion of lactic acid to pyruvic acid (Fig. 20.11).

$$
\begin{array}{ccc}
CH_3 & & CH_3 \\
| & \text{lactic} & | \\
HC - OH + DPN \rightleftharpoons & & C = O + DPNH \\
| & \text{dehydrogenase} & | \\
COOH & & COOH \\
\text{Lactic acid} & & \text{Pyruvic acid}
\end{array}
$$

Fig. 20.11 : Biochemistry of lactic dehydrogenase

This enzyme is found in varying concentration in all the tissues of the body, namely in decreasing order-liver, skeletal muscle, kidney, heart muscle, lung, serum etc.

LDH rise is usually noted within the first 12 to 24 hours after myocardial infarction, peak is reached in two to four days and gradual return to normal is seen from the eighth to the fourteenth day. The peak elevations in LDH are roughly proportional to the extent of injury to the myocardial tissue. **In myocardial infarction, LDH elevations above 3,000 units suggest a grave prognosis.**

The disadvantage of LDH determinations is that this enzyme is also relatively non-specific for myocardial tissue. It is so widespread in body cells that coexistent disease processes in other organ systems

> LDH levels get increased in megaloblastic anaemia, carcinomatosis, acute leukaemia, granulocytic leukaemia, heart failure, pulmonary infarction, renal necrosis, muscle disease and sickle cell anaemia. Less pronounced LDH increases are seen in inflammatory hepatic disease.

can cause elevations.

Isoenzymes of Lactic Dehydrogenase (LD)

Mammalian lactic (lactate) dehydrogenases are tetramers composed of two types of subunits, designated as M (the major form found in muscle or liver) and H (the major form found in heart). Five combinations of subunits are possible i.e.,

HHHH (H_4)
HHHM (H_3M)
HHMM (H_2M_2)
HMMM (HM_3)
MMMM (M_4)

The possible combinations can be separated by electrophoresis as shown in Fig. 20.12.

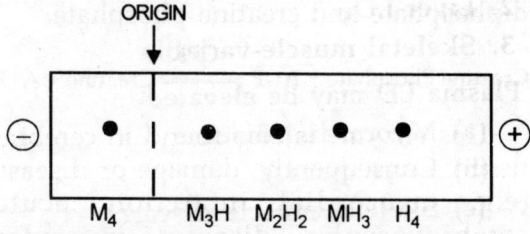

Fig. 20.12: Electrophoresis of lactate dehydrogenase isoenzymes at pH 8.6

It is clear from the Fig 20.12 that the net charge on the isozyme differs, those with an increasing content of the H subunit have an increasingly larger negative charge, while M_4 isozyme has a slightly positive net charge. These five forms of lactate dehydrogenase are isozymes that catalyze the same reactions, but they are found to different extents in different tissues. In man, the context of the several isozymes differs in heart and liver. Although the reason for this is not yet known, use is made of the fact in diagnostic differentiation of various diseases of liver and myocardium (heart). In both types of disease states, LD leaks out of the damaged · cell and increases the concentration of the enzyme in blood serum.

In liver and heart muscle the predominant isozyme has subunit composition H_4 whereas in skeletal muscle, the predominant isozyme is M_4. The H_4 and M_4 isozymes have different K_m values for pyruvate. **Raised levels of LD_1 and LD_2 are characteristic of myocardial infarction; whereas LD_4 and LD_5 get elevated in liver disorders.**

Five isoenzymes of LD are known to exist:

LD_1 LD_2, LD_3, LD_4 and LD_5 **(based on electrophoretic mobility)**

1. **Heart-LD_1 and LD_2**
2. **Liver-LD_5**
3. **Skeletal muscle-variable**

Plasma LD may be elevated in:
   (a) **Myocardial disease**
   (b) **Liver disease**
   (c) **Skeletal muscle disease**
   (d) **Miscellaneous**

LDH of serum and various tissues consists of five different components which are separable by electrophoresis. These fractions are known as isoenzymes because they catalyze the same chemical reaction, i.e; the reduction of pyruvate to lactate.

Cellular damage to tissues such as myocardium and liver results in characteristic abnormalities in the relative proportions of various isoenzymes, demonstrable by electrophoresis. The plasma of normal adults contains five plasma isoenzymes, i.e. LDH_1, LDH_2, LDH_3, LDH_4 and LDH_5. These isoenzymes may be differentiated by physical (thermal stability), chemical (mobility on starch gel) and immunological characteristics.

LDH_1 and LDH_2 fractions of lactic dehydrogenase become predominated in cases of myocardial infarction during electrophoresis. These isoenzyme changes occur earlier in the course of infarction and persist longer than the total plasma LDH enzyme activity.

Haemolyzed specimens cannot be used and the amount of serum subjected to electrophoresis must contain an adequate amount of enzyme activity.

Normal range

It differs with the method employed. For the spectrophotometric method, Wroblewski has given the normal range as 200-650 units (85-300 I.U. per litre), Elliot and Wilkinson as 150-500 units (72 to 240 I.U. per litre) whereas King, using his own method as 70-240 I.U. per litre.

There is a marked increase in the proportion of LD_1 in serum in myocardial infarction and LD_5 in liver disease.

An increase in the level of lactate dehydrogenase activity in cerebrospinal fluid has been reported in cases of tumours of the Central Nervous System. The normal range has been given as 10-25 I.U./l by King and as 3-20 by Wroblewski.

Antienzymes

Antienzymes may be referred to as the enzymes possessing antagonistic property to the proteolytic enzymes of the human system. Such enzymes are synthesized within our body. **Because of the availability of such enzymes, the wall of**

> **Some well known antienzymes are:**
> 1. Anti-trypsin
> 2. Anti-pepsin
> 3. Anti-rennin
> 4. Anti-urease etc.

the alimentary canal is not digested itself by its own proteolytic enzymes. Likewise, intestinal parasites (which are very common especially amongst children for example round-worms, hook-worms, pinworms, etc.) are also not digested by the proteolytic enzymes present in the alimentary canal. **Reports are also available regarding production of antienzymes in the serum when certain enzyme preparations are given parenterally.** The mucous membrane is also believed to contain anti-proteolytic enzymes. **Ascaris has been shown to contain anti-trypsin and anti-pepsin activity.**

> **Radioimmunoassay can also be used to measure serum trypsin activity in suspected cases of cystic fibrosis.**

CLINICAL APPLICATIONS OF ENZYMES OR THERAPEUTIC USES OF ENZYMES

Several enzymes are known today which have got beneficial important role in several disorders/diseases so as to make the sick person better one. These are being used in medicine without any hesitation. Their use in medicine is on increase day by day. More and more researches are going on in this direction. Since, the enzymes are inactivated in gastrointestinal tract, hence these are administered parenterally. Some of the important examples of such enzymes are as follows:

Trypsin

This has proved to be of value in the treatment of several clinical conditions. The purified enzyme has been administered parenterally, orally and intramuscularly. **In the treatment of acute thrombophlebitis (a blood clot and inflammation in a vein), small recurrent injections have been beneficial in many patients.**

Some types of ulcers have responded well to trypsin therapy, as have some specific traumatic injuries, such as boxers' black-eye and a number of other injuries to athletes and others.

Streptokinase

It is a bacterial enzyme obtained principally from β-hemolytic streptococci. **It causes fibrinolysis and dissolution of clot. It is used in the treatment of haemothorax and haematoma.**

Hyaluronidase

It is prepared from mammalian testes. It acts by depolymerizing hyaluronic acid and increasing tissue permeability. **It is used in the treatment of traumatic or postoperative edema.**

Pepsin

It is obtained from hog stomach. It is used in the treatment of gastric achylia (congenitally undeveloped gastric glands).

Thromboplastin

This is prepared by lysis of blood platelets and is used for blood coagulation.

Urokinase

It is prepared from human urine and is used in the treatment of pulmonary embolism and in myocardial infarction

to dissolve the clot.

Fibrinolysin

It is prepared by activating fibrinolysinogen by streptokinase and is used in the treatment of venous thrombosis, pulmonary and arterial embolism.

Rennin

It is obtained from the glandular layer of calf stomach and is used in the therapy of gastric achylia.

Table 20.3 : Enzymes of diagnostic importance with principal conditions involved

Enzymes	Principal conditions in which level of activity in serum gets elevated
Amylase	Acute pancreatitis
Acid phosphatase (optimum pH 5)	Prostatic carcinoma *
Alkaline phosphatase of (optimum pH 10)	Diagnosis of liver diseases, especially biliary obstruction and detection osteoblastic bone disease, e.g. rickets.
Aspartate transaminase (AST-previously GOT)	Myocardial infarction. Liver diseases, especially with liver cell damage.
Alanine transaminase (ALT-previously GPT)	Liver diseases especially with liver cell damage.
Lactate dehydrogenase (LDH or LD)	Myocardial infarction, but also increased in many other diseases (liver disease, some blood diseases).
Creatine phosphokinase dystrophy, (CPK) or Creatine kinase (CK)	Myocardial infarction and skeletal muscle diseases (muscular dermatomyositis).
γ-glutamyl transferase alcoholism. (γ-GT) **	Diagnosis of liver diseases, particularly biliary obstruction and
Urinary Elevation of N -acetyl glucosaminidase in Urine can be used to indicate renal transplant rejection.	

* Determination by radioimmunoassay technique which gives good results, is the choice of estimation these days, therefore, it should be carried at least in cases of suspected **prostatic carcinoma**.

** γ - GT is elevated in the plasma of **alcoholics**, and also of **epileptics** taking barbiturates. This is because consumption of alcohol or barbiturates causes considerable proliferation of the endoplasmic reticulum inducing high levels of the enzyme.

Diagnostic importance of enzymes (at a glance)

The assay of serum enzymes is used as an important aid to diagnosis. The level of enzymic activity of a number of enzymes gets raised in different pathological conditions. With the advancement of 'Biochemistry', it is now preferable to take into account the level of serum enzymes in certain diseases before starting the treatment. Timely enzymic investigations are of great value and significance to the physicians/surgeons.

Some enzymes of diagnostic importance with principal conditions involved are as follows: (in alphabetical order, Table 20.3).

The great significance of enzymes is that the thousands of chemical transformations going on continually in living matter would not be possible without enzymes, which are the most important tools of the living cell. For the hydrolysis or the oxidation of such substances like fats and proteins, in the laboratory we commonly employ strong acids or alkalies or oxidizing agents and high temperatures.

Enzymes are organic catalysts produced by living organisms. They are generally soluble and colloidal substances, characterized by great activity, specificity and susceptibility to the influence of pH, temperature, and other environmental changes.

All the enzymes which have been isolated in pure condition to date are proteins. (The converse of this statement, i.e., that all proteins are necessarily enzymatically active is, however, not true).

All enzymes are proteins in nature does not hold true 100% as now there do exist few enzymes that are made up of RNA; **such enzymes are called as ribozymes. Thomas Cech** and **Sidney Altman** discovered ribozymes for which they were awarded Nobel Prize in Physiology and Medicine in the year **1989**.

CHAPTER 21

HUMAN NUTRITION/BALANCE DIET

> Who is not aware of the tremendous value of us? If you consume us taking certain nutritious and calories precautions, then we always try our best in your favour and do not allow you to go to a doctor.
>
> Longer the belt, shorter the life; few people die by taking less calories but many times more from excess. Check the obesity from the very begining of life, do not depend upon fast foods, do atleast moderate exercise/yoga daily and enjoy the life till the last respiration.

Nutrition deals with the needs of the organism for sustenance. Food is the basic requirement for all the living beings whether microorganisms or plants or animals, without which the existence of life is not possible. The modern science of nutrition deals mainly with the requirement of the body, both in kind and amount, and the choice of food to meet these needs. **Main three functions of food are to:**

(a) Supply energy

(b) Form (or maintain) body tissues and

(c) Preserve a suitable internal environment so that enzymes bringing about hundreds of metabolic reactions and the hormones regulating various processes might function properly.

Following is the nutritional requirement of human beings:

(a) **Carbohydrates** (b) **Lipids**

(c) **Proteins** (d) **Minerals**

(e) **Vitamins, and** (f) **Sufficient amount of water**

Excess intake of such foods should be taken care of which contain various food toxins (Table 21.1).

ENERGY REQUIREMENT

The energy requirement of the animal body may be divided into two functional classifications, viz., **that for basal metabolism and that for active work. (Table 21.2). Basal metabolism includes the energy expended in respiration, blood circulation, intestinal contractions, activities of various organs, maintenance of muscular tonus, thermal equilibrium,**

Table 21.1 : Various food toxins found in routine edibles.

Sl. No.	Food toxin	Source(s)
1.	5-dehydroxytryptamine	Banana and some other fruits
2.	Tyramine	Some cheeses
3.	Cyanide	Almonds, cassava* and other plants
4.	Cycasin	Cycad nuts
5.	Nitrosamines	Some fishes, meat or cheese
6.	Sanguinarine	Mustard oil
7.	Hemagglutinins	Legumes
8.	Oxalate	Rhubarb
9.	Solanine	Green potatoes
10.	Various mycotoxins	Fungi
11.	Aflatoxin B_1	Produced by the species of fusarium
12.	Aflatoxin G_1	

etc. The basal metabolic rate is influenced by the amount of active protoplasmic mass (hence by height, weight, surface area, age, sex, composition of the tissues, etc.) and is governed by endocrine organs, particularly the thyroid and pituitary glands.

The energy consumed in work, play and

Table 21.2 : Energy requirement for basal metabolism and active work.

Energy Requirement	
Basal metabolism	**Active work**
(It covers involuntary actions like respiration, blood circulation, intestinal contractions, activities of various organs, maintenance of muscular tonus, thermal equilibrium, etc.)	(It covers voluntary actions like playing, running, swimming, walking, pulling rikshaw, ploughing fields manually, wood-cutting manually, etc.)

a south american plant with thick roots that is grown for food; its roots are used as food; synonym: tapioca

indeed all forms of voluntary activity, imposes an additional requirement for fuel over the basal which depends upon the nature and extent of the muscular work. Whereas an average man expends about 100 Cal per hour while sitting at rest, his/her metabolism may increase to as high as six times this value with extreme physical effort.

Mary, Swartz and Rose summarised the hourly expenditure of calories of an average 70 kg man under various conditions as follows :

1.	Sleeping	: 65
2.	Awake lying still	: 77
3.	Sitting at Rest	: 100
4.	Standing relaxed	: 105
5.	Dish washing	: 144
6.	Light exercise	: 170
7.	Walking slowly to moderately fast	: 200–300
8.	Carpentry or painting	: 240
9.	Active exercise	: 290
10.	Walking down stairs	: 364
11.	Sawing wood	: 480
12.	Swimming	: 500
13.	Running 5.3 miles per hour	: 570
14.	Very severe exercise	: 600
15.	Walking up stairs	: 1100

From the above estimates one may predict the calorie requirement of the individuals. **The total energy requirement for different types of workers ranges from:**

(a) a minimum of **2000 to 2500** Cal per day {White - collar workers Table 21.3 (c)}.

Break-up of calories per day by a normal adult individual may be considered as:

(i) Carbohydrates

(400 g) x 4 = 1600 Calories

(ii) Lipids

(80 g) x 9 = 720 Calories

(iii) Proteins

(45 g) x 4 = 180 Calories

2500 Calories

(b) **to a maximum of 4000 to 6000 (lumbermen, excavators, etc),** of which about 1400 to 1900 Cal are consumed in basal metabolism and the balance in various forms of activity.

Calorie intake must be adjusted to specific needs. The proper allowance is that which will maintain body weight and rate of growth at the desired levels over extended periods. **When disease is present, calorie supply must provide energy for tissue repair, for the immunological mechanisms and for the wasting effects of fever.**

The Food and Nutrition Board, National Research Council, recommended daily calorie intake as given in Tables 9.3 (a & b) The calorie allowances apply to the individual normally engaged in moderate physical activity, under usual environmental stresses.

For a long time, emphasis in the study of nutrition was laid on calorie requirements. **Animal calorimeter was developed by Atwater, Rosa and Benedict. Human calorimeter developed by Du Bois revealed that a normal 70 kg man expends, on an average, energy equivalent to about 3,000 calories per day.** There is yet another calorimeter which is known as Bomb calorimeter; this can be used to determine the caloric value of various foods. Composition and energy content of various common food stuffs are as given in Table 9.4.

On the basis of the definition of a large calorie (Cal or kcal), the quantity of heat necessary to raise the temperature of 1kg of water through $1^{\circ}C$, the following values are obtained:

1 gm of carbohydrate = 4.1 kcal

1 gm of fat (lipid) = 9.4 kcal

1 gm of protein = 5.6 kcal

However, in the body, protein is not completely utilized, although carbohydrates and lipids are. On this basis, the following round figures are commonly used in Medicine/Science.

1 gm of carbohydrate = 4 kcal

1 gm of fat = 9 kcal

1 gm of protein = 4 kcal

Daily Requirement

The average normal man needs 2,,500 to 3,000 calories (see above break-up of calories) per day and the normal woman somewhat less, usually, 1,700 to 2,100 calories per day. Recommended daily- dietary allowance for various categories of human beings is given in Table 21.3 (a and b).

Following is the nutritional requirement of human beings:

(a) Carbohydrates

(b) Lipids

High fat consumption has been found to be associated with **cancer of breast and colon.**

The main sources of saturated fat in the human diet are the meat of ruminants, dairy products and hard margarine. Cholesterol is found only in foods of animal origin, particularly in egg yolk.

Table 9.3 (a) : Recommended daily calories intake and other dietary allowances for different categories

	Age years	Weight kg (lbs)	Height cm (In)	Cal-ories	Protein 'g'	Calcium 'g'	Iron 'mg'	Vitamin 'A' 'I.U.'	Thia-mine 'mg'	Ribo-flavin 'mg'	Equiv. Niacin 'mg'	Vita-min 'C"mg'	Vita-min 'D"I.U.'
Men	18-35	70(154)	175 (69)	2906	70	0.8	10	5000	1.2	1.7	19	70	
	35-55	70(154)	175 (69)	2600	70	0.8	10	5000	1.0	1.6	17	70	
	55-75	70(154)	175 (69)	2200	70	0.8	10	5000	0.9	1.3	15	70	
Women	18-35	58(128)	163 (64)	2100	58	0.8	15	5000	0.8	1.3	14	70	
	35-55	58(128)	163 (64)	1900	58	0.8	15	5000	0.8	1.2	13	70	
	55-75	58(128)	163 (64)	1600	58	0.8	10	5000	0.8	1.2	13	70	
Infants	0-1	8 (18)		kg×11.5 ± 15	kg×2.5 ± 0.5	0.7	kg × 1.0	1500	0.4	0.6	6	30	400
Children	1-3	13 (29)	87 (34)	1300	32	0.8	8	2000	0.5	0.8	9	40	400
	3-6	18 (40)	107 (42)	1600	40	0.8	10	2500	0.6	1.0	.11	50	400
	6-9	24 (53)	124 (49)	2100	52	0.8	12	3500	0.8	1.3	14	60	400
Boys	9-12	33 (72)	140 (55)	2400	60	1.1	15	4500	1.0	1.4	16	70	400
	12-15	45(98)	156(61)	3000	75	1.4	15	5000	1.2	1.8	20	80	400
	15-18	61 (134)	172(68)	3400	85	1.4	15	5000	1.4	2.0	22	80	400
Girls	9-12	33 (72)	140 (55)	2200	55	1.1	15	4500	0.9	1.3	15	80	400
	12-15	47 (103)	158 (62)	2500	62	1.3.	15	5000	1.0	1.5	17	80	400
	15-18	53 (117)	163 (64)	2300	58	1.3	15	5000	0.9	1.3	15	70	400

Table 9.3 (b) : Important daily allowances of nutrients for expectant and nursing mothers

Nutrient	Normal Women			Pregnant	Lactating
	Seden-tary	Moderately active	Very active		
Calories (Cal)	1900	2200	3000	+ 300	+ 500 to 700
Proteins (g)	45	45	45	55	65
Calcium (g)	0.4-0.5	0.4-0.5	0.4 - 0.5	1.0	1.0
Iron (mg)	30	30	30	40	30
Vitamin 'A' as					
(i) retinol (µg)	750	750	750	750	1150
(ii) carotene (µg)	3,000	3,000	3,000	3,000	4,600
Thiamine (mg)	1.0	1.1	1.5	+ 0.2	+ 0.4
Riboflavin (mg)	1.0	1.2	1.7	+ 0.2	+ 0.4
Folic acid (µg)	100	100	100	150-300	150

Table 21.3 (c) Calories requirement for men

	Sedentary	Moderately active	Very active*
Calories	2500	2900	3900

* May require more subject to nature of work e.q., rickshaw pullers, gymnasts, athletes etc. between 4000 - 6000 or even more.

Table 9.4 : Composition and energy content of various common foodstuffs

Sl. No.	Food Foodstuff	Food energy (calories/ 100 gm)	Water %	Protein 'gm'	Fat 'gm'	Carbohy-drate 'gm'	Calcium 'mg'	Phosphorus 'mg'
1.	Bread, white	275	34.7	8.5	3.2	51.8	79	92
2.	Bread, toasted	313	25.5	9.7	3.7	59.0	90	105
3.	Whole wheat	240	36.6	9.3	2.6	49.0	96	263
4.	Barley	349	11.1	8.2	1.0	78.8	16	189
5.	Millet	350	9-13	7-13	2.2 $\pm$	73.0	-	-
6.	Rice (brown, raw)	360	12.0	7.5	1.7	77.0	39	303
7.	Rice (milled, cooked)	119	70.5	2.5	0.1	26.2	8.0	45
8.	Wheat flour (whole)	333	12.0	13.3	2.0	71.0	41	372
9.	Wheat germ	361	11.0	25.2	10.0	49.5	84	1096
10.	Butter	720	15.5	0.6	81.0	0.4	20	16
11.	Cheese	398	37.0	25.0	32.2	2.1	725	495
12.	Milk (cow's whole)	69	87.0	3.5	3.9	4.9	118	93
13.	Milk (cow's skimmed)	36	90.5	3.5	0.1	5.1	123	97
14.	Eggs, fresh, whole	165	74.0	12.8	11.5	0.7	54	210
15.	Eggs, fresh, white	50	87.8	10.8	0	0.8	6.0	17
16.	Eggs, fresh, yolk	361	49.4	16.3	31.9	0.7	147	586
17.	Apple	66	84.1	0.3	0.4	14.9	6.0	10
18.	Banana	88-132	74.8	1.2	0.2	23.0	8.0	28
19.	Orange	45	87.2	0.9	0.2	11.2	33	23
20.	Peach	46	86.9	0.5	0.1	12.0	8.0	22
21.	Carrots, raw	42	88.2	1.2	0.3	9.3	39	37
22.	Poatoes, peeled, boiled	83	77.8	2.0	0.1	19.1	11	56
23.	Tomatoes, raw	20	94.1	1.0	0.3	4.0	11	27
24.	Almonds	600	4.7	18.6	54.1	19.6	254	475
25.	Groundnuts (roasted)	560	2.6	26.9	44.2	23.6	74	393
26.	Walnuts	650	3.3	15.0	64.4	15.6	83	380

(c) Proteins
(d) Minerals
(e) Vitamins, and
(f) Sufficient amount of water

Carbohydrates

Principal carbohydrates in the human diet are the starches and the sugars. Grains and vegetables constitute the primary sources of the starches, while fruits of sugars. Carbohydrates make up some 40-80 per cent of total calories furnished by the diet. Less than 1 percent of the carbohydrate intake is found in the tissues, emphasizing its ready utilization as a source of energy or its conversion to fat stores in adipose tissues as a potential energy source.

When ingested in amount in excess of that required to produce energy, carbohydrate is converted to fat, e.g., glycogen, a principal carbohydrate of the human body, gets firstly converted to pyruvic acid **via 'glycolysis' and then to acetyl CoA which is the precursor for the biosynthesis of fatty acids vis-a-vis fats in the human body.**

No definite amount of the intake of carbohydrates is known today but it has been established so far that at least **100 grams of carbohydrates are required per day by a normal healthy adult in order to avoid ketosis, excessive protein catabolism and other undesirable responses.** These carbohydrates remain confined to almost all kinds of foodstuffs which we consume daily in a normal course i.e., all types of vegetables (potatoes, carrots, chillies, arums, beans, pumpkin etc.), spices, condiments, corns (wheat, maize, oat, millet, gram, etc.), pulses, meat, egg, milk, fish etc.

The paper with which we come across daily is a form of cellulose, which, chemically has got as much glucose in it as starch has, but this paper can not be digested by the human beings because of the lacking of the corresponding enzyme i.e. **'cellulase'** in the digestive tract. On the other hand, this enzyme remains present in ruminants, therefore, they are able to digest cellulose which is found in abundance in their diet. Be it known that the main food of the ruminants is different types of grasses.

Potato consists of starch granules surrounded by an envelope of cellulose. If a raw potato is eaten, even if it is chewed thoroughly, it will pass as such through the digestive tract without yielding any calories and appear undigested in the faeces. **A raw potato, therefore, has got no food value. On the other hand, if the potato is heated, then the cellulose envelope will burst, and the content is then available for digestion. This is an**

Table 20.5 : Calorie values of some important common foods

1.	Cow's milk	: 69 Cal/100 ml
2.	Buffalo's milk	: 109 Cal/100 ml
3.	Human milk	: 67 Cal/100 ml
4.	Butter	: 720 Cal/100 g
5.	Desi ghee	: 830-890 Cal/100g
6.	Fishes	: 50-150 Cal/100g
7.	Meats	: 100-450 Cal/100g
8.	Egg	: 165 Cal/100g
9.	Curd (cow's)	: 69 Cal/100 ml
10.	Curd (buffalo's)	: 109 Cal/100 ml
11.	Apple, one medium size	: 66 Cal
12.	Banana, one	: 88-132 Cal
13.	Potato, boiled, 1 medium size	: 83 Cal
14.	Tomato, raw, 1 medium size	: 20 Cal
15.	Peas, green, cooked, 1/2 cup	: 56 Cal

example of a food which has got no food value in the raw state, but has a very high food value in the cooked state. Calorie values of some of the important routine items (foods) are as mentioned in Table 21.5.

Lipids

Lipids are the principal energy yielding substances and the per unit heat production from lipids (fats) is more than double in comparison to carbohydrates and proteins which are other two major food stuffs for the human beings. Fat is rather slowly digested and the large amounts of it in a meal tend to slow down the digestion process of other foods as well.

There is no rule for the proportion of fat and carbohydrate in a diet. For a normal person, 80gm fat is recommended. Of course, the essential fatty acids(Table 21.6) must be supplied, the requirement of which is small and these fatty acids are found in many food oils. The deficiency of the so called essential fatty acids in the diet of rats causes retarded growth, scaly skin, kidney lesions, and bloody urine formation (haematuria). **These fatty acids are also believed to control the rate of cholesterol**

biosynthesis in animals.

Linoleic, linolenic and arachidonic acids are considered to be essential fatty acids (EFA) in the mammals as they are not synthesized in them, hence, must be supplied in the diet. They all are poly-unsaturated fatty acids.

Although, the synthesis of fatty acids from intermediates in the catabolism of carbohydrates and amino acids has been demonstrated in many species of animals and plants, most mammals are unable to synthesize in adequate amounts fatty acids containing more than one double bond in the carbon chain. When rats are fed a diet not containing polyunsaturated fatty acids for two to three months, they develop deficiency symptoms, characterized by scaliness of the skin, desquamation and sloughing of the tail, lesions in the kidneys, and ultimately death. All these symptoms can be prevented or cured by the addition of 10 drops of lard oil or a small amount of linoleic acid to the diet. Other polyunsaturated fatty acids are also curative, **but linoleic acid is considered to be the essential fatty acid, since it cannot be synthesized but is the precursor for the biosynthesis of other polyunsaturated fatty acids.**

Although the deficiency of linoleic acid in the diet of humans is very rare, there have been reported some cases of dermatitis in infants and animals that responded to the addition of a few drops of lard oil to the diet (Fig. 21.1).

Polyunsaturated fatty acids also decrease the biosynthesis of cholesterol from either saturated fatty acids or nonfat sources. As little as 2 to 3 grams of fats per day like cottonseed, corn, and safflower (Kusumbh) oils will inhibit the cholesterol-promoting effect of 1 gram of fat consisting of saturated fatty acids, such as beef tallow

Table 9.6: Essential fatty acids	
Sl No. Name	Sources
1. Linoleic acid	linseed oil, cottonseed oil, peanut oil, corn oil, soyabean oil, egg-yolk, etc.
2. Linolenic acid	linseed oil, rapeseed oil, soybean oil, fish viscera, etc.
3. Arachidonic acid	lecithin*, cephalin*

* these are phospholipids which are found both in plants and animal tissues, viz; plant seeds (soyabean etc.), egg yolk etc.

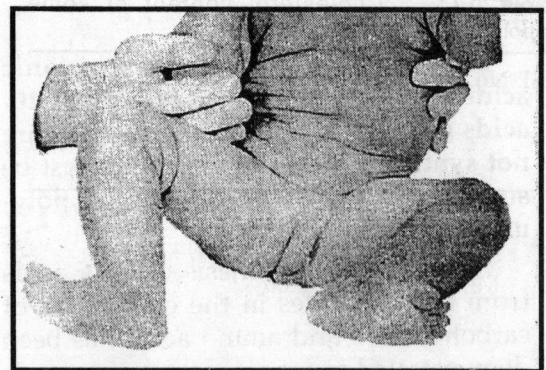

Fig 21.1 : Essential fatty acid deficiency

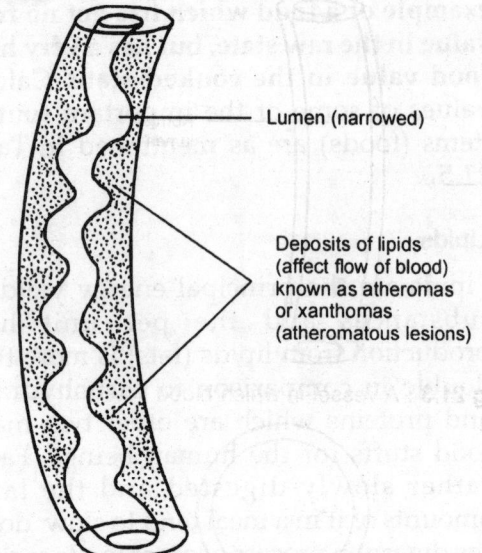

Fig 21.2 : A vessel in which lumen has become narrow due to haphazard deposit of lipids (cholesterol, TG etc.). Sick artery / vessel.

(animal fat melted down) or butter.

The hydrogenation of fats, which is carried out extensively in order to convert liquid oils into a more solid state, **results into considerable reduction in the amount of essential unsaturated fatty acids.**

An outstanding problem of lipid nutrition these days is the relationship of dietary fat to hypercholesterolaemia and that of hypercholesterol-aemia to atherosclerosis which remains unclear even to day.

Atherosclerosis is a disease primarily concerned with the integral layer of the artery and is characterized by the thickening and loss of elasticity of the arterial wall by the excessive deposits of cholesterol and other lipids. When narrowing of a vessel occurs (Figures 21.2, 21.3, 21.4 and 21.5), serious impairment of the blood supply to important structures may result. **Atherosclerosis, for instance, in the coronary arteries, is responsible for angina pectoris (pain in the heart i.e., heart attack), and in the cerebral arteries for many mental changes in the old age.** In the vessels of the legs it may be responsible for intermittent claudication (limping,

lameness). Complete obstruction of blood flow, usually due to thrombosis results in cardiac infarction, hemiplegia or senile gangrene.

> **Streptokinase and urokinase are the enzymes being used to disintegrate thrombus (clots) in the cardiac arteries and elsewhere.**

Normal amount of the cholesterol in serum is in the range 0f 150-250 mg. It's still on safer side if the level of cholesterol is maintained between **150 to 200 mg%** in blood as per the latest recommendations of the Nutrition Board of U.S.A. which is of the opinion that such people possess the least risk of cardiac disorders.

In order to keep away from hyper-cholesterolaemia and atherosclerosis one should avoid excess intake of those foodstuffs which are known to possess high amount of cholesterol (Table 20.7).

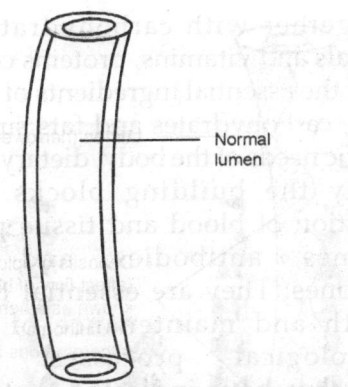

Fig 21.3 : A vessel in which blood flow is normal

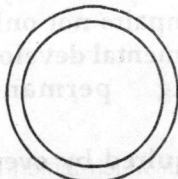

Fig. 21.4 : A normal vessel in which blood flow is normal

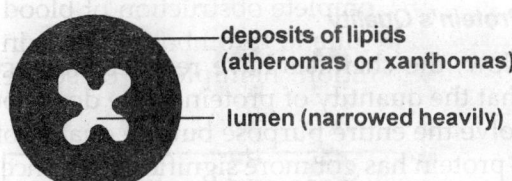

Fig. 21.5 : An affected vessel

Table 20.7 : Cholesterol content of some important human foods

Sl. No.	Food/item	Cholesterol (mg per 100 gm edible portion)
1.	Vegetable oils	nil
2.	Margarine (imitation butter)	nil
3.	Milk, cow's skimmed	3
4.	Milk, cow's whole	11
5.	Chicken	60
6.	Fish	70
7.	Pork	70
8.	Beef	70
9.	Cheese	100
10.	Butter	250
11.	Liver	300
12.	Kidney	375
13.	Egg, whole	550
14.	Egg, yolk	1,500
15.	Brain	2,000

Another problem in lipid metabolism is the role of essential unsaturated fatty acids in the diet. It has been established that vegetable oils, e.g. sunflower oil, groundnut oil, soyabean oil, til oil, etc. have a tendency to reduce serum cholesterol level in human beings in contrast to the effect of dietary animal fat i.e. desi ghee etc.

Habitual consumption of too much mustard oil is also not good for the heart, according to the researches conducted by the Indian Council of Medical Research (ICMR) as it causes myocardial fibrosis (growth of fibrous tissue). The mechanism by which mustard oil leads to '**myocardial fibrosis**' is not clear but the agent suspected is erucic acid, which is a major component of mustard oil. The ICMR bulletin says, it may be necessary to cultivate mustard varieties with low levels of erucic acid or no erucic acid. Consumption of too much coconut oil and mustard oil can lead to an increase in the level of blood cholesterol; contrarily gingily oil (til oil) can actually reduce cholesterol content.

Percentage of linoleic acid, the so called essential fatty acid in fats and oils of plant and animal origin is as follows :

1. Safflower oil (Kusumbh) 80%
2. Sunflower oil 70%
3. Corn oil 55%
4. Soyabean oil 50%

5. Cottonseed oil   45%
6. Sesame oil (Til oil)   45%
7. Peanut oil   30%
8. Coconut oil   5%

Those having a tendency of obesity/ family history of obesity or hypercholesterolaemia should avoid the food items summarised in `box'.

FAT CONTROLLED DIET: FOODS TO BE AVOIDED

Whole milk, ice cream sour cream, cheese, commercial biscuits, beef, pork, chicken, lamb, kidney, brain, liver, butter, lard, coconut oil, olive oil, chocolate, custards, puddings, etc.

Lipids play an important role in the diet by helping in the absorption of fat soluble vitamins i.e. A,D, E and K. Lecithins prevent development of fatty livers. **Nutritional cirrhosis of liver is caused due to the deficiency of dietary choline which remains present in lecithin.**

Lipids serve as the more important source of energy in the diet of the hard workers such as wrestlers, athletes, labourers, wood-cutters, etc. Ordinarily, excess fat intake should be avoided because this causes an increase in adiposity, hypercholesterolaemia, ketosis, etc. which all are undesirable.

Proteins

Nature of Proteins and their role in nutrition

Proteins are complex nitrogenous substances present in all living tissues. They are built up of simpler molecules called **'amino acids'**. There are **22** different amino acids which occur in an infinite variety of combinations in proteins.

Together with carbohydrates, fats, minerals and vitamins, proteins constitute one of the essential ingredients of our diet. While, carbohydrates and fats supply the calorific needs of the body, dietary proteins supply the building blocks for the formation of blood and tissue proteins, enzymes, antibodies, and certain hormones. They are essential for body growth and maintenance of normal physiological processes. **Recent researches have indicated that protein deficiency in infancy and early childhood (upto 5 years) impairs not only physical growth but also mental development, the damage being permanent and irreversible.**

Protein is required by every cell and is the basis of protoplasm. Moreover, it is the most expensive of the foodstuffs.

Protein's Quality

Now, the chemists have reached the fact that the quantity of protein alone does not solve the entire purpose but the quality of a protein has got more significance, hence, one must give emphasis on the quality of a protein. By the quality of a protein, we mean that it must comprise of essential amino acids in it. This came about with the realization by chemists that proteins from various sources differ widely in their amino acid make up and that their value in nutrition depends largely upon the presence of specific amino acids.

It should be known that the requirement of animals and man is not for proteins, but for specific amount of specific amino acids, the so called essential, or indispensable amino acids.

Casein of milk has been respected as a complete biological protein. It supplies sufficient quantity of all the amino acids required for growth and other needs of the body (Table 21.8). Proteins have been classified into two categories i.e. adequate and inadequate (Table 21.9).

Table 21.8 : Nutritive classification of the amino acids

Essential (Indispensable)	Semi-essential (semi-indispensable)	Non-essential (dispensable)
1. Lysine	1. Arginine	1. Glutamic acid
2. Leucine	2. Tyrosine	2. Aspartic acid
3. Isoleucine	3. Cystine	3. Alanine
4. Methionine	4. Glycine	4. Proline
5. Valine	5. Serine	5. Hydroxyproline,
6. Phenylalanine	6. Histidine*	etc.
7. Tryptophan		
8. Threonine		

* It's treated to be an essential amino acid for the infants

The adult human body can maintain nitrogenous equilibrium on a mixture of eight pure amino acids as its sole source of nitrogen. These eight are as given in Table 21.7. **For growth in infants, histidine is also needed.**

Table 21.9 : Proteins for the growth of rats

Sl. No.	Adequate (Sufficient)	Sl. No.	Inadequate (insufficient)
Animal Proteins			
1.	Casein of milk	1.	Gliadin of wheat
2.	Lactalbumin of milk	2.	Legumin of pea
3.	Ovalbumin of egg	3.	Zein of corn
Vegetable Proteins		4.	Hordein of barley
4.	Globulin of cottonseed	5.	Gelatin of horn
5.	Glutenin of wheat	6.	Legumelin of
6.	Edestin of hempseed		soyabean
7.	Excelsin of Brazil nut		

Are all dietary proteins equally good?

No, it is a common fallacy to consider all dietary proteins to be equally good. Actually, proteins differ widely in their nutritional value. The variations are due to differences in digestibility and more particularly the amino acids' composition (Figures 21.6 and 21.7). The nutritive value

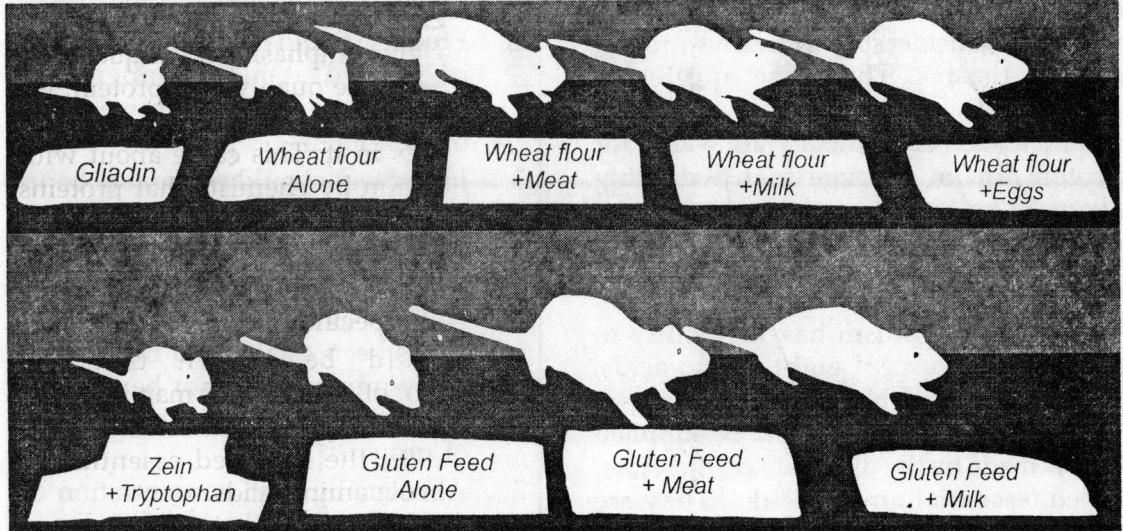

Fig. 21.6 : These rats were all of the same age and had been fed for the same length of time on diets containing the same proportion of protein. The variation in size is due to differences in the chemical constitution of the proteins eaten.

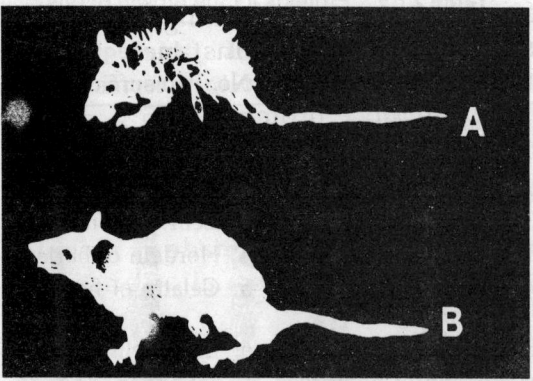

Fig. 21.7 : Essential amino acid deficiency in the growing rat. A. A rat fed a mixture of amino acids lacking valine. B. The same rat after receiving valine added to the amino acid mixture.

of a protein is largely determined by the relative concentrations of the 'essential amino acids' it contains.

Studies of various investigators have shown that an intake of about 0.9 gm of protein per kg body weight is adequate for all ordinary needs in the normal adult. In childhood, this allowance must be increased considerably to permit growth of new tissues. The same applies in pregnancy and lactation. The recommended daily dietary allowance for protein for an average man weighing about 70 kg is 70 g and for an average woman 58 grams.

What are 'essential' amino acids?

The human organism has the ability to synthesize all except **eight** amino acids, utilizing the available sources of nitrogen. The **eight** amino acids should be supplied ready- made by the diet and are, therefore, called 'essential amino acids'. **They are the following: Tryptophan, Lysine, Methionine, Threonine, Phenylalanine, Leucine, Isoleucine and Valine (Table 21.9).**

Can the deficiency of one protein be made good by another?

Yes, this is known as mutual complementation between proteins. Although one protein is deficient in one essential amino acid 'X', it may contain an excess of another essential amino acid 'Y'. If such a protein in mixed with another protein which is deficient in 'Y' but rich in 'X', the NPU of the combination is considerably higher than that of either individual protein. This explains the general recommendation for the

1. Protein content of the product should be sufficiently high to facilitate the administration of atleast 10-20 grams of protein daily.
2. Nutritive value of the protein should be high. Adequate (first class proteins) are given in table 9.9.
3. Product should be palatable enough to enable the easy administration of the required quantity of protein.
4. Product should not have been baked or toasted at high temperature which damages the nutritive value of the protein.
5. Its protein should preferably be in intact condition and not predigested, i.e. not in the form of protein hydrolysate or mixture of amino acids.
6. It has been established that amino acids mixture cannnot be utilized as efficiently as equivalent amount of proteins.
7. Abnormally high concentration of amino acids in the intestines may also provoke diarrhoea while the elevated blood amino acids levels may cause nausea and vomiting.

consumption of cereals (low in lysine but rich in methionine) together with pulses (rich in lysine but low in methionine).

Relation between calorie intake and protein utilization

Carbohydrates and fats are the main sources of energy (i.e. calories). Proteins are primarily of value in the formation and regeneration of tissues but they too can serve as a source of energy. When the calorie needs of the body are not adequately met from the intake of carbohydrates and fats, part of the dietary protein is diverted towards energy production. To prevent such wastage of proteins, therefore, care should be taken to raise the intake of carbohydrates and fats to the required levels when offering protein supplements to cover a dietary protein gap.

Protein foods in slimming regimens

The sheet anchor of any weight reduction course consists in reducing the carbohydrates' content of the diet and limiting the calorie intake by restricting the quantity of the diet. As protein has a high satiety value, protein-rich foods with low carbohydrate content find an important place in slimming regimens.

Daily Protein Requirements

The protein requirements of an individual depend upon the age, sex and body-weight. Primarily, it is expressed in terms of the "ideal reference protein". Infants, whether breast-fed or bottle- fed, receive only the reference protein (NPU = 75-100) until they are weaned. But the mixed proteins of the diets of children and adults are of lower quality and, therefore, due allowance should be made

for this factor in calculating the protein requirements. For instance, if the requirement of an adult, in terms of the ideal reference protein, is 0.5 g. per kg bodyweight, it will be 1 g per kg in terms of a dietary protein with an NPU of 50. This is the basis of the official recommendations made recently regarding the dietary allowances for Indian subjects.

Recommended Dietary Protein Allowances for Indians

The following are the daily protein allowances for Indians recommended by the Expert Group of th Indian Council of Medical Research.

Category	Description	Daily protein allowance (g)	Nature of diet
Man	Body weight 55 kg	55	
Woman	Body weight 45 kg	45	Mainly cereals
Woman	2nd half of pregnancy	55	and pulses NPU = 65*
Woman	Lactation upto 1 year	65	
Infants	0-3 months	2.3/kg	Entirely milk
Infants	3-6 months	1.8/kg	NPU = 75-100
Infants	6-9 months	1.8/kg	Milk, cereals and
Infants	9-12 months	1.5/kg	pulses;NPU= 65
Children	1 year	17	
Children	2 years	18	
Children	3 years	20	
Children	4-6 years	22	Mostly cereals
Children	7 -9 years	33	and pulses
Children	10-12 years	41	NPU = 50*
Adolescents: Boys 13-15 years		55	
Adolescents: Boys 16-18 years		60	
Adolescents: Girls 13-18 years		50	

* The essential amino acid requirements of adults are less exacting than those of infants and children. Therefore, the same diet has a higher NPU for adults than for children

Nature of the "Protein Gap" in India

The considered opinion of nutrition authorities is that the protein content of the average Indian diet is adequate but the actual quantity of food consumed by the majority is insufficient. An increased consumption of the normal diets would serve to make up the calorie deficit and also ensure a satisfactory level of protein intake. However, this does not apply to some cases, e.g. weaned infants, pre-school children and pregnant or lactating mothers, whose protein needs in both quality and quantity are considerably higher than those of the general adult population. For such vulnerable groups, the average diets consisting mostly of cereals and pulses cannot satisfy the needs, as the persons find it inconvenient or physically difficult to eat enough of such diets. Therefore, they need more concentrated sources of proteins as dietary supplements.

Effect of Heat on Protein Quality

Under normal condition of cooking, the digestibility of food proteins is generally improved and no damage occurs to the availability of the amino acids. **In the raw state, some vegetable foodstuffs, e.g. peas and beans, contain trypsin-inhibitors which lower the digestibility of their proteins.** Mild heating destroys these inhibitors and improves the protein digestibility and thereby the nutritive value.

However, proteins suffer serious damage in nutritive value when they are subjected to drastic conditions of heating, especially in presence of sugars and other carbohydrates in the dry state, as in the baking of biscuits. **The damage is due to the formation of an indigestible linkage between the essential amino acid lysine and a reducing sugar.** The deterioration can be detected only by biological tests but not by chemical analysis. As lysine is the most limiting essential amino acid in cereal proteins, even a slight reduction in its availability results in a conspicuous fall in the nutritive value af cereal-based products. It is, therefore, imperative to avoid any drastic process of heating such as baking or toasting in the manufacture of protein foods.

How Useful are Protein Hydrolysates and Amino Acid Preparations for Oral Administration?

The practical value of 'oral" amino acid preparations (predigested proteins) has been seriously overemphasized. Their use was originally based on a misconception, concerning the digestive capacities of the human gastrointestinal tract. **Actual feeding trials have proved that, even in extreme starvation or diseases like peptic ulcer, ulcerative colitis or regional enteritis,** protein digestion and amino acid absorption are normal and the use of hydrolysed protein seems unnecessary. **It was observed that being unpalatable, protein digests were often rejected and vomited by the patients.** It is also established that amino acid mixtures cannot be utilized as efficiently as equivalent amounts of proteins. The main reason for such poor utilization seems to be the extremely rapid absorption of free amino acids and the consequent flooding of the tissues with excessive amounts af amino acids which cannot be utilized equally rapidly and are therefore partially wasted. The abnormally high concentration of amino acids in the intestines may also provoke diarrhoea while the elevated blood amino acid levels may cause nausea and vomiting. On the other hand, in the course of normal protein digestion, the amino acids are released in a slow and regulated manner, keeping pace with absorption and utilization, there being neither accumulation of amino acids in the intestines nor unduly high level in the blood.

The recent craze for the addition of lysine to multivitamin and mineral preparations intended as supplement to children has no rational basis. Being in the free form, it is rapidly absorbed but is largely wasted as the other essential amino acids are not supplied simultaneously. Further, although lysine content of cereals is low, **the most limiting essential amino acid in the average mixed diets consumed in our country may be either methionine, threonine or tryptophan but not lysine.**

Increased Protein Needs of Diabetics and the Elderly

Additional protein upto 0.5 g per kg body weight per day is recommended to diabetics because it has a more sustained effect in maintaining blood sugar than carbohydrate. A protein rich snack at bed time serves as a precaution against morning hypoglycaemia.

In old age, the calorie requirements are considerably reduced but not those of proteins and other nutrients. **Owing to the increased proneness to illness with the resulting tissue breakdown and negative nitrogen balance, speedy recovery demands a higher protein intake than that provided by the normal diet. Therefore, the elderly should receive, protein-rich foods fortified with minerals and vitamins:**

Conclusion

In view of the scientific data presented in the earlier pages, the following consideration should be borne in mind while selecting a protein food as a dietary supplement.

1. The protein content of the product should be sufficiently high to facilitate the administration of at least 10-20 grams of protein daily.

2. The nutritive value of the protein should be high equivalent to a Net Protein Utilization of at least 60.

3. The product should be palatable enough to enable the easy administration of the required quantity of protein.

4. The product should not have been baked or toasted at high temperatures which damage the nutritive value of the protein.

5. Its protein should preferably be in the intact condition and not predigested, i.e. not in the form of protein hydrolysate of mixture of amino acids.

Kwashiorkor

It is mainly a disease of rural areas, occurring in the second year of life. It occurs most commonly in the infants after weaning (breast feeding) when the diet which replaces the mother's milk is markedly deficient in protein (Figures 21.8 & 21.9) but high in carbohydrate. Kwashiorkor disease has its highest incidence between the age group of 1 to 4 years when the need for essential amino acids for tissue synthesis is great. No age is immune, but in elders, clinical manifestations not so obvious and usually less severe, because both protein and energy requirements are relatively reduced as age advances.

The disease is characterized by growth

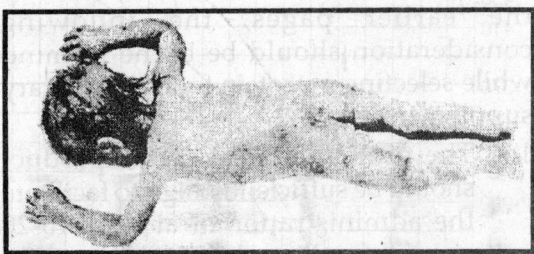

Fig. 21.8 : Symptoms of protein deficiency : Boy, 2 years 1 month old on admission. Note widespread distribution of skin lesions and edema.

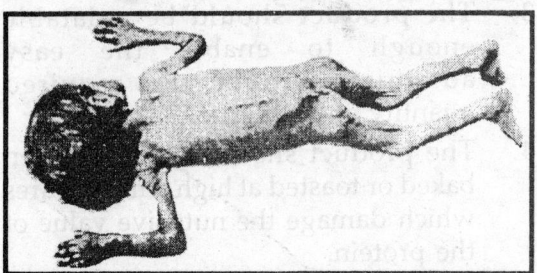

Fig. 21.9 : Same child two weeks after starting the treatment, showing disappearance of the edema and improvement in the skin lesions. Note the degree of muscular wasting, which had been concealed by the edema.

failure, retarded development, loss of appetite, mental apathy, hypoalbuminemia leading to edema, diarrhoea, pellagrous skin lesions, low plasma amino acids, lipids, glucose and potassium. Gastrointestinal disturbances, dermatosis, fatty liver infiltration and mental disturbances are also frequent. The condition is usually complicated by dietary deficiencies other than protein and calories. It has been observed in children that protein malnutrition causes a reduction of the circumference of the head which may lead to impaired growth of the brain and its development and mental retardation. Malnutrition may likewise reduce resistance to infection. Treatment consists in instituting more adequate diet, with special reference to protein and correction of electrolyte and water balance.

Marasmus

Marasmus literally means **"to waste"**. It results from a continued severe deficiency of both **dietary proteins** and the **calories** i.e. **energy**. It generally occurs in the children below 1 year of age. **The symptoms include growth retardation, muscle wasting, anaemia, weakness, and repeated infections. Attitude is irritable.** Skin is shrunken, dry and atrophic.

A marasmic child does not show edema on decreased concentration of plasma albumin **(usual level in them is 2 to 3g/dl whereas in kwashiorkor cases it is always less than 2g/dl)** and the level of cortisol in serum gets increased in marasmic child whereas decreased in kwashiorkor.

> Marasmus is predominantly due to the **deficiency of calories**. This is usually observed in children given watery gruels (of cereals) to supplement the mother's breast milk.

Soyabean (Glycine hispida - a very good source of proteins for vegetarians).

Soyabean is being eaten in China for several thousands of years. The whole dry grain contains about **40-43 percent of protein** (twice as much as in most other pulses) and also upto **20% fat**. Soyabean forms the basis of the great variety of the sauces and pastes with which Chinese cooks garnish their food. Contrarily, in India and Europe the people have not yet been attracted by it because of its peculiar bitter flavour.

It has been observed that the nutritive value of the wheat flour is increased by several folds if the soyabean flour is mixed with it in the ratio of 50:50. Such a flour has been proved to be very useful for the growing children. Effect of a single protein on the growth of rats has been shown in figure 21.10, whereas supplementation effect (supplemented with amino acids and protein) has been shown in Figures 21.11 and 21.12 respectively.

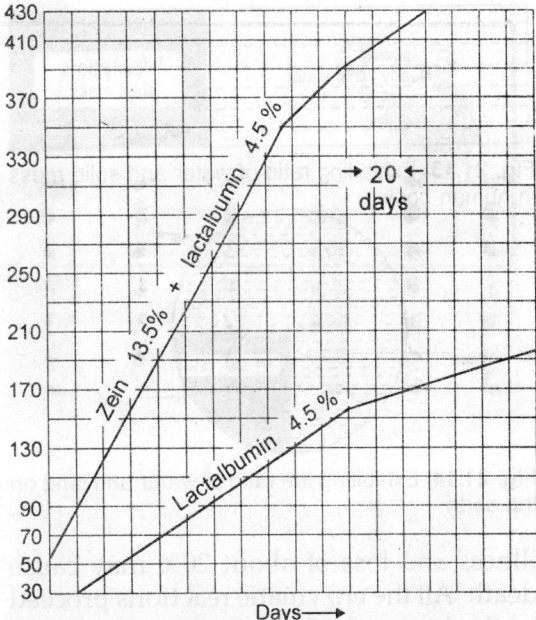

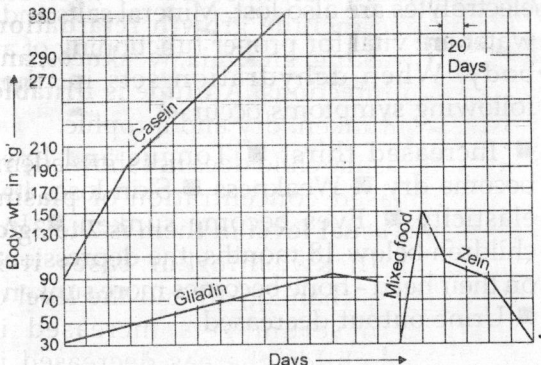

Fig. 21.10: Growth curve of rats maintained on diets containing a single protein. Poor growth is observed with gliadin as the protein (lysine deficient), and with zein (lysine and tryptophan deficient). Excellent growth is obtained with a casein diet.

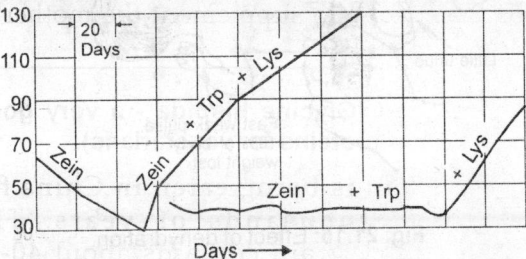

Fig. 21.11: Graph showing supplementation effect. When zein supplemented with tryptophan and lysine, excellent growth is obtained. With tryptophan as the only supplement, body weight alone is maintained, there is no remarkable gain in body weight; growth takes place only after further addition of lysine.

Minerals

These have equally important role in the human body for proper growth and maintenance. Living organisms contain at least 29 elements. among these, **13 are non metals** i.e. C, H, O, N, S, P, Cl, F, Br, I, B, Si

Fig. 21.12: Supplementation effect. Effect on rat growth after supplementing a zein diet with lactalbumin. Excellent growth is observed with the combination proteins.

and As. The metals are Ca, Mg, Na, K, Fe, Cu, Zn, Ni, Co, Mn, Al, Pb, Sn, Mo, V and Ti.

Among the elements needed in quantities **greater than 100 mg daily are** Ca, Mg, Na, K, P, and Cl; these are called the **macroelements**. The others are needed in very minute quantities (less than 100 mg daily) and are termed as **microelements or oligoelements or trace elements.**

Water

It constitutes nearly 70% of the total body weight and may be roughly compared to the ratio of water and land on the earth (Figures 21.13 and 21.14) where again water covers nearly 75% of the total area of the earth, thus emphasizing the contribution of water in the human body and on the earth.

Loss of about 10% of body water causes

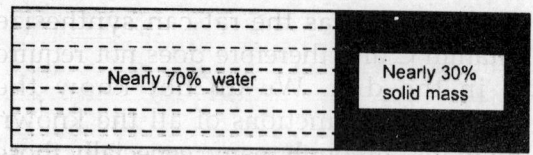

Fig. 21.13: Exhibiting ratio of water and solid mass in human body

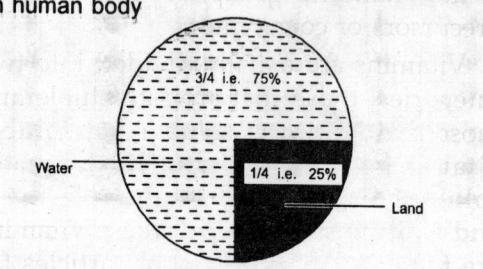

Fig. 21.14: Exhibiting the ratio of water and land on the earth

illness and loss of about 20% may cause death. All the enzymatic reactions proceed in the human body in an aqueous phase of which water is the important component. Nearly 75% of the total diseases of the infants are caused due to giving them deficient and uncleaned water.

Diarrhoea and oral rehydration

Young children in our country suffer from various health problems. **Malnutrition and diarrhoeal diseases cause a large proportion of illness and death in young children.** Repeated attacks of diarrhoea often produce and worsen malnutrition.

What is diarrhoeal disease?

When a person passes liquid watery stools more than three times in 24 hours, he or she is said to have diarrhoea. It is very often accompanied by vomiting, fever and loss of appetite. This disease is caused by a variety of bacterial and viral agents which usually come from unclean surroundings. **Food, water, dirty hands and clothing carry these bacterial and viral agents.**

The immediate danger of diarrhoea is that it leads to dehydration (Fig 9.15) which may result in death if not corrected promptly. **Dehydration means loss of water.** When a person repeatedly vomits or passes watery stools, his body loses lot of water. Along with water, various important mineral salts, known as electrolytes are also lost. Mineral salts and water are vital for proper functioning of a body. When dehydration sets in, the following symptoms occur:

■ Increased thirst ■ Tongue and lips become dry ■ Weakness ■ Skin loses its elasticity ■ Eyes become sunken ■ In children below 18 months, the depression on their head - bone becomes more sunken ■ Urine output decreased

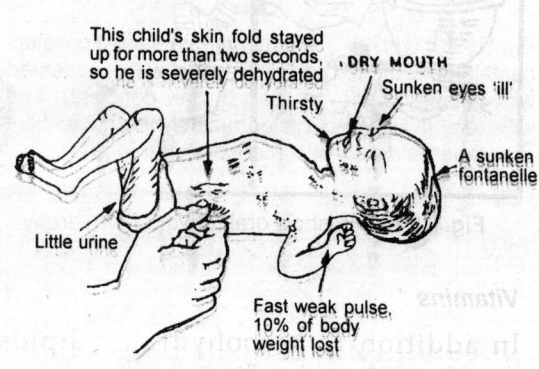

Fig. 21.15: Effect of dehydration

In diarrhoea in children, oral rehydration therapy (a mixture of pinch of sugar and salt in a cup of boiled and cooled water) should be started immediately (Fig 21.16) without any delay.

When liquid from the body is lost in large quantities and rapidly, particularly in very young children, dehydration can be very severe. This can lead to sudden death.

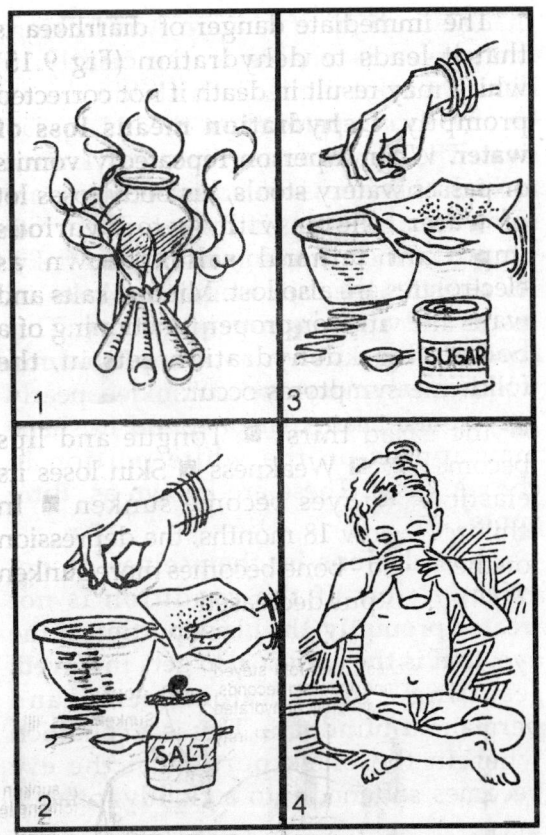

Fig. 21.16 : To show oral rehydration therapy

Vitamins

In addition to carbohydrates, lipids, proteins, inorganic salts and water, normal growth and good health in the mammals require the presence of additional compounds in the diet. These are organic in nature and are called vitamins. Not all living organisms require vitamins (some bacteria do not), nor do they necessarily need the same number or kind, since some vitamins can be synthesized by the organism. **For example, the guinea pig, man and other primates cannot synthesize vitamin C (ascorbic acid) due to the absence of enzyme L-gulono-oxidase and are therefore susceptible to** scurvy, whereas the rat can synthesize vitamin C and therefore does not require it in the diet. We do not know the biochemical functions of all the known vitamins, although many, especially those of the vitamin B group, are known to be precursors of coenzymes.

Vitamins are usually divided into two categories: those that are fat soluble and those that are water soluble. **Fat soluble vitamins are A, D, E and K; the water soluble vitamins are members of the B and C groups.** Nearly, all these vitamins are found in the consumable articles for instance vegetables, milk, meat, fish, pulses, corns(wheat, millet, gram, etc), fruits, cereals, etc.

Intestinal organisms play a role in the vitamin quota available to the animal or man. They may synthesize vitamins in significant amount. Vitamin K is an important example of a vitamin synthesized by intestinal organisms. Folic acid, nicotinic acid, pyridoxine, biotin, thiamine and riboflavin are other examples. These may be absorbed to varying extents and utilized.

Less intake of vitamins in the diet causes avitaminosis in animals and man. Likewise, hypervitaminosis has also been observed in those cases who consume large doses of vitamins.

Preventable Blindness- Vitamin A deficiency

It has been estimated that there are about nine million blind persons in India. Some reports state that every fifth blind person in the world is an Indian. About 20% of the blindness in India can easily be classified as preventable blindness which is the result of nutritional deficiencies.

Man needs vitamin A for normal health,

growth, for the resistance against diseases and for reproduction. The most serious result of the deficiency of vitamin A is the loss of eye sight. {Fig. 21.17 (a and b)}.

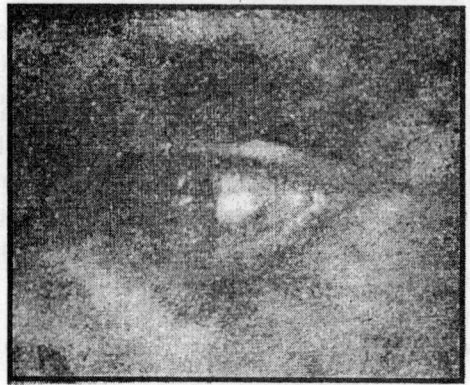

Fig. 21.17 (a) : Preventable Blindness - vitamin A deficiency

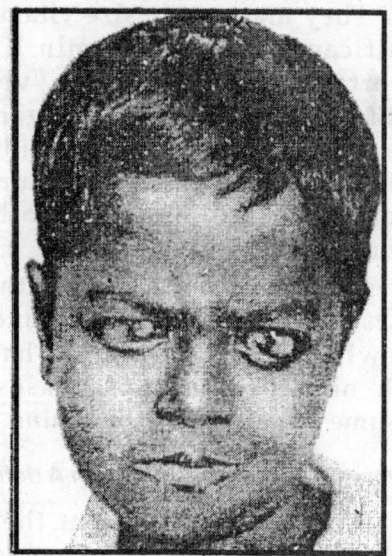

Fig. 21.17 (b) : To show the effect of vitamin A deficiency

Signs and Symptoms

One of the earliest symptoms is **night-blindness.** Vitamin A is necessary for the eye to respond or become sensitive to changes in light. If vitamin A is lacking, the person is unable to see clearly in dimlight or at night. Such children may be able to see perfectly well during day time. The condition is commonly known as night blindness. In addition, there are some visual changes in the eye. The white portion of the eye becomes dry and flaky. As a result, the thin membrane loses its lustre and appears rough and dry. This condition is known as **xerophthalmia** which means **'dry-eye'.** Wrinkled pearly grey spots, triangular or round in shape may appear on the white portion in chronic cases. These are known as **'Bitot spots'.**

These lesions by themselves do not affect vision. If the condition is not treated promptly, the black portion of the eye, that is the cornea also gets involved, resulting in keratomalacia and permanent blindness. This is a condition wherein the black portion of the eye becomes softened into a cloudy, opaque mass.

In India, we have abundant sources of vitamin A that are easily and cheaply available. These include foods such as carrot, green leafy vegetables, namely drumstick leaves, amaranth, spinach and fruits like mango and papaya. Studies conducted by National Institute of Nutrition have shown that **if 40 g of green leafy vegetables are added to the existing diet, the child would get the required amount of vitamin A. This is because leafy vegetables are good sources of carotene which can be converted into vitamin A in the body.**

Causes

However, intake of vitamin A by children as well as women is very low. In some areas, it is believed that children should not be given green leafy vegetables as it may cause diarrhoea. Others believe that pregnant women should not eat papaya; Thus, some of the rich sources of this vitamin are denied to those who need it most.

A well - nourished mother provides adequate vitamin A to her baby to be stored in its liver. After birth, the infant obtains vitamin A through the mother's milk. Therefore, a healthy mother provides enough vitamin A to her baby before birth as well as after birth.

Colostrum is the thick milky secretion of the breast in the first few days after child birth. This is a very rich source of vitamin A. Infants fed colostrum have better reserves of vitamin A. The practice of feeding colostrum should be encouraged.

During acute infections, vitamin A status of the child deteriorates. It has been shown that measles- common childhood infection is one of the important causes of keratomalacia. Acute respiratory and gastrointestinal infections also aggravate vitamin A deficiency. Intestinal parasites, especially round worms are common among children belonging to poor communities. **Incidence of vitamin A deficiency is higher among the children having round worms in their gastrointestinal tracts.**

Prevention and treatment

Even the most severe cases of vitamin A deficiency can be successfully treated. **The usual practice is to administer intramuscular injections of 30,000 µg of vitamin A for 2 or 3 consecutive days.** This is followed by oral doses for a few more days till the body reserves are built up.

Conjunctival lesions and night blindness respond well to relatively small doses of vitamin A. **Oral administration of 1,000 µg daily for about a week usually reverses the changes.**

Corneal lesions should be treated as a medical emergency. **30,000 µg of water miscible vitamin A can be injected intramuscularly followed by 1000 µg of vitamin A orally for a period of 15 days. This helps in rapid clinical and biochemical improvement. Oil soluble vitamin A should not be injected as the absorption of this compound from the site of injection is poor.**

Diet improvement

The most logical method of prevention would be to improve the diet of the vulnerable groups.

Consumption of adequate amount of vitamin A is essential to keep the eyes bright. Drumstick leaves, spinach, amaranth, carrots and pumpkin contain large quantities of carotene. The substance is converted into vitamin A in our body. Even children suffering from mild forms of malnutrition are able to absorb carotene from amaranth. The presence of even small amount of fat helps in the absorption. Carotene is also present in large quantities in fruits like mango and papaya. **Consumption of such food [Fig. 21.18 (a & b)] should be encouraged.** Particularly pregnant and lactating women should eat sufficient quantities of foods rich in vitamin A. They can meet requirements easily if they eat atleast one medium sized bowl full of cooked greens every day.

As a short- term measure, periodical oral administration of vitamin A has been suggested for the prevention of vitamin A

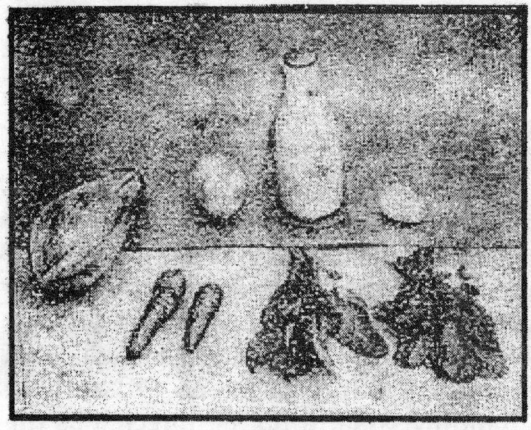

(a)

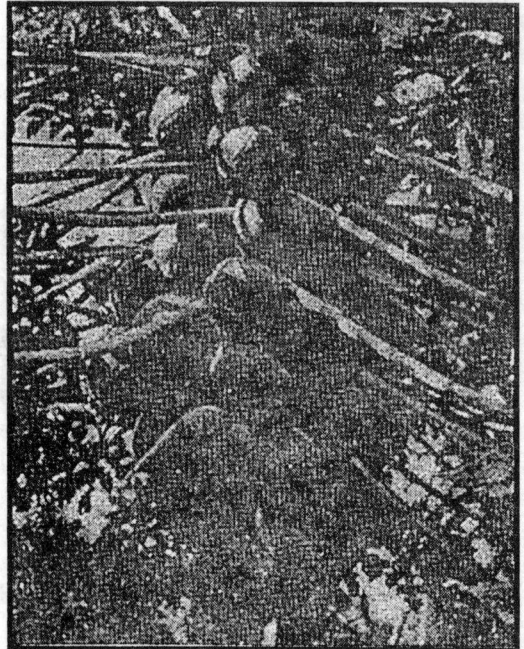

Fig. 21.18 (a & b) : Treatment part of vitamin 'A' deficiency

deficiency in children.

Based on the recommendations of the National Institute of Nutrition (NIN),

Hyderabad, **the Government of India has launched a massive prophylaxis programme against vitamin A deficiency from 1970 in several states. In this programme children between 1-5 years are being given an oral dose of 2,00000 I.U. of vitamin A once in six months.** The programme is implemented through the existing public health set up. Evaluation carried out in some states has shown a significant reduction in the incidence of xerophthalmia wherever the programme was well implemented.

A few paise spent on inexpensive foods rich in vitamin A can make all the difference between **good vision and no vision** (Fig. 21.19).

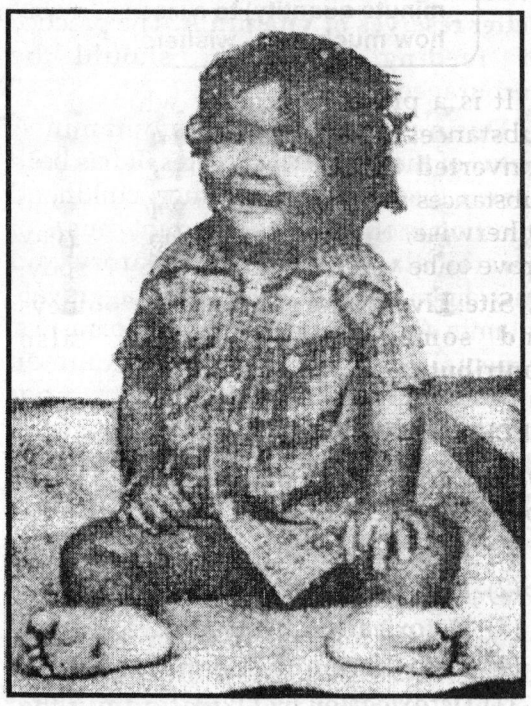

Fig. 21.19 : Normal child with good vision

CHAPTER 22

DETOXICATION (BIOTRANSFORMATION)

> **Ours mechanisms have got a special favour for the body as they convert toxic substances into less toxic or non - harmful substances and ultimately eliminate them. Ours mechanisms are so strong that they can even convert the most dreadful substance i.e., potassium cyanide (if consumed in micrograms or via natural eatables as it remains present in them in very minute quantity) to a less toxic substance. Now, you can very well imagine, how much well - wishers are ours mechanisms to the human body.**

It is a phenomenon by which toxic substances taken by an individual are converted to less harmful or nontoxic substances which are eventually excreted. Otherwise, these toxic substances may prove to be very fatal to the human body.

Site: Liver is the main site but kidneys and some other tissues do also contribute.

MECHANISM OF DETOXICATION

Detoxication takes place by the following mechanisms:
   (1) **Detoxication by Oxidation**
   (2) **Detoxication by Reduction**
   (3) **Detoxication by Hydrolysis**
   (4) **Detoxication by Conjugation**

(1) *Detoxication by Oxidation:* It is the most important mechanism for the disposal of toxic substances. Oxidation reactions are mostly carried out by a group of *'mixed function oxidases'* in the liver which in the final step involve a cytochrome P - 450 haemoprotein, NADPH and O_2.

For various types of substances/ compounds, detoxication by oxidation is as follows:

(i) *Aromatic hydrocarbons:* On oxidation, these are converted to phenol, e.g.

$$C_6H_6 \longrightarrow C_6H_5OH \longrightarrow \text{conjugation later}$$
benzene   phenol   on

(ii) *Alcohols and aldehydes:* These are converted into acids:

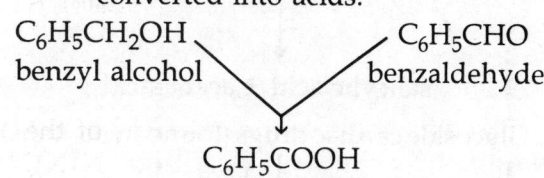

$C_6H_5CH_2OH$ C_6H_5CHO
benzyl alcohol   benzaldehyde

C_6H_5COOH
benzoic acid
↓
Conjugation later on

(iii) *Amines* : Many primary aliphatic amines undergo oxidation to the corresponding acids as a result of which nitrogen is converted to urea according to the general reaction:

$R - CH_2NH_2 \rightarrow R - COOH + NH_2CONH_2$

$C_6H_5CH_2NH_2 \rightarrow C_6H_5COOH \rightarrow$ Conjugation

benzylamine   benzoic acid   later on

(iv) *Drugs:* Meprobamate (tranquilizer used for the control of anxiety, tension and muscle spasm) is hydroxylated during its metabolism.

Meprobamate

↓ hydroxylation

hydroxy meprobamate

(2) *Detoxication by Reduction:* In human beings, this mechanism is less common than the oxidation. Many nitrocompounds are reduced i n the body to amino compounds, e.g.

Picric acid $\longrightarrow$ picramic acid

p - Nitrobenzene $\longrightarrow$ p - Nitrophenol

Dibenzyldisulfides $\longrightarrow$ sulphhydryl derivatives

(3) *Detoxication by Hydrolysis:* The hydrolytic cleavage of ester, amide, glucoside and other linkages causes molecular alteration of foreign molecules, e.g.

Atropine $\xrightarrow{\text{atropine esterase}}$ tropic acid + tropine

Acetylsalicylic acid (aspirin)

↓

salicylic acid + acetic acid

Glucoside cardiac drugs (found in digitalis)

↓

sugars + aglucone

(4) Detoxication by Conjugation

Conjugation reactions cause foreign compounds to become more soluble as a result of which they are more readily excretable. Conjugating agents are glucuronic acid, glycine, sulfuric acid, acetic acid, glutamine, ornithine, cysteine, etc.

(i) Conjugation with glucuronic acid

This is the most common type of conjugation reaction which is carried out by the enzyme *glucoronyl tarnsferase*,

Phenol $\longrightarrow$ phenol glucuronide

Benzoic acid $\longrightarrow$ benzoyl glucuronide

Chloramphenicol $\rightarrow$ chloramphenicol glucuronide

Bilirubin $\longrightarrow$ bilirubin glucuronide (excreted in bile)

(ii) Conjugation with glycine

benzoic acid

↓ CoA.SH, ATP

benzoyl coenzyme A

↓ glycine

hippuric acid

> The best known and most frequently used test for knowing the protective functions of liver is the detoxication of benzoic acid by conjugation with glycine. The test also measures the metabolic functions of the liver since the rate of formation of hippuric acid also depends upon the concentration and the amount of glycine available.

Nicotinic acid $\xrightarrow{\text{glycine}}$ nicotinuric acid

Salicylic acid $\xrightarrow{\text{glycine}}$ salicyluric acid

(iii) Conjugation with sulfuric acid

Phenol $\xrightarrow{\text{sulfuric acid}}$ phenyl sulfuric acid

(iv) Conjugation with acetic acid

p - aminobenzoic acid

$\downarrow$ acetic acid

p- acetylaminobenzoic acid

(v) Conjugation with cysteine

Cysteine is first acetylated to form N-acetylcysteine which then reacts with benzene to give phenylmercapturic acid which is excreted in urine. Similar reactions are used for the disposal of other aromatic compounds.

Benzene + N - acetylcysteine

$\downarrow$

phenyl mercapturic acid
(aromatic compound)

(vi) Conjugation with ornithine

Chickens, etc. detoxify phenylacetic acid by conjugation with ornithine.

(vii) Conjugation with glutamine

Phenylacetic acid is cojugated with glutamine.

PRODUCTION AND METABOLISM OF FOREIGN COMPOUNDS IN LARGE INTESTINE

Bacterial enzyme system in the large intestine brings about several biochemical alterations of the unabsorbed food molecules. In a few instances, the substances such produced have a degree of toxicity. After absorption, they are metabolized in various ways as described earlier so that their elimination occurs afterwards, for example, neutral fats are hydrolyzed by bacterial action and the products so formed are normal to gut, however, the choline fraction of phospholipids may yield an abnormal amine *neurine* which has a low order of toxicity.

Choline $\longrightarrow$ neurine

Many amino acids undergo decarboxylation as a result of the action of intestinal bacteria to produce toxic amines (ptomaines)

Amino acid $\xrightarrow[\text{CO}_2]{}$ ptomaine

Detoxication of Cyanides

Although the cyanide radical (CN^-) is very poisonous to the body, even then, very small quantities of it may be harmless. The CN^- radical is converted to relatively nontoxic thiocyanate radical- SCN^-, and excreted as salts of this acid radical, this reaction is catalysed by an enzyme known as *rhodanese* in the presence of thiosulfate as shown below:

$HCN + Na_2S_2O_3$

$\downarrow$ rhodanese

$NaHSO_3 + NaCNS$

Enzyme *'rhodanese'* is of considerable significance in the animals that eat foods containing 'cyanogenic substances'.

BIOCHEMICAL VALUES

Sl. No	Constituent	Normal Range	High in	Low in
DIABETES MELLITUS				
1.	(a) Blood sugar (fasting) (b) Serum glucose (SI unit)	70-100 mg/dl 4.2-6.1 mmol/l	Diabetes mellitus, hyperthyroidism, adrenocortical hyperactivity, hyperpituitarism etc.	Hyperinsulinism, hypothyroidism (myxoedema, cretinism), hypopituitarism (for example, Simmond's disease), and hypoadrenalism (Addison's disease), with values well down in the hypoglycaemic range in severe cases of the last two of these conditions.
	(c) Glucose (random)	80-120 mg/dl	-do-	-do-
2.	Blood sugar (P.P. i.e., after 2 hrs of 75 g glucose or routine full meal)	Less than 140 mg/dl	-do-	-do-
3.	Glycosylated or glycated haemoglobin (HbA$_1$)	upto 7.5%	Diabetes mellitus (upto 20%)	
RENAL FUNCTION TESTS				
1.	(a) Blood urea (b) Blood urea (SI units) (c) Urea Nitrogen	14-43 mg/dl 2.2-7.2 mmol/l 6-20 mg/dl	Glomerulonephritis, chronic pyelonephritis, nephrotic syndromes, massive gasro-intestinal hemorrhage, severe dehydration, obstruction in the urinary tract due to benign hyperplasia of the prostate, bilateral ureteral obstruction due to carcinoma or calculus in the urinary bladder.	Nephrosis

Contd

SI. No	Constituent	Normal Range	High in	Low in
2.	(a) Serum creatinine (b) Serum creatinine (SI units)	0.1-1.2 mg/dl 44-124 μmol/l	Renal failure, congestive heart failure, shock and mechanical obstruction of the urinary tract.	-

LIVER FUNCTION TESTS

SI. No	Constituent	Normal Range	High in	Low in
1.	Serum bilirubin	0.2-1.0 mg/dl	Obstructive jaundice, hemolytic jaundice, neonatal jaundice, and hepatitis.	-
2.	Direct (conjugated) bilirubin	0.0-0.2 mg/dl	Hepatitis	
3.	Indirect (unconjugated) bilirubin = Total bilirubin-direct i.e., conjugated bilirubin	0.2-0.8 mg/dl	Haemolytic jaundice and neonatal jaundice	-
4	(a) Serum cholesterol (total)	150-200mg/dl (3.9-5.2 mmol/l in S.I units)	Diabetes mellitus, hypothyroidism, obstructive jaundice, cirrhosis of liver, nephrotic syndrome, atherosclerosis, etc	Acute hepatitis, malnutrition anaemia, occasionally in hyperthyroidism and Gaucher's disease
	(b) Free cholesterol	25-30% of the total cholesterol	Xanthomatous biliary cirrhosis	-
	(c) Esterified cholesterol	70-75% of the total cholesterol,		Liver diseases, infective hepatitis, acute hepatic necrosis
5.	GOT (AST)*; Glutamic oxalacetic transaminase (Aspartate transaminase) **(Peak in 4-6 hrs after MI)**	8-40 units/ml or 4-17 IU/l	Myocardial infarction, liver disorders, skeletal muscle trauma or regeneration, etc	-
6	GPT (ALT)*; Glutamic pyruvic transaminase (Alanine transaminase)	5-35 units/ml or 3-15 IU/l	Liver disorders and the increase is significantly higher than SGOT. Determination of SGPT can be useful in showing the severity and prognosis of the disease.	-
7.	Alkaline phosphatase*	4-11 KA units or 60-160 IU/l	Diseases of the liver primarily with destructive or obstructive pathology (e.g., hepatitis, cirrhosis, chemical toxicity, gall-stones, biliary duct obstructions, and primary or metastatic or 'space occupying' lesions of the liver), bony lesions (e.g. osteogenic sarcoma, metastatic carcinomas, rickets, Paget's disease) and also with primary and secondary parathyroidism.	Scurvy, severe anemia, malnutrition, achondroplasia, cretinism, hypophosphatasia

Contd

Sl. No	Constituent	Normal Range	High in	Low in
8	(a) Serum total proteins (b) Serum total proteins (S.I. units)	6.0-8.0 g/dl 60-80 g/l	Multiple myeloma and conditions associated with high globulin concentration.	Different clinical conditions associated with nephrotic syndromes, neoplastic disease, malnutrition, Kwashiorkor syndrome, cirrhosis of liver and other liver disorders.
9.	(a) Serum albumin (b) Serum albumin (S.I. units)	3.5-5.0 g/dl 35-50 g/l	Pathological conditions associated with increased levels of serum albumin are not known.	Different conditions such as cirrhosis of liver, other liver disorders, nephrotic syndromes, malnutrition, malignancies, chronic protracted conditions like ulcerative colitis.
10.	Serum globulins	2.3-3.6 g/dl	Advanced liver diseases	-
11.	Fibrinogen (plasma)	0.3-0.6 g/dl	Infections	Cirrhosis of liver, acute hepatic necrosis, poisoning by carbon tetrachloride, etc,
12.	Albumin/Globulins ratio (ratio gets reversed in advanced liver diseases)	1.2-1.5	-	Less than 1 in infective hepatitis
13.	Gamma glutamyl transferase (γ-GT)*	11-50 IU/l (men) 7-32 IU/l (women)	Biliary obstruction and alcoholism	

PANCREATIC FUNCTION TESTS

1.	Amylase*	80-180 Somogyi units	Pancreatitis, stone and cancer in biliary duct	
2.	Serum lipase	Less than 150 U/l	Pancreatitis, cancer in pancreas, cirrhosis, hepatitis, duodenal ulcer, diseases of the biliary tract, etc.	

LIPID PROFILE

1.	(a) Serum cholesterol (total)	150-200mg/dl (3.9-5.2 mmol/l in S.I. units)	Diabetes mellitus, hypothyroidism, obstructive jaundice, cirrhosis of liver, nephrotic syndrome, atherosclerosis, etc.	Acute hepatitis, malnutrition anaemia, occasionally in hyperthyroidism and Gaucher's disease
	(b) HDL cholesterol	30-63 mg/dl (men) 35-75 mg/dl (women)	The combined risk factor of coronary heart disease (CHD) can be determined following the estimations of serum cholesterol and HDL - cholesterol	-
	(c) LDL - cholesterol**	upto 150 mg/dl	The ratio of cholesterol to HDL cholesterol has predictive value in	-

---

* in serum

Contd

SI. No	Constituent	Normal Range	High in	Low in
			determining the risk of CHD more accurately. **For normal males the ratio of 5:1 and for normal females the ratio of 4.5:1 are considered as average risk.** Lower ratios significantly reduce the risk, whereas ratios 9.5:1 and 7:1 for males and females respectively, are believed to double the risk of CHD. An inverse relationship has been observed between the risk of CHD and the concentration of HDL - cholesterol. HDL cholesterol represents approximately 20-25% of the total cholesterol in serum.	
	(d) VLDL	upto 28 mg/dl	Hyperlipidaemia	
	(e) Lipoprotein (a)	0-30 mg/dl	-	
	(f) Free cholesterol	25-30% of the total cholesterol	Xanthomatous biliary cirrhosis	
	(g) Esterified cholesterol	70-75% of the total cholesterol		Liver diseases, infective hepatitis, acute hepatic necrosis
2.	Triglycerides*	30-140 mg/dl	Hyperlipidemia, atherosclerosis, diabetes mellitus; nephrosis, biliary obstruction and metabolic disorders associated with certain endocrine diseases.	
3.	Total lipids *	360-820 mg/dl	Diabetes mellitus, biliary cirrhosis, late pregnancy, nephrosis and hypothyroidism.	Hyperthyroidism

STOMACH FUNCTION TEST

1.	Fractional test meals (FTM) i.e., gastric analysis	Free acidity 0.0-40 meq/l Total acidity 20-55 meq/l	Duodenal ulcer and gastric ulcer	Hypochlorhydria (hypoacidity)

ANAEMIA

1.	(a) Haemoglobin (males)	14-18 g/dl	Polycythaemias,	Anaemias of different

Contd

* in serum

** $\underline{\text{Plasma (serum) triglycerides}}$ = VLDL
   5

   (Total serum cholesterol - HDL) - (VLDL) = LDL

Note: **Hypercholesterolaemia is known to be associated with an increased risk of coronary heart disease (CHD)**

SI. No	Constituent	Normal Range	High in	Low in
	(b) Haemoglobin (females)	11-16 g/dl	congenital cyanotic heart disease, and in haemoconcentration due to various clinical causes e.g., heatstroke and dehydration.	kind resulting from haemorrhage or from deficiency of iron, vitamin B_{12} or folic acid. Red cell haemolysis resulting from auto-immune process or due to enzyme abnormality (G-6-PD) may result in anaemia. The defective globin chain synthesis as in thalassemias or structural abnormalities of the haemoglobin molecule as in abnormal haemoglobins may result in severe anaemia.

CARDIAC ENZYMES

SI. No	Constituent	Normal Range	High in	Low in
1.	GOT (AST)*; Glutamic oxalacetic transaminase (Aspartate transaminase) **(Peak in 4-6 hrs after MI)**	8-40 units/ml or 4-17 IU/l	Myocardial infarction, liver disorders, skeletal muscle trauma or regeneration, etc	-
2.	Serum lactic dehydrogenase (LDH) **(Peak in 8-10 hrs after MI)**	230 - 460 IU/l	Myocardial infarction, infective hepatitis, toxic jaundice, etc.	-
3.	Serum creatine phosphokinase (CPK or CK) **(Peak in 24-36 hrs after MI)**	20-50 IU/l (men) 10-37 IU/l (women)	Myocardial infarction and progressive muscular dystrophy of Duchenne type. In MI, CPK is increased earlier than GOT and LDH, beginning within 6 hrs, and at peak on an average at 24 hrs. and returning to the normal within 2-3 days. Increased levels may also be found in polymyositis and other muscular dystrophies, etc.	-

CARDIAC MARKERS

SI. No	Constituent	Normal Range	High in	Low in
1.	Troponin - T (c Tn T)	0 - 0.1 µg/L	Myocardial Infarction	-
2.	Troponin - I (c Tn I)		Myocordial Infarction	
3.	Homocysteine	4.0 -12 µmol/L	Myocardial Infarction	Pregnancy
4.	Myoglobin	19-92 µg/L (M) 12-76 µg/L (F)	Myocardial Infarction (a relatively early marker, elevation after 4-6 hrs of AMI)	

THYROID FUNCTION TESTS

SI. No	Constituent	Normal Range	High in	Low in
1.	Triiodothyronine (T_3)	60 - 190 ng/dl (RIA mehtod)	Pregnancy, hyperthyroidism	Hypothyroidism

* in serum

Contd

SI. No	Constituent	Normal Range	High in	Low in
2.	Thyroxine (T$_4$)	1.5 - 4.0 ng/dl (RIA mehtod)	Hyperthyroidism	Hypothyroidism
3.	TSH	0.3 - 6.0 µU/ml	Hypothyroidism	Hyperthyroidism
4.	Thyroid Binding Globulin (TBG)	2.0 - 4.8 ng/dl	Pregnancy, Acute Liver Disease Thyrotoxicosis	Major illness, Nephrosis,
5.	Protein Bound Iodine	4 - 8 µg/dl (PBI)	Hyperthyroidism	Hypothyroidism, Nephrosis, etc.

HORMONES

1.	Insulin	5 - 20 µU/ml (Adult Fasting)	Hypoglycemia, Insulinoma	Diabetes Mellitus
2.	Testosterone	350-1000 ng/dl , (Males)		Hypogonadism (Males)
		20 - 70 ng /dl, (Females)	Elevated (females)-Adrenal or Ovarian Tumors	
3.	Thyrocalcitonin	20 - 400 pg / ml	Medullary Carcinoma of the Thyroid	
4.	Human Chorionic Gonadotropin (HCG)	2,000-40,000 IU/l	Detectable level confirms pregnancy	Threatened pregnancy
5.	**Gastrin**	< 300 pg/ml	**Stomach or Duodenal Ulcer, Zollinger Ellison Syndrome**	

MISCELLANEOUS

1.	Ketone bodies (blood)	upto 3 mg%	Diabetes mellitus	
2.	(a) Acid phosphatase (Total)* (b) Acid phosphatase (Prostatic)	1-0-4.0 KA units 0.0-0.8 KA units	Carcinoma of prostrate gland, Paget's disease and hyperparathy- roidism	
3.	Serum uric acid	2.5-7.0 mg/dl (men) 1.5-6.0 mg/dl (women)	Gout, renal failure, uremia, leukae- mia and following radiotherapy of lymphomas.	Wilson's disease, Fanconi syndrome, some cases of Acromegaly and following the usage of uricosuric drugs.
4.	(a) Serum calcium	8.5-10.5 mg/dl	Hyperparathyroidism,	Tetany, hypoparathyroidism,

Contd

* in serum

SI. No	Constituent	Normal Range	High in	Low in
	(b) Serum calcium (S.I. units)	2.1-2.6 mmol/l	hypervitaminosis-D and associated with increased levels of thyrocalcitonin.	rickets, osteomalacia, etc.
5.	(a) Inorganic phosphorus (Adults)* (b) Inorganic phosphorus * (Children)	2.5-4.8 mg/dl (0.8-1.6 mmol/l) 4.0-7.0 mg/dl (1.3-2.3 mmol/l)	Hypoparathyroidism, renal failure, hypervitaminosis-D, etc	Rickets, hyperparathyroidism, Fanconi syndrome, etc.
6.	Renal threshold value for glucose	160-180 mg/dl	-	-
7.	Magnesium*	1-3 mg/dl	-	Vomiting and diarrhoea
8.	Lithium *	Absent or in traces	-	-
9.	Sodium*	137-148 meq/l	-	Diabetic acidosis, excessive diarrhoea, pernicious vomiting, extreme sweating over a long period
10.	Potassium*	3.6-5.4 meq/l	Pneumonia, acute infections and uremia.	Muscle weakeness, tiredness, paralysis mental confusion, polyuria, chronic diarrhoea, repeated vomiting, etc

* in serum

DESIRED LIPID PROFILE

Risk Category	Total Cholesterol mg / dl	HDL Cholesterol mg /dl	LDL Cholesterol mg / dl	Triglycerides mg / dl
DESIRABLE	<200	>=35	<130	<200
BORDERLINE HIGH	200 - 239	...	130 - 159	200 - 400
WORRISOME	>=240	<35	>=160	401 - 1000

IMPORTANT TUMOR MARKERS

Sl. No	TUMOR MARKERS	ASSOCIATED CANCER
1.	Carcino Embryonic Antigen (CEA)	Colon, Lung, Breast, Pancreas
2.	Alpha Fetoprotein (AFP)	Liver, Gonadal Germ Cell Tumor
3.	Prostate - Specific Antigen (PSA)	Prostate Cancer
4.	Prostatic - Acid Phosphatase (PAP)	Prostate Cancer
5.	Lactic Dehydrogenase (LDH)	Lymphoma, Ewing's Syndrome
6.	Calcitonin (CT)	Medullary Cancer of the Thyroid
7.	Human Chorionic Gonadotropin (HCG)	Trophoblast, Gonadal Germ Cell Tumor

APPENDIX - II

CSF in Differential Diagnosis

Disease	Appearance	Cells/cmm	Protein (mg%)	Glucose (mg%)
Normal pH (7.35-7.4)	-	-	-	-
Normal case	Crystal clear	< 5 cells, all lymphocytes	15-45	50-80
Acute purulent meningitis	Opalescent to purulent clot	500-20,000 mostly poly's	45 - 100 +	0 - 45
Tuberculous meningitis	Opalescent fibrin web, pellicle	10-500 mostly lympho's	45-500 +	0 - 45
Early, acute syphilitic meningitis	Clear to turbid, Occasional clot	25-2,000 mostly lympho's	45-400 +	15-75
Late CNS syphilis	Normal	Normal or ↑	Normal or ↑	Normal
Viral encephalitis (arthropod borne)	Normal	0-100 mostly lympho's	Normal or increased	45-100
Viral meningoencephalitis	Normal	0-2000+ mostly lympho's	Normal or ↑	Normal

APPENDIX - III

Table showing anticancerous sources, phytochemical present etc.

Sl. No.	Fruit/Vegetable/ Spices	Phytochemical Present	Biochemical basis of its/their action	Comments
1.	(i) Citrus fruits like orange, lemon amla, malta, kino, etc. are rich in vitamin C, folate and fibres.	Limonin	Limonin increases the level of natural enzymes by increasing their synthesis which have got the capability to disintegrate the cancer causing substances and then eliminates them from body.	(i) Various organs are protected from cancer
	(ii) Cardamom and aniseed (saunf)			(ii) Are also anticancer
2.	Grapes (black grapes are richer in phenolics than the green).	(i) Allomic acid (ii) Flavonoids (especially phenolics)	Inhibit the enzymes which may otherwise help biochemical reactions causing cancer	(i) Various organs are protected (ii) In the countries where grapes-wine is used in abundance for e.g., France, incidence of heart ailments is less.
3.	Apple. strawberry, plum (Ber)	(i) Antioxidants (ii) Phenols (iii) Raveratol		(i) Various organs are protected. (ii) **Raveratol has got the property to control the level of bad cholesterol (LDL-cholesterol) as well in blood.**
4.	Watermelon	**Carotenoids especially cantalop**		(i) Various organs are protected (ii) It also contains an anticoagulant named **adenosine which protects from heart ailments.**
5.	Tomato, papaya, watermelon, carrot strawberry, apricot, etc.	(i) Vitamin 'C' (ii) Lycopene	Prevents biochemical changes of DNA of the cell.	Protects from the cancers of prostate glands, lungs, stomach, etc.

	Source	Active principle	Mode of action	Benefits
6.	Chillies	Capsenin	(i) Checks the possible damage of **gene** by creating interruption which may be caused by the cancerous agents present in the smoke of cigarettes	(i) Protects from the lung cancer (ii) **More bitter the chillies-more is the capsenin in them.**
7.	Garlic and onion	Alicin	(i) Increases the synthesis of enzymes which have got the capability to disintegrate the cancerous substances. (ii) Gives more energy to immune cells	(i) Protects from the cancer of oesophagus (ii) Regular intake of garlic also protects from the cancer of anus as per the latest findings published in the American Journal of Clinical Nutrition. (iii) Regular intake of garlic also controls the level of cholesterol in blood. (iv) Garlic also contains antibiotics.
8.	Cauliflower, cabbage, radish, mustard	Indole-3-carbinol	Increases the synthesis of enzymes responsible for degarding cancerous substances	Protects from the cancer of stomach, lungs and breasts.
9.	Carrots	β-Carotene	Antioxidant property	(i) Protects from the cancer of lungs, stomach (ii) Also lowers down the level of cholesterol in blood.
10.	Soyabean, groundnut and germinating alfa-alfa	Genistin	Interrupts the blood supply to the cancerous cells	(i) Estrogen hormone found in the females induces the cancerous cells whereas genistin protects from the cancer of breast and ovaries.
11.	Spinach, fenugreek, greeen leaves of mustard, chaurai	(i) Leutein (ii) Geoxanthine		Protects from loss of eye sight and blindness as well.
12.	Tea leaves (especially green leaves)	Polyphenols	(i) Antioxidant property (ii) Controls the multiplication of cancerous cells. (iii) Eliminates cancerous substances from the body	Protects from the cancer of oesophagus.

Table - I : Commonly Used Anticoagulants

S.No.	Anticoagulant	mg/ml Blood	Use	Mode of Action
1.	Heparin	0.2	Procedures requiring whole blood or plasma especially useful when intact erythrocytes are desired	Inhibits conversion of prothrombin to thrombin
2.	Ethylenediamine - tetraacetic acid (EDTA)	1	Procedures requiring whole blood or plasma	Chelates ionic calcium
3.	Oxalates (a) Lithium (b) Sodium (c) Potassium (d) Ammonium	1 - 2	Procedures requiring whole blood or plasma. Causes shrinkage of cell volume, should not be used in haematological procedures.	Forms unionized calcium oxalate complex; reduces level of ionized calcium below that required for clotting
4.	Sodium Citrate	5	As for oxalates	Forms unionized complex with calcium
5.	Sodium Fluoride	10	**Combination anticoagulant and preservative for blood glucose determination by inhibiting blood enzymes causing glycolysis;** causes erythrocyte shrinkage. Combined with thymol **(1mg +10 mg NaF)** for effective control of microbial growth in stored blood samples.	Forms unionized calcium fluoride complex

INDEX